Student Resources

Online Student Resources are included with this textbook.
Visit http://nursing.pearsonhighered.com for the following assets and activities:

- Learning Outcomes
- Chapter Review Questions
- Case Studies
- Appendices and additional content updates
- Weblinks
- Links to additional nursing resources

PEARSON

ALWAYS LEARNING

Instructor Resources—Redefined!

PEARSON NURSING CLASS PREPARATION RESOURCES

New and Unique!

- Use this preparation tool to find animations, videos, images, and other media resources that cross the nursing curriculum! Organized by topic and fully searchable by resource type and key word, this easy-to-use platform allows you to:
  - Search through the media library of assets
  - Upload your own resources
  - Export to PowerPoint™ or HTML pages

Use this tool to find and review other unique instructor resources:

Correlation Guide to Nursing Standards

- Links learning outcomes of core textbooks to nursing standards such as the 2010 ANA Scope and Standards of Practice, QSEN Competencies, National Patient Safety Goals, AACN, Essentials of Baccalaureate Education and more!

Pearson Nursing Lecture Series

- Highly visual, fully narrated and animated, these short lectures focus on topics that are traditionally difficult to teach and difficult for students to grasp
- All lectures accompanied by case studies and classroom response questions for greater interactivity within even the largest classroom
- Use as lecture tools, remediation material, homework assignments and more!

MYTEST AND ONLINE TESTING

- Test questions even **more accessible** now with both pencil and paper (MyTest) and online delivery options (Online Testing)
- **NCLEX®-style** questions
- **All New!** Approximately 30% of all questions are in alternative-item format
- **Complete rationales** for correct and incorrect answers mapped to learning outcomes

BOOK-SPECIFIC RESOURCES

Also available to instructors:

- **Instructor's Manual and Resource Guide** organized by learning outcome
- Comprehensive **PowerPoint™** presentations integrating lecture notes and images
- **Image library**
- **Classroom Response Questions**
- **Online course management systems** complete with instructor tools and student activities

mynursinglab

- **Proven Results:** Pearson's MyLab/Mastering platform has helped millions of students
- Provide your students with a one-of-a-kind guided learning path and personalized study plan! An engaging **REVIEW**, **REMEMBER**, and **APPLY** approach moves students from memorization to true understanding through application with:
  - Even more alternate-item format questions
  - More analysis and application level questions
  - An interactive eText (also available via iPad®) with multimedia resources built right in
- **Trusted Partner:** A network of customer experience managers and faculty advocates are available to help instructors maximize learning gains with MyNursingLab.

REAL NURSING SIMULATIONS

- 25 simulation scenarios that span the nursing curriculum
- Consistent format includes learning objectives, case flow, set-up instructions, debriefing questions and more!
- Companion online course cartridge with student pre-and post-simulation activities, videos, skill checklists and reflective discussion questions

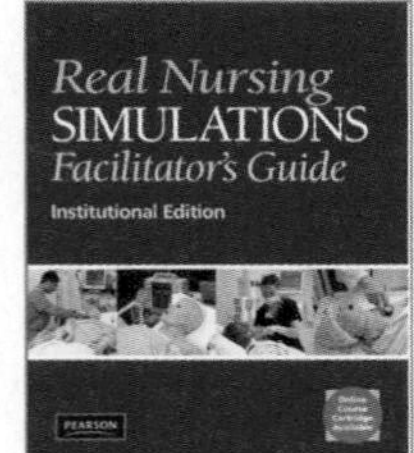

Genetics and Genomics for Nursing

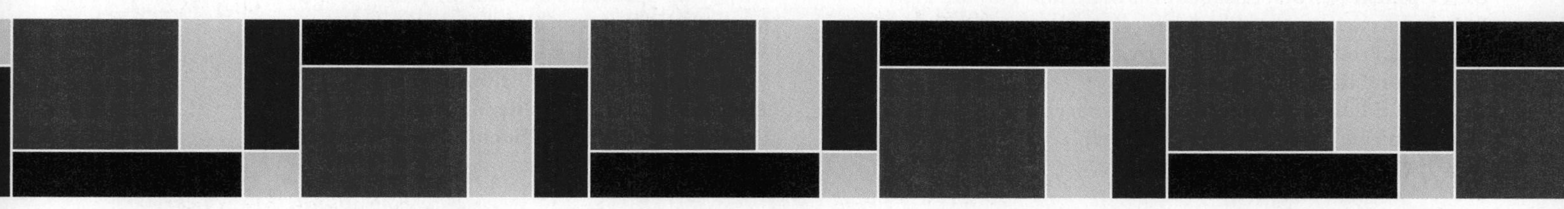

Carole Kenner, PhD, RNC-NIC, FAAN
Dean/Professor, School of Nursing
Associate Dean, Bouvé College of Health Sciences
Northeastern University
Boston, Massachusetts

Judith A. Lewis, PhD, RN, WHNP-BC, FAAN
Professor Emerita, School of Nursing
Virginia Commonwealth University
Richmond, Virginia

PEARSON

Boston Columbus Indianapolis New York San Francisco Upper Saddle River
Amsterdam Cape Town Dubai London Madrid Milan Munich Paris Montréal Toronto
Delhi Mexico City São Paulo Sydney Hong Kong Seoul Singapore Taipei Tokyo

Publisher: Julie Levin Alexander
Publisher's Assistant: Regina Bruno
Executive Acquisitions Editor: Pamela Fuller
Development Editors: Elisabeth Garofalo and Barbara Price
Editorial Assistant: Cynthia Gates
Managing Production Editor: Patrick Walsh
Production Liaison: Cathy O'Connell
Production Editor: GEX Publishing Services
Manufacturing Manager: Lisa McDowell
Art Director: Laura Gardner
Cover and Interior Designer: Symmetre Design Group
Director of Marketing: David Gesell
Marketing Manager: Phoenix Harvey and Debi Doyle
Marketing Specialist: Michael Sirinides
Marketing Assistant: Crystal Gonzalez
Media Product Manager: Travis Moses-Westphal
Composition: GEX Publishing Services
Printer/Binder: Courier/Kendallville
Cover Printer: LeHigh Phoenix Color/Hagerstown

Credits and acknowledgments for content borrowed from other sources and reproduced, with permission, in this textbook appear on appropriate page within text.

Library of Congress Cataloging-in-Publication Data
Kenner, Carole.
Genetics and genomics for nursing / Carole Kenner, Judith A. Lewis.
p. ; cm.
Includes bibliographical references.
ISBN-13: 978-0-13-217407-7 (pbk.)
ISBN-10: 0-13-217407-3 (pbk.)
I. Lewis, Judith A., II. Title.
[DNLM: 1. Genetics, Medical--Nurses' Instruction. 2. Genetic Phenomena--Nurses' Instruction.
3. Genomics—Nurses' Instruction. QZ 50] LC Classification not assigned
616'042—dc23

2012034146

10 9 8 7 6 5 4 3 2 1

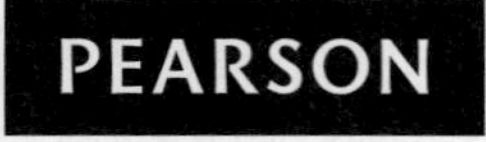

ISBN-10: 0-13-217407-3
ISBN-13: 978-0-13-217407-7

Dedication

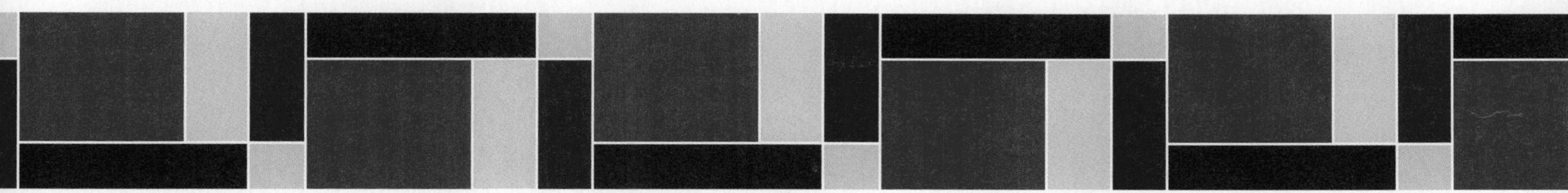

This book is dedicated to students and nurses who are committed to excellence in patient care and nursing education.

About the Authors

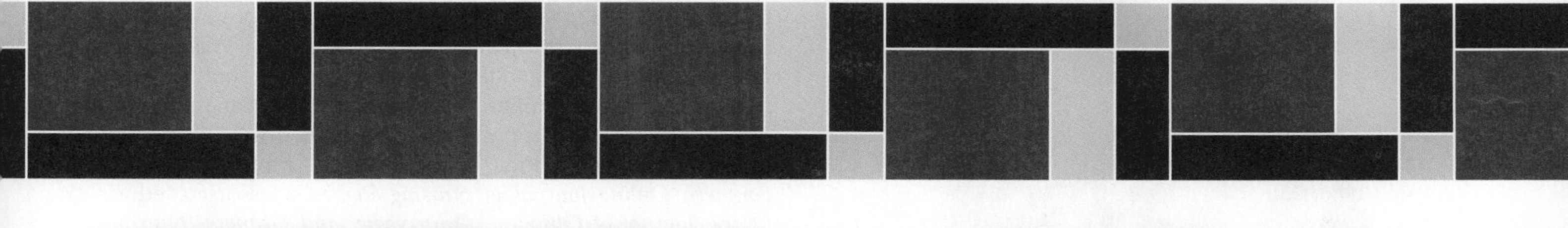

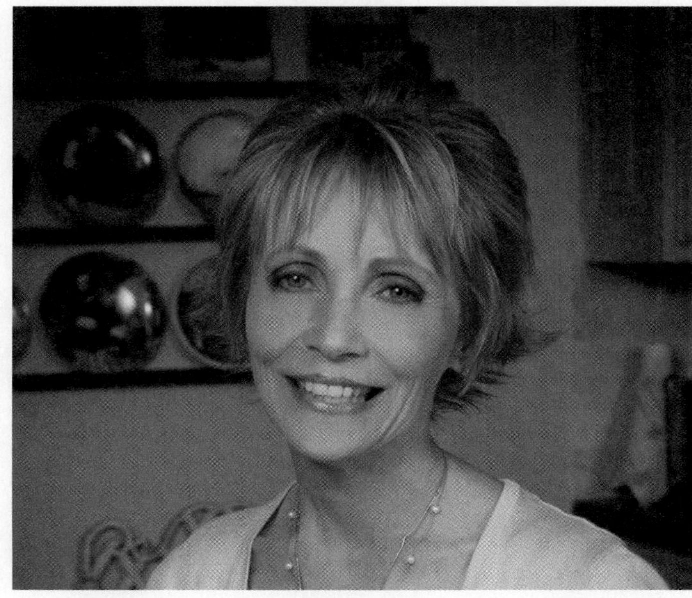

Carole Kenner, PhD, RNC-NIC, FAAN

Dr. Carole Kenner is the Dean in the School of Nursing and Associate Dean of the Bouvé College of Health Sciences at Northeastern University. Dr. Kenner received a Bachelor of Science in Nursing from the University of Cincinnati and her master's and doctorate in nursing from Indiana University. She specialized in neonatal/perinatal nursing for her master's degree and obtained a PhD in nursing with a minor in higher education for her doctorate. She has almost 30 years' experience in teaching, with 20 of those years in higher education administration. She has served as a Chiron Mentor for nurses through Sigma Theta Tau International, a nursing honor society. She also has served as a mentor for new deans and assistant deans through the American Association of Colleges of Nursing. Dr. Kenner has authored more than 100 journal articles and 20 textbooks.

Dr. Kenner's career is dedicated to nursing education and to the health of neonates and their families, as well as to the educational and professional development of health care practices in neonatology. Her dedication includes providing a health care standard for educating neonatal nurses nationally and internationally. Her passion led her to begin the journal *Newborn and Infant Nursing Reviews,* for which she now serves as international column editor. She serves on the *Consensus Committee of Newborn Intensive Care Design Standards* (which sets recommendations for Neonatal Intensive Care Unit designs), as well as on the March of Dimes Nursing Advisory Committee. Dr. Kenner is a fellow of the American Academy of Nursing (FAAN), past president of the National Association of Neonatal Nurses (NANN), and Founder and President of the Council of International Neonatal Nurses (COINN), the first international organization representing neonatal nursing. She is the 2011 recipient of the Audrey Hepburn Award for Contributions to the Health and Welfare of Children internationally. Her book *Developmental Care of Newborns & Infants,* second edition, which she coedited with Dr. Jacqueline McGrath, won the 2011 American Journal of Nursing Book of the Year Award. She coauthored the book *Teaching the IOM* with Anita Finkelman, which is now in its second edition and won an award for merit from the Society for Technical Communication, Washington, DC. Dr. Kenner was also one of the founders of the 501C Institute for Oklahoma Nursing Education (IONE), which addresses building capacity in the workforce in the state of Oklahoma. She has been involved in genetics her entire career—at the University of Cincinnati, she headed one of the first master's degree in nursing programs that had a minor in genetics. She represented the National Association of Neonatal Nurses to the National Coalition of Health Professions Education in Genetics (NCHPEG) for over 10 years. She also helped develop the nursing competencies in genetics through her work with NCHPEG and the American Nurses Association. In addition, Dr. Kenner headed an NIH grant that focused on the family context of clinical genetics. She is a member of the International Society of Nurses in Genetics and the American Academy of Nursing's Expert Panel on Genetics.

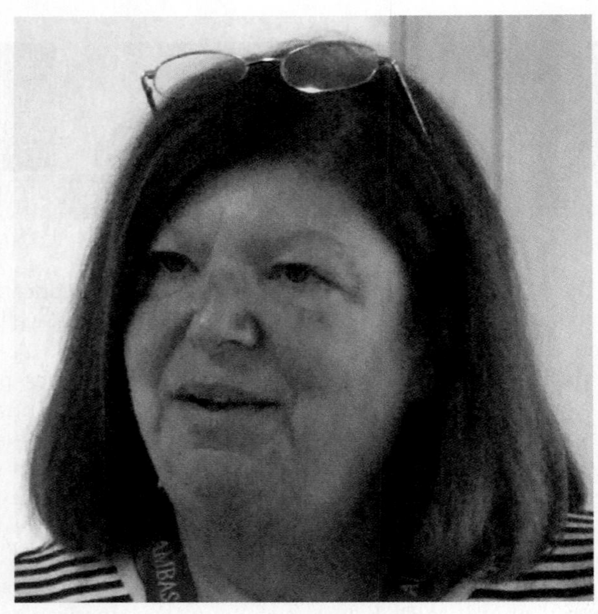

Judith A. Lewis, PhD, RN, WHNP-BC, FAAN

Judith A. Lewis is Professor Emerita at Virginia Commonwealth University in Richmond, VA. She is a certified women's health nurse practitioner and has completed postdoctoral education in genetics through the Web-Based Genetics Institute at Cincinnati Children's Medical Center and the Summer Genetics Institute sponsored by the National Institutes of Health, National Institute of Nursing Research, and Georgetown University.

Dr. Lewis received an AB in English and American Literature from Brandeis University, a BS in Nursing from Boston University, an MS in Nursing from the University of California at San Francisco, and a PhD in Health Policy and Social Welfare from the Heller School at Brandeis University. She also holds a post-master's certificate in Online Teaching from UCLA Extension.

Dr. Lewis has served in leadership roles in several professional associations. She has been the editor of the *Southern Online Journal of Nursing Research*, associate editor of the *Journal of Obstetric, Gynecologic, and Neonatal Nursing*, the founding editor of *Issues in Interdisciplinary Care*, and president of the International Society of Nurses in Genetics. She was appointed by Donna Shalala to the Secretary's Advisory Committee on Genetic Testing, and served as a member for the entire length of the Committee's tenure. She has received AWHONN's Distinguished Professional Service Award, the National Academies of Practice's Nicholas Andrew Cummings Annual Award, and the ISONG Founder's Award for Service. She served as a member of the Steering Committee for the Essential Nursing Competencies and Curricula Guidelines for Genetics and Genomics. Currently, Dr. Lewis is a member the American Academy of Nursing's Expert Panel in Genetics, the Academy's Expert Panel in Women's Health, the Editorial Board of *MCN: The American Journal of Maternal Child Nursing*, and the March of Dimes National Nurse Advisory Council. She is widely published and has given numerous lectures nationally and internationally on public policy in genetics and the integration of genetics into nursing education and practice. Dr. Lewis is actively involved in nursing education and serves as an adjunct faculty member in the School of Nursing and the department of Gender, Sexuality, and Women's Studies at Virginia Commonwealth University, and as a Term Lecturer in the School of Nursing at MGH Institute of Health Professions in Boston, MA.

Thank You

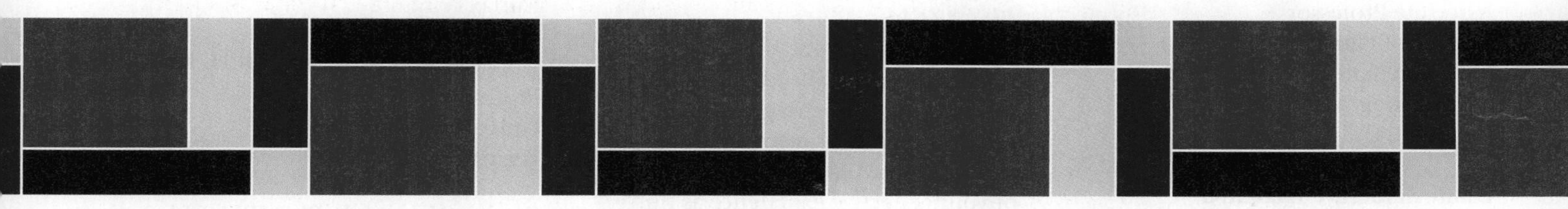

We extend a heartfelt thanks to our contributors, who gave their time, effort, and expertise so tirelessly to the development and writing of chapters and resources that helped foster our goal of preparing student nurses for evidence-based practice.

Text Contributors

Michelle Beauchesne, DNSc, RN, CPNP, FAAN
Associate Professor
Northeastern University
Boston, Massachusetts
Chapter 11: Newborn Screening and Genetic Testing: Ethical Considerations

Linda K. Bennington, MSN, RNC
Senior Lecturer
Nursing Department
Old Dominion University
Norfolk, Virginia
Chapter 6: Mosaicism
Chapter 15: Immunogenetics

Marina V. Boykova, PhD (c), RN
Doctoral Student
University of Oklahoma College of Nursing
Oklahoma City, Oklahoma
Chapter 3: Family Context of Clinical Genetics

Linda Callahan, CRNA, PhD, PMHNP
Professor Emeritus
School of Nursing
California State University,
Long Beach, California
Chapter 20: Depression and Genetic Linkages

Michele DeGrazia, PhD, RN, NNP
Neonatal Nurse Practitioner
Nurse Scientist
Children's Hospital Boston
Boston, Massachusetts
Chapter 11: Newborn Screening and Genetic Testing: Ethical Considerations

Robert M. Fineman, MD, PhD
Dean, Health and Human Services
North Seattle Community College and Clinical Professor of Pediatrics
University of Washington
Seattle, Washington
Chapter 2: Basic Concepts in Genetics and Genomics: Part of Every Type of Nursing Practice
Chapter 17: Impact of Environment on Health: Interaction with Genes

Ellen Giarelli, EdD, RN, MS, CRNP
Associate Professor
Division of Graduate Nursing
Drexel University
Philadelphia, Pennsylvania
Chapter 22: Autism

Cynthia L. Little, PhD, RN
Assistant Clinical Professor of Nursing
College of Nursing and Health Professions
Drexel University
Philadelphia, Pennsylvania
Chapter 8: Genetics and Fetal Development
Chapter 13: Family History Tool

Ann Maradiegue, PhD, CRNP-BC
Assistant Professor, School of Nursing, College of Health and Human Services
George Mason University
Fairfax, Virginia
Chapter 14: Risk Assessment

Cheryl A. Mele, MSN, RN
Assistant Clinical Professor
Division of Graduate Nursing
Nurse Practitioner, MSN Program
Drexel University
Philadelphia, Pennsylvania
Chapter 7: Mendelian Inheritance

Cindy L. Munro, PhD, RN, ANP-C, FAAN
Associate Dean for Research and Innovation, Professor
University of South Florida College of Nursing
Tampa, Florida
Chapter 18: Common Diseases with Genetic Linkages

Sharon J Olsen, PhD, RN, AOCN
Assistant Professor
Johns Hopkins University School of Nursing
Baltimore, Maryland
Chapter 16: Cancer Genetics

Alexandra Paul-Simon, PhD, RN
Assistant Director for the Accelerated BSN Program
Clinical Associate Professor
MGH Institute of Health Professions
Boston, Massachusetts
Chapter 4: Meiosis and Mitosis

Cindy Prows, MSN, RN, FAAN
Clinical Nurse Specialist
Cincinnati Children's Hospital
Division of Human Genetics
Cincinnati, Ohio
Chapter 23: Pharmacogenomics

Houry Puzantian PhD, BSN
Lecturer in Pharmacology,
University of Pennsylvania
School of Nursing, Claire M. Fagin Hall
Philadelphia, Pennsylvania
Research Fellow/MTR Program, School of Medicine
Institute for Translational Medicine & Therapeutics
Chapter 23: Pharmacogenomics

Debra Schutte, PhD, RN
Associate Professor
College of Nursing
Michigan State University
East Lansing, Michigan
Chapter 24: Genetics and Aging

Diane Seibert, PhD, CRNP
Program Director
Family Nurse Practitioner Program
Graduate School of Nursing
Uniformed Services University of the Health Sciences
Bethesda, Maryland
Chapter 14: Risk Assessment

Matthew R. Sorenson, PhD, RN
Department of Nursing
DePaul University
Chicago, Illinois
Chapter 5: Aneuploidy
Chapter 19: Bipolar Disorder and Genetic Linkages

Sharon Terry, MA
President and Chief Executive Officer
Genetic Alliance
Washington, DC
Chapter 12: Genetic Information Nondiscrimination Act Legislations

Eileen Trigoboff, RN, PMHCNS-BC, DNS, DABFN, CIP
Director, Program Evaluation
Buffalo Psychiatric Center
State University of New York at Buffalo
Research Instructor,
School of Medicine
Department of Psychiatry
State University of New York at Buffalo
Adjunct Faculty,
School of Rehabilitation & Social Work
Buffalo, New York
Chapter 21: Addictive Behaviors and Genetic Linkages

Reviewers

Our heartfelt thanks go out to our colleagues from schools of nursing across the country who have given their time generously to help us create this exciting new edition. We have reaped the benefit of your collective experience as nurses and teachers, and we have made many improvements due to your efforts. Among those who gave us their encouragement and comments are as follows:

Sheila A. Alexander, PhD, RN
Assistant Professor
University of Pittsburgh
Pittsburgh, Pennsylvania

Nancy R. Bowers, MSN, RN, CNS
Professor
University of Cincinnati
Cincinnati, Ohio

Elisabeth Chismark, PhD, RN
Adjunct Professor
Clemson University
Clemson, South Carolina

Julie Eggert, PhD, GNP-BC, AOCN(R)
Associate Professor
Clemson University
Clemson, South Carolina

Lori Sholders Farmer, ARNP, MSN, MS, APNG
Adjunct Professor
Pensacola State College
Pensacola, Florida

Dale Halsey Lea, MPH, RN, CGC, FAAN
Consultant, Public Health Genomics
Maine Genetics Program
Augusta, Maine

Ann Maradiegue, PhD, BC-FNP, FAANP
Assistant Professor
George Mason University
Fairfax, Virginia

Gia Mudd Martin, PhD, MPH, RN
Professor
University of Kentucky
Lexington, Kentucky

Patricia Newcomb, PhD, RN, CPNP
Assistant Professor, Director, Genomics Translational Research Lab
University of Texas at Arlington
Arlington, Texas

Carmen T. Paniagua, EdD, MSN, RN, CPC, ANP, ACNP-BC, APNG, FAANP
Associate Professor
University of Arkansas for Medical Sciences
Little Rock, Arkansas

Lynn Rew, EdD, RN, AHN-BC, FAAN
Professor
University of Texas at Austin
Austin, Texas

Marie E. Twal, DrPH, CPNP
Professor
Indiana University of Pennsylvania
Indiana, Pennsylvania

Suzanne W. Van Orden, MSEd, MSN, RN
Professor
Old Dominion University
Norfolk, Virginia

Marcia Van Riper, PhD, RN, FAAN
Professor
University of North Carolina at Chapel Hill
Chapel Hill, North Carolina

Linda D. Ward, PhD, ARNP
Assistant Professor
Washington State University
Spokane, Washington

Preface

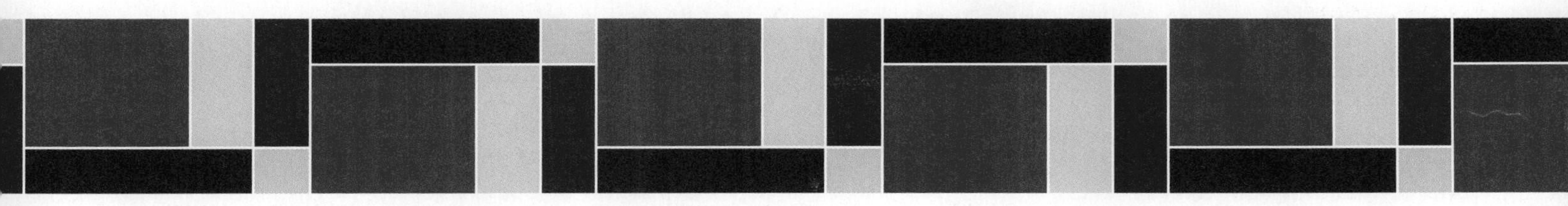

The sequencing of the human genome was a watershed event that ushered in a new understanding of the mechanisms of health promotion, disease prevention, and illness. Nurses and other health care professionals are expected to understand the basic principles of genetics and genomics and how these principles influence health care delivery to individuals, families, and communities.

Purpose of the Text

This book was developed to ensure that nursing students and practicing nurses had access to information necessary for safe and effective nursing care in the genomic era. The book is designed to present information in small, discrete units to enhance understanding. Each chapter includes pretests, section quizzes, and posttests, with answers provided so that learners can ensure their comprehension of content. The book can be used in its entirety or as a modularized learning tool that can support content in many different courses.

The chapters focus on basic genetic information and its relationship to nursing practice. The goals of the book are to

1. present critical information in a practical, easy-to-understand fashion.
2. delineate the competencies necessary for effective nursing practice, regardless of clinical specialty or nursing role.

While the primary audience for this book is undergraduate nursing students, it also will be useful for other levels of nursing education. Practicing nurses who received their education in the pregenomic era will find the book helpful in reviewing basic concepts and applications of genetics and genomics to clinical practice. It will be a valuable reference for nursing educators in academic and clinical settings.

Organization of the Text

The book consists of 24 discrete chapters. Part I, "Back to the Basics," places genetics and genomics into context. Part II, "Basic Genetics Concepts," provides the reader with knowledge of current genetics and genomics concepts that will enable the reader to have a firm understanding of the basic science of genetics. Part III, "Ethical, Legal, and Social Implications," provides the reader with information on the social, ethical, and legal implications of genetics and genomics, including important public policy implications of genomic health care, newborn screening and prenatal genetics, and will provide examples of how these concepts are relevant in health care today. Part IV, "Assessment," describes the importance of the family history and the concept of risk assessment. Part V, "Genetics of Cancer," contains information about immunogenetics and cancer genetics that is important for understanding the contributions genomic science has made to the field of cancer prevention and treatment. Part VI, "Public Health Genetics," describes the importance of genetics in health promotion and in the diagnosis, prevention, and treatment of complex health problems that have a significant public health importance. Part VII, "Psychiatric Disorders," focuses on the contributions genetics and genomics have made to our understanding of mental health issues, including depression, addictions, and autism. The final section, Part VIII, "Special Topics," is devoted to special topics such as pharmacogenomics and the role genetic knowledge plays in our understanding of aging.

The book includes a comprehensive glossary and a list of abbreviations. It also includes an exhaustive compendium of Internet resources that will provide the reader with the most up-to-date information available in this rapidly developing field. Each chapter includes features such as Emerging Evidence and Critical Thinking Checkpoints that encourage the reader to apply chapter content to clinical practice. The comprehensive reference list will allow readers to expand their knowledge in areas relevant to their personal area of interest. The ultimate goal of the book is to ensure genetic and genomic literacy for the nursing workforce of the 21st century.

Acknowledgments

We would like to thank Pamela Fuller, Executive Acquisitions Editor at Pearson Education, and Elisabeth Garofalo and Barbara Price, the developmental editors, for their support and encouragement during the project. We also would like to thank the contributors who have generously shared their expert knowledge, and the reviewers who provided feedback and validation for our work. We would like to acknowledge our families, who often only saw us for brief minutes during the book's writing and production: Lester Kenner, Arthur Lewis, and Jonathan Lewis.

Contents

PART 1

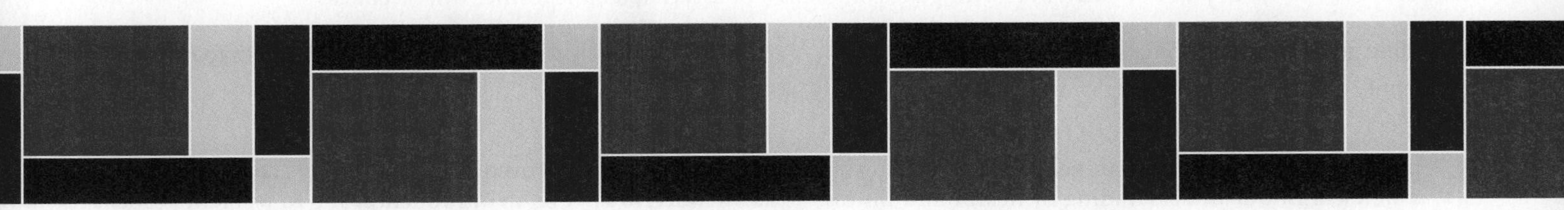

Back to the Basics

CHAPTER

1 Genetics and Genomics: Definitions and Trends

Judith A. Lewis

LEARNING OUTCOMES Following the completion of this chapter, the learner will be able to

1. Define genetics and genomics.
2. Identify current trends in genetics and genomics.
3. Discuss the relevance of genetics and genomics to nursing practice.

The sequencing of the human genome has ushered in a new era in our understanding of health and illness. The purpose of this chapter is to introduce the reader to the human genome and provide some basic definitions. Material will not be covered in depth in this chapter; rather, it is intended to serve as an introduction and to whet the reader's appetite for the subject.

PRETEST

1. Genetics is the study of
   A. human heredity.
   B. individual genes.
   C. the transmission of health and illness.
   D. mitosis and meiosis.
2. The Human Genome Project
   A. was designed to identify the hereditary causes of health and illness.
   B. is an ongoing effort of the U.S. Department of Health and Human Services.
   C. focused solely on the science of genetics.
   D. successfully mapped the entire complement of genes in humans.
3. The relevance of genetics to nursing practice
   A. is marginal at best.
   B. is limited to advanced practice nurses.
   C. is important to all nurses, regardless of level of education or site of practice.
   D. is complex and difficult to describe.
4. Nurses need to know about genetics because
   A. they may have patients who ask questions that are hard to answer.
   B. they may be working in places where there are no medical geneticists.
   C. they have a special interest in genetics.
   D. genetics knowledge is a core competency for nursing practice.
5. Illnesses that have a genetic component are limited to
   A. those syndromes identified by newborn screening.
   B. certain forms of cancer, including breast cancer.
   C. hereditary conditions.
   D. essentially all issues affecting health and illness.
6. Which of the following diagnoses does NOT have a genetic component?
   A. Type 2 diabetes mellitus
   B. Acute trauma
   C. Cystic fibrosis
   D. Rheumatoid arthritis
7. Which statement is true?
   A. There are significant genetic differences between races.
   B. There is more genetic variation within racial groups than between racial groups.
   C. Some races are genetically inferior to other races.
   D. Mental retardation has a large racial component that is genetically determined.
8. Multifactorial genetic inheritance
   A. includes environmental factors.
   B. is a result of climate change.
   C. is found in individuals who have sickle cell anemia.
   D. is only found in conditions transmitted from mother to son.

9. The Human Genome Project
   A. was conducted solely by the U.S. Government.
   B. has been completed and has no further relevance for scientific research.
   C. continues to be the foundation for our understanding of health and illness.
   D. resulted in the controversy over the use of stem cell therapy.

10. The most valuable information to determine an individual's risk for a condition with a genetic component is
    A. the sequencing of the breast cancer gene.
    B. the test for cystic fibrosis carriers.
    C. maternal serum screening for alpha fetoprotein.
    D. the family history.

Pretest answers are located in the Appendix.

SECTION ONE: Definitions

The term **genetics** originated from a Greek term that referred to the scientific branch of biology focusing on genes and heredity. In the mid-1800s, Greg Mendel popularized inheritance pattern theory when he conducted scientific experiments. This activity was considered the application of genetics. The term *genetics* continued to gain prominence for the next few decades. In 1953, Watson and Crick first described the structure of the **DNA** (**deoxyribonucleic acid**) molecule. (Watson & Crick, 1953). This was the beginning of a new era of scientific advancement—one that changed forever our understanding of health and illness. Exactly 50 years later, Dr. Francis Collins announced that the entire **human genome** had been sequenced (Collins, 2003). This event meant that the entire gene composition of humans was sequenced and known.

There have been very few events that have had the same transformative effect on health care as **sequencing** of the human genome. The 19th century saw the invention of anesthesia and the evolution of medical asepsis. The 20th century will be remembered for innovations such as the development of immunizations for diseases such as polio and the discovery of antibiotics. The 21st century promises to be memorable for **genomic health care** and personalized approaches to health promotion and disease treatment.

The sequencing of the human genome, along with the sequencing of other organisms, provides us with valuable information regarding health and illness. We have learned that almost all conditions adversely affecting health and illness have both genetic and environmental causes, often referred to as **genomics**. Some conditions, such as human immunodeficiency virus (HIV), are caused by environment, but there still is a genetic component that helps explain why two individuals with the same **viral load**, or amount of virus present, respond so differently to the disease and to disease treatment. Other conditions, such as cystic fibrosis, are largely due to genetics, but environmental influences may be responsible for the differences in the course of the illness in individuals who have the same mutation.

It is important to remember, however, that genetics and genomics do not exist in isolation. It is tempting to believe that genetics is an absolute science, and that all phenomena are reducible to the sequencing of the **genetic code**. Genes interact with the environment and may be expressed differently in different situations. At the turn of the 20th century, respected men who studied what was then cutting-edge science made pronouncements in the name of **eugenics** that caused great pain and suffering. Eugenics science was used to provide the rationale for mental hygiene movements that denigrated those considered "feeble minded," and the concept of eugenics was central to Adolph Hitler's belief that the Aryan race was superior to others. It is important that the limitations of genetics and genomics be acknowledged and respected.

SECTION ONE REVIEW

1. Watson and Crick
   A. described the structure of DNA
   B. were the fathers of genetic science.
   C. developed the human genome.
   D. worked in the science of eugenics.
2. Eugenics
   A. is the basis of human variation.
   B. provides us with valuable information about the superiority of one race over the other.
   C. is a current theory of human evolution.
   D. provided the rationale for the inappropriate treatment of those who had developmental disabilities.
3. The father of human genetics was
   A. Adolph Hitler.
   B. Gregor Mendel.
   C. James Watson.
   D. Francis Collins.

Answers: 1. A; 2. D; 3. B

SECTION TWO: Trends and Innovations

There are many exciting innovations that already have shown great promise. **Pharmacogenomics** allows our knowledge of genetic variation to help tailor drug therapy to an individual's genetic response. Oncologists can determine which chemotherapy protocol will yield the best therapeutic outcomes with the fewest side effects. Individuals who have hypertension are able to reduce their blood pressure while controlling those side effects that adversely affect adherence to drug regimens. And individuals who have mental illness have the opportunity to have their symptoms managed effectively without having to undergo the trial-and-error process when searching for the optimal medication regime!

The sequencing of the human genome has provided us with information that allows for the testing for various forms of genes. **Genetic testing** shows great promise. Used wisely, genetic testing allows individuals to have information about their genetic makeup that helps them make informed decisions about reproductive options, health screening, and behavioral modifications to reduce the risk of developing certain diseases. Why is it that some smokers develop lung cancer and some do not? Why do some overweight people develop Type 2 diabetes while others maintain normal glucose levels? Why do some women and men develop certain types of cancer while others do not? In some cases, the information gleaned from genetic testing helps individuals reduces their risk of developing certain conditions; in other cases, the rationale for a more aggressive screening protocol is suggested.

People are bombarded daily with information from the public and scientific media about the relationship of certain personal behaviors with increased risk of certain diseases. Does smoking increase the risk of bladder cancer in all individuals, or is there a genetic mediation to the relationship? What about coffee consumption? Moderate alcohol use? Exercise? As our knowledge of genetic factors that influence these relationships continues to increase, individuals are able to better understand how their personal genetic makeup puts them at greater or lesser risk for certain conditions. Coupled with a robust knowledge of their family history, individuals are able to tailor a personal plan that makes sense for them individually. While it is impossible to avoid all risk, knowing which health-promoting behaviors have the greatest chance of return on personal investment helps individuals make healthy choices for themselves and their family members. Nurses are experts at obtaining information regarding individual and family histories. The family history is a key component of understanding the role genetic information has in helping individuals and family members understand their personal risk factors. This will be discussed in detail in Chapter 13.

Emerging Evidence

The National Institutes of Health (**NIH**) have listed several research priorities that relate to research and health professions education in genetics. The website http://www.genome.gov is the place to visit to be up to date on the emerging evidence related to genetics and genomics. Another important website, http://www.cdc.gov/genomics, provides information from the Centers for Disease Control and Prevention (**CDC**) in the area of public health genomics.

SECTION TWO REVIEW

1. The work of the Human Genome Project
   - A. created the rationale for genetic determinism.
   - B. provided us with the basis for personalized health care.
   - C. dictates which drugs will be most effective in treating cancer.
   - D. allows scientists to prove which individuals are healthiest.
2. Pharmacogenomics will allow health care providers to
   - A. avoid prescribing medications that have any side effects.
   - B. tailor drug therapy to enhance drug effectiveness.
   - C. decrease the number of medications an individual needs.
   - D. decrease the cost of medications.
3. One of the uses of genetic testing is
   - A. to totally prevent the transmission of genetic conditions.
   - B. to provide information to individuals so they can make decisions about their personal health.
   - C. to tell people how to lead healthy lives.
   - D. to help people focus on the genetic basis of all illness.

Answers: 1. B; 2. B; 3. B

SECTION THREE: Importance of Genetics for Nurses

All nurses need to have a working knowledge of genetics and genomics. In 2005, members of over 40 professional nursing organizations, along with several schools of nursing and consumer advocacy groups, endorsed a document outlining the essentials of genetic nursing competencies and curricula guidelines (ANA, 2005); in 2009, the outcome indicators were published. A full discussion of the specific competencies will be presented in Chapter 2. These documents note that genetic and genomic literacy are a core competency for all nurses, regardless of their level of education, clinical specialty, professional role, or site of practice. The scope and standards of practice for nurses related to genetics have been jointly published by **ISONG** (The International Society of Nurses in Genetics) and the American Nurses Association (**ANA**). These standards delineate the scope and standards of practice for those nurses whose practice is in the field of genetics/genomics nursing at both the basic and advanced practice level.

The American Association of Colleges of Nursing (**AACN**) has identified genetics/genomics knowledge as a part of the essential competencies for baccalaureate education at the undergraduate level (AACN, 2008). The newest version of the *Essentials of Master's Education for Advanced Practice Nursing by AACN (2011)* states that advanced practice nurses need a working knowledge of genetics. Accreditation for nursing programs will include standards that ensure that nurses are educated appropriately to be prepared to practice professional nursing in the genetic/genomic era of health care.

It is clear from the movement within nursing leadership that all nurses will need a level of genetic literacy. There are basic concepts that all nurses will need to know, and specific knowledge and competencies that will be required in specific practice areas. No nurse will be exempt from these expectations. Those who do not have the basic knowledge will find a myriad of print and electronic resources available to assist them in acquiring this knowledge. Resources such as this booktext will provide essential knowledge to students and practicing clinicians as well. The web-based resources found within the book will allow for nurses to stay up to date in a field that is rapidly changing and developing.

SECTION THREE REVIEW

1. The essential competencies for nursing practice in genetics/genomics
   A. were endorsed by over 40 professional nursing associations.
   B. were developed by geneticists who were experts in the field.
   C. are required by accrediting organizations.
   D. apply only to those nurses who specialize in genetics.
2. Those nurses who are required to have basic genetic literacy include
   A. advanced practice nurses.
   B. nurses who practice in specialty areas.
   C. nurses who practice in medical-surgical nursing.
   D. all nurses, regardless of practice area, clinical specialty, or level of education.

Answers: 1. A; 2. D

POSTTEST

1. The most important source of genetic information can be gleaned from
   A. the results of genetic testing.
   B. newborn screening test results.
   C. buccal swabs.
   D. the family history.
2. Public health genetics/genomics information can be obtained from which website?
   A. CDC
   B. ANA
   C. ISONG
   D. NIH
3. The standards for nursing education in genetics for professional nursing programs are promulgated by:
   A. American Association of Colleges of Nursing
   B. National Institutes of Health
   C. Centers for Disease Control and Prevention
   D. American Medical Association
4. The interaction of medications and an individual's genetic makeup is the study of
   A. eugenics.
   B. genomics.
   C. pharmacogenomics.
   D. pharmacology.
5. The belief that all human responses to health and illness is caused by genetics is
   A. eugenics.
   B. genetic determinism.
   C. pharmacogenomics.
   D. genomics.

Posttest answers are located in the Appendix.

CHAPTER SUMMARY

The area of genetics and genomics is an important area for nursing practice. Essentially all conditions have a genetic component, and the interaction between genetic material and environmental influences is equally important. While genetics is a key factor in predicting the occurrence of disease, it must be remembered that each of us is more than our genes. While we must respect the important contribution made by the science of genetics and genomics, we must also remember that genes are but one factor that makes us who we are. The dangers of genetic determinism (the belief that our genes dictate our future) must be tempered with humanism and humanity. The dangers of **genetic determinism** have been well documented in the shortcomings of the eugenic movement. These important lessons also are portrayed in the movie, *GATTACA*.

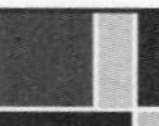

CRITICAL THINKING CHECKPOINT

A newly graduated professional nurse is working on a busy medical-surgical unit. She has a postoperative patient who is at risk for thrombus formation. This patient, who currently is receiving low-dose molecular heparin, is scheduled to be discharged on warfarin (Coumadin) therapy. The nurse has heard of the importance of genetic testing before implementing Coumadin therapy, but there are no such medical orders for this testing. How should the nurse proceed?

Answers are provided in the Appendix

ONLINE RESOURCES

Association of Colleges of Nursing: http://www.aacn.nche.edu

Centers for Disease Control and Prevention's Public Health Genomics Center: http://www.cdc.gov/genomics

International Society of Nurses in Genetics: http://www.isong.org

NIH National Human Genome Research Institute: http://www.genome.gov

REFERENCES

American Association of Colleges of Nursing. (2011). *The essentials of master's education for the advanced practice nurses.* Washington, DC: Author.

American Association of Colleges of Nursing. (2008). *The essentials of baccalaureate education for professional nursing practice.* Washington, DC: Author.

Collins, F. S. (2003, April 14). *Opening remarks.* Presented at the From Double Helix to Human Sequence and Beyond Symposium, Bethesda, MD.

Consensus Panel on Genetic/Genomic Nursing Competencies. (2009). *Essentials of genetic and genomic nursing: Competencies, curricula guidelines, and outcome indicators* (2nd ed.). Silver Spring, MD: American Nurses Association.

International Society of Nurses in Genetics and American Nursing Association. (2007). *Genetics/genomics nursing: Scope and standards of practice.* Silver Spring, MD: American Nurses Association.

Watson, J. D., & Crick, F. H. C. (1953). Molecular structure of nucleic acids: A structure for deoxyribose nucleic acid. *Nature, 171,* 737–738.

CHAPTER

2 Basic Concepts in Genetics and Genomics: Part of Every Type of Nursing Practice

Robert M. Fineman

LEARNING OUTCOMES

Following the completion of this chapter, the learner will be able to

1. Outline basic concepts of genetics and genomics in nursing practice.
2. Identify differences in the knowledge base and skills needed to incorporate basic concepts in genetics and genomics into every type of nursing practice.
3. Identify intervention strategies that promote health and/or prevent disease in genetically high-risk populations.

This chapter emphasizes the importance of integrating genetics and genomics into every kind of nursing practice regardless of academic preparation, practice setting, role, or specialty. The chapter describes competencies regarding genetics and genomics that need to be incorporated into nursing practice. These particulars form the fundamental basis for the roles and responsibilities nurses assume in the complex health care systems of the United States and elsewhere.

PRETEST

1. Genetic/genomic bio-banking refers to the collection and storage of biological materials for research and other purposes including, but not limited to, clinical diagnosis, treatment and/or the prognosis of genetic diseases, and other genetic health-related issues.
   A. True
   B. False
2. Community health nurse practice refers to nursing practice that emphasizes both personal health care practice and public health nurse practice.
   A. True
   B. False
3. The [three words] refers to a multiyear, multibillion dollar, international research project, completed in 2003, whose primary aim was to determine the sequence of the chemical base pairs that make up human DNA, and to identify and map the approximately 25,000 genes in the human genome from a physical and functional standpoint. What are three words are missing from the preceding sentence?
4. Epidemiology refers to the
   A. study of the distribution of health-related events and states.
   B. frequency of health-related events and states.
   C. determinants of health-related events and states.
   D. control and/or prevention of health-related problems.
   E. All of the above
5. Essential competencies, curricula guidelines, and outcome indicators for all registered nurses in the United States have been developed by an independent panel of nurse leaders from clinical, research, and academic settings whose goal was to establish the minimum basis by which to prepare the nursing workforce to deliver competent genetic- and genomic-focused nursing care.
   A. True
   B. False
6. Primary prevention refers to efforts aimed at
   A. reducing the incidence of specific disorders, injury, and disability, including birth defects.

B. minimizing the clinical manifestations of specific disorders, injury, and/or disability, including birth defects, through disease management.
C. averting and/or preventing social, financial, ethical, and legal burdens and situations including, for example, stigmatization, discrimination, and/or bias against affected patients, families, and communities.
D. All of the above

7. Registered nurses treat and educate patients, families, and communities; record medical histories; perform physical examinations; order tests and analyze their results; utilize equipment; administer treatments including medications; and help patients and families with follow-up care.
A. True
B. False

8. Genetic counseling refers to a communication process that helps individuals, families, and communities understand and adapt to which of the following implications of the genetic contributions to disease?
A. Biological
B. Medical
C. Psychological
D. Financial
E. Ethical
F. Legal
G. Social
H. All of the above

9. Genetic testing refers to
A. a diagnostic evaluation to determine if a genetic condition is present.
B. analyzing a population to determine which individuals are at risk for a genetic disease or for transmitting one
C. Both A and B

10. Health literacy refers to which of the following?
A. Cultural and conceptual knowledge
B. Listening and speaking skills
C. Writing and reading skills
D. The ability to understand and work with numbers (numeracy), as they pertain to health and health care
E. All of the above
F. B and C, above

Pretest answers are located in the Appendix.

SECTION ONE: Genetic and Genomic Competencies for RNs

A monograph containing essential competencies, curricula guidelines, and outcome indicators for all **registered nurses** in the United States, regardless of their academic preparation, practice setting, role, or specialty, was developed by an independent panel of nurse leaders from clinical, research, and academic settings. The goal was to establish the minimum basis by which to prepare the nursing workforce to deliver competent genetic- and genomic-focused nursing care (American Nurses Association, 2009).

Since all diseases and health conditions have some genetic or genomic component, the 27 competencies described in the monograph and subdivided into five major categories form an excellent foundation for any further discussion involving the inclusion of genetics and genomics into all nursing practice.

Professional Responsibilities

Registered nurses are expected to:

- Recognize when one's own attitudes and values related to genetic and genomic science may affect care provided to clients.
- Advocate for clients' access to desired genetic/genomic services and/or resources, including support groups.
- Examine competency of practice on a regular basis, identifying areas of strength, as well as areas in which professional development related to genetics and genomics would be beneficial.
- Incorporate genetic and genomic technologies and information into registered nurse practice.
- Demonstrate in practice the importance of tailoring genetic and genomic information and services to clients based on their culture, religion, knowledge level, literacy, and preferred language.
- Advocate for the rights of all clients for autonomous, informed genetic- and genomic-related decision-making and voluntary action.

Nursing Assessment

The registered nurse:

- Demonstrates an understanding of the relationship of genetics and genomics to health, prevention, screening, diagnostics, prognostics, selection of treatment, and monitoring of treatment effectiveness.
- Demonstrates ability to elicit a minimum of three-generation family health history information.
- Constructs a pedigree from collected family history information using standardized symbols and terminology.
- Collects personal, health, and developmental histories that consider genetic, environmental, and genomic influences and risks.
- Conducts comprehensive health and physical assessments that incorporate knowledge about genetic, environmental, and genomic influences and risk factors.
- Critically analyzes the history and physical assessment findings for genetic, environmental, and genomic influences and risk factors.
- Assesses clients' knowledge, perceptions, and responses to genetic and genomic information.
- Develops a plan of care that incorporates genetic and genomic assessment information.

Emerging Evidence

Competencies, like the ones described here, are vital in defining professional roles, duties, qualifications, responsibilities, and/or accountabilities. Oftentimes, these terms are used interchangeably in job descriptions, advertisements for positions, grant and contract proposals and renewals, and in many other human resource–related ways. Therefore, the information described here should help integrate genetics and genomics into nursing practice well into the 21st century in a variety of ways.

Identification

The registered nurse:

- Identifies clients who may benefit from specific genetic and genomic information and/or services based on assessment data.
- Identifies credible, accurate, appropriate, and current genetic and genomic information, resources, services, and/or technologies specific to given clients.
- Identifies ethical, ethnic/ancestral, cultural, religious, legal, fiscal, and societal issues related to genetic and genomic information and technologies.
- Defines issues that undermine the rights of all clients for autonomous, informed genetic- and genomic-related decision-making and voluntary action.

Referral Activities

The registered nurse:

- Facilitates referrals for specialized genetic and genomic services for clients as needed.

Education, Care, and Support

The registered nurse:

- Provides clients with interpretation of selective genetic and genomic information or services.
- Provides clients with credible, accurate, appropriate, and current genetic and genomic information, resources, services, and/or technologies that facilitate decision making.
- Uses health promotion and disease prevention practices that
    - consider genetic and genomic influences on personal and environmental risk factors.
    - incorporate knowledge of genetic and/or genomic risk factors (e.g., a client with a genetic predisposition for high cholesterol who can benefit from a change in lifestyle that will decrease the likelihood that the genetic risk will be expressed).
- Uses genetic- and genomic-based interventions and information to improve clients' outcomes.
- Collaborates with health care providers in providing genetic and genomic health care.
- Collaborates with insurance providers/payers (and other financial resources) to facilitate reimbursement for genetic and genomic health care services.
- Performs interventions/treatments appropriate to clients' genetic and genomic health care needs.
- Evaluates impact and effectiveness of genetic and genomic technology, information, interventions, and treatments against clients' outcome.

SECTION ONE REVIEW

1. Regarding health promotion and disease prevention practices, the registered nurse should
    A. consider genetic and genomic influences pertaining to personal and environmental risk factors.
    B. incorporate knowledge of genetic and/or genomic risk factors into the care plan of the client/patient.
    C. explain to the client/patient how she or he would handle the situation if she or he were in their shoes.
    D. All of the above
    E. A and B, above
2. The registered nurse should facilitate referrals for specialized genetic and genomic services for clients as needed.
    A. True
    B. False
3. It is acceptable for a registered nurse to ignore a client's decisions/decision-making process if the client's decisions or process are counter to the nurse's religious and/or cultural beliefs.
    A. True
    B. False

Answers: 1. E; 2. A; 3. B

SECTION TWO: Nursing Competencies for Community Health (PCH)

To be considered a nurse who can effectively integrate genetics and genomics into **PCH** practice, strong leadership, organizational, and management skills are required, as well as a minimum foundation of knowledge, including:

- Cellular and molecular biology, genetic variation, and inheritance.
- Interactions among genes, environmental factors, and behavioral factors that contribute to health and disease; i.e., the **determinants of health** and illness.
- Epidemiological and statistical methods used to study genetic risk factors, diseases, and protective factors.
- Genetic/genomic **core functions and health care services**.
- Factors, strategies, and programs that contribute to health promotion and disease prevention.
- Defining, assessing, and understanding the health status of individuals, families, and communities/populations.
- **Primary**, **secondary**, and **tertiary prevention**.
- Systems development/program planning, implementation, and evaluation including collecting, analyzing, and summarizing data relevant to **genetic/genomic health care** issues or problems; understanding relevant local, state, and federal laws and regulations; identifying policy and/or legislative options; writing clear and concise policy statements, bills, or regulations; articulating the economic, ethical, legal, social, political, and administrative implications of policy decisions (e.g., legislative and executive options/actions); and utilizing methods of monitoring and evaluating quality and effectiveness of health care systems and/or programs (**quality assurance**).
- Financial planning and systems management including the development and dissemination of budget information; managing problems and/or issues within budgetary constraints; creating, implementing, and analyzing program **performance measures**; writing and overseeing grant proposals and contracts; and hiring, managing (including team building, scheduling, and conflict resolution), and evaluating personnel.
- Cultural awareness, competence, and sensitivity regarding **diversity** in individuals and communities.
- Privacy, confidentiality, discrimination, bias, stigmatization, autonomy, beneficence, nonmaleficence, and equity.
- The structure and function of local, state, and national public and private health agencies and organizations.
- Issues and/or problems regarding access to accessible, available, high-quality, culturally competent, community-based, family-oriented, affordable, effective, and efficient services and education.
- Relevant technologies including, but not limited to, genetic testing, screening, and genetic/genomic bio-banking.
- Mobilizing community partnerships involving data collectors/analyzers, policy makers, health care providers, families, the general public, and others to identify and solve patient, family, and community-related problems and issues.
- Support for research and training that demonstrates new insights and innovative solutions to genetic/genomic health and health care problems/issues.
- Efforts that ensure a public and personal health care workforce that is competent in genetics and genomics health/health care.

The PCH genetic/genomic **core competencies** described here are an up-to-date version of competencies described previously (Fineman, Qualifications of public health geneticists? Community Genet 2(2-3): 113-4. Reprinted by permission of Karger.). They are applicable to all health care providers (nurses, doctors, genetic counselors or others) who regularly participate in genetic/genomic PCH-related activities regardless of academic preparation, practice setting, role, or specialty (Grason and Guyer, 1995; **ASTHO** 2001).

SECTION TWO REVIEW

1. What types of nurses are the competencies in Section Two most relevant to compared to the kinds of nurses and the competencies in Section One?
2. Nurses who perform PCH-related activities need to be very knowledgeable about the structure and function of relevant local, state, and national public and private health agencies and organizations.
   A. True
   B. False
3. Nurses who perform PCH-related activities need to be very knowledgeable about access to accessible, available, high-quality, culturally competent, community-based, family-oriented, affordable, effective, and efficient services and education of clients, families, and communities.
   A. True
   B. False

Answers: 1. The competencies in Section One are aimed at all registered nurses while the competencies in Section Two are aimed more so at those who participate in PCH-related activities; 2. A; 3. A.

POSTTEST

1. The public health core functions include three specific types of activities. Name them. Educate, Care, Support
2. Which of the following are considered to be essential public health services?
   A. Monitor health status to identify community health problems.
   B. Inform, educate, and empower people about health issues.
   C. Diagnose and investigate health problems in a community.
   D. Develop policies and practices that support individual and community health efforts.
   E. Evaluate effectiveness, accessibility, and quality of personal and population-based health services.
   F. All of the above
3. The human genome contains approximately
   A. 15,000 genes
   B. 25,000 genes
   C. 50,000 genes
   D. 100,000 genes
4. Which of the following are determinants of health and illness?
   A. Genetic/genomic factors
   B. Environmental factors
   C. Behavioral factors
   D. All of the above
   E. A and B, above
5. Systems development/program planning, implementation, and evaluation could include which of the following?
   A. Collecting, analyzing, and summarizing data relevant to genetic/genomic health care issues or problems
   B. Understanding relevant local, state, and federal laws and regulations
   C. Identifying policy and/or legislative options
   D. Articulating the economic, ethical, legal, social, political, and administrative implications of policy decisions; e.g., legislative and executive options/actions
   E. Utilizing methods of monitoring and evaluating quality and effectiveness of health care systems and/or programs (quality assurance)
   F. All of the above
6. Diversity refers to differences that distinguish individuals and/or groups from one another.
   A. True
   B. False
7. When performing a nursing assessment, registered nurses should be able to elicit a minimum, three-generation family health history and also construct a pedigree from that information using standardized symbols and terminology.
   A. True
   B. False
8. Financial planning and systems management could include which of the following?
   A. Development and dissemination of budget information
   B. Managing problems and/or issues within budgetary constraints
   C. Creating, implementing, and analyzing program performance measures
   D. Writing and overseeing grant proposals and contracts
   E. Hiring, managing (including team building, scheduling, and conflict resolution) and evaluating personnel
   F. All of the above
9. Registered nurses need not recognize their own attitudes and values related to genetic and genomic services and information when providing care to clients.
   A. True
   B. False
10. Regardless of academic preparation, practice setting, role, or specialty, there are numerous opportunities for registered nurses to utilize genetics/genomics services and information to understand and promote health and well- being, lower morbidity and mortality, and prevent diseases and disability.
   A. True
   B. False

Posttest answers are located in the Appendix.

CHAPTER SUMMARY

Advances in genetics/genomics in the past 20+ years have and will continue to present numerous opportunities for understanding and promoting health and well-being, lowering morbidity and mortality, and preventing diseases and disability.

Nurses, regardless of their academic preparation, practice setting, role, or specialty, have and will continue to play an important role in the creation of new genetics/genomics knowledge, in health care provider education and training, and in the integration of genetics/genomics information, technologies, and education into virtually every aspect of our health care systems. They also help to "fulfill society's interest in assuring conditions in which [all] people can be healthy" (Institute of Medicine, 1988).

The competencies described in Section One relate to accountabilities that should be part of the job description of virtually every registered nurse in the United States. Those described in Section Two are aimed at nurses who work primarily in PCH. Numerous opportunities will continue to exist for many years to come for nurses to participate in the exciting fields of genetic/genomic health and health care.

CRITICAL THINKING CHECKPOINT

Mrs. John Smith delivered a baby with obvious signs and symptoms of Down syndrome. The baby died several minutes after birth. The causes of death listed in the death certificate were congenital heart disease and Down syndrome. Neither an autopsy nor a chromosome study was performed. Mrs. Smith and her husband, both 25-years-old, live in a rural setting. Pregnancy, labor, and the delivery at home (planned) were normal. No prenatal screening or testing procedures were done. Mrs. Smith had two previous miscarriages at 9 or 10 weeks' gestation. The abbreviated family medical history, obtained by their primary care provider, revealed that Mr. Smith was adopted, and he knew very little about his biological parents or his family medical history. Mrs. Smith is an only child. Her mother had a few miscarriages before and after she was born. Almost all of Mrs. Smith's relatives live several thousand miles away on the east coast of the United States, and she has a cousin in Florida (who she never met) who is "not right." In fact, unbeknownst to the Smiths, the cousin has Down syndrome.

No one, not even their primary care provider, suggested to Mrs. Smith that she delve further into her family medical history. When she asked her primary care provider about her chance of having another child with Down syndrome, he responded "practically nil." Eighteen months later Mrs. Smith had another child with Down syndrome. Once again, prenatal testing and/or screening were not done. The Smiths were very angry and upset, especially with their primary care provider. If he had encouraged Mrs. Smith to obtain additional family medical history information, she easily would have found she has two maternal cousins, one living in Florida and the other in Pennsylvania, who have Down syndrome, and that several relatives on her mother's side of the family have had multiple miscarriages. This was all due to a 14/21 balanced translocation chromosome anomaly in Mrs. Smith's mother's side of the family. Both of the Smith children inherited an unbalanced 14/21 translocation form of Down syndrome!

1. Which of the competencies listed in Section One apply to this case report?
2. Should a chromosome study have been performed on the first Smith baby?
3. Would a complete three-generation family history have helped this family?
4. Did the Smiths ever receive standard of care genetic counseling?
5. Should options such as prenatal testing and/or screening have been offered to the Smiths?

Answers are provided in the Appendix

Pearson Nursing Student Resources

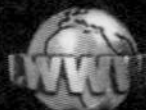

Find additional review materials at nursing.pearsonhighered.com

Prepare for success with additional NCLEX®-style practice questions, interactive assignments and activities, web links, animations, videos, and more!

ONLINE RESOURCES

Alliance of Genetic Support Groups: http://www.geneticalliance.org

American Association of Occupational Health Nurses, Inc.: http://www.aaohn.org

American College of Medical Genetics: http://www.acmg.net//AM/Template.cfm?Section=Home3

American Nurses Association: http://www.nursingworld.org and http://www.nursingworld.org/SpecialPages/Search?SearchMode=1&SearchPhrase=genetics+and+nursing

American Public Health Association – Environmental Public Health: http://www.apha.org/programs/environment/

American Public Health Association - Genetics and Public Health: http://www.apha.org/advocacy/policy/policysearch/default.htm?id=1161

American Public Health Association – Occupational Health & Safety: http://www.apha.org/membergroups/sections/aphasections/occupational/

American Society of Human Genetics: http://www.ashg.org

Association of State and Territorial Health Officials: http://www.astho.org

Centers for Disease Control and Prevention – National Center for Environmental Health: http://www.cdc.gov/nceh/

Centers for Disease Control and Prevention – Public Health Genomics: http://www.cdc.gov/genomics/default.htm

Centers for Disease Control and Prevention – Public Health Organizations and Associations: http://wwwn.cdc.gov/dls/links/links_pa.aspx

Environmental Health - Medline Plus: http://www.nlm.nih.gov/medlineplus/environmentalhealth.html

Environmental Health & Toxicology: http://sis.nlm.nih.gov/enviro.html

Gene Tests: http://www.ncbi.nlm.nih.gov/sites/GeneTests/?db=GeneTests

Geneticalliance UK: http://www.geneticalliance.org.uk

Genetic Nursing Credentialing Commission: www.geneticnurse.org

Genetic Services Branch – Maternal Child Health Bureau: http://mchb.hrsa.gov/programs/geneticservices/index.html

International Society of Nurses in Genetics (ISONG): http://www.isong.org

National Association of County & City Health Officials: http://www.naccho.org

National Coalition for Health Professional Education in Genetics: http://www.nchpeg.org

National Environmental Health Association: http://www.neha.org/index.shtml

National Human Genome Research Institute: http://www.genome.gov

National Human Genome Research Institute – Online Genetics Education Resources: http://www.genome.gov/10000464

National Society of Genetic Counselors: http://www.nsgc.org

Nursing Organization Links: http://www.nurse.org/orgs.shtml

Occupational Safety and Health Administration: http://www.osha.gov

Online Mendelian Inheritance in Man: http://www.ncbi.nlm.nih.gov/omim

Organization of Teratology Information Specialists: http://www.otispregnancy.org

Teratology Society: http://www.teratology.org

University of Iowa Public Health Genetics Program: http://registrar.uiowa.edu/registrar/catalog/publichealth/publichealthgenetics/

University of Michigan Public Health Genetics Program: http://www.sph.umich.edu/genetics/

University of Pennsylvania Graduate School Program in Public Health Genetics: http://www.publichealth.med.upenn.edu/course_listing.shtml#Genetics

University of Pittsburgh Graduate Programs in Human Genetics: http://www.hgen.pitt.edu/handbook/handbook_september_2007.pdf

University of Washington Public Health Genetics Program: http://depts.washington.edu/phgen/

World Health Organization – Genetics: http://www.who.int/topics/genetics/en/

World Health Organization – Environmental Health: http://www.who.int/topics/environmental_health/en/

World of Genetics Societies: http://genetics.faseb.org/genetics/

REFERENCES

American Nurses Association. (2009). Consensus Panel on Genetic/Genomic Nursing Competencies. *Essentials of genetic and genomic nursing: Competencies, curricula guidelines, and outcome indicators* (2nd ed.). Silver Spring, MD. Retrieved June 12, 2012, from http://www.genome.gov/Pages/Careers/HealthProfessionalEducation/geneticscompetency.pdf

ASTHO. (2001). *Framework for public health genetics policies and practices in state and local health agencies.* Retrieved June 12, 2012, from http://www.ct.gov/dph/LIB/dph/Genomics/astho.pdf

Fineman, R. M. (1999). Qualifications of public health geneticists? *Community Genet, 2*(2–3), 113–4.

Grason, H. A., & Guyer, B. (1995). *Public MCH program functions framework: Essential public health services to promote maternal and child health in America.* Johns Hopkins University Child and Adolescent Policy Center. Baltimore, retrieved June 12, 2012, from http://www.jhsph.edu/bin/i/j/pubmchfx.pdf

Institute of Medicine. Committee for the Study of the Future of Public Health, Division of Health Services. (1988). *The future of public health.* Washington, D.C.: National Academy Press.

CHAPTER

3 Family Context of Clinical Genetics

Carole Kenner, Marina Boykova

LEARNING OUTCOMES

Following the completion of this chapter, the learner will be able to

1. Define family context in relation to having a family member with present or possible genetic conditions.
2. Describe why the practical application of genetics in a clinical setting must include the family.
3. Explain the nurse's role in ensuring the consideration of the family when applying genetics to practice.

This self-study chapter presents the definitions of family, family context, and clinical genetics. The chapter will describe the importance of the consideration of the family when a nurse is applying genetics knowledge and information in a clinical setting. It provides a brief overview of what a family context means when genetic conditions are present or possible and describes how this can be applied in a clinical setting. In addition, this chapter summarizes the nurse's role within the interdisciplinary team in order to ensure the inclusion of the family with possible or actual genetic conditions across the lifespan.

PRETEST

1. Family refers to the members of
   - A. the immediate household unit.
   - B. a unit related by marriage, blood, or adoption.
   - C. a group that are considered by themselves to be related.
   - D. Both B and C
2. The family context is important when discussing a genetic condition because it
   - A. frames the perception of the situation.
   - B. takes into account the cultural beliefs and values.
   - C. provides important information to the health professional.
   - D. All of the above
3. Family functioning is defined as the ability to
   - A. work outside the home.
   - B. carry out tasks of daily living.
   - C. carry out roles according cultural beliefs.
   - D. Both B and C
4. Once a proband is identified as having a positive genetic condition, other family members should
   - A. be given the option to be tested if the proband wishes to reveal the information.
   - B. be given the option to be tested whether or not the proband wishes to reveal the information.
   - C. never be told about the genetic problem and their risk even if the proband grants permission.
   - D. be given no information.
5. Genetic testing is the same as genetic screening.
   - A. True
   - B. False
6. Newborn screening is diagnostic.
   - A. True
   - B. False
7. A visible birth defect is an example of a
   - A. genotype.
   - B. karyotype.
   - C. phenotype.
   - D. zenotype.
8. The family perception of having a family member with a genetic condition is influenced by
   - A. cultural values and beliefs.
   - B. religious views.
   - C. health professionals' support.
   - D. All of the above
   - E. None of the above
   - F. B only
9. Transitions are associated with
   - A. information needs.
   - B. role development.
   - C. stress and coping.
   - D. social support.
   - E. All of the above

10. The nurse's role in genetic screening and testing is
   A. advocating.
   B. Information giving.
   C. teaching.
   D. managing.
   E. All of the above.
   F. None of the above
   G. B and C only

Pretest answers are located in the Appendix.

SECTION ONE: What Is the Family Context?

A **family**, for the purposes of this chapter, refers to the members of a social group living together or perceiving themselves as living together; members of a unit that are considered by that unit to be related and provide caregiving, nurturing, and development to the children or other family members of the household. The family, for the purposes of a pedigree or family history, is generally defined as those members of a group related by marriage, blood, or adoption.These members may or may not be blood relatives (more correctly referred to as first-, second-, or third-degree–related family members), but defined as a family by themselves. First-degree relatives are parents, siblings, and children. Second-degree relatives are grandparents, grandchildren, aunts, uncles, nephews, nieces, and half-siblings; and third-degree relatives are two generations removed from the person that is being examined. In other words, first-degree relatives share 50% genes, second-degree relatives share 25% of the gene pool, and third-degree relatives share around 10%. The family context will be considered differently if the members are blood relatives versus those considered by the family as unit members. Why? Because those that have a blood relationship share a gene pool while other non-blood relatives do not. Yet, within the social context of the family, all members are important if they are considered important by the family unit. **Family context**, when caring for patients with a present or possible genetic condition, refers to the consideration of the family's beliefs, culture, traditions, support systems, functioning, and experiences with health care system. Often, the family's role in health care decision-making in terms of genetic screening, genetic testing, or treatment varies within the individual families and must be considered by health care professionals.

Genetic screening refers to a test that determines the possibility of having a heritable disease or condition. It is not a 100% confirmation of the diagnosis and it must be followed by specific genetic tests. For example, newborn screening tests that are aimed at determining if an infant has inherited a disease such as phenylketonuria, maple syrup urine disease, or beta thalassemia must be followed by additional tests and examinations. Screening tests do not determine definitively that these diseases are present even if the screening test is positive; false-positive test results can also occur when tests show that the disease exists but, in reality, there is no disease present. Once a positive screening test result is received, more diagnostic, specific testing must be done to reach a diagnosis. Genetic testing is the more precise diagnostic workup on the gene level to determine if a genetic disease or susceptibility is present. In the case of susceptibility, this does not mean that the person will ever actually develop the disease. Some experts refer to this as DNA or biological marker examination (i.e., specific proteins or enzymes). DNA mutations are identified by genetic testing while biological markers identify the biochemical or hematological changes. Mistakenly, the terms *screening* and *testing* are used by health professionals and lay public interchangeably. This mistake occurs because most screening is for genetic diseases.

Attitudes Toward Genetic Testing

Family attitudes to and perception of the genetic diagnosis, screening, and testing can vary. For example, some African-American families distrust the health care system and do not want to participate in genetic screening or testing due to past unethical experiments that were performed on their race. The roots of such behavior are associated with the Tuskegee experiment on syphilis that was sanctioned by the government and public health care services (Centers for Disease Control and Prevention, 2009). While this was not a genetic condition, it led some African-Americans to question any form of governmental sanctioned testing or research participation (Bussey-Jones et al., 2010; Haga, 2010). Another example is sickle cell anemia and its testing. Because this disease is primarily found in African-Americans and those of Mediterranean descent, it is often considered another potential source of discriminatory testing. Since the 1970s, sickle cell screening has been feared as a source of health insurance discrimination and potential loss of a job. This is just one reason some people are afraid of genetic screening. African-American patients often believe that clinical trials regarding genetic factors may be dangerous and unethical yet they view the government as protective when it comes to genomic factors such as environmental influences (Achter, Parrott, & Silk, 2004). Other cultural and ethnic group members may have other views, depending on their cultural norms and religious beliefs (i.e., Native American or Asian). These statements in no way imply these views apply to all members of a certain ethic group. The point is that health professionals need to be sensitive to cultural values and beliefs that impact the meaning that genetic screening, testing, and diagnoses may have on them.

There are other reasons for a person's reluctance to undergo genetic testing or participate in research such as ethical and moral dilemmas that are often related to a genetic condition. For example, a woman who is diagnosed with breast cancer may be tested for the breast cancer (**BRCA**-breast cancer susceptibility gene 1 and BRCA 2 forms) gene. The prevalence of the BRCA-1 gene in women with early onset breast cancer is about 3.5–6.2% while BRCA-2 mutation or change is 2.1–3.4% (Robson, 2002). If the test is positive, it is then up to the woman whether or not to tell her daughters that they may have the gene too. This situation may create potential stress for the whole family, such as fears of developing the disease in the future, feelings of guilt for being a carrier of the cancer gene, thus influencing all family members and affecting relationships and life course. For instance, if the daughter is a carrier, she may decide to have an elective **oophorectomy** (removal of the ovaries) and removal of the fallopian tubes as well as a bilateral mastectomy. Some families decide that minor children should make the decision of genetic testing for themselves (McConkie-Rosell & Spiridigliozzi, 2004). However, this decision is not clear-cut, as families are often encouraged by health professionals to have a minor tested if there is a clear medical reason that will be potentially improved if a condition is discovered early (McConkie-Rosell & Spiridigliozzi, 2004). This improvement may be in the form of physical or psychological health (McConkie-Rosell & Spiridigliozzi, 2004). In the case of the BRCA genes, this indication is not as apparent when or if the condition will appear and health care interventions or family expectations may not be feasible or realistic. While having this gene puts the girl or woman at risk for ovarian cancer prior to menopause, the risk is not immediate (Levy-Lahad & Friedman, 2007). One must not forget that paternal genes can contribute to the inheritance of this gene (McCuaig et al., 2011). The BRCA 1 gene also puts men at risk for breast cancer and possibly pancreatic, prostatic, and testicular cancers (Levy-Lahad & Friedman, 2007). The BRCA 2 gene is also related to these cancers. These forms of cancer may not strike until a person is in their 20s or beyond. It also must be remembered that in some individuals several genes are responsible for the development of breast or ovarian cancer. BRCA genes are just indicators of susceptibility for breast and/or ovarian cancer and not predictors that a person will ever have these diseases. Another example of a genetic disease is Huntington disease, an autosomal dominant neurological disease that diminishes the affected patient's ability to walk, talk, and reason, may not show signs of a problem until the person is in their 40s (Huntington's Disease Society of America, 2011). This condition is linked to chromosome 4 and is noted to have CAG (trinucleotide or base sequence) repeats of more than 36 times in the HTT gene. It is a result of a mutation in the HTT gene that is involved in the production of the protein huntingtin, hence the name *Huntington disease*. Current research involves the development of biological markers for the disease (Weir, Sturrock, & Leavitt, 2011). Another example of a genetically inherited disease with an adult onset is Alzheimer disease, which occurs in the later life. This particular disease is very complex in that only a very small percentage of cases of Alzheimer's is considered genetically linked. There are several genes involved in this condition so at the present time there is no one genetic test available. The ethical and moral dilemmas for families—whether or not to test their children while the children are without symptoms (presymptomatically) or to let their children decide for themselves—are also reflected in health professionals' community, with existing controversies in health care worker's attitudes and professional guidelines (Elger & Harding, 2006; Toufexis & Gieron-Korthals, 2010). The testing for Huntington disease, for example, may also depend on a country's whole culture and attitudes to genetic problems (Elger & Harding, 2006). Another instance is differences between health care institutions that do newborn screening as part of the hospital consent to treat form and those that require informed consent, which is not always obtained (Tarini, Burke, Scott, & Wilfond, 2008). Each state has different newborn screening rules; some have panels who decide the type of testing. The other major issue is that parents often do not know that the testing is being done, or, if they are aware of it, they have the option to refuse it. This situation is a point of controversy in genetics and varies from country to country (Dhondt, 2005; Tarini et al., 2010).

A family's response to having a family member diagnosed with a genetic condition can also differ due to the culture, values, beliefs, experiences, and the family's understanding of the disease or inheritance patterns. In some cases, whether this is a disease that results in a change inphenotype (observable difference), genotype (the arrangement of the genes at the basic or gene level, which may or may not be visible to the naked eye), or only in the karyotype (chromosomal level) does make a difference in the family's response. In some Asian families, any birth defect that impairs the visual appearance of the child makes the child of less value (Hughes et al., 2009). In other cultures, such as Hmong, birth defects can be considered a blessing from God and not preventable (Fadiman, 1997; Viste, 2007). Genetic conditions can add a burden to the family but be perceived as a gain as well—in other words, it brings a richness to the family life and makes them closer and stronger due their religious beliefs (Dura-Vila, Dein, & Hodes, 2010). Another challenge is the geriatric population. Elders who have an illness linked to a genetic or genomic cause may not seek aggressive treatment as they feel they have lived their lives. The family may feel differently as they wish to hold on as long as possible. The important aspect here is whether or not the disease has implications for other family members: Is this a genetic condition that may be preventable, or that at least has preventable complications if other family members are tested? Often, the roles within the family become reversed: Children have to care about the parent with a genetically linked disease while it should be opposite. In some cultures, it is the expectation that children will care for the parents when there is a need. Thus, the family roles and acceptance of who should provide care within the family context is culturally influenced.

Another possible response of the family to having a member with genetic condition is influenced by the knowledge and competencies of the health care professional that should be able to answer the questions family has. Stark and colleagues (2010) found that sometimes pediatricians may not have a full understanding of a particular condition and the results of what a positive or negative screening test means in relationship to carrier detection (Stark, Lang, & Ross, 2010). Health professionals may not give genetic testing information to the family if they themselves do not understand the genetic linkages; thus the family members may not know what options they have or what action they should take regarding further diagnostic tests, future childbearing, or long-term health consequences. While genetic counseling is always nondirective, laying out the options and giving as much information as possible, not telling or directing family towards a certain test or treatment, there are unintended consequences when the health professional does not have enough knowledge of the genetic linkages. Another consequence of this lack of information is that parents may not allow their newborn's screening samples to be used for future research if they do not have an explanation of the rationale for the need for such study. Yet when parents' permission is sought and thorough explanations are given for the need for such research, the parents will generally grant such usage (Tarini, et al., 2010). This is an area of concern and a reason why all health professionals need genetic knowledge. Otherwise the health professional's lack of knowledge may add to the burden of the family who has a family member with a genetic disease or predisposition to a genetic problem.

The family's ability to perform the tasks associated with family life must be considered when there is a family member, no matter what the age of the affected person, who is diagnosed with an inheritable problem. **Family functioning** refers to the ability of the persons who make up a family unit to perform expected (or perceived/accepted) tasks or roles of that family/social unit. In other words, family functioning is the ability of the members of a unit—either blood or those considered relatives by the unit or household occupants—to carry out activities of daily living or cultural tasks. The influences on the family's functioning are numerous when it comes to a genetic condition. Emotional, psychological burdens as well as financial and social ones should be considered when dealing with families who have a member affected by a genetic disease. For instance, a family with a child who has a congenital genetic problem can be stigmatized (inappropriate labeling of the child and his or her disease), which may lead to social isolation and deepen the emotional and psychological burden that the family already has (Bailey, Skinner, Davis, Whitmarsh, & Powell, 2008). A referral to social support groups, counseling, and church services may be needed as well as recommendations for the special services or respite care facilities, depending on the family's needs. However, there are other factors to consider. For example, parents who are deaf, due to causes that may or may not be genetic, would view a hearing child as no different from a nonhearing one. This situation is referred to as deaf culture, where hearing loss is not viewed as a disability (Shuman, Byrd, Kileny, & Kileny, 2011). Thus it is important to find out the attitude and perception of the family about a genetic condition. If the family wishes help, there are special social and learning disabilities' services as well as foundations that offer assistanec. Foundations such as the March of Dimes Foundation (**MOD**) and national Huntington and Alzheimer disease organizations can provide valuable support for families and patients. Certain personal and religious beliefs may also help patients and family members to copy with an incurable genetic diagnosis or caregiver burden and can enhance the level of perceived social support (Newton & McIntosh, 2010; Smith, 2009; Ward, Clark le, & Heidrich, 2009). Again, the response of the family will depend on the culture and many other factors that influence a family's life. In order to provide the most adequate care for a patient and a family, the benefits of both parties must be considered. The family context—those influencing factors that impact family functioning and decision-making—is crucial to understand if the health professional is to guide and advocate appropriately for the proband (the first person to be identified with genetic health condition in the family). Advocacy for other members of the family is also necessitated in terms of needed genetic consultation, genetic screening, and testing.

It is important to consider the lifestage of the family when screening and testing is done. In other words, is this a family that is of childbearing age and must make reproductive decisions? Or is this a family that is past childbearing but is concerned for their children or grandchildren if they are diagnosed with a genetically linked condition in their own adult lives and now recognize there is a risk for their relatives? The application of the family context within the clinical setting is the next consideration.

SECTION ONE REVIEW

1. _____ is a diagnostic workup to determine if a genetic condition is present.
   A. Genetic testing
   B. Genetic screening
   C. Health assessment
   D. Physical examination
2. The family's role in health care decision making in terms of genetic screening varies according to
   A. cultural beliefs.
   B. knowledge of the condition.
   C. trust of the health care system.
   D. All of the above
3. Minor children who are at risk for developing a genetic condition later in life should always be tested.
   A. True
   B. False
4. Presymptomatic testing is available for Huntington disease.
   A. True
   B. False

Answers: 1. A; 2. D; 3. B; 4. A

SECTION TWO: Application of the Family Context Within the Clinical Setting

The previous section discussed the role of the family in genetic screening and testing and the various influences that may impact the perception of a potential or real genetic condition. The implications of cultural awareness for health professionals are that, for instance, teaching about folic acid supplementation in the Hmong population to prevent neural tube defects is not useful unless the cultural context of the message is considered (Viste, 2007). It has also been shown that in order to increase the chances of participation in research or to allow genetic testing, understandable explanations about the research and expected outcomes facilitated trust (White, Koehly, Omogbehin, & McBride, 2010). There are also certain periods of time when a patient and family are in need for the increased professional and social support. Beattie and colleagues (2009) found the median time for the elective surgery after a patient is confirmed a carrier of the breast cancer gene is four months from the time of testing—the time that is critical for support (Beattie, Crawford, Lin, Vittinghoff, & Ziegler, 2009). In these four months patients may undergo feelings of anger, sorrow, and difficulties in continuing their life routines as they are trying to make a difficult decision.

Many people fear genetic testing. Patients and families must understand the risks as well as the benefits of genetic testing and newborn screening in order to overcome their fears; this is the area where nurses can play a very important role (Andermann & Blancquaert, 2010). Genetic knowledge in family members can impact reproductive decisions. For example, Fragile X is one of the leading causes of mental retardation and is linked to autism, a growing problem (Hantash, 2010; Hersh, 2011). This condition can be determined prenatally and even prior to conception, as can the carrier state (Hantash, 2010). The carriers, as is the case in most carrier states, will have minimal or no disease symptoms. So some families will be in shock when a health professional suggests testing or that a child may be suffering from Fragile X. This is not a condition whose routine screening and testing is mandated yet, and some families that do test prior to having a child affected by a genetic disease can make reproductive decisions (Hantash, 2010; Hill, Archibald, Cohen, & Metcalfe, 2010). Another related issue is that Fragile X, when present, often is not diagnosed until the child is about three years old (Hantash, 2010). By this time the family may already be concerned about behavior issues or developmental delays. It has been shown that parents suffer from increased parenting stress when providing care and nurturing for the child affected by a genetic disease (Waisbren, Rones, Read, Marsden, & Levy, 2004). It is important that the disabilities associated with a genetic disease may be lessened with early intervention. So, the question becomes what impact does making the screening available have on a family's decisions to have children, seek genetic counseling, seek early intervention services, or add to parental stress? It has been argued that the applicability of the genetic tests for health professionals is not well established, and predictive value of genetic tests can be low (van El & Cornel, 2011). There are no easy or uniform answers to any of these questions. As noted in the previous section of this chapter, in large part the impact depends on the family's understanding of the disease, its progression, their cultural beliefs and values, the information they can get from health professionals, and their fear of discrimination if a genetic condition is found (Hantash, 2010; Miller, 2007; Musci & Moyer, 2010; van El & Cornel, 2011).

Role of the Health Professional

Health professionals also influence a family's ability to cope with the news of a possible or actual genetic condition. Social supports that are available to families also influence the ways families manage genetic information. No matter what the age of the family member that has a potential or actual genetic condition, the family members undergo a transition from the view of a well family to one with a problem. **Transition**, a passage from one stage in life to another or from one circumstances to another (Meleis, 2010; Naylor & Keating, 2008), has been associated with the presence of informational needs, role development challenges (the new role of a person with an illness or of a family with a member who may be ill), grief over the loss of what was the familiar or anticipated, social support, and stress and coping (Kenner & Lott, 1990). Kenner's Transition Model (Kenner & Lott, 1990) identified these five categories as important for the transition of families after discharge of an infant from a newborn intensive care unit (Flandermeyer, Kenner, Spaite, & Hostiuck, 1992; Kenner & Lott, 1990). Another group concerned about families and transitions is the Southeast Regional Newborn Screening and Genetics Collaborative (http://southeastgenetics.org/about.php). These categories of transitional problems and experiences can be applied to any circumstance that creates a major change for a family or its member. When there has been a loss of the image of the perfect baby or child, or the loss of envisioned future, the grief and sadness occurs. This grief can turn into **chronic sorrow** (Fraley, 1990). Chronic sorrow refers to unresolved grief that can last a lifetime, whether or not the child/family member dies (Fraley, 1990). This sorrow must be defined by the family or within the family context. It is often not continual or continuous but rather was evoked or exacerbated by developmental milestones or experiences (Wikler, Wasow, & Hatfield, 1981). These researchers found 10 distinct development crisis points when grief and sorrow could be evoked. Two of these included the onset of puberty and the child's 21st birthday (Wikler, Wasow, & Hatfield, 1981). A few examples of conditions that can lead to a change in family functioning, a transition, or chronic sorrow are cystic fibrosis, Tay Sachs, Trisomy 21, and ambiguous genitalia. The knowledge of these conditions coupled with better ways to examine the impact a genetic disease has on the person and families affected by the disease has led to changes in genetic testing and screening. Preconception and prenatal testing has expanded in the last few years, leading to many actual or carrier conditions being identified early, even before a pregnancy occurs (Norton, 2008). However, with this knowledge comes moral and ethical dilemmas. Who should be tested? When? Should the screening/testing be mandated? In 2008 the Genetic Information Nondiscrimination Act (**GINA**) legislation was passed. (For more in-depth information please refer to Chapter 9). This legislation is aimed at protecting individuals and families from use of genetic information to impact employment or insurance decisions. Until this legislation was passed many families feared genetic testing because if the results were discovered their insurance coverage for the entire family or their own employment chances could be affected even if the member was a child who was affected. Other aspects of this law include the ability to ensure that benefits are available to the family for services, medication, and other special needs. For example, if a child needs a special diet because of an error of metabolism, then GINA ensures that this benefit and use of flexible spending account funds are available. If GINA does not exist then the family may be denied such benefits. The family history and GINA is inextricably linked, leading to concerns about testing, treatment needs, and the accompanying benefits even today (Scott, 2010).

The other aspect of this situation is how much the family function is affected. There are many instruments that measure family functioning that are often used by nurses in practice. Some of the tools of family functioning measure parental distress or adjustment, interactions of family member's, resiliency, and dimensions of value or personal growth, interpersonal relationships, and how family systems are maintained and a chronic health condition is managed (Bloom, 1985; K. Knafl et al., 2009; Moos & Moos, 1994). The examples are the Moos and Moos Scale, called the Family Environment Scale (Moos & Moos, 1994); Feetham's Family Functioning scale (Gallo, Angst, Knafl, Twomey, & Hadley, 2010); and the Family Management Measure (K. Knafl, et al., 2009). These are just a few examples of the many scales that can be used to determine how well a family is able to carry out family obligations. There are also theories and models developed for better understanding of the family functioning; for instance, the Family Management Style Framework that describes and explains the family's ability to cope with chronic illnesses in their children (K. Knafl et al., 2009). It measures the normalization or **normalcy** of the family or the view of the family member's condition as part of the fabric of the family (K. A. Knafl, Darney, Gallo, & Angst, 2010). Findings from studies that use this instrument show that health care providers, especially nurses, can facilitate normalization through advocacy, education, and care coordination.

Another movement that is impacting both families and health professionals is the action by the Surgeon General and the Department of Health and Human Services to promote the development and use of a family history tool. The result of this action was the creation of a website, *My Family Health Portrait,* where family members can use a tool to build their own family history and transport it to health visits (https://familyhistory.hhs.gov/fhh-web/home.action). A recent study indicates that use of this tool in pediatric practices can facilitate positive health promotion (Kanetzke, Lynch, Prows, Siegel, & Myers, 2011). While this study focused on the pediatric population, the same is true for the tool's use across the lifespan. However, more research is needed to support the use in other populations. Nonetheless, the use of this toolkit provides another opportunity for nurses and other health professionals to determine the risk for genetically linked conditions and therefore potentially intervene early for the sake of the health of the family. If this tool is not used, then health professionals must elicit family history information with special emphasis on recurring health problems found in families, causes of death or illnesses of family members, and any genetically linked diseases that are known. Health professionals must be knowledgeable about the genetics involved in such conditions so that they may advocate for the families and make sure referrals are made to appropriate resources, either for genetic counseling or for treatment. Thorough consideration should be given to the all aspects of the genetic testing as well as to interactions between genetic and environmental factors. This aspect of genetic conditions merits further studies, especially of the families.

Emerging Evidence

There is emerging evidence to support the genetics of eating behaviors. These behaviors—part of the genomics or environment—can lead to obesity, hypertension, and cardiovascular disease (Grimm & Steinle, 2011). Understanding the context with a genetic lens increases the ability to account for the genetics of taste and how this impacts eating and long-term obesity and its complications. Why is this important? It is important because the increasing morbidity and mortality in the United States is for the most part related to these conditions that may be mediated within the genetic context. It is important within the family context because the interactions between family members often sets the tone for the value food has on the family as well as for what is considered typical foods supported by their cultural values and beliefs. Health promotion and disease prevention measures will incorporate the family and the knowledge of the "genetics" of eating behaviors and how these can be modified to promote a healthy lifestyle and improve outcomes.

There is also emerging evidence related to atopic dermatitis. This condition has a genetic foundation and is linked to genomics—the interplay of the environment and genes (Barnes, 2010). This condition is very common but is rarely considered to be genetic. It is often linked to allergy by the lay public and some health professionals. Knowledge that the underlying genesis of this condition is genetics changes the health promotion approaches and disease prevention plan of care. Inclusion of the family members in the treatment plan by educating them about the relationship between genes, environmental exposures, and atopic dermatitis is another important aspect of the plan of care.

Evidence is emerging every day. Now there is a belief that any kind of disease can be related to genetics. Future evidence is still to come that will change the health care of most diseases.

SECTION TWO REVIEW

1. The Moos and Moos Scale measures
   A. family functioning only.
   B. family functioning and environment.
   C. family coping only.
   D. family stress only.
2. Family-functioning refers to the person's ability to perform the task of the unit. This ability can be measured by
   A. evidence-based tools.
   B. a health professional's assessment.
   C. Both A and B
   D. the family themselves.
3. GINA legislation affords a family some protection against indiscriminate use of genetic formation.
   A. True
   B. False
4. Chronic sorrow occurs when
   A. there has been an actual death of a family member.
   B. there is a perceived loss of the image of the family member.
   C. there is a perceived or actual loss of a family member.
   D. there are unresolved feelings about a perceived or actual loss.
5. A transition is a change in
   A. capabilities of a family unit.
   B. employment of a family member.
   C. role of a family member.
   D. All of the above
   E. None of the above

Answers: 1. B; 2. C; 3. A; 4. D; 5. D

SECTION THREE: The Nurse's Role Within the Interdisciplinary Team

Any time there is a possible genetic condition that is present or undergoing testing, there needs to be a team approach. The nurse is the key person who brokers the information between the interdisciplinary health care team members (physicians, nurses, social workers, geneticists, and so on) and the patient and his or her family—i.e., the nurse is the patient's collaborator. Nurses in the past could be certified as genetic counselors, but this is a very specific role that requires additional knowledge. Today, Advanced Practice Nurses in Genetics or **APNG** are those that hold a master's degree and have specialized training in genetics. There is also a route for bachelor's degree prepared nurses to obtain the Genetic Clinical Nurse (GCN) title. See http://www.geneticnurse.org for more information. The competencies that nurses must possess in genetics have been identified (Calzone, Jenkins, Prows, & Masny, 2011; Consensus Panel, 2009). These competencies were supported by the American Nurses Association and the National Coalition for Health Professionals Education in Genetics. However, the general nurse also has a role to provide the best care for the patient and family including enough knowledge of genetics and genomics to interpret information for them. In relation to the family context, the nurse generally spends more time with the patient and family than does any other health professional. In the case with Fragile X syndrome, for example, knowledgeable nurses can help identify those children earlier as they may know the family better than other health professionals; thus, nurses have the ability to improve the child's and family's life and health outcomes by referring to early intervention services, learning disability services, and so on. The nurse oftentimes will be the first one to know the fears and misinformation, the lifestyle, and the cultural or financial context that a family has, and will be able to incorporate this information in the plan of care. The nurse is and must be the best advocate for the family, as well as help the family members incorporate the condition into their life and reach normalcy. The nurse can transfer the family information to the other team members; for example, what the family does or does not understand about the disease, what resources the family has, or the family's attitude towards screening, testing, and treatments. Also the nurse can help the family members understand the information they have received from other health professionals and simplify the complicated terminology, thus promoting the family's understanding of the condition. The interpreter of information is another critical role as health professionals tend to talk in medical terms and forget the family may not understand. The nurse may be the one to know that there is another family member with a related condition. The family may not have thought to tell the physician but will tell the nurse. The nurse may be the one to find out that the insurance does not cover genetic counseling or disabilities services. This must be conveyed to the other health care team members.

The nurse's role is complex when it comes to families with a member that is affected by a genetic condition. It encompasses ethical, psychological, and professional practice issues. The role of care coordination, advocacy, and support is essential. The nurse may be the frontline person who can assess the family functioning, determine how effectively the family is making the transition to becoming a unit that has an actual or potential problem, and how the family is managing changes that have occurred. A key ingredient to all of this is the family and patient. The family and patient set the tone and direction for the care, and they should be an integral part of the health professional's team in all decision making, planning, and care.

SECTION THREE REVIEW

1. The nurse is part of a larger health care team. The role of the nurse in genetic testing and screening is
   A. a small part of the team's approach.
   B. an essential part of the team's approach.
   C. not important to the overall care.
   D. limited to advocacy.
2. The family oftentimes does not understand the genetic implications of a disease.
   A. True
   B. False
3. A key ingredient to the genetic care plan is
   A. the family.
   B. the geneticist.
   C. the nurse.
   D. the physician.
4. An interdisciplinary team approach requires
   A. communication between all team members.
   B. inclusion of the patient and family in the plan.
   C. nurse-driven planning.
   D. physician-driven planning.
5. Normalcy regarding family management of a chronic condition refers to
   A. usual pattern of functioning without regard for condition.
   B. incorporation of a condition into family life.
   C. lack of recognition of seriousness of condition.
   D. viewing the member's condition as unimportant.

Answers: 1. B; 2, A; 3. A; 4. A; 5. B

POSTTEST

1. When a family member is diagnosed with a genetic condition, the family member's role as the primary caregiver can be reversed.
   A. True
   B. False
2. Genetic testing and screening can be used in
   A. adolescents.
   B. infants.
   C. adults.
   D. All of the above
3. Genetic testing of a minor child considers
   A. only the age of the child.
   B. only the wishes of the parents.
   C. only the impact on the physical health.
   D. the impact on physical and psychological health.
4. The Family History Portrait tool is
   A. for use by lay public.
   B. for use by health professionals.
   C. for use by parents.
   D. All of the above
5. Family functioning refers to
   A. the ability of the family to carry out tasks of daily living.
   B. the coping ability of the family.
   C. the family's view of the genetic condition.
   D. the family's earning capacity.
6. Informed consent is always required for newborn screening.
   A. True
   B. False
7. The nurse's role in assisting in family functioning, genetic screening and testing, and care is
   A. advocacy.
   B. coordination.
   C. educator.
   D. All of the above
8. Family functioning is influenced by
   A. attitudes about a condition.
   B. cultural values and beliefs.
   C. knowledge about the condition.
   D. All of the above
9. The major aim of the nursing intervention and use of the family history is to
   A. change the prognosis of the condition.
   B. individualize care plans for families.
   C. treat the condition.
   D. obtain informed consent.
10. Race and ethnicity oftentimes influence consent to undergo genetic testing due to
    A. fear of violation of privacy.
    B. fear of discrimination.
    C. A and B
    D. None of the above

Posttest answers are located in the Appendix.

CHAPTER SUMMARY

Family is more than blood relatives (first-, second-, or third-degree–related members). It may encompass individuals living together or those considered related by social ties. Family context refers to all factors that influence the unit's functioning and decision making; i.e., culture, beliefs, values, psychological, moral, and financial issues. Family is the most important element in carrying out the tasks/roles of the family unit. The roles within the family may be altered when there is an actual or potential genetic disease.

Genetic testing and *newborn screening* are terms that often are used interchangeably by some health professionals as well as the lay public because most if not all newborn screening is for genetic conditions. They are not the same and should not be used interchangeably.

There are resources for families with a member affected by a genetic disease, but the role of the nurse is crucial. It is multifaceted in support of the family undergoing genetic screening and testing and is critical to the success of the family functioning.

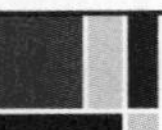

CRITICAL THINKING CHECKPOINT

Olivia is a 39-year-old, Caucasian woman who recently got pregnant. She believes she is about 10 weeks pregnant. Olivia is not married and wants to keep the pregnancy despite her advanced maternal age. She recently learned that there were two persons in her family who had Fragile X syndrome. She does not have all the information about the disease, and she fears that she might be a carrier of the gene and that her unborn baby can be affected. Olivia starts to consider genetic testing but is afraid that it is too late. She is also worried about her insurance not covering the cost of testing and losing her job if the information about her being affected is available to the employer or if she has a child that has a genetic disease. Her close family members who hold strict Catholic religious beliefs are not supportive of her pregnancy but would not support an abortion. For that reason they are against Olivia being tested either for Trisomy 21 (which her advanced age puts her at risk for) or for the Fragile X condition that is noted to be present in her family.

1. Is genetic testing appropriate for this woman?
2. Who should be involved in making decisions about testing and pregnancy?
3. Who should be part of the interdisciplinary team for this case?
4. What information should be available for this woman's best interests and future?
5. Will GINA legislation protect this woman?

Answers are provided in the Appendix

Pearson Nursing Student Resources

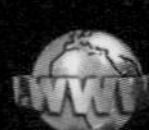

Find additional review materials at nursing.pearsonhighered.com

Prepare for success with additional NCLEX®-style practice questions, interactive assignments and activities, web links, animations, videos, and more!

ONLINE RESOURCES

Alzheimer's Foundation of America: http://www.alzfdn.org/AboutAlzheimers/research.html

Cystic Fibrosis Foundation: http://www.cff.org/research/ResearchMilestones/

Genetic Alliance: http://www.geneticalliance.org

Genetic Counseling: http://www.marchofdimes.com/pregnancy/trying_geneticcounseling.html

Genetic Home Reference: Your Guide to Understanding Genetic Conditions: http://ghr.nlm.nih.gov

GINA or Genetic Information Nondiscrimination Act: http://www.ginahelp.org

Huntington's Disease Society of America: http://www.hdsa.org

March of Dimes Birth Defects Foundation: http://www.marchofdimes.com/?gclid=COH6wICtpqkCFRG4KgodEhwWtg

March of Dimes Loss and Grieving in Pregnancy and the First Year of Life Online Course: http://www.marchofdimes.com/nursing/modnemedia/perinataltests/loss_grieving.pdf

March of Dimes Newborn Screening: What Caregviers Need to Know Online Course: http://www.marchofdimes.com/professionals/education_newbornscreening.html

My Family Health Portrait: https://familyhistory.hhs.gov/fhh-web/home.action

National Cancer Institute: http://www.cancer.gov/cancertopics/pdq/genetics/overview/healthprofessional/page5

Online Genetics Education Resources: http://www.genome.gov/10000464

Parent and Family Resources: http://genes-r-us.uthscsa.edu/parentpage.htm

Southeast Regional Newborn Screening and Genetics Collaborative: http://southeastgenetics.org/about.php

REFERENCES

Achter, P., Parrott, R., & Silk, K. (2004). African Americans' opinions about human-genetics research. *Politics and the life sciences: The journal of the association for politics and the life sciences, 23*(1), 60–66.

Andermann, A., & Blancquaert, I. (2010). Genetic screening: A primer for primary care. *Canadian Family Physician, 56*(4), 333–339.

Bailey, D. B., Jr., Skinner, D., Davis, A. M., Whitmarsh, I., & Powell, C. (2008). Ethical, legal, and social concerns about expanded newborn screening: Fragile X syndrome as a prototype for emerging issues. *Pediatrics, 121*(3), e693–704.

Barnes, K. C. (2010). An update on the genetics of atopic dermatitis: Scratching the surface in 2009. *Journal of Allergy and Clinical Immunology, 125*(1), 16–29 e11–11. doi: 10.1016/j.jaci.2009.11.008

Beattie, M. S., Crawford, B., Lin, F., Vittinghoff, E., & Ziegler, J. (2009). Uptake, time course, and predictors of risk-reducing surgeries in BRCA carriers. *Genetic Testing and Molecular Biomarkers, 13*(1), 51–56. doi: 10.1089/gtmb.2008.0067

Bloom, B. L. (1985). A factor analysis of self-report measures of family functioning. *Family Process, 24*(2), 225–239.

Bussey-Jones, J., Garrett, J., Henderson, G., Moloney, M., Blumenthal, C., & Corbie-Smith, G. (2010). The role of race and trust in tissue/blood donation for genetic research. *Genetics in Medicine: Official journal of the American College of Medical Genetics, 12*(2), 116–121. doi: 10.1097/GIM.0b013e3181cd6689

Calzone, K. A., Jenkins, J., Prows, C. A., & Masny, A. (2011). Establishing the outcome indicators for the essential nursing competencies and curricula guidelines for genetics and genomics. *Journal of Professional Nursing, 27*(3), 179–191. doi: 10.1016/j.profnurs.2011.01.001

Centers for Disease Control and Prevention. (2009). U.S. Public Health Service Syphilis Study at Tuskegee. Retrieved May 24, 2011, from http://www.cdc.gov/tuskegee/timeline.htm#

Consensus Panel on Genetic/Genomic Nursing Competencies. (2009). *Essentials of genetic and genomic nursing competencies, curricula guidelines and outcome indicators* (2nd ed.). Silver Spring, MD: American Nurses Association.

Dhondt, J. L. (2005). Implementation of informed consent for a cystic fibrosis newborn screening program in France: Low refusal rates for optional testing. *The Journal of Pediatrics, 147*(3), S106–108. doi: 10.1016/j.jpeds.2005.08.008

Dura-Vila, G., Dein, S., & Hodes, M. (2010). Children with intellectual disability: A gain not a loss: Parental beliefs and family life. *Clinical Child Psychology and Psychiatry, 15*(2), 171–184. doi: 10.1177/1359104509341009

Elger, B. S., & Harding, T. W. (2006). Should children and adolescents be tested for Huntington's disease? Attitudes of future lawyers and physicians in Switzerland. *Bioethics, 20*(3), 158–167. doi: 10.1111/j.1467-8519.2006.00489.x

Fadiman, A. (1997). *The spirit catches you and you fall down: A Hmong child, her American doctors, and the collision of two cultures*. New York: Farrar, Straus, and Giroux.

Flandermeyer, A., Kenner, C., Spaite, M. E., & Hostiuck, J. (1992). Transition from hospital to home: Part III. *Neonatal Network, 11*(6), 84–85.

Fraley, A. M. (1990). Chronic sorrow: A parental response. *Journal of Pediatric Nursing, 5*(4), 268–273.

Gallo, A. M., Angst, D. B., Knafl, K. A., Twomey, J. G., & Hadley, E. (2010). Health care professionals' views of sharing information with families who have a child with a genetic condition. *Journal of Genetic Counseling, 19*(3), 296–304. doi: 10.1007/s10897-010-9286-0

Grimm, E. R., & Steinle, N. I. (2011). Genetics of eating behavior: Established and emerging concepts. *Nutrition Reviews, 69*(1), 52–60. doi: 10.1111/j.1753-4887.2010.00361.x

Haga, S. B. (2010). Impact of limited population diversity of genome-wide association studies. *Genetics in Medicine, 12*(2), 81–84. doi: 10.1097/GIM.0b013e3181ca2bbf

Hantash, F. M. (2010). Fragile X syndrome: Is now the time for population screening? *Medical Laboratory Observer, 42*(5), 20–22.

Hersh, J. H. (2011). Difficult diagnosis: AAP report offers updated age-related health supervision guidelines for Fragile X syndrome. *AAP News, 32*(5). Retrieved May 22, 2011, from http://aapnews.aappublications.org/cgi/content/full/32/5/32

Hill, M. K., Archibald, A. D., Cohen, J., & Metcalfe, S. A. (2010). A systematic review of population screening for fragile X syndrome. *Genetics in Medicine, 12*(7), 396–410. doi: 10.1097/GIM.0b013e3181e38fb6

Hughes, J., Naqvi, H., Saul, K., Williamson, H., Jonson, M. R. D., Rumsey, N., & Charlton, R. (2009). South Asian community views about individuals with a disfigurement. *Diversity in Health and Care, 6*(4), 241–253.

Huntington's Disease Society of America. (2011). *Family care: Living at risk*. Retrieved May 24, 2011, from http://www.hdsa.org/living-with-huntingtons/family-care/living-at-risk.html#Testing

Kanetzke, E. E., Lynch, J., Prows, C. A., Siegel, R. M., & Myers, M. F. (2011). Perceived utility of parent-generated family health history as a health promotion tool in pediatric practice. *Clinical Pediatrics*. doi: 10.1177/0009922811403301

Kenner, C., & Lott, J. W. (1990). Parent transition after discharge from the NICU. *Neonatal Network, 9*(2), 31–37.

Knafl, K. A., Darney, B. G., Gallo, A. M., & Angst, D. B. (2010). Parental perceptions of the outcome and meaning of normalization. *Research in Nursing and Health, 33*(2), 87–98. doi: 10.1002/nur.20367

Knafl, K., Deatrick, J. A., Gallo, A., Dixon, J., Grey, M., Knafl, G., & O'Malley, J. (2009). Assessment of the psychometric properties of the family management measure. *Journal of Pediatric Psychology*, 1–12. doi: 10.1093/jpepsy/jsp034

Levy-Lahad, E., & Friedman, E. (2007). Cancer risks among BRCA1 and BRCA2 mutation carriers. *British Journal of Cancer, 96*(1), 11–15. doi: 10.1038/sj.bjc.6603535

McConkie-Rosell, A., & Spiridigliozzi, G. (2004). "Family Matters": A conceptual framework for genetic testing in children. *Journal of Genetic Counseling, 13*(1), 9–29. doi: 10.1023/B:JOGC.0000013379.90587.ef

McCuaig, J. M., Greenwood, C. M., Shuman, C., Chitayat, D., Murphy, K. J., Rosen, B., & Armel, S. R. (2011). Breast and ovarian cancer: The forgotten paternal contribution. *Journal of Genetic Counselling, 20*(5), 442–449. doi: 10.1007/s10897-011-9368-7

Meleis, A. I. (Ed.) (2010). *Transitions theory: Middle-range and situation specific theories in nursing research and practice*. New York: Springer Publishing Company.

Miller, P. S. (2007). Genetic testing and the future of disability insurance: Thinking about discrimination in the genetic age. *The Journal of Law, Medicine and Ethics, 35*(2 Suppl), 47–51.

Moos, R., & Moos, B. (1994). *Family enviornment scale manual: Development, applications, research* (3rd ed.). Palo Alto: Consulting Psychologist Press.

Musci, T. J., & Moyer, K. (2010). Prenatal carrier testing for fragile X: Counseling issues and challenges. *Obstetrics and Gynecology Clinics of North America, 37*(1), 61–70. doi: 10.1016/j.ogc.2010.03.004

Naylor, M., & Keating, S. A. (2008). Transitional care. *American Journal of Nursing, 108*(9 Suppl), 58–63.

Newton, A. T., & McIntosh, D. N. (2010). Specific religious beliefs in a cognitive appraisal model of stress and coping. *International Journal for the Psychology of Religion, 20*(1), 39–58.

Norton, M. E. (2008). Genetic screening and counseling. *Current Opinion in Obstetrics and Gynecology, 20*(2), 157–163. doi: 10.1097/GCO.0b013e3282f73230

Robson, M. (2002). Risk for hereditary breast and ovarian cancer: Prevalence of BRCA1 and BRCA2 mutations. *Medscape Today*. Retrived December 27, 2011, from http://www.medscape.com/viewarticle/447546_3

Scott, M. (2010). Family history and GINA. *Psychiatric Services, 61*(6), 634. doi: 10.1176/appi.ps.61.6.634

Shuman, A.G., Byrd, S., Kileny, S., & Kileny, P.R. (2011). *The right not to hear: The ethics of parental refusal of hearing rehabilitation*. Ann Arbor, MI: University of Michigan Health System. Retrieved June 15, 2012, from http://cbssm.org/downloads/Shuman.pdf

Smith, D. H. (2009). Christianity, health, and genetics. *American Journal of Medical Genetics, Part C, 151C*(1), 77–80.

Stark, A. P., Lang, C. W., & Ross, L. F. (2010). A pilot study to evaluate knowledge and attitudes of Illinois pediatricians toward newborn screening for sickle cell disease and cystic fibrosis. *American Journal of Perinatology, 23*(3), 169–176. doi: 10.1055/s-0030-1265828

Tarini, B. A., Burke, W., Scott, C. R., & Wilfond, B. S. (2008). Waiving informed consent in newborn screening research: balancing social value and respect. *Amercan Journal of Medical Genetics, Part C, 148C*(1), 23–30. doi: 10.1002/ajmg.c.30164

Tarini, B. A., Goldenberg, A., Singer, D., Clark, S. J., Butchart, A., & Davis, M. M. (2010). Not without my permission: Parents' willingness to permit use of newborn screening samples for research. *Public Health Genomics, 13*(3), 125–130.

Toufexis, M., & Gieron-Korthals, M. (2010). Early testing for Huntington disease in children: Pros and cons. *Journal of Child Neurology, 25*(4), 482–484. doi: 10.1177/0883073809343315

van El, C. G., & Cornel, M. C. (2011). Genetic testing and common disorders in a public health framework. *European Journal of Human Genetics, 19*, 377–381. doi: 10.1038/ejhg.2010.176

Viste, J. (2007). Communicating (birth defects) prevention information to a Hmong population in Wisconsin: A study of cultural relevance. *Substance Use and Misuse, 42*(4), 753–774. doi: 10.1080/10826080701202577

Waisbren, S. E., Rones, M., Read, C. Y., Marsden, D., & Levy, H. L. (2004). Predictors of parenting stress among parents of children with biochemical genetic disorders. *Journal of Pediatric Psychology, 29*(7), 565–570. doi: 10.1093/jpepsy/jsh058

Ward, E. C., Clark le, O., & Heidrich, S. (2009). African American women's beliefs, coping behaviors, and barriers to seeking mental health services. *Qualitative Health Research, 19*(11), 1589–1601. doi: 10.1177/1049732309350686

Weir, D. W., Sturrock, A., & Leavitt, B. R. (2011). Development of biomarkers for Huntington's disease. *Lancet Neurology, 10*(6), 573–590. doi: 10.1016/S1474-4422(11)70070-9

White, D. B., Koehly, L. M., Omogbehin, A., & McBride, C. M. (2010). African Americans' responses to genetic explanations of lung cancer disparities and their willingness to participate in clinical genetics research. *Genetics in Medicine, 12*(8), 496–502. doi: 10.1097/GIM.0b013e3181e5e513

Wikler, L., Wasow, M., & Hatfield, E. (1981). Chronic sorrow revisted: Parent vs. professional depiction of the adjustment of parents of mentally retarded children. *American Journal of Othopsychiatry, 51*(1), 63–67.

PART 2

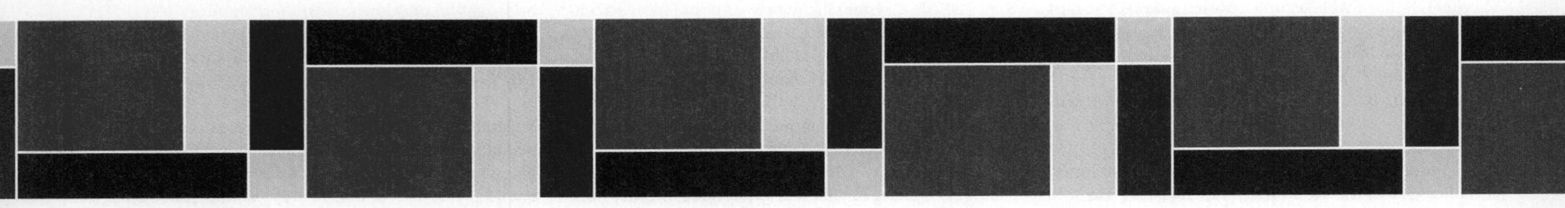

Basic Genetic Concepts

CHAPTER

4 Meiosis and Mitosis

Judith A. Lewis, Alexandra R. Paul-Simon

LEARNING OUTCOMES

Following the completion of this chapter, the learner will be able to

1. Describe the structure and function of DNA, genes, and chromosomes.
2. Describe the life cycle of a cell.
3. Discuss the mechanisms of meiosis and mitosis.
4. Identify mechanisms of genetic variation.

This chapter will discuss the structure and function of DNA, **RNA**, **genes**, and **chromosomes**. The process of DNA replication, RNA **transcription**, and protein synthesis will be described, as well as the roles of genes and chromosomes. The life cycle of a cell will also be discussed. In order for an organism to survive, cells must grow and duplicate. Cell growth, division, and programmed cell death are all parts of the natural progression of life.

PRETEST

1. Cell division is
   A. an orderly sequence.
   B. identical for all cells in an organism.
   C. regulated by the hypothalamus.
   D. a random event.
2. The process of creating germ cells occurs during
   A. mitosis.
   B. meiosis.
   C. apoptosis.
   D. translocation.
3. The planned sequence for cell death is called
   A. mitosis.
   B. meiosis.
   C. translocation.
   D. apoptosis.
4. The longest phase of the cell cycle is
   A. mitosis.
   B. meiosis.
   C. cytokinesis.
   D. interphase.
5. Which is not present in DNA?
   A. Adenine
   B. Guanine
   C. Cytosine
   D. Uracil
6. When the orderly process of cell division is interrupted, the result can lead to cancer.
   A. True
   B. False
7. The process for division of cells into two daughter cells is called
   A. meiosis.
   B. mitosis.
   C. translocation.
   D. interphase.
8. Genetic variation occurs during
   A. crossing over.
   B. mitosis.
   C. interphase.
   D. cytokinesis.
9. A germ cell is
   A. diploid.
   B. haploid.
   C. aneuploidy.
   D. mutated.
10. Genetic variation is
    A. important for species survival.
    B. the result of unwanted mutations.
    C. caused by apoptosis.
    D. caused by human manipulation.

Pretest answers are located in the Appendix.

SECTION ONE: DNA, RNA, and Protein Synthesis

The central dogma of molecular genetics, how DNA provides the codes for **proteins**, was first described by Crick (1958; 1970). The process is two steps: 1. *Transcription* is the term used for the process by which DNA makes RNA, and 2. **Translation** is the step for the actual formation of proteins. This decoding process is unidirectional: Information flows from DNA to RNA to proteins, and the process never occurs in reverse (Hartl & Jones, 2001).

The structure of DNA, as shown in Figure 4–1 ■, is that of a double helix. This structure resembles a spiral staircase, in which the strands of DNA are the banisters. The chemical bonds, which are made from the bases of adenine, cytosine, guanine, and thymine, form the risers that connect the banisters to each other. Adenine always pairs with thymine and guanine pairs with cytosine. DNA replicates itself as the double helix "unzips"—the bonds between the base pairs loosen, and a complementary strand forms as adenine pairs up with thymine and cytosine is paired with guanine (Lewis, 2010).

Transcription is the first step in the formation of proteins. One single strand of separated DNA serves as a template, and messenger RNA (mRNA) serves as an intermediary. It is formed in the same way that DNA replication takes place, except uracil replaces thymine and bonds with adenine. This process allows the genetic information to be transported to the places in the cell where protein is formed. The strand of mRNA is read in its sequence and in a specific order. The process of reading the mRNA goes in a predetermined direction.

The process of protein formation is called translation. As the mRNA is read, a three-base pair sequence codes for a specific protein. There are 20 amino acids and 64 possible DNA combinations (four possibilities at each of the three positions, so $4^3 = 64$) so there is considerable opportunity for redundancy. Table 4–1 displays the genetic code for the various proteins. Note that UAA and UAG are termination sequences. These sequences, called *stop codons*, inform the process that protein sequencing is complete. The translation stops at this point and the completed polypeptide chain is then released (Lewis, 2010). Figure 4–2 ■ is a pictorial representation of this process.

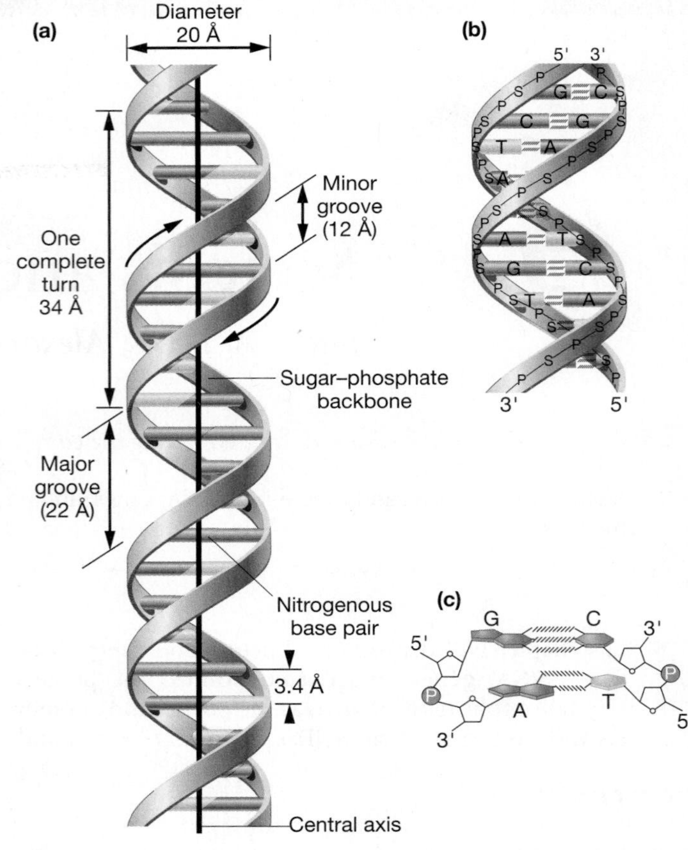

Figure 4–1 ■ Double helix

Source: Klug, William S.; Cummings, Michael R.; Spencer, Charlotte A.; Palladino, Michael A., Concepts Of Genetics, 9th, ©2009. Printed and Electronically reproduced by permission of Pearson Education, Inc., Upper Saddle River, New Jersey.

TABLE 4–1: The Standard Genetic Code

UUU Phenylalanine	UCU Serine	UAU Tyrosine	UGU Cysteine
UUC Phenylalanine	UCC Serine	UAC Tyrosine	UGC Cysteine
UUA Leucine	UCA Serine	UAA *Termination*	UGA *Termination*
UUG Leucine	UCG Serine	UAG *Termination*	UCG Tryptophan
CUU Leucine	CCU Proline	CAU Histidine	CCU Arginine
CUC Leucine	CCC Proline	CAC Histadine	CGC Arginine
CUA Leucine	CCA Proline	CAA Glutamine	CGA Arginine
CUG Leucine	CCG Proline	CAG Glutamine	CGG Arginine
AUU Isoleucine	ACU Threonine	AAU Asparagine	AGU Serine
AUC Isoleucine	ACC Threonine	AAC Asparagine	ACG Serine
AUA Isoleucine	ACA Threonine	AAA Lysine	AGA Arginine
AUG Methionine	ACG Threonine	AAG Lysine	AGG Arginine
GUU Valine	GCU Alanine	GAU Aspartic acid	GGU Glycine
GUC Valine	GCC Alanine	GAC Aspartic acid	GGC Glycine
GUA Valine	GCA Alanine	GAA Glutamic acid	GGA Glycine
GUG Valine	GCG Alanine	GAG Glutamic acid	GGG Glycine

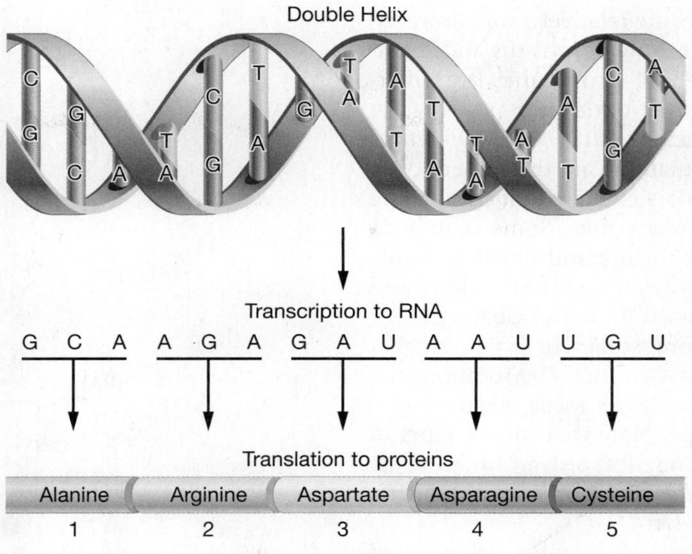

Figure 4–2 ■ DNA genetic code dictates amino acid identity and order

SECTION ONE REVIEW

1. The process of RNA formation from DNA is called
   A. transcription.
   B. translocation.
   C. translation.
   D. protein synthesis
2. The genetic code for the protein glycine is
   A. GGA.
   B. CCC.
   C. AGU.
   D. UCG.
3. The number of amino acids is
   A. 3.
   B. 4.
   C. 20.
   D. 64.
4. The completion of protein synthesis is signaled by a
   A. break in a DNA strand.
   B. lack of base pairs matching up.
   C. mutation.
   D. stop codon.

Answers: 1. A; 2. A; 3. C; 4. D

SECTION TWO: Genes and Chromosomes

The basic unit of heredity is a gene: a segment of DNA that contains the information necessary to create a specific protein. Genes are located on chromosomes, in specific spots, and in specific sequences. The goal of the Human Genome Project was to map the location of genes along each of the 23 chromosomes. It was originally thought that the human genome contained hundreds of thousands of genes. In reality, there are between 20,000 and 25,000 genes comprising the human genome, many fewer than originally thought (U.S. Department of Energy, 2009).

Each cell contains identical genetic material and the same DNA code, but not all DNA code is active in all cells.

Emerging Evidence

As knowledge of the structure of the human genome is complete, attention has turned to the complex issues of function. To ensure that the science keeps pace with technology and new developments, the NIH Office of the Human Genome is undergoing reorganization. Keep up to date with current scientific developments at http://www.genome.gov/reorg/.

The structure and function of each cell is determined by which genes are expressed within the cell.

As noted earlier, there are many possible spelling variations for each protein. Even so, with the volume of DNA replication, some spelling errors may occur, regardless of the redundancy built into the system. These errors are relatively rare; however, some errors do make a difference. Polymorphisms and mutations are the result of these spelling errors—they are differences that occur in the genetic code during the processes of transcription and translation (Lewis, 2010). The differences between polymorphisms and mutations are the frequency of their occurrence. Polymorphisms are changes that occur more frequently, while mutations are rare events. Some mutations are known to cause changes in structure and function, while the cause of others is yet to be determined. Mutations and changes in genetic code are discussed further in Chapter 18.

Genes are arranged on chromosomes in a pattern that has been mapped by the Human Genome. The location of a gene on a chromosome is known as its locus. Figure 4–3 ■ displays a normal male karyotype. Note that the 23 pairs of chromosomes are displayed in numerical order. Chromosome 1 is the longest, and the size of the chromosomes diminishes as the number of the pair gets higher.

Each normal somatic cell has 46 chromosomes: 23 of which came from each parent. Thus, the cell has two copies of each gene, known as alleles. The relationship between these alleles and the function of the pairs of genes will be further discussed in Chapter 6.

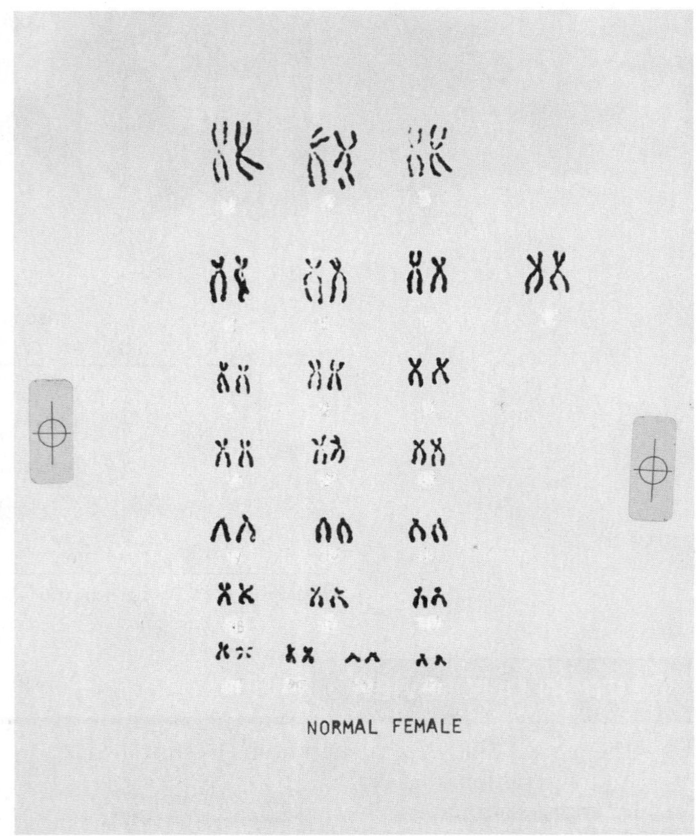

Figure 4–3 ■ Normal karyotype
Leonard Lessin / Photo Researchers, Inc.

SECTION TWO REVIEW

1. A change in genetic code that is a common spelling error is known as a
   A. mutation.
   B. translocation.
   C. polymorphism.
   D. structural anomaly.
2. The two copies of a gene found within a cell are known as
   A. mutations.
   B. polymorphisms.
   C. alleles.
   D. translocations.
3. Genes are comprised of
   A. proteins.
   B. chromosomes.
   C. mutations.
   D. mRNA.
4. The human genome is comprised of
   A. approximately 24,000 genes.
   B. over 100,000 genes.
   C. a great many mutations and errors.
   D. material that has very little in common with that of other living organisms.

Answers: 1. B; 2. C; 3. A; 4. A

SECTION THREE: The Cell Cycle and Mitosis

The **cell cycle** is a process that occurs in all body cells. It is comprised of two states: nondivision and division. Figure 4–4 ■ is a graphic depiction of the cell cycle. The length of the cell cycle can vary from several minutes to several years, depending on the specific type of cell and the placement within the human life cycle. The cell cycle consists of three parts: interphase, mitosis, and cytokinesis. When cells depart from the orderly process of the cell cycle, they can become cancerous. This orderly process is a part of the natural rhythm of life.

Shortly after cell division is completed, the cell enters interphase, the resting cell between cell division. Interphase consists of three parts: G1 (Gap 1), S (Synthesis), and G2 (Gap 2). Interphase is by far the longest period of time in the life cycle of a cell, and it is the time that is most variable. Rapidly dividing

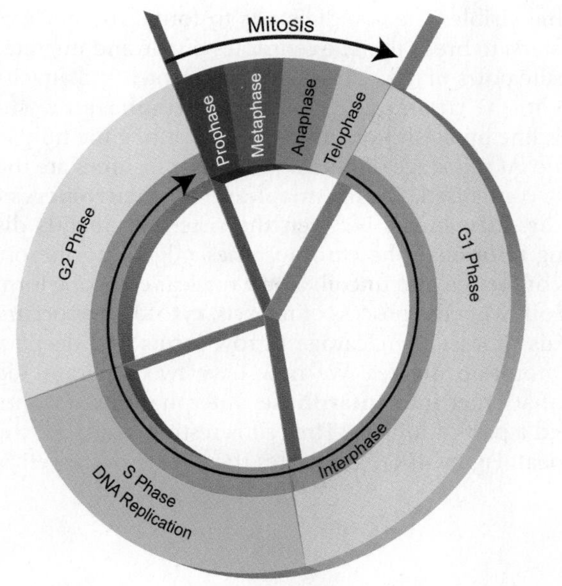

Figure 4–4 ■ Cell cycle
Source: Darryl Leja, National Human Genome Research Institute

cells, such as bone marrow cells, pass through interphase rather quickly while other cells may remain in interphase for months or years. There are some cells that enter a permanent resting stage, called G0, and undergo no further cell division. G1, the stage immediately following mitosis, is the time when all cell metabolic activity occurs. This is the stage of interphase that is most variable in length, ranging from minutes to years. Following G1, the cell enters into S (Synthesis). This is the stage of the cell cycle when DNA replication occurs and the chromosomes become double stranded. The rate of DNA replication is about 50 base pairs per second. This phase lasts about six hours (Mange & Mange, 1999). At the end of this phase, the sister **chromatids**, joined by the centriole, are visible. During the G2 phase, which lasts about 3 to 4 hours, the mitochondria divide. The precursors of the spindle fibers become visible.

Mitosis is the stage of the cell cycle where a parent cell divides, giving rise to two daughter cells, each of which will have a complete set of 46 chromosomes (see Figure 4–5 ■). Mitosis is a fluid, continuous process, but has been described in four stages: prophase, metaphase, anaphase, and telophase. During **prophase**, the chromosomes shorten and thicken. They

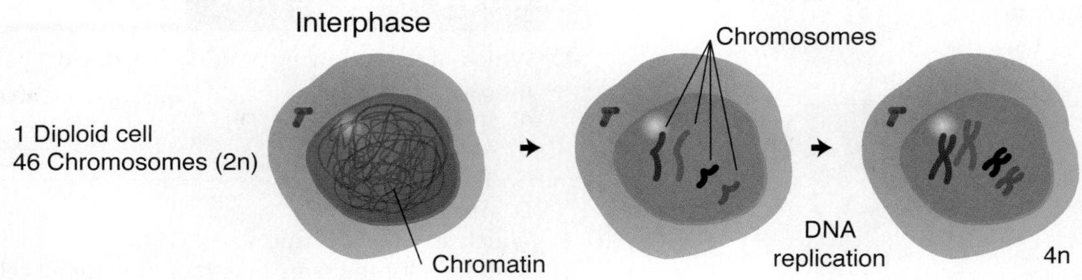

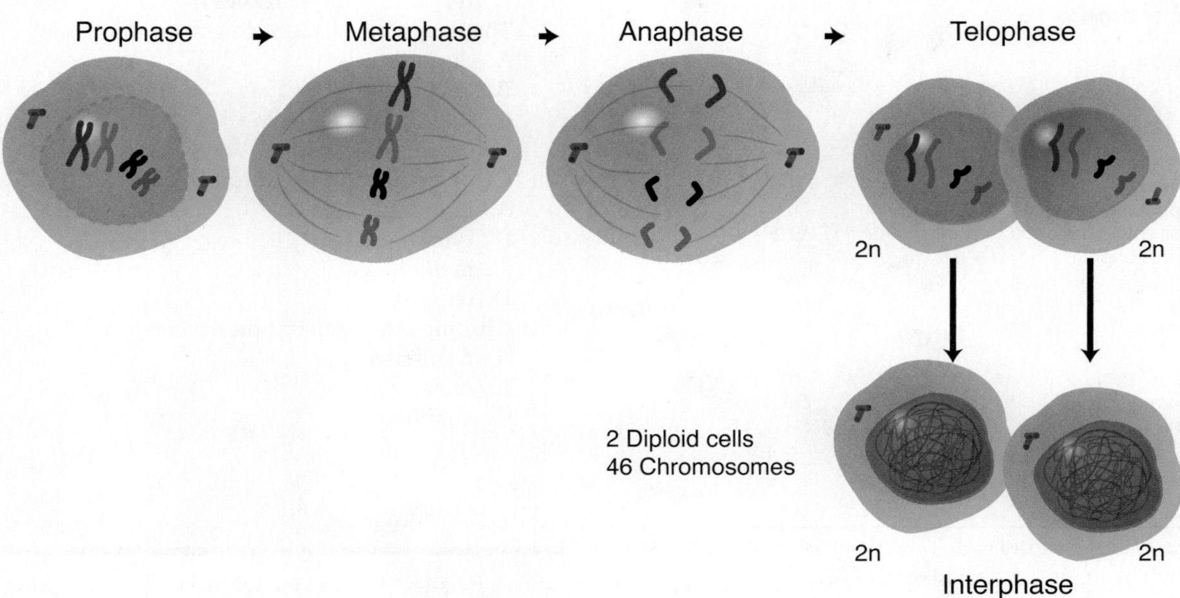

Figure 4–5 ■ Mitosis
Source: Darryl Leja, National Human Genome Research Institute.

Interphase

Gap 1
- Stage begins immediately after mitosis.
- RNA, protein, and other molecules are synthesized.

Synthesis
- DNA is replicated.
- Chromosomes become double stranded.

Gap 2
- Mitochondria divide.
- Precursors of spindle fibers are synthesized.

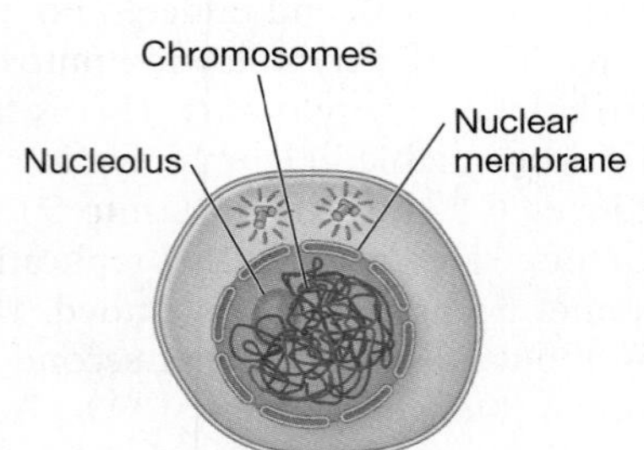

Mitosis

Prophase
- Chromosomes condense.
- Nuclear envelope disappears.
- Centrioles divide and migrate to opposite poles of the dividing cell.
- Spindle fibers form and attach to chromosomes.

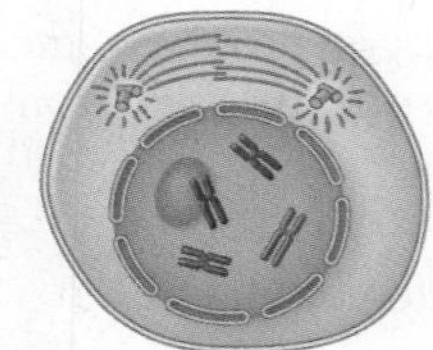

Metaphase
- Chromosomes line up on the midline of the dividing cell.

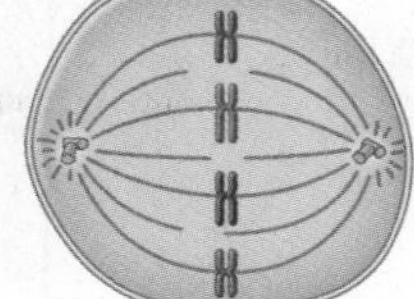

Anaphase
- Chromosomes begin to separate.

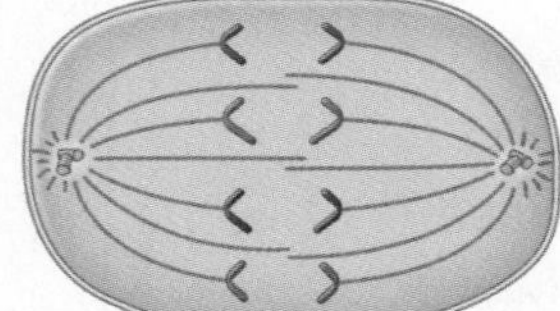

Telophase
- Chromosomes migrate or are pulled to opposite poles.
- New nuclear envelope forms.
- Chromosomes uncoil.

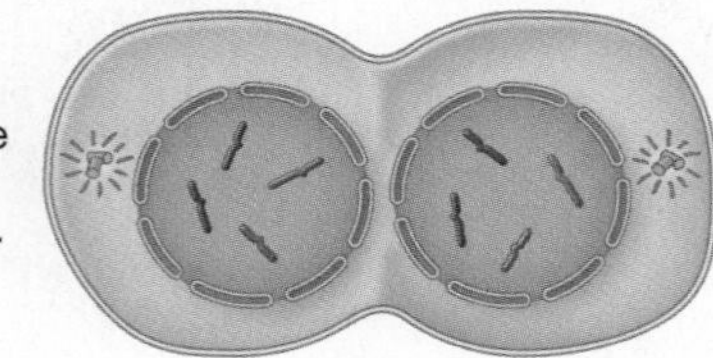

Cytokinesis
- Cleavage furrow forms and deepens.
- Cytoplasm divides.

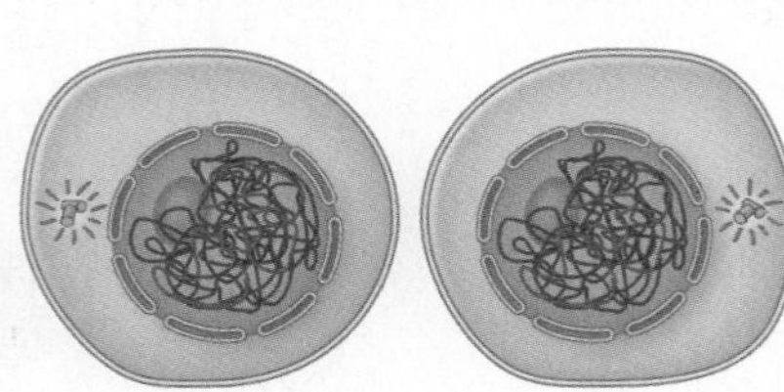

Figure 4–6 ■ Phases of the Cell Cycle

become visible. The spindle starts to form. The nuclear envelope starts to break up. The centrioles divide and migrate to the opposite poles of the cell. Spindle fibers form and attach themselves to the chromosomes. During **metaphase** the chromosomes line up at the equator of the cell, along the fully formed spindle. At this stage of mitosis, the chromosomes are the most tightly condensed. During **anaphase**, the **centromeres** divide and the attachments between the sister chromatids dissolve. During **telophase** the chromosomes migrate to the opposite poles of the cell and uncoil; a new nuclear envelope forms.

Following the process of mitosis, **cytokinesis** occurs. During this process the cleavage furrow forms and deepens, and the cytoplasm divides. We now have two separate, identical cells that enter into **interphase**. Interphase itself is not considered a part of mitosis. The cell is resting, ready for the cycle to repeat. Figure 4–6 ■ illustrates the phases of the cell cycle.

SECTION THREE REVIEW

1. Which of the following is NOT considered a part of mitosis?
   A. Interphase
   B. Metaphase
   C. Telophase
   D. Anaphase
2. Which statement is true about G1?
   A. It lasts for the same length of time for all cells.
   B. It is the phase of the cell cycle where cellular metabolic activity occurs.
   C. It is when the chromosomes are most tightly coiled.
   D. It is when the centrioles divide.
3. The daughter cells resulting from mitosis are
   A. diploid.
   B. aneuploid.
   C. haploid.
   D. germ cells.
4. Cytoplasmic division into two cells occurs during
   A. interphase.
   B. cytokinesis.
   C. metaphase.
   D. telophase.
5. Chromosomal separation occurs during
   A. prophase.
   B. metaphase.
   C. anaphase.
   D. telophase.

Answers: 1. A; 2. B; 3. A; 4. B; 5. C

SECTION FOUR: Meiosis and Gametogenesis

Meiosis is the process by which germ cells, eggs, and sperm are formed. Where cells that divide during mitosis have the same number of chromosomes (46) that were found in the parent cell, eggs and sperm have half the number of chromosomes (23). When fertilization occurs as the result of the union of egg and sperm, the resulting zygote then has a full complement (46) of chromosomes. Thus meiosis maintains a constant chromosome number from generation to generation. Figure 4–7 ■ illustrates the process of meiosis. Each cell that results from meiosis has one chromosome from each of the 23 pairs of chromosomes. If the germ cell does not contain the correct number of chromosomes, then the resulting zygote will contain fewer or greater than 23 pairs of chromosomes. The vast majority of these zygotes will not survive and develop. The chapter on aneuploidy (Chapter 5) provides an in-depth discussion of those conditions that do occur.

Meiosis actually consists of two separate rounds of cell division. During the first division, Meiosis I, the number of chromosomes is reduced from the diploid number of 46 to the haploid number of 23 (see Figure 4–8 ■). During Interphase I, chromosomal replication takes place. During Prophase 1, the chromosomes become visible and the homologous chromosomes pair. This process is called synapsis. The four sister chromatids are close to each other and genetic material is exchanged among the sister chromatids, a process called *crossing over,* which is depicted in Figure 4–9 ■. The sister chromatids stay closely aligned until Anaphase I. Any interruption to the crossing over process may lead to nondisjunction and to gametes with fewer or more than 23 chromosomes at the end of the process. The chapter on aneuploidy (Chapter 5) will discuss the anomalies that may occur as a result.

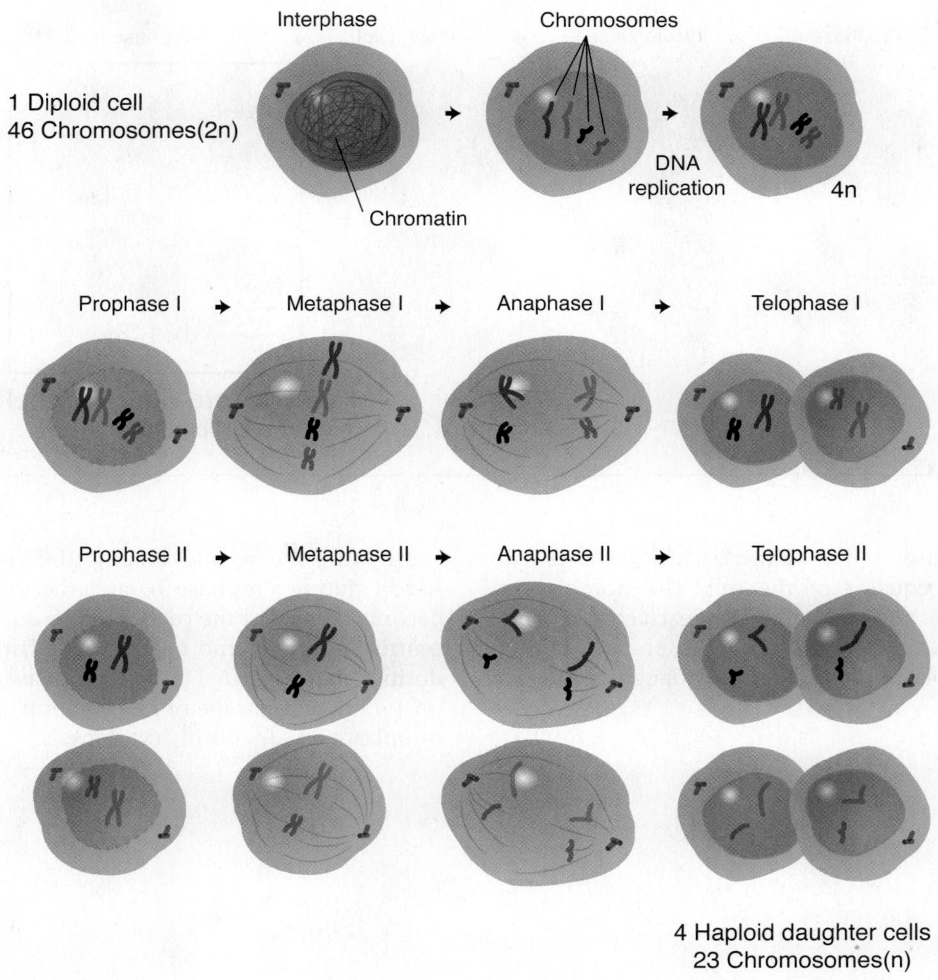

Figure 4–7 ■ Meiosis
Source: Darryl Leja, National Human Genome Research Institute.

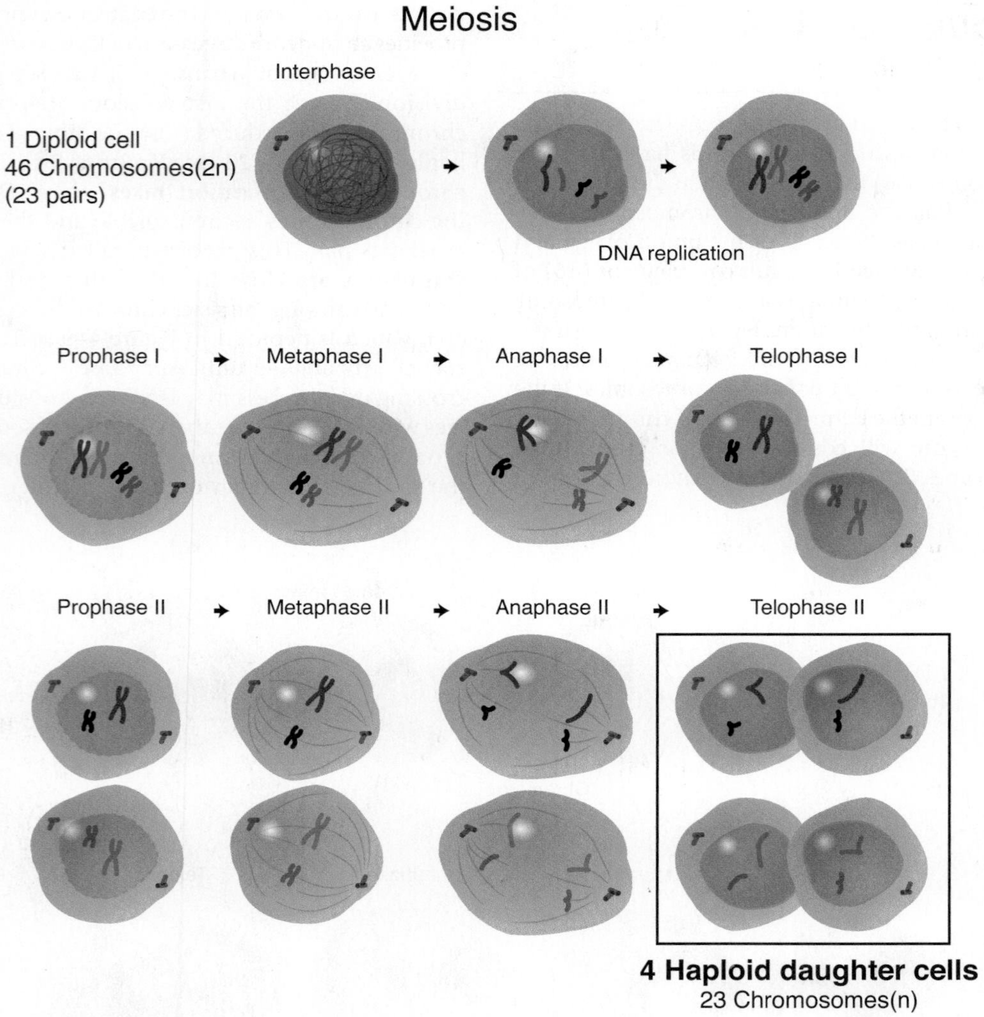

Meiosis

Interphase

1 Diploid cell
46 Chromosomes(2n)
(23 pairs)

DNA replication

Prophase I → Metaphase I → Anaphase I → Telophase I

Prophase II → Metaphase II → Anaphase II → Telophase II

4 Haploid daughter cells
23 Chromosomes(n)

Figure 4–8 ■ Haploid

During Metaphase I the paired chromosomes are seen aligned at the equator of the cell. The homologous chromosomes separate and the members of each chromosome pair move to opposite cell poles during Anaphase I. During Telophase I the cytoplasm divides and two daughter cells are produced.

During the second meiotic division, the chromosomes re-coil during Prophase II, and the unpaired chromosomes become aligned at the cell's equator during Metaphase II. The centrosomes split and the daughter chromosomes pull apart during Anaphase II. During Telophase II the chromosomes uncoil, the nuclear membranes reform, and meiosis ends. The cytoplasm divides during cytokinesis.

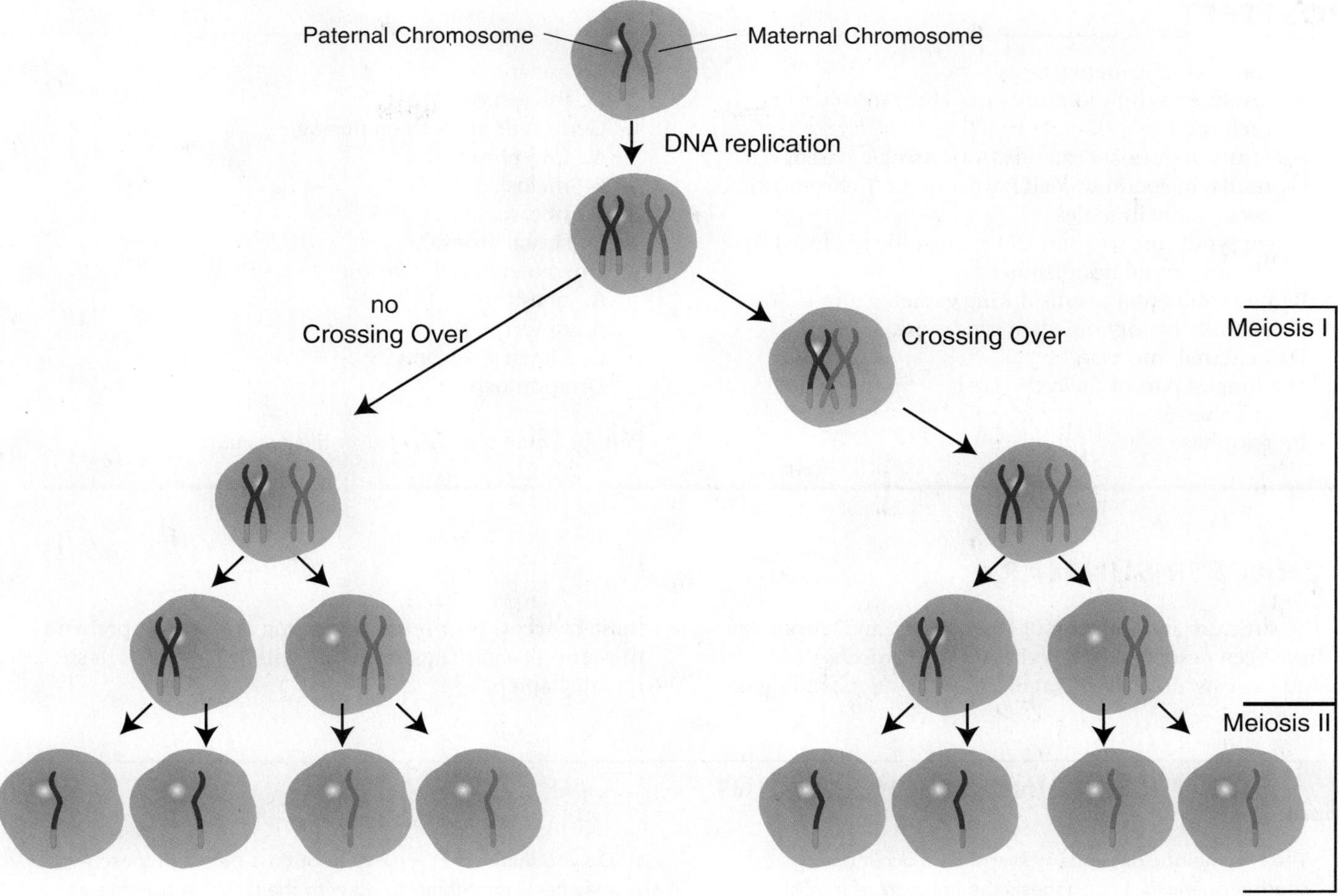

Figure 4–9 ■ Crossing over

SECTION FOUR REVIEW

1. Which cell division is considered the reduction division?
   A. Meiosis I
   B. Meiosis II
   C. Mitosis
   D. Interphase
2. The result of chromosomal nondisjunction can lead to
   A. monosomy.
   B. aneuploidy.
   C. triploidy.
   D. All of the above
3. Meiosis is the process by which
   A. cancer cells are allowed to duplicate unchecked.
   B. somatic cells divide.
   C. germ cells are formed.
   D. fertilization occurs.
4. At the end of the first meiotic division, each daughter cell has
   A. 23 chromosomes.
   B. 46 chromosomes.
   C. both an X and a Y chromosome.
   D. an unknown number of chromosomes.
5. The process by which genetic variation is created is called
   A. nondisjunction.
   B. cell division.
   C. asexual reproduction.
   D. crossing over.

Answers: 1. A; 2. D; 3. C; 4. A; 5. D

POSTTEST

1. The process of gametogenesis
   A. results in a diploid number of chromosomes in each cell.
   B. results in four spermatids from a single parent cell.
   C. results in sperm that all have a single Y chromosome.
   D. occurs only in males.
2. Down syndrome [trisomy 21] is most likely caused by
   A. chromosomal nondisjunction.
   B. environmental insults during gametogenesis.
   C. a family history of Down syndrome.
   D. maternal infection.
3. The longest part of the cell cycle is
   A. anaphase.
   B. telophase.
   C. metaphase.
   D. interphase.
4. Germ cells are formed during
   A. interphase.
   B. meiosis.
   C. mitosis.
   D. sexual arousal.
5. Unregulated cell division can result in
   A. obesity.
   B. cancer.
   C. Down syndrome.
   D. apoptosis.

Posttest answers are located in the Appendix.

CHAPTER SUMMARY

The structure and function of DNA, genes, and chromosomes have been described in this chapter. The processes of mitosis and meiosis also have been discussed. Understanding of these concepts is important to being able to comprehend the concepts and constructs that will be described in subsequent chapters.

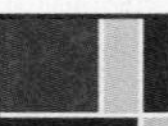

CRITICAL THINKING CHECKPOINT

The two meiotic divisions in sperm cells occur during spermatogenesis. In oogenesis the first part of meiosis occurs during fetal development, and meiosis is completed after puberty.

1. Do you think that the amount of time between these events may have something to do with the fact that the rate of infants born with chromosomal abnormalities increases with maternal age?

Answers are provided in the Appendix

Pearson Nursing Student Resources

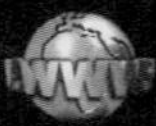

Find additional review materials at nursing.pearsonhighered.com

Prepare for success with additional NCLEX®-style practice questions, interactive assignments and activities, web links, animations, videos, and more!

ONLINE RESOURCES

National Human Genome Research Institute: http://www.genome.gov

Online Mendelian Inheritance in Man: (OMIM): http:// http://www.ncbi.nlm.nih.gov/omim/

REFERENCES

Crick, F. (1958). On protein synthesis. *Symposia for the Society of Experimental Biology, XII,* 139–163.

Crick, F. (1970). Central dogma of molecular biology. *Nature, 227,* 561–563.

Cummings, M. R. (2006). *Human heredity: Principles and issues* (7th Ed.). Belmont. CA: Thomson Brooks/Cole.

Hartl, D. L., & Jones, E. W. (2001). *Genetics: Analysis of genes and genomes.* Sudbury, MA: Jones & Bartlett.

Lewis, J. A. (2010). Genetics and genomics. (3rd ed.). White Plains, NY: March of Dimes.

Lewis, R. (2007). *Human genetics: Concepts and applications* (7th ed.). Boston: McGraw-Hill.

Mange, E. J., & Mange, A. P. (1999). *Basic human genetics* (2nd ed.). Sunderland, MA: Sinauer Associates, Inc.

U.S. Department of Energy, Office of Science (2009). *Human genome project information.* Retrieved from http://www.ornl.gov/sci/techresources/Human_Genome/home.shtml

CHAPTER

5 Aneuploidy

Matthew Sorenson

LEARNING OUTCOMES

Following the completion of this chapter, the learner will be able to

1. Define aneuploidy and the differing forms.
2. Discuss the relevance of aneuploidy for nursing.
3. Summarize the connection between maternal age and aneuploidy.

This chapter reviews the concept of aneuploidy. It provides chromosomal information regarding the incidence of aneuploidy and resultant conditions and explores aneuploidy from the perspective of missing chromosomal segments—particularly nullisomy and monosomy. It also examines chromosomal additions, such as trisomy and **tetrasomy**, and their relevance for health. This chapter also reviews the relationship between aneuploidy and maternal age.

PRETEST

1. Aneuploidy is the presence of
   A. telomere shortening.
   B. telomere lengthening.
   C. an abnormal number of chromosomes.
   D. a lack of normative nullisomy.
2. Aneuploidy is believed to be caused by
   A. low levels of steroidal hormones.
   B. carcinogens.
   C. maternal age under 18.
   D. paternal age under 18.
3. Nullisomy is the
   A. loss of one chromosome.
   B. loss of two chromosomes.
   C. addition of one chromosome.
   D. addition of two chromosomes.
4. Monosomy is the
   A. loss of one chromosome.
   B. loss of two chromosomes.
   C. addition of one chromosome.
   D. addition of two chromosomes.
5. Down syndrome is an example of
   A. nullisomy.
   B. monosomy.
   C. tetrasomy.
   D. trisomy.
6. Autosomes are best described as
   A. sex chromosomes.
   B. chromosomes related to autoimmune processes.
   C. chromosomes associated with brain and spinal cord development.
   D. those chromosomes responsible for aneuploidy.
7. Disjunction refers to a process that occurs during cell
   A. apoptosis.
   B. meiosis.
   C. nullisomy.
   D. trisomy.
8. Humans normally have how many chromosomal pairs?
   A. 8
   B. 19
   C. 23
   D. 46
9. Trisomy is the
   A. loss of one chromosome.
   B. loss of two chromosomes.
   C. addition of one chromosome.
   D. addition of two chromosomes.
10. The development of cancer could be considered a form of
    A. nonrandom aneuploidy.
    B. random aneuploidy.
    C. parsimony.
    D. tetrasomy.

Pretest answers are located in the Appendix.

SECTION ONE: Overview of Aneuploidy

Chromosomes provide encoding for thousands of genes necessary for development and continued health. At times, the development of these chromosomes can be altered, with pieces missing or added, or a particular chromosomal segment may be missing. When this occurs, the ability to encode, or produce, the genes associated with the missing segments is lost. Such chromosomal variations are often associated with cognitive and structural deficits, often due to the loss of genes that are necessary for fetal development. Ultimately, chromosomal variation results in changes in gene expression, either a loss of expression or an excess (Nussbaum, McInnes, & Hungtington, 2004).

There are two main mechanisms through which chromosomal variation can occur. Chromosomal segments can be duplicated, relocated, or inverted. If pieces, or segments, of chromosomes are being rearranged, the term *translocation* is often used. Such rearrangements can occur with equal amounts of chromosomal material and are then referred to as reciprocal. When rearrangements occur with unequal amounts of chromosomal material, they are referred to as unbalanced translocations and often lead to missing genes (Nussbaum et al., 2004). Another means of variation is through the addition or subtraction of complete chromosomes or chromosomal segments. This results in duplicate or triplicate copies of a chromosome or segment and has adverse consequences for health. For example, an individual with Down syndrome has an extra chromosome (Chromosome 21), while an individual with Turner syndrome is missing a chromosome (X chromosome). The process through which this occurs is identified as **aneuploidy**, which means there has been a change in the number of individual chromosomes or chromosomal segments.

The term *ploidy* refers to the presence of a normative number of sets or pairs of chromosomes. To be **aneuploid** means there is an incorrect number of chromosomes. This process can occur through either the addition or subtraction of chromosomes, and it takes place prenatally or develops later in life. Aneuploidy often occurs during meiosis, which is the process leading to the production of sperm and egg cells (Nussbaum et al., 2004). A related term is **mosaicism** (see Chapter 6), which refers to variations or mutations that occur after conception, and affects a select group of cells such as blood cells.

There can be a lack of clarity sometimes between aneuploidy and mosaicism. At times, some authors use the terms in a somewhat interchangeable manner. Basically, aneuploidy is concerned with changes in the number of chromosomes due to improper separation of chromosomes during cell division. Aneuploidy can occur with both autosomal and sex chromosomes. **Autosomes** are those chromosomes that are not associated with the development of sex characteristics. Many of these chromosomes are instead involved in the development of the brain and spinal cord. Several forms of autosomal aneuploidy result in spontaneous abortion as these deficits can be incompatible with life. Those infants with autosomal aneuploidy that survive are often born with significant defects in cognition and mental function. The most well-known form of autosomal aneuploidy is Down syndrome. The loss or gain of a sex chromosome is more compatible with life, and often these infants survive. Turner syndrome and Klinefelter syndrome are examples of sex chromosome aneuploidy.

In terms of naming the forms of aneuploidy, chromosomal addition is traditionally referred to as trisomy or tetrasomy. **Trisomy** is the addition of a single chromosome, while the addition of two homologous chromosomes is referred to as tetrasomy. Chromosomal subtraction is traditionally referred to as nullisomy or monosomy. **Nullisomy** is loss of two chromosomes, while the loss of a single chromosome is referred to as **monosomy**.

Aneuploidy is associated with the development of several disease states and is considered the leading cause of spontaneous abortion. It has been reported that up to 30% of all aneuploid pregnancies result in spontaneous abortion, often long before the mother is aware of the pregnancy. Aneuploidy is considered to account for up to 50% of these abortions due to the presence of chromosomal abnormalities that are incompatible with life (Menasha, Levy, Hirschhorn, & Kardon, 2005; Suzumori & Sugiura-Ogasawara, 2010). Most of these abortions would be considered autosomal aneuploidy. An additional consideration is that aneuploidy is not only manifest in those with birth defects and developmental delay. It is also the main mechanism through which most cancers develop (Fang & Zhang, 2011).

Potential Causes

The causes of aneuploidy are not well understood. Carcinogens and toxins are believed to be associated with the chromosomal abnormalities reflected in cases of aneuploidy primarily through effects on **gametes** (sperm or egg) (Duesberg, Fabarius, & Hehlmann, 2004). Should the chromosomes in the cell fail to divide properly during meiosis, then a nondisjunction abnormality may occur. Should a gamete encounter another gamete and join to it, the process leads to trisomy, with the addition of another chromosome. Partial forms of aneuploidy can occur through translocation of chromosomal segments (Nussbaum et al., 2004).

Nondisjunction

Nondisjunction refers to chromosomal abnormality that occurs during a period of cell division. During meiosis I, the homologous chromosomes disjoin, or separate. With nondisjunction, a pair of chromosomes may not separate. This nondisjunction can then result in a group of cells that share the same chromosomal abnormality, while other cells may be spared this abnormality. For example, blood cells could display an abnormality while neurons may not. This failure of the chromosomes to properly separate during cell division serves as the basis for mosaicism (Nussbaum et al., 2004). As discussed in the chapter on meiosis, there are periods during the cell cycle that serve as checkpoints and ensure the integrity of cell division and structure. If there is damage to one of these important regulatory checkpoints, then chromosomal abnormalities may develop that lead to aneuploidy.

Random and Nonrandom

Most prenatal forms of aneuploidy would best be considered as occurring through random variation of a chromosome. However, certain processes and toxins may contribute to the development of specific chromosomal abnormalities. This is best represented by the chromosomal theory of cancer. In this theoretical model, an individual could be placed at risk for the development of cancer due to the presence of specific chromosomal abnormalities at birth, or through a process of carcinogenetic damage that influences a specific chromosome (S. Thompson & Compton, 2011; S. L. Thompson, Bakhoum, & Compton, 2010). There is also a strong relationship between maternal age and aneuploidy, one that has been speculated to occur through elevation in gonadotropin levels either in association with aging or the use of artificial reproductive procedures (Dursun, Gultekin, Yuce, & Ayhan, 2006).

SECTION ONE REVIEW

1. Autosomal aneuploidy can result in
   A. Turner syndrome.
   B. Down syndrome.
   C. translocative nullisomy.
   D. Klinefelter syndrome.
2. Nondisjunction means that a pair of chromosomes
   A. separated prematurely.
   B. separated late.
   C. did not separate.
   D. fused together within one particular group of cells.
3. Those infants with experienced autosomal aneuploidy are born with significant defects in
   A. secondary sex characteristics.
   B. cardiovascular and respiratory function.
   C. cognition and mental function.
   D. personality and mood.
4. Aneuploidy is believed to account for approximately what percentage of spontaneous abortions?
   A. 5
   B. 10
   C. 25
   D. 50
5. Trisomy is defined as
   A. the addition of one chromosome.
   B. the addition of two chromosomes.
   C. the subtraction of one chromosome.
   D. the addition of two chromosomes.

Answers: 1. B; 2. C; 3. C; 4. D; 5. A

SECTION TWO: Scope

The frequency of aneuploidy varies greatly both in terms of incidence and symptom severity. In general, the survivable forms of aneuploidy include trisomy and monosomy. Select forms of tetrasomy exist, but are rare and while considered aneuploid conditions, they more accurately reflect mosaicism. Nullisomy is generally not considered a condition supportable with fetal life and is a leading cause of spontaneous abortion. More common are partial forms of aneuploidy in which select chromosomal segments have been relocated. These conditions still result in significant congenital birth defects but overall are considered to be more survivable. Additionally, the relocation or absence of chromosomal segments tends to influence multiple genes, resulting in deficits across several bodily systems. The loss or addition of even a small chromosomal segment can influence hundreds of proteins that are necessary for human development.

Overall, aneuploidy has been estimated to occur as frequently as in 1 of every 160 live births. For autosomal aneuploidy, the most common conditions involve trisomy of chromosomes 13, 18, and 21. (For a list of common conditions, see Table 5–1). Out of those conditions, those infants with Down syndrome are most likely to survive to adulthood even with significant deficits. Out of those with trisomy 13 or 18, it has been estimated that only 10% will reach their first

TABLE 5–1: Common Conditions Associated with Survivable Aneuploidy

Condition	Incidence per Live Births	Chromosomal Variation
1p36 Syndrome	1:10,000	Deletion of short arm of chromosome one.
DiGeorge Syndrome	1:4,000	Deletion occurring in location 11.2 of chromosome 22.
Down Syndrome (Trisomy 21)	1:691	Addition of chromosome 21.
Edwards Syndrome (Trisomy 18)	1:3,762	Additional of chromosome 18.
Klinefelter Syndrome	1:650 (males)	Addition of an X chromosome.
Patau Syndrome (Trisomy 13)	1:7,906	Addition of chromosome 13.
Turner Syndrome	1:2,000 (females)	Deletion of an X chromosome.

Note: Data derived from Canfield et al. (2006); Parker et al. (2010).

Emerging Evidence

- Studies are beginning to examine not only the frequency of chromosomal variation in association with disease, but also treatment responsiveness in relation to such variation (Fischer et al., 2011).
- There are several aspects to the transcription of DNA and RNA. In terms of processes associated with aneuploidy, the presence of certain transcription factors appears to be necessary to ensure appropriate transcription without chromosomal variation during fetal development. Some of these factors also appear to play a role in tumor suppression, highlighting the interplay between cancer and aneuploidy (Iotti et al., 2011).
- New procedures and techniques are being developed to provide accurate prenatal screening for aneuploidy that provide a means of screening for microdeletions as well as large chromosomal changes (Shaffer et al., 2011).
- The relationship between common disease states and aneuploidy continues to demonstrate the complex nature amongst genetic variables and health. A recent study demonstrated a possible connection between Type 1 diabetes and the probability of aneuploidy, concluding that mothers with Type 1 diabetes require closer monitoring and tighter glycemic control (Madsen et al., 2011).
- The potential effect of hormones on aneuploidy has been supported by work finding that administration of dehydroepiandrosterone reduces the incidence of aneuploidy (Gleicher, Weghofer, & Barad, 2010a).

birthday. It has been speculated that the length of these chromosomes ultimately is one of the reasons that these conditions are survivable in the face of chromosomal variation. Chromosomes 13, 18, and 21 are the smallest of all the chromosomes in respect to the number of genes that they encode for (Torres, Williams, & Amon, 2008); thus a deficit of these particular chromosomes may enhance survivability.

Aneuploidy is a major source of birth defects, of which several recognizable patterns exist. Of those, perhaps the most common malformations are cardiac in nature. The incidence of congenital heart defects has been estimated to occur in 30% of all children with chromosomal abnormalities, and it occurs more frequently in certain syndromes. For example, almost all children with trisomy 18 exhibit congenital heart defects (Pierpont et al., 2007). Physical growth retardation is also a common characteristic usually accompanied by a small skull (microcephaly), other facial changes, and neurologic deficits usually in terms of hypotonicity and an increased risk for seizure activity (Torres et al., 2008).

Ultimately, questions arise about the source of aneuploidy. While numerous etiologic factors have been investigated, ranging from caloric intake to toxins, little consistent supporting evidence has been found for one cause over another. One of the major factors thought to be involved in aneuploidy is pesticides. A review of the literature concluded that an association exists between pesticides and nondisjunction in sperm, but that the evidence remains lacking (Perry, 2008). It has also been speculated that aneuploidy merely serves the stage for autoimmune processes, which then contribute to congenital deficits and spontaneous abortion (Gleicher, Weghofer, & Barad, 2010b).

SECTION TWO REVIEW

1. Of those with Edwards syndrome, how many are expected to reach age 10?
   A. 50%
   B. 40%
   C. 20%
   D. 10%
2. Which syndrome is most likely to occur in those with aneuploidy?
   A. Down
   B. Edwards
   C. Patau
   D. Turner
3. Trisomy is most likely to involve which chromosomes?
   A. 13, 18
   B. 5, 7
   C. 13, 25
   D. 5, 8
4. The evidence for paternal involvement in aneuploidy is
   A. strong.
   B. inconsistent.
   C. unequivocal.
   D. No research has been done.
5. Aneuploidy has been estimated to occur in approximately every 1 out of every __________ live births.
   A. 10
   B. 100
   C. 150
   D. 200

Answers: 1. D; 2, A; 3. A; 4. B; 5. C

SECTION THREE: Chromosomal Deletion: Monosomy and Nullisomy

The primary chromosomal deletions are monosomy and nullisomy. In monosomy there is just a single chromosome present, and in nullisomy two chromosomes or chromosomal segments are lost.

Monosomy

Monosomy is the loss of one chromosome and is often depicted by the equation 2n–1. In this equation, n refers to the number of chromosomes. So, humans with a normal number of 23 paired chromosomes would display 2n, or 46 chromosomes. In monosomy there is a loss of a chromosome, resulting in 45 chromosomes. So, there is then only a single copy of a particular chromosome, or a chromosomal segment.

Syndromes Known to be Associated with Monosomy

Turner syndrome and Klinefelter syndrome are examples of sex chromosome aneuploidy. Monosomy of the X chromosome can result in Turner syndrome. Females possess two X chromosomes, and in the case of Turner syndrome (45, XO), are missing one of the two. This form of aneuploidy accounts for approximately 50–60% of all cases of Turner syndrome. There is a form of partial monosomy of the X chromosome that can manifest as Turner mosaicism, which also accounts for a number of cases (Oliveira et al., 2009). Klinefelter syndrome occurs in males and is a form of trisomy with the presence of an extra X chromosome (Wikstrom & Dunkel, 2011).

Clinically, Turner syndrome is characterized by short stature and skeletal malformations. Cardiovascular complications such as coarctation of the aorta and defects of the ventricular septum are common. There is often a loss of secondary sex characteristics, and those with Turner syndrome often are infertile. Due to a lack of reproductive development and resultant endocrine deficiencies, women with Turner syndrome may not experience menses (Oliveira et al., 2009). Learning disabilities are common, along with sleep apnea and low bone density (Davenport, 2010).

Nullisomy

Nullisomy is the loss of two chromosomes or deletion of two chromosomal segments, and is often depicted by the equation 2n–2. In this equation, n refers to the number of chromosomes. So, in humans with a normal number of 23 paired chromosomes there should be 2n, or 46 chromosomes. In nullisomy there can be a loss of a pair of chromosomes, resulting in 44 chromosomes. However, nullisomy can also refer to the loss of chromosomal segments in different groups of cells. In such a case, an individual could have experienced a deletion of two different chromosomal segments. This condition is traditionally referred to as mosaicism, although many authors and sources also refer to it as nullisomy. As an example, studies of autism have referred to a mosaic aneuploidy (Yurov et al., 2007).

Nullisomy is often not considered compatible with human life, and most fetuses with this condition would undergo spontaneous abortion. There are several forms of partial nullisomy that are associated with medical conditions.

Syndromes Associated with Nullisomy: Autosomal and Sex Chromosome Based

Individuals with autism are believed to be missing two segments on the X chromosome (Xp22). While this deletion has traditionally been thought to influence males, there are case reports of females with autism displaying the same pattern of deletion (Shinawi et al., 2009). Deletions in this area of the X chromosome are believed to be associated with intellectual disability (Filges et al., 2011), leading to the possibility of this sequence playing a role in the development of autism and other disorders of cognition and intellect.

SECTION THREE REVIEW

1. Nullisomy results in how many chromosomes?
   A. 44
   B. 45
   C. 46
   D. 47
2. Monosomy refers to
   A. a missing chromosome.
   B. two missing chromosomes.
   C. an extra chromosome.
   D. two extra chromosomes.
3. In Turner syndrome, there is a(n)
   A. additional X chromosome.
   B. loss of an X chromosome.
   C. extra Y chromosome.
4. The outcome of nullisomy is often
   A. an extra X chromosome.
   B. Klinefelter syndrome.
   C. spontaneous abortion.
   D. Turner syndrome.
5. Those with autism are believed to be missing segments on what chromosome?
   A. The 4th chromosome.
   B. The 8th chromosome.
   C. The 21st chromosome.
   D. The X chromosome.

Answers: 1. A; 2. A; 3. B; 4. C; 5. D

SECTION FOUR: Chromosomal Additions: Trisomy and Tetrasomy

The primary chromosomal additions are trisomy and tetrasomy. In trisomy, there is an added chromosome, or chromosomal segment. With tetrasomy there are two additional copies.

Trisomy

Trisomy is the addition of a chromosome or chromosomal segment and is often depicted by the equation 2n+1. In this equation, n refers to the number of chromosomes. So, humans with a normal number of 23 paired chromosomes would display 2n, or 46 chromosomes. In trisomy there is then an additional chromosome. Trisomy can occur with any chromosome, but with certain ones this would result in spontaneous abortion. With other chromosomes, however, the fetus survives, most likely due to a smaller number of genes in relation to other chromosomes. With trisomy there is upregulation of gene expression due to the presence of the extra chromosome, or chromosomal segment. This increased gene expression is most often associated with the development of congenital growth deficits and cognitive delay. The most common forms of trisomy are trisomy 18 (Edwards syndrome) and trisomy 21 (Down syndrome). Trisomy 13 (Papau) is less common, with a high incidence of first-year mortality often due to cardiovascular defects (Rios, Furdon, Adams, & Clark, 2004).

Associated Syndromes: Trisomy 21

In Down syndrome, the infant usually has three copies of chromosome 21. There is a partial form of trisomy 21, in which part of the chromosome has been added. Symptom presentation is less severe in partial forms of trisomy 21. Children with Down syndrome exhibit a particular set of facial characteristics that include a protruding tongue, upward slanting (almond shaped) eyes, and a smaller skull (microcephaly) than expected for age. In terms of other physical findings and characteristics, these children display hypotonicity and excessive flexibility due to ligamental laxity as well as short, stubby fingers and broad hands.

As with Down syndrome, Edwards syndrome is a trisomy except this time the involved chromosome is the 18th. Edwards syndrome shares many of the same physical defects as Down syndrome. Those with Edwards syndrome often display microcephaly, misshaped ears, and cleft palate along with cardiac defects. As with Down syndrome, the risk of Edwards syndrome increases in relation to maternal age.

Klinefelter syndrome occurs in males and is a form of trisomy with the presence of an extra X chromosome. It is characterized by the presence of infertility and decreased testicular size, along with decreased facial and pubic hair. A reduction in muscle strength and metabolic syndrome also occurs in a significant percentage of those with the condition (Wikstrom & Dunkel, 2011).

Tetrasomy

Tetrasomy is often depicted by the equation 2n+2. In tetrasomy, there is then an addition of two additional copies of a chromosome or part of a chromosome. Tetrasomy tends to be rare, partly due to the presence of significant, life-threatening defects that can occur in the presence of two additional copies of a chromosome. One condition that has been identified is Pallister-Killian syndrome. In this condition, the infant has two identical arms of the short arm of chromosome 12. For most survivable cases of tetrasomy, the replicated genetic material is in one of the chromosomal arms, and it is provided four copies of the genes located in that region, rather than a complete insertion of a full chromosome. Some sources refer to this condition as a mosaic syndrome, in that some cells will have four copies of the genes present on the short arm of chromosome 12, while other cells may not. As with other chromosomal variations, a range of disability may be seen. Generally, a lack of muscle tone is present accompanied by cognitive deficits, patchy hyperpigmentation of the skin, cardiac defects, and extra fingers or toes. These infants are considered at high risk for the development of seizure activity.

A similar clinical picture is seen in those with tetrasomy 18p, in which the replicated chromosomal segments are again located on the short arm of the chromosome. An even rarer condition is tetrasomy 9p, which can present in a similar fashion to Klinefelter syndrome. In tetrasomy 9p there is also the presence of significant cognitive deficits along with cleft palate and abnormalities of the ear (Ogino et al., 2007). In all of these forms of tetrasomy, abnormalities of the genitalia may also be seen.

SECTION FOUR REVIEW

1. Tetrasomy is
   A. a relatively common condition.
   B. a relatively rare condition.
   C. a condition with little significance on functional ability.
   D. a leading cause of cancer in the developed world.
2. Edwards syndrome is a
   A. trisomy of chromosome 13.
   B. trisomy of chromosome 18.
   C. trisomy of chromosome 21.
   D. tetrasomy of chromosome 9p.
3. Pallister–Killian syndrome is an example of
   A. trisomy 13.
   B. trisomy 18.
   C. trisomy 21.
   D. tetrasomy.
4. Trisomy is the
   A. addition of a single chromosome.
   B. addition of two chromosomes.
   C. deletion of a single chromosome.
   D. deletion of two chromosomes.
5. The shape of the skull in children with trisomy 18 and 21 is best described as
   A. macrocephaly.
   B. microcephaly.
   C. anencephaly.
   D. craniostenosis.

Answers: 1. B; 2. D; 3. D; 4. A; 5. B

SECTION FIVE: Aneupliody and Aging

There are strong relationships between parental age and aneuploidy, particularly in terms of maternal age. For example, the primary risk factor identified for the development of Down syndrome is maternal age. At the age of 35, the maternal risk of having a child with Down syndrome is 1 in 400. At age 45, the risk rises to 1 in 24 (Resta, 2005). Several theories have been proposed regarding the association between maternal age and aneuploidy. The major operative premise is that increased maternal age is associated with increased episodes of nondisjunction: The older the mother, the greater the probability that chromosomes in the egg will not divide properly during meiosis. This then contributes to abnormal combinations or loss of chromosomes that can result in birth defects. This relationship has been demonstrated to exist even with in vitro fertilization procedures (Spandorfer, Davis, Barmat, Chung, & Rosenwaks, 2004).

Several mechanisms have been studied in terms of maternal age and aneuploidy. It has been speculated that increased levels of gonadotropin levels may well be associated with the increase in chromosomal abnormalities in association with aging (Dursun et al., 2006). Other work has suggested that advanced maternal age may be associated with an increase in proteins that result in nondisjunction (Eichenlaub-Ritter, Staubach, & Trapphoff, 2010). Animal studies have demonstrated that significant caloric restriction has been able to prevent age-associated changes in several meiotic structures (Selesniemi, Lee, Muhlhauser, & Tilly, 2011). This caloric reduction is thought to influence metabolic pathways that may otherwise produce hormones and other mediators that affect the meiotic spindle and other components of meiosis.

On the paternal side, some authors have speculated that aging can have adverse effects on sperm quality and have investigated the role of paternal age in aneuploidy. At this point the evidence appears inconclusive, although a recent review of the field suggested that there is no paternal role in association with age (Fonseka & Griffin, 2011).

The Elderly and Natural Aneuploidy: Relevance for Disease

It is also possible that aneuploidy reflects age-associated decay in other cell mechanisms, a type of programmed senescence. The increasing incidence in cancer associated with age implies defects in immune surveillance and points to a potential role of immunosenescence. In other words, older cells do not work as effectively, and early aneuploidy-induced deficits may appear later in life and contribute to the development of cancer. Aneuploidic theories of cancer fit with several findings that imply that many cancers that are not heritable develop over long periods of time and are often characterized by chromosomal abnormalities that lead to cell growth that is not necessary for homeostasis (Duesberg et al., 2004). The presence of chromosomal disruptions affects numerous proteins that all play a role in growth and development. Dysregulation of these proteins can lead to changes in cellular mechanisms and a loss of tumor suppressive elements that over time set the stage of the development of cancer.

SECTION FIVE REVIEW

1. Increased maternal age is associated with a(n) __________ risk of having an infant with Down syndrome.
   A. decreased
   B. increased
   C. equivalent
   D. decreased (but only in cases of monosomy).
2. The incidence of cancer __________ with increased age.
   A. decreases
   B. increases
   C. remains the same
   D. decreases (but only in cases of monosomy).
3. At the age of 35, the maternal risk of having a child with Down syndrome is 1 in __________.
   A. 4
   B. 40
   C. 400
   D. 4,000
4. At age 45, the maternal risk of having a child with Down syndrome is 1 in __________.
   A. 2
   B. 12
   C. 24
   D. 48
5. The risk of aneuploidy increases in association with age.
   A. True
   B. False

Answers: 1. B; 2. B; 3. C; 4. C; 5. A

POSTTEST

1. Which of the following is a reliable risk factor for the development of aneuploidy?
   A. Cigarette smoking
   B. Maternal age
   C. Paternal age
   D. Smog
2. How many chromosomes would be found in a patient with tetrasomy?
   A. 44
   B. 46
   C. 48
   D. 50
3. Aneuploidy has relevance for human health due to the potential to
   A. be an inheritable condition.
   B. be difficult to detect prenatally.
   C. lead to congenital defects that result in spontaneous abortion.
   D. lead to a loss or excess of gene production.
4. The addition of two chromosomes is referred to as
   A. trisomy.
   B. monosomy.
   C. tetrasomy.
   D. mosaicism.
5. Which of the following forms of aneuploidy is most likely to result in survival of the fetus?
   A. Nullisomy
   B. Trisomy
   C. Tetrasomy
   D. Tetrasomy 9p
6. Nondisjunction is most likely to occur during
   A. Meiosis I.
   B. Meiosis II.
   C. mitosis.
7. Which of the following is a syndrome associated with sex chromosomal aneuploidy?
   A. Down syndrome
   B. Edwards syndrome
   C. Klinefelter syndrome
   D. Patau syndrome
8. Nullisomy is the
   A. loss of one chromosome.
   B. loss of two chromosomes.
   C. addition of one chromosome.
   D. addition of two chromosomes.
9. The most common form of trisomy encountered in clinical practice is most likely to be
   A. Down syndrome
   B. Edwards syndrome
   C. Patau syndrome
   D. Turner syndrome
10. The development of cancer could be considered a form of
    A. nonrandom aneuploidy.
    B. random aneuploidy.
    C. parsimony.
    D. tetrasomy.

Posttest answers are located in the Appendix.

CHAPTER SUMMARY

Aneuploidy is a serious condition that can be identified through prenatal screening for obvious cases. The potential role of aneuploidy's effects on immune function and cancer imply less obvious processes that take years to develop. Research is still continuing in terms of identifying the potential pathways and mechanisms between aneuploidy and other disease states. Unfortunately, little consistent evidence exists as to the possible causes of aneuploidy itself, with maternal age and a previous pregnancy resulting in a trisomy being the only consistent predictors. The literature implies that caloric restriction and ensuring adequate nutrition may be means of helping to prevent aneuploidy. Nursing then needs to provide consistent education to family members regarding nutrition and the avoidance of potential toxic mutagens. As well, education needs to be provided to family members regarding the potential defects present in those with aneuploidy in order to ensure a prepared family environment.

CRITICAL THINKING CHECKPOINT

T. J. is a 8-year-old male who presents with a small chin, round face with protruding tongue, an almond shape to his eyes, and shorter-than-expected extremities. His speech is halting and cognition appears impaired. His parents have brought him in for evaluation of a rapid heart rate with occasional pain behaviors centered on his chest (holding chest while rocking accompanied by moaning) over the past week. His mother reports that he often appears to experience heartburn after eating, and she is expressing concern about the possibility of long-term medical complications. His father reports that they have been thinking about having another child but are concerned about the possibility of having another child with significant deficits.

1. Which condition are these symptoms most compatible with?
2. What form of aneuploidy is Down syndrome associated with?
3. What are the most common risk factors associated with aneuploidy that may be relevant to this case?
4. How would you respond to the father regarding the possibility of having another child?

Answers are provided in the Appendix

ONLINE RESOURCES

Genetic and Rare Diseases (GARD) Information Center: http://rarediseases.info.nih.gov/GARD/

International WAGR Syndrome Association (11p Deletion Syndrome): http://www.wagr.org

Living with Trisomy 13: http://www.livingwithtrisomy13.org

March of Dimes, particularly the site page on birth defects: http://www.marchofdimes.com

Support Organization for Trisomy 18, 13, and Related Disorders: http://www.trisomy.org

The Prader-Willi Syndrome Association: http://www.pwsausa.org

The Ring Chromosome 20 Foundation: http://www.ring20.org

REFERENCES

Canfield, M. A., Honein, M. A., Yuskiv, N., Xing, J., Mai, C. T., Collins, J. S., et al. (2006). National estimates and race/ethnic-specific variation of selected birth defects in the United States, 1999-2001. Birth defects research, Part A. *Clinical and Molecular Teratology, 76*(11), 747–756.

Davenport, M. L. (2010). Approach to the patient with Turner syndrome. *The Journal of Clinical Endocrinology & Metabolism, 95*(4), 1487–1495.

Duesberg, P., Fabarius, A., & Hehlmann, R. (2004). Aneuploidy, the primary cause of the multilateral genomic instability of neoplastic and preneoplastic cells. *IUBMB Life, 56*(2), 65–81.

Dursun, P., Gultekin, M., Yuce, K., & Ayhan, A. (2006). What is the underlying cause of aneuploidy associated with increasing maternal age? Is it associated with elevated levels of gonadotropins? *Medical Hypotheses, 66*(1), 143–147.

Eichenlaub-Ritter, U., Staubach, N., & Trapphoff, T. (2010). Chromosomal and cytoplasmic context determines predisposition to maternal age-related aneuploidy: Brief overview and update on MCAK in mammalian oocytes. *Biochemical Society Transactions, 38*(6), 1681–1686.

Fang, X., & Zhang, P. (2011). Aneuploidy and tumorigenesis. *Seminars in Cell & Developmental Biology.*

Filges, I., Röthlisberger, B., Blattner, A., Boesch, N., Demougin, P., Wenzel, F., et al. (2011). Deletion in Xp22.11: PTCHD1 is a candidate gene for X-linked intellectual disability with or without autism. *Clinical Genetics, 79*(1), 79–85.

Fischer, K., Cramer, P., Busch, R., Stilgenbauer, S., Bahlo, J., Schweighofer, C. D., et al. (2011). Bendamustine combined with rituximab in patients with relapsed and/or refractory chronic lymphocytic leukemia: A multicenter phase II trial of the German Chronic Lymphocytic Leukemia Study Group. *Journal of Clinical Oncology, 29*, 3559–3566.

Fonseka, K. G., & Griffin, D. K. (2011). Is there a paternal age effect for aneuploidy? *Cytogenetic and Genome Research, 133*, 269–279

Gleicher, N., Weghofer, A., & Barad, D. H. (2010a). Dehydroepiandrosterone (DHEA) reduces embryo aneuploidy: Direct evidence from preimplantation genetic screening (PGS). *Reproductive Biology and Endocrinology, 8*, 140.

Gleicher, N., Weghofer, A., & Barad, D. H. (2010b). Do chromosomally abnormal pregnancies really preclude autoimmune etiologies of spontaneous miscarriages? *Autoimmunity Reviews, 10*(6), 361–363.

Iotti, G., Longobardi, E., Masella, S., Dardaei, L., De Santis, F., Micali, N., et al. (2011). Homeodomain transcription factor and tumor suppressor Prep1 is required to maintain genomic stability. *Proceedings of the National Academy of Sciences of the United States of America, 108*(33), E314–E322.

Madsen, H. N., Ekelund, C. K., Torring, N., Ovesen, P. G., Friis-Hansen, L., Ringholm, L., et al. (2012). Impact of type 1 diabetes and glycemic control on fetal aneuploidy biochemical markers. *Acta Obstetricia et Gynecologica Scandinavica, 91*, 57–61.

Menasha, J., Levy, B., Hirschhorn, K., & Kardon, N. B. (2005). Incidence and spectrum of chromosome abnormalities in spontaneous abortions: New insights from a 12-year study. *Genetics in Medicine, 7*(4), 251–263.

Nussbaum, R. L., McInnes, R. R., & Hungtington, F. W. (2004). *Thompson & Thompson genetics in medicine*. Philadelphia: Saunders.

Ogino, W., Takeshima, Y., Nishiyama, A., Yagi, M., Oka, N., & Matsuo, M. (2007). Mosaic Tetrasomy 9p case with the phenotype mimicking Klinefelter syndrome and hyporesponse of gonadotropin-dtimulated testosterone production. *Kobe Journal of Medical Science, 53*(4), 143–150.

Oliveira, R. M., Verreschi, I. T., Lipay, M. V., Eca, L. P., Guedes, A. D., & Bianco, B. (2009). Y chromosome in Turner syndrome: Review of the literature. *Sao Paulo Medical Journal, Revista Paulista de Medicina, 127*(6), 373–378.

Parker, S. E., Mai, C. T., Canfield, M. A., Rickard, R., Wang, Y., Meyer, R. E., et al. (2010). Updated National Birth Prevalence estimates for selected birth defects in the United States, 2004-2006. Birth defects research, Part A. *Clinical and Molecular Teratology, 88*(12), 1008–1016.

Perry, M. J. (2008). Effects of environmental and occupational pesticide exposure on human sperm: a systematic review. *Human Reproduction Update, 14*(3), 233–242.

Pierpont, M. E., Basson, C. T., Benson, D. W., Jr., Gelb, B. D., Giglia, T. M., Goldmuntz, E., et al. (2007). Genetic basis for congenital heart defects: Current knowledge: A scientific statement from the American Heart Association Congenital Cardiac Defects Committee, Council on Cardiovascular Disease in the Young: Endorsed by the American Academy of Pediatrics. *Circulation, 115*(23), 3015–3038.

Resta, R. G. (2005). Changing demographics of advanced maternal age (AMA) and the impact on the predicted incidence of Down syndrome in the United States: Implications for prenatal screening and genetic counseling. *American Journal of Medical Genetics. Part A, 133A*(1), 31–36.

Rios, A., Furdon, S. A., Adams, D., & Clark, D. A. (2004). Recognizing the clinical features of Trisomy 13 syndrome. *Advances in Neonatal Care, 4*(6), 332–343.

Selesniemi, K., Lee, H., Muhlhauser, A., & Tilly, J. L. (2011). Prevention of maternal aging-associated oocyte aneuploidy and meiotic spindle defects in mice by dietary and genetic strategies. *Proceedings of the National Academy of Sciences of the United States of America, 108*, 12319–12324.

Shaffer, L. G., Coppinger, J., Morton, S. A., Alliman, S., Burleson, J., Traylor, R., et al. (2011). The development of a rapid assay for prenatal testing of common aneuploidies and microdeletion syndromes. *Prenatal Diagnosis, 31*(8), 778–787.

Shinawi, M., Patel, A., Panichkul, P., Zascavage, R., Peters, S. U., & Scaglia, F. (2009). The Xp contiguous deletion syndrome and autism. *American Journal of Medical Genetics. Part A, 149A*(6), 1138–1148.

Spandorfer, S. D., Davis, O. K., Barmat, L. I., Chung, P. H., & Rosenwaks, Z. (2004). Relationship between maternal age and aneuploidy in in vitro fertilization pregnancy loss. *Fertility and Sterility, 81*(5), 1265–1269.

Suzumori, N., & Sugiura-Ogasawara, M. (2010). Genetic factors as a cause of miscarriage. *Current Medicinal Chemistry, 17*(29), 3431–3437.

Thompson, S., & Compton, D. (2011). Chromosomes and cancer cells. *Chromosome Research, 19*(3), 433–444.

Torres, E. M., Williams, B. R., & Amon, A. (2008). Aneuploidy: Cells losing their balance. *Genetics, 179*(2), 737–746.

Wikstrom, A. M., & Dunkel, L. (2011). Klinefelter syndrome. *Best Practice & Research Clinical Endocrinology & Metabolism, 25*, 239–250.

Yurov, Y. B., Vorsanova, S. G., Iourov, I. Y., Demidova, I. A., Beresheva, A. K., Kravetz, V. S., et al. (2007). Unexplained autism is frequently associated with low-level mosaic aneuploidy. *Journal of Medical Genetics, 44*, 521–525.

CHAPTER

6 Mosaicism

Linda K. Bennington

LEARNING OUTCOMES

Following the completion of this chapter, the learner will be able to

1. Explore the basics of chromosomes to clarify the definition of mosaicism.
2. Discuss the theoretical concepts of the development of mosaicism.
3. Describe and define chromosomal mosaicism.
4. Explain the ways mosaicism can occur.
5. Review the implications of mosaicism in pregnancy.

This chapter presents the definitions of terms related to normal chromosomal functioning and the deviations that can cause changes in physiological appearance as well as physiological functioning. To this end, this chapter provides a brief overview of the functioning of chromosomal activity and elaborates on the formation of trisomies. This chapter also focuses on the origins of Mosaicism and discusses the factors affecting the clinical presentation of mosaicism. In addition, this chapter presents the implications of mosaicism in pregnancy as to possible outcomes.

PRETEST

1. DNA is stored in what organelle?
   A. Ribosome
   B. Nucleus
   C. Cytoskeleton
   D. Mitochondria
2. Which of the following is NOT an example of a base used to form DNA?
   A. Guanine
   B. Adenine
   C. Cytosine
   D. Uracil
3. This is the structural and functional unit of all known living organisms.
   A. The cell
   B. Organelles
   C. Nucleolus
   D. RNA
4. The double helix is a structure formed from what molecule?
   A. DNA
   B. RNA
   C. Protein
   D. None of the above
5. Mutations, or changes in the DNA, can be which of the following?
   A. Advantageous
   B. Deleterious
   C. Have no effect
   D. All of the above
6. The occurrence of one or more extra or missing chromosomes, leading to an unbalanced chromosome complement, is known as
   A. diploidy.
   B. polyploidy.
   C. aneuploidy.
   D. tetraploidy.
7. The loss of a part of the chromosome or DNA sequence is referred to as
   A. insertion.
   B. deletion.
   C. substitution.
   D. addition.
8. The production of multiple copies of a region of DNA that contains a gene is referred to as
   A. deletion.
   B. insertion.
   C. duplication/amplification.
   D. addition.

9. When a piece of chromosome breaks off and reattaches in the reverse direction it is referred to as
   A. chromosomal deletion.
   B. chromosomal translocation.
   C. chromosomal inversion.
   D. chromosomal substitution.

10. Which of the following is the central dogma?
    A. RNA to DNA to protein
    B. DNA to RNA to protein
    C. Protein to RNA to DNA
    D. RNA to protein to DNA

Pretest answers are located in the Appendix.

SECTION ONE: Chromosomal Basics

In a manner similar to a central information storage system, the nucleus of human **eukaryote cells** contains long strands of deoxyribonucleic acid (DNA) that encode an individual's genetic information. Named from its chemical composition, it consists of a deoxyribose sugar and a phosphate backbone linking **nucleotides** that contain alternating patterns of four bases: adenine, cytosine, tyrosine, and guanine (ACTG). Its double helix molecular structure is often described as two strands winding around each other like a twisted ladder, with the phosphate backbone maintaining its stability. **Replication** is the process of linking structures to create DNA while RNA is created through transcription.

An individual's **genotype** is determined at the gene level as long stretches of DNA are repeatedly coiled in a number of complex ways to facilitate packing into a chromosome. The fundamental building blocks of that coiling are nucleosomes, which are blocks of small spheres of histone proteins resembling beads. These histones are a special class of proteins contained within the nucleic acid mixture—i.e., **chromatin**—that perform two specific functions: 1. They assist in making the chromosome more compact so it can properly fit in the nucleus and thus provide structural support (see Figure 6–1 ■). 2. They regulate the transcription of the DNA that makes up the chromosome by virtue of their presence and absence. When present, those areas of the chromosomes are transcribed; if not present, no transcription occurs.

Fundamentally, a chromosome contains a single, long DNA molecule of which only a portion corresponds to a single gene; or equally, a gene could be thought of as a working subunit of DNA. Mitochondria, the energy centers of the cell, also contain DNA but it is present as one long string of genes not arranged as chromosomes. Approximately 25,000 genes are arranged on human chromosomes and alternative forms or versions of a gene are referred to as an **allele**. One allele is inherited for each autosomal gene from each parent. The alleles are generally lumped into categories as normal or wild type alleles and abnormal or mutated alleles. *Locus,* or *loci,* is the term used to describe where on a chromosome a specific gene is—the physical location of the gene.

Ribonucleic acid (RNA) is structurally similar to DNA, although it is composed of a single strand, a different sugar, ribose, and a phosphate backbone with the same bases (except uracil, which substitutes for tyrosine). RNA performs a number of different cellular tasks via messenger RNA (**mRNA**), a nucleic acid information molecule that transcribes codes from the genome into proteins by the process of translation. The transferred code is represented by a **codon**, which is a trinucleotide sequence of DNA or RNA that corresponds to a specific amino acid. This genetic code describes the relationship between the sequence of DNA bases (A, C, G, and T) in a gene and the corresponding protein sequence that it encodes. The cell reads the sequence of the gene in these groups of three bases. There are 64 different codons: 61 specify amino acids while the remaining 3 are used as stop signals. Transfer RNA (**tRNA**) is a nonprotein-encoding molecule that physically carries amino acids to the translation site and facilitates their assembly into proteins. In the cell cytoplasm, the ribosome can be thought of as a docking station that binds to mRNA and reads the coded sequence in groups of three bases for tRNA, which, in turn, contains the amino acid that will become part of the growing polypeptide chain that eventually becomes a specific protein. The **endoplasmic reticulum** is the network of membranes in the cell through which the different forms of RNA act and is essentially the protein-generating factory of the cell.

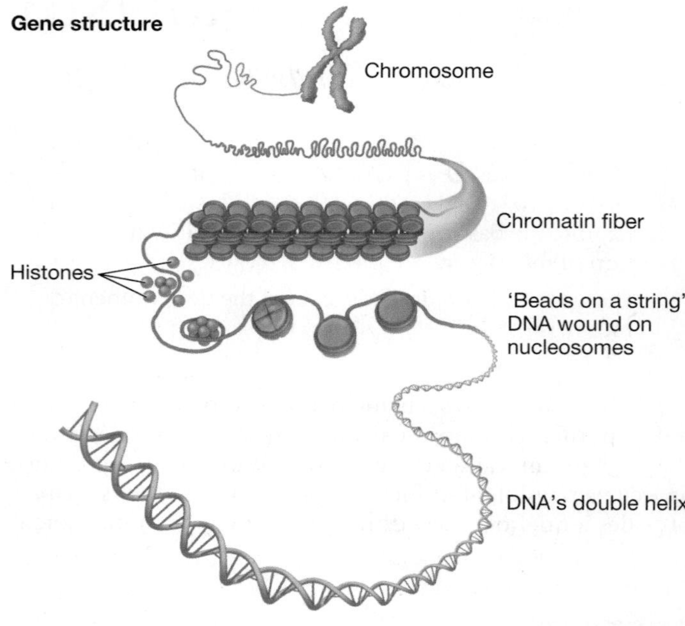

Figure 6–1 ■ Structure of a gene
Source: Darryl Leja, National Human Genome Research Institute

Teleologically we begin with one cell and end up with trillions by virtue of the process of cell division, which requires perfect copying of the cellular information. DNA is a molecule that can be replicated to make almost perfect copies through the use of enzymes called DNA polymerases. Since there are about 3 billion base pairs of DNA to be copied, the replication of the entire DNA in a single human cell can take several hours. Once completed, a **daughter cell** containing twice the amount of DNA is formed. The resultant **phenotype** leads to observable traits that come not from DNA alone but from the RNA that is made from the DNA and the proteins that are made

Emerging Evidence

- The determination of the presence of cell-free fetal DNA in the plasma of pregnant women has led to the feasibility of diagnosing fetal genetic disorders prenatally in a noninvasive way. A process of genome-wide scanning was used to examine the fetal and maternal genomes, which were found to be represented at a constant relative proportion in maternal plasma (Lo et al, 2010).
- Approximately 98% of invasive diagnostic procedures could be avoided if pooled maternal plasma DNA sequencing analysis is used to rule out fetal trisomy 21 among high risk pregnancies (Chiu, 2011).

from the RNA. The central dogma of molecular biology is considered to be the flow of information from DNA to RNA to proteins (see Chapter 4 for an in-depth review of cell division).

Changes in Chromosome Number

Human somatic cells are **diploid**, having 23 pairs of chromosomes for a total of 46 chromosomes in each cell. Human sex cells (egg and sperm cells) contain a single set of chromosomes and are known as **haploid**. Meiosis is a critical transition period in humans that permits the reduction of chromosomes from diploid to haploid for the creation of eggs or sperm. These haploid cells have the duplicated identical nuclei of each parent; during reproduction and fertilization, they come together to form a zygote, which is essentially a reconstituted diploid cell of newly combined genetic material. The chromosomes are numbered from 1–22 according to size from the largest to the smallest, and there are two sex chromosomes, X and Y.

Although there are individuals born with differing numbers of chromosomes, the correct number and structure of chromosomes is important for the proper growth and development of a fetus. In humans, abnormalities of chromosome number usually occur during meiosis and are the leading cause of birth defects and miscarriages. A gain or loss of chromosomes from the normal 46 is called aneuploidy, whereas **polyploidy** refers to the gain of whole sets of chromosomes. Monosomy refers to the status of an autosomal gene when normally two copies are supposed to be present but only one is. It also refers to multiple genes or segments, or to an entire chromosome, where an individual is supposed to have two copies but only has one.

A **marker** is a simple concept that could be related to being a signpost along the road map of DNA. It is essentially a DNA sequence with a known physical location on a chromosome that comes from a variety of sources, typically from variations in DNA sequence or a single variation of DNA sequence referred to as a **single nucleotide polymorphism (SNP)**. Sets of closely linked genes or DNA polymorphisms inherited as a unit are referred to as **haplotypes**. Markers offer insight into linking an inherited disease with the responsible genes since it is also known that DNA segments close to each other on a chromosome tend to be inherited together. Markers can also be used to track the inheritance of a nearby gene that has not yet been identified but whose approximate location is known. Interestingly, the marker itself may be a part of a gene or may have no known function.

The normal structure of a chromosome includes a single constriction point called the centromere, which separates the chromosome into the long (p) and short (q) arms. The centromere is an area that consists of very tightly coiled DNA and is used as a reference point in cytogenetics to distinguish the appearance of the chromosome structure for genetic testing. During cell division this is the place where the chromosomes, when undergoing replication, are held together to prevent the loss of their sister chromatin.

The structural changes that can occur during egg or sperm cell formation, early fetal development, or in any cell after birth include pieces of DNA that can be rearranged within one chromosome or transferred between two or more chromosomes. The effects of structural changes depend on their size and location and whether any genetic material is gained or lost. The most commonly known changes include translocation, **inversion**, **deletion**, and **duplication**. Translocation involves a break in one particular chromosome that then fuses to a different chromosome to create a fusion product or gene fusion. This type of reorganization is described as balanced if no genetic material is gained or lost in the cell and unbalanced if there is a gain or loss of genetic material. It is called an inversion if it involves the same chromosome. An inversion that involves the chromosome's constriction point (centromere) is called a pericentric inversion. An inversion that occurs in the long (q) arm or short (p) arm and does not involve the centromere is called a paracentric inversion (Figures 6–2, 6–3, and Figure 6–4 ■).

Deletion is a type of mutation involving the loss of genetic material. It can be small, involving a single missing DNA base pair, or large, involving part of a gene, or even larger involving an entire chromosome (Figure 6–5 ■). Different deletions can lead to different findings. They can affect just behavior or affect how a person looks, as to eye color or weight or height of a person or a deformity so severe that an infant will die soon after birth.

Duplications occur when there is more than one copy of a specific stretch of DNA or of a gene or a region of a chromosome. The end result is extra copies of genetic material from the duplicated segment (Figure 6–6 ■). Gene duplication is an important mechanism involved with evolution.

An **isochromosome** is a chromosome with two identical arms. Rather than having the one long (q) arm and one short (p) arm, it has two long arms or two short arms. As a result, these abnormal chromosomes have extra copies of some genes and are missing copies of others (Figure 6–7 ■).

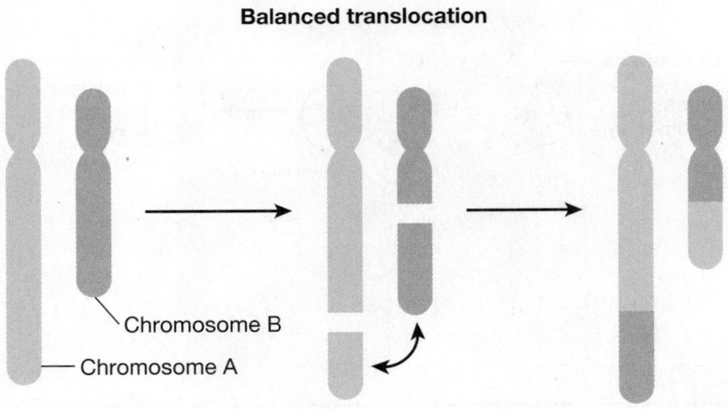

Balanced translocation

Chromosome B

Chromosome A

Figure 6–2 ■ Balanced translocation

Source: U.S. National Library of Medicine

Unbalanced translocation

Normal chromosomes of Parent 1

Chromosomes of Parent 2 with balanced translocation

Figure 6–3 ■ Unbalanced translocation
Source: U.S. National Library of Medicine

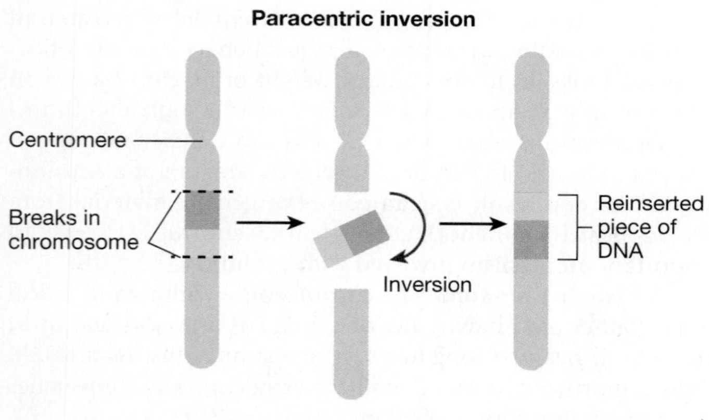

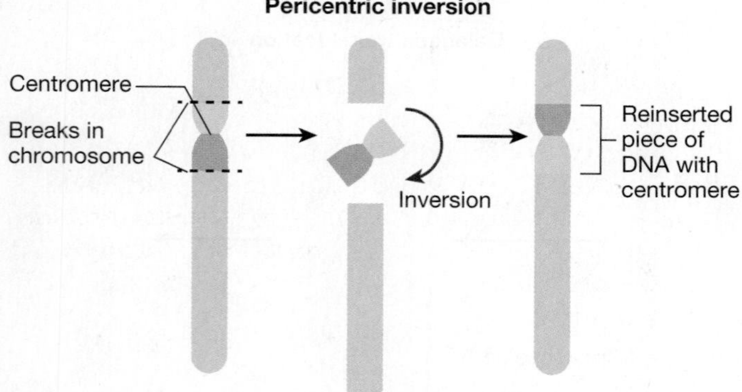

Figure 6–4 ■ Inversion
Source: U.S. National Library of Medicine

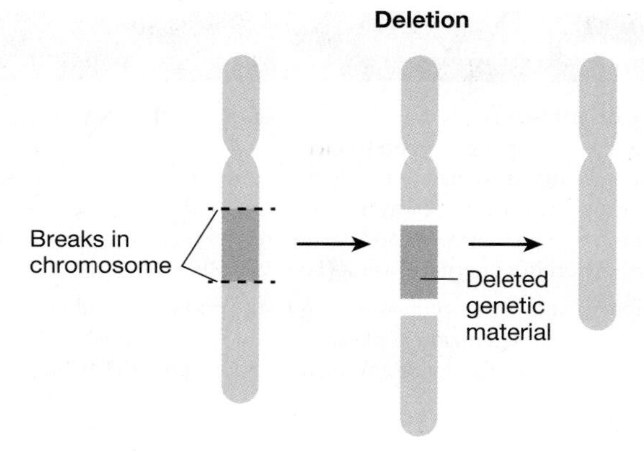

Figure 6–5 ■ Deletion
Source: U.S. National Library of Medicine

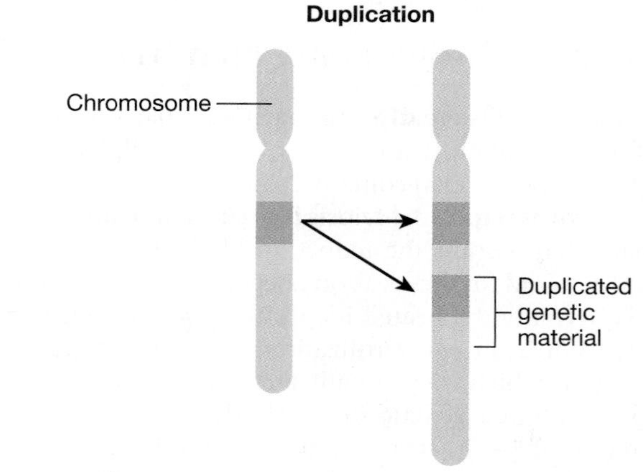

Figure 6–6 ■ Duplication
Source: U.S. National Library of Medicine

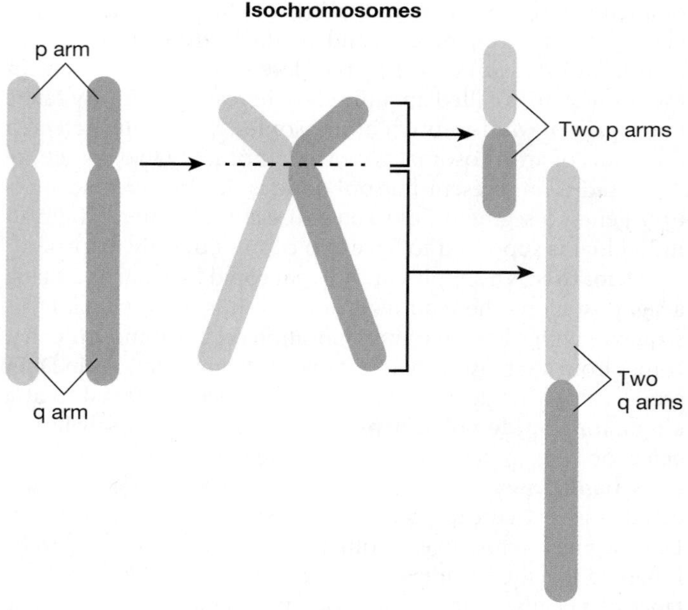

Figure 6–7 ■ Isochromosome
Source: U.S. National Library of Medicine

Dicentric chromosomes, unlike normal chromosomes, contain two centromeres and are the result of the abnormal fusion of two chromosome pieces, each of which includes a centromere. These structures are unstable and often involve a loss of some genetic material (Figure 6–8 ■).

Ring chromosomes usually occur when a chromosome breaks in two places and the ends of the chromosome arms fuse together to form a circular structure. The ring may or may not include the chromosome's centromere and frequently, genetic material near the ends of the chromosome is lost (Figure 6–9 ■).

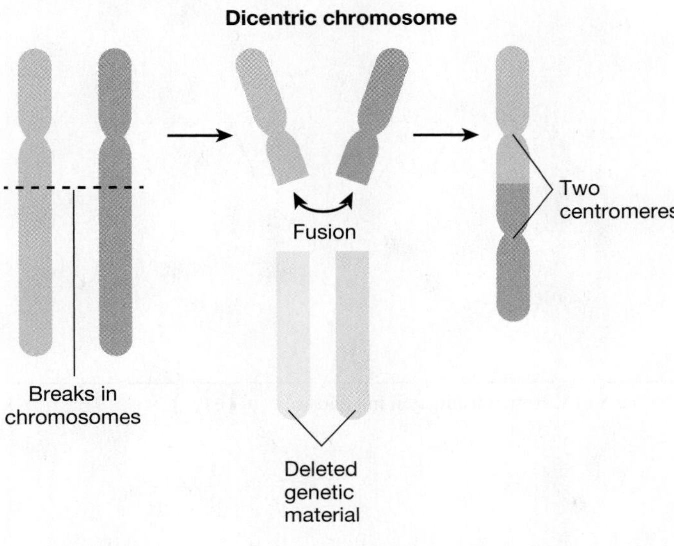

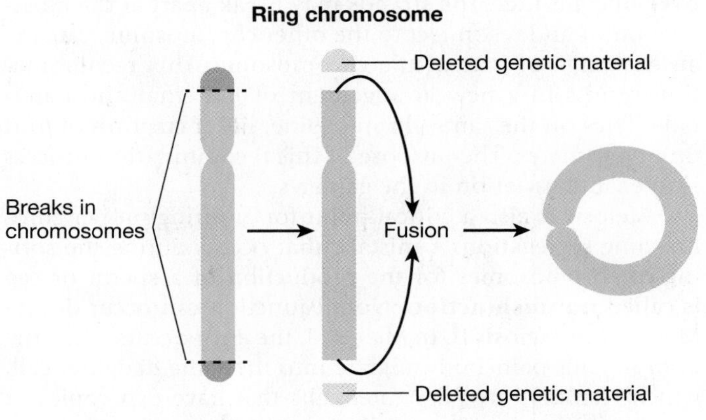

Figure 6–8 ■ Dicentric chromosome
Source: U.S. National Library of Medicine

Ring chromosome

Deleted genetic material

Breaks in chromosomes

Fusion

Deleted genetic material

Figure 6–9 ■ Ring chromosome
Source: U.S. National Library of Medicine

SECTION ONE REVIEW

1. Which word describes the organized structure of DNA in the nucleus of a cell? (Human beings have 23 pairs of these.)
   A. Genome
   B. Codon
   C. Chromosome
   D. Gene
2. What membrane bound organelle contains the cell's chromosomes?
   A. Golgi body
   B. Nucleus
   C. Lysosome
   D. Endoplasmic reticulum
3. Which of the following refers to the sex cells (eggs and sperm) that are used by sexually reproducing organisms to pass on genes from one generation to the next?
   A. Autosome
   B. Bacteria
   C. Germ line
   D. Carrier
4. An important class of macromolecules that is found in all cells and viruses with the function of storing and expressing genetic information is
   A. Protein.
   B. Amino acid.
   C. Nucleic acid.
   D. Hemogloblin.
5. What is a set of DNA variations that tends to be inherited together and refers to an allele combination or a set of single nucleotide polymorphisms (SNPs) found on the same chromosome?
   A. Gene pool
   B. Locus
   C. Haplotype
   D. Phenotype

Answers: 1. C; 2. B; 3. C; 4. C; 5. C

SECTION TWO: Aneuploidy Formations

Gametes are haploid cells created during the two stages of the meiotic process for the purpose of reproduction. The first stage is distinguished for being known as the reduction division stage because it is the division in which the chromosome number is reduced from diploid to haploid. It is also notable as the stage during which two strands of a chromosome pair may physically accomplish **crossing over** one another. The strands may break apart at the crossover point and reconnect to the other chromosome, causing an exchange of part of the chromosome. This recombination results in a new arrangement of maternal and paternal alleles on the same chromosome; i.e., a creation of four unique gametes. The purpose of this recombination process is to ensure variation in the gametes.

Meiosis is also a critical point for ensuring proper chromosome segregation. A mistake that occurs during the sorting of chromosomes for the production of a sperm or egg is called **nondisjunction**. Nondisjunction can occur during Meiosis I or Meiosis II. In Meiosis I, the error occurs when the homologous pairs both migrate into the same daughter cell, which results in two daughter cells that have two copies of the chromosome and two cells that are missing that chromosome (Figure 6–10 ■). In Meiosis II, the error occurs when the sister chromatids will not separate and thus migrate into the same daughter cell (Figure 6–11 ■). This failure to recombine properly is a frequent cause of chromosome abnormalities. These changes are not inherited, but occur as errors in cell division to create reproductive cells with an abnormal number of chromosomes. If one of these dissimilar reproductive cells contributes to the genetic makeup of a zygote, an infant will have an extra or missing chromosome in the body's cells. The cause of nondisjunction is not known; however, it is known that it occurs more frequently in the eggs of women as they get older.

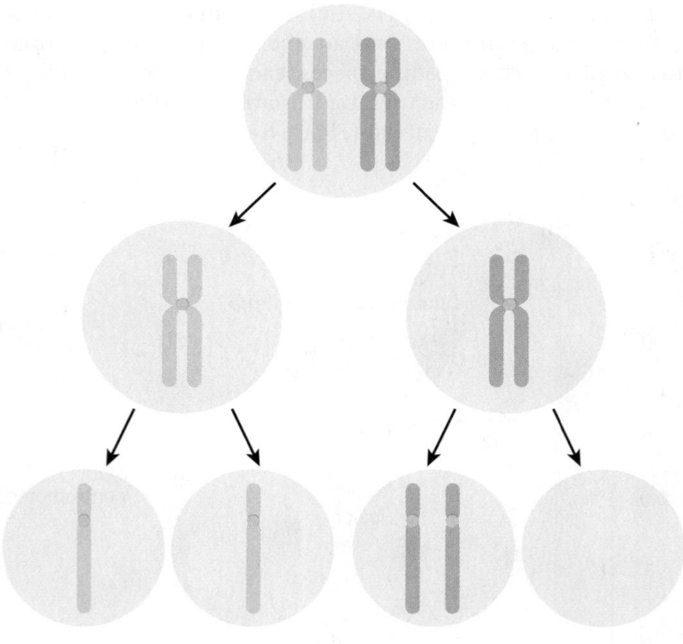

Figure 6–11 ■ Nondisjunction in Meiosis II

Typically at fertilization the egg and the sperm each contribute 23 chromosomes that fuse to create a zygote with 46 chromosomes. If the egg or sperm carries an extra copy of one of the chromosomes due to nondisjunction with Meiosis I or II, there will be a total of 24 chromosomes instead of the normal 23 in the reproductive cell. Subsequently if this particular gamete is fertilized by a normal gamete the result will be a total of 47 chromosomes instead of 46, and a **trisomy** zygote will form.

If the trisomy is created as a result of errors in Meiosis I, the zygote receives three different chromosomes because the egg contributed both a maternal copy and a paternal copy of homologous chromosomes (Figure 6–12 ■). If the trisomy is the result of errors in Meiosis II, two similar chromosomes are contributed (Figure 6–13 ■).

By the same token, if one of the empty appearing reproductive cells is fertilized by a normal gamete, the result is a monosomy chromosome. Monosomy is defined as having only one copy of a chromosome that is normally present in two copies. Thus the gamete cell contains one less chromosome, or 22 chromosomes, and when fertilized results in a total of 45 chromosomes. In most cases, the loss of a chromosome is incompatible with life but the loss of an X or Y chromosome results in a condition known as monosomy X or Turner syndrome, which means there are 45 chromosomes present.

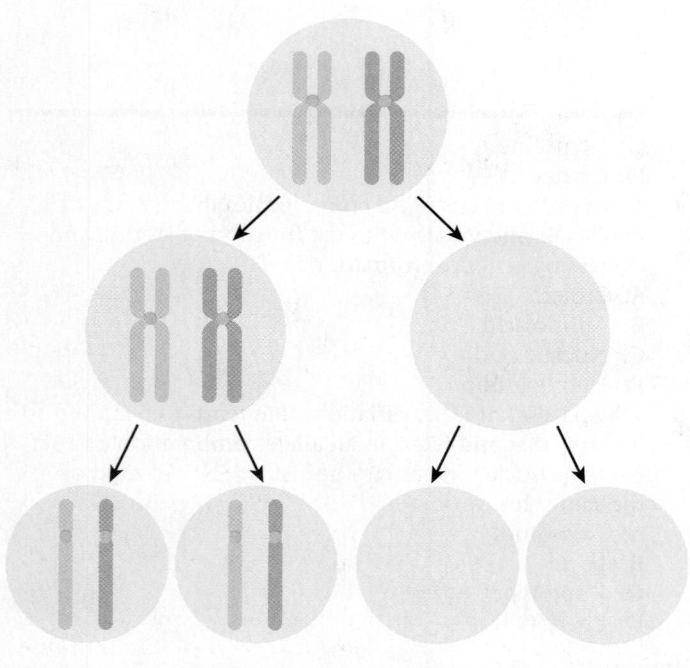

Figure 6–10 ■ Nondisjunction in Meiosis I

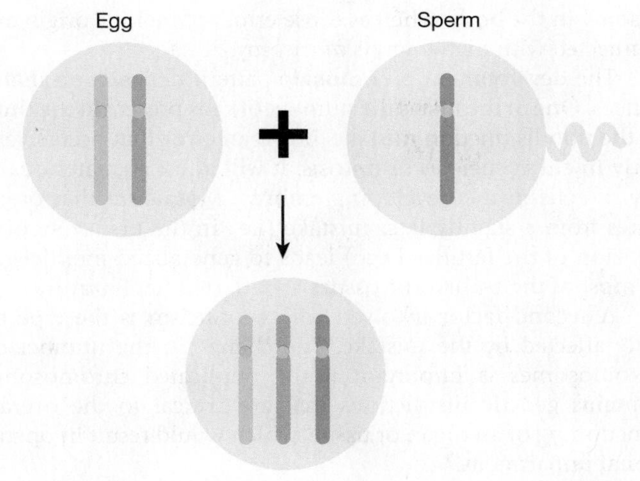

Figure 6–12 ■ Meiosis I error

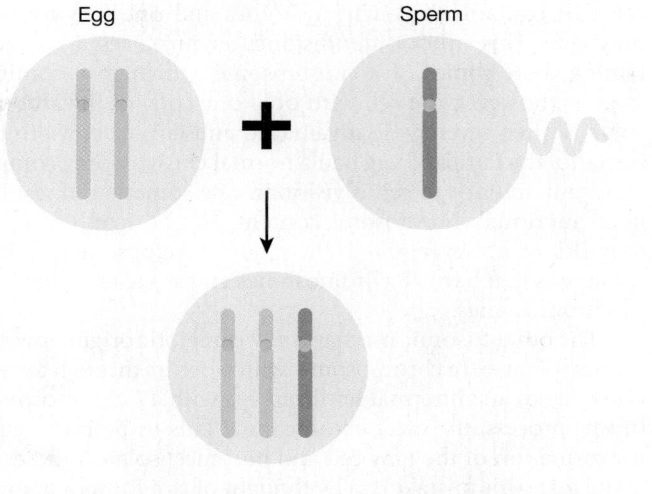

Egg

Sperm

Figure 6–13 ■ Meiosis II error

SECTION TWO REVIEW

1. An individual inherits two of these for each gene, one from each parent. What are these gene variations called?
   A. Cell
   B. Amino acid
   C. Allele
   D. Nucleotide
2. This refers to a swapping of genetic material that occurs in the germ line:
   A. Recombinant DNA
   B. Polymorphism
   C. Crossing over
   D. Bioinformatics
3. This refers to a nondisjunction error occurring during Meiosis I or II to create extra genetic material in a fertilized zygote:
   A. Monosomy
   B. Trisomy
   C. Polymorphism
   D. Allele
4. This refers to a nondisjunction error occurring during Meiosis I or II resulting in a lack of genetic material in a fertilized zygote:
   A. Polymorphism
   B. Recombinant DNA
   C. Monosomy
   D. Trisomy
5. The two components that make up a duplicated chromosome are called
   A. homologues.
   B. sister chromatids.
   C. translation.
   D. karyotype.

Answers: 1. C; 2. C; 3. B; 4. C; 5. B

SECTION THREE: Chromosomal Mosaicism

Following the formation of a single celled zygote with 46 chromosomes, a period of rapid growth, called *cleavage*, begins that involves the process of mitosis. During mitosis the 46 chromosomes make identical copies of themselves and each pair of replicated chromosomes pull away from each other to form daughter cells. The purpose of mitosis is to pass on a complete copy of genetic material to the daughter cells for the ultimate formation of a new body. As with meiosis, there can be mistakes during mitosis that involve the separation or segregation of chromosomes. Two sister chromatids may migrate into the same daughter cell, or a malfunction in chromosome sorting may find two identical chromosomes in the same daughter cell. These errors in proper chromosome segregation are called nondisjunction. This was previously discussed as it related to meiosis with development of the sperm and egg; however, nondisjunction in the zygote is called post-zygotic nondisjunction or mitotic nondisjunction. **Anaphase lag** is a term related to another mechanism where one chromosome simply fails to get incorporated into the nucleus of a daughter cell; it is probably the most common mechanism for trisomy mosaicism formation.

Trisomy mosaicism can occur in one of two ways: via somatic origin or via meiotic origin. Mitotic nondisjunction in the cell of a fertilized egg with the typical 46 chromosomes leads to a different cell line with an additional chromosome. During mitotic replication two new daughter cells are formed that in turn replicate. This replication can result in a daughter cell that contains three chromosomes and one that contains only one. This mitotic nondisjunction produces a cell containing three copies of a chromosome, which may continue to grow; however, the cell with only one copy of the chromosome is often severely disadvantaged and fails to grow. In this scenario, the fertilized egg had a normal chromosome complement but an error in cell division in one somatic cell resulted in an abnormal chromosome content. All of the cells continue to multiply, however, and as the zygote develops, there will be some cells that have 46 chromosomes and some cells that have 47 chromosomes.

The other trisomic mechanism, via meiotic origin, involves the loss of an extra chromosome, which occurs through an anaphase lag in an abnormal fertilized egg with 47 chromosomes. In this process, the extra chromosome fails to be included in the formation of the new cell and becomes isolated and eventually lost. This mistake can be thought of as a form of trisomic "rescue" because it is, in essence, a correction to the trisomic fertilized egg. Depending on how early this occurrence takes place determines the outcome. If a **trisomic rescue** occurs early in the post-zygotic divisions and involves the cells destined to be the embryo, then the abnormal chromosomal content will be decreased. In both situations of mitotic nondisjunction and meiotic nondisjunction, it is the timing of the nondisjunction that influences the end result. In general, errors resulting from somatic origin are linked with lower levels of trisomy in the body, whereas those errors of meiotic origin are connected with higher levels of trisomy.

The development of a **mosaic** pattern depends on many factors. One of the first is the number of cells present at the time of the nondisjunction mistake. If it is an error that occurs very early in either meiosis or mitosis, it will affect a greater quantity of cells in the developing embryo. Mosaicism that originates from a slightly later mistake (i.e., in the first or second division of the fertilized egg) leads to generalized mosaicism, as most of the embryonic tissues are affected haphazardly.

A second factor involved with mosaicism is the type of cells affected by the mistake. The change in the number of chromosomes is important if the duplicated chromosome contains genetic instructions that are critical to the overall functioning of an organ or tissue, which would result in operational impairment.

A third factor that contributes to the mosaicism patterning is the survival of trisomic cells. Cytogenetic studies of cell cultures have suggested that trisomic cells usually divide less quickly and undergo cell death more commonly than diploid cells (Robinson, 2007). Thus, the outcome with mosaicism can be determined to some extent on the ability of the abnormal cells to survive. The particular chromosome involved appears to play a role in the survival of the cells such that the abnormal trisomic cells are prevented from reproducing, which in turn minimizes or eliminates the effect of the original nondisjunction error.

SECTION THREE REVIEW

1. Which of the following is NOT a function of mitosis in humans?
   A. Repair of wounds
   B. Growth
   C. Production of gametes from diploid cells
   D. Replacement of dead or damaged cells
2. Which cells of the human body are made through the process of meiosis?
   A. Gametes
   B. Somatic cells
   C. All cells of the body
   D. X and Y chromosomes
3. The development of mosaicism depends on what stage of meiosis or mitosis that the trisomy first appeared?
   A. True
   B. False
4. ____________ is more likely to contribute to a higher incidence of mosaicism within an individual.
   A. DNA replication
   B. Meiotic nondisjunction
   C. Chromosomal duplication
   D. Mitotic nondisjunction
5. Trisomic rescue is essentially a correction of a trisomic cell.
   A. True
   B. False

Answers: 1. C; 2. A; 3. A; 4. B; 5. A

SECTION FOUR: Factors Affecting Clinical Presentation of Chromosomal Mosaicism

Prenatal diagnosis for chromosomal abnormalities typically consists of either having chorionic villus sampling (**CVS**) or amniocentesis (see Chapter 10 for prenatal testing). CVS involves analyzing the chromosomes in the placenta whereas amniocentesis involves the analysis of fetal cells present in the amniotic fluid. The method of detection that results in a diagnosis of chromosomal mosaicism provides guidance as to what tissues are affected. The presence of trisomy with CVS indicates that it is definitely present in the placenta and its presence in amniotic fluid indicates that at least one fetal tissue is affected by trisomy.

When considering the implications of trisomy presence in CVS, it is important to remember that the fetus is derived from only a few cells (1–5 cells) of the 64-celled **blastocyst**. The majority of the cells in the blastocyst contribute to the placental formation; therefore, if an error occurs in a cell at the blastocyst stage it is more likely to be one that is a part of the placenta than one destined to be the fetus. Recent research has corroborated that the karyotype of the placenta can differ from that of the fetus. In approximately 1–2% of pregnancies, the placenta will be mosaic (i.e., contain two distinct cell lines) despite an entirely **euploid** fetal karyotype (Wapner, 2010). This is referred to as confined placental mosaicism (**CPM**) and it can occur via two mechanisms.

The first mechanism involves mitotic nondisjunction occurring in the early development of the zygote, which leads to a trisomic population of daughter cells. During blastula development with CPM these cells segregate exclusively into the extra fetal compartments, leaving a chromosomally normal fetus. In the second mechanism, a meiotic error occurs during gametogenesis resulting in a trisomic zygote, which would usually result in a miscarriage. If, however, a second error in the anaphase lag occurs during early mitotic divisions a disomic cell line will result rescuing the potentially lethal embryo (trisomic rescue). The morula will then contain both euploid and aneuploid cells and again, by chance, the aneuploid cells may segregate entirely into the trophoblast. As meiotic errors occur more frequently with advancing maternal age, it would be expected that this mechanism for CPM occurs more frequently in older mothers (Wapner, 2010).

Altered perinatal outcomes occur in up to 20% of cases with CPM. It is associated with stillbirth, an increase in the risk of first and second trimester losses as well as intrauterine growth restriction. Its significance in any particular pregnancy depends on a number of factors that include the specific chromosome involved and the percentage of cells affected. Those chromosomes associated with a poor outcome include 13, 16, and 17, but chromosomes 2, 3, 9, 14, 15, 16, and 18 have the highest risk. Approximately one in five pregnancies diagnosed by CVS in the first trimester having a normal fetal karyotype and CPM for chromosome 16 results in a stillbirth. Moreover, preterm birth, early pregnancy loss, and intrauterine growth restriction occur more frequently with this CPM. Robinson (2007) maintains a website that is continually updated regarding the potential outcomes of mosaicism according to specific chromosomes. She has noted a greater percentage correlation with placental mosaicism and fetal mosaicism.

Potential clinical outcomes with mosaicism are strongly dependent upon the specific chromosome involved and the number of trisomic cells in the fetus and the placenta. The proportions of chromosomally altered cells and normal cells can be quite inconstant and may vary between the cells of different body tissues. For instance, an individual who is mosaic for trisomy 21 may have the chromosomal change in 60% of their skin cells and in only 5% of their blood cells. Theoretically, an increased number of trisomic cells would be more likely to be associated with an abnormal outcome than those with a decreased proportion; however, an accurate determination of the proportion of trisomic cells present is virtually impossible to determine in a living person, much less prenatally. The exact proportion can only be determined on autopsy.

Since it is unlikely that an outcome can be predicted based upon the results of CVS or an amniocentesis, high resolution ultrasounds can be used to determine fetal morphology, nuchal translucency, and growth and development. A severely abnormal trisomic mosaicism would more than likely demonstrate intrauterine growth restriction early on in a pregnancy because abnormal cells tend not to grow or develop properly. It is difficult for a pregnant woman to deal with this kind of diagnosis since, on the surface, it appears to be so equivocal. Obtaining more information from reports of chromosomal mosaicism is necessary to prepare and counsel the woman who receives a diagnosis of mosaicism so that a greater understanding of potential outcomes can be clarified.

Lastly, another possible outcome of trisomy is that of **uniparental disomy (UPD)**, which arises when an individual inherits two copies of a chromosome pair from one parent and no copy from the other parent. Three possible mechanisms have been considered in the development of this occurrence. The first involves the loss of a chromosome from a trisomic zygote, previously referred to as "trisomic rescue." Second is the possible duplication of a chromosome from a monosomic zygote or a "monosomic rescue." Third is the fertilization of a gamete with two copies of a chromosome by a gamete with no copies of the same chromosome, which is referred to as "gamete complementation." All of these mechanisms require two consecutive errors. The incidence of UPD seems to be associated with the type of confined placental mosaicism, the chromosome involved, and the origin of the trisomy (mitotic or meiotic).

The issue with UPD relates to the expression of genes. Like chromosomes, there are two copies of each gene, one from the mother and one from the father. Expressed genes actively give instructions to create proteins and interestingly, some genes are only expressed when inherited from the father while others are only expressed when inherited from the mother. This phenomenon of differential gene expression depending on the parent of origin is called **imprinting**, and it occurs in each generation. The concern with UPD is related to the circumstance of only inheriting either maternal copies of a chromosome or paternal copies. With paternal UPD or maternal UPD, a chromosome may contain genes or regions of chromosomes that have been switched off, which means this individual will have no working copies of these genes. Additionally, if an autosomal recessive gene is present in the UPD parent of origin, it will be expressed as the disease with which it is associated since two copies are inherited. It is difficult to determine if an abnormal outcome associated with UPD is due to the effects of UPD itself (i.e., imprinting effects or homozygosity for recessive traits) or to an excess of trisomy cells in the placenta and/or undetected trisomy in the fetus because a meiotic origin correlates with high levels of trisomy in both placental cell lineages and UPD. Additional research is ongoing in an effort to sort out cause and effect.

SECTION FOUR REVIEW

1. Chorionic villus sampling is conclusive with regards to the presence of a trisomic zygote.
   A. True
   B. False
2. A maternal autosomal recessive trait is inherited and expressed with maternal uniparental disomy.
   A. True
   B. False
3. Trisomy mosaicism can be the result of ___________.
   A. meiotic nondisjunction alone
   B. mitotic nondisjunction alone
   C. either meiotic or mitotic nondisjunction
   D. translocation alone
4. Clinical outcomes with trisomy mosaicism are always abnormal.
   A. True
   B. False
5. Amniocentesis provides a definitive result for the extent of trisomy mosaicism in the fetus.
   A. True
   B. False

Answers: 1. B; 2. A; 3. C; 4. B; 5. B

SECTION FIVE: Implications of Mosaicism in Pregnancy

Due to new methods of detecting genetic anomalies, the statistics on percentage of pregnancy losses or stillbirths resulting from this are continuously changing. Presently, it is estimated that genetic changes are responsible for 50% to 70% of spontaneous abortions (SAB), with the most common abnormalities being autosomal trisomies (60%), monosomy X (20%), and polyploidy (20%). The most common trisomy is trisomy 16, accounting for 20% to 30% of all trisomies seen in abortus specimens (Warren & Silver, 2008). To date no data has been gathered on whether any of these SABs involved mosaicism, primarily due to the difficulty of analyzing the specimens.

The proportion of abnormal karyotypes in abortus specimens is highest earlier in gestation with more unusual aneuploidies being noted during that stage. Although the rate of anomalies does decrease with increasing gestational age, the karyotypes of fetal deaths at later gestations are similar to those seen in live newborns with trisomies 21, 18, and 13 making up the majority of these abnormalities. Moreover, chromosomal abnormalities do exist in at least 6% to 12% of stillbirths at or beyond 20 weeks. For anembryonic specimens (blighted ovum), the reported rates of chromosomal abnormalities are up to 90% with approximately 50% at 8 to 11 weeks gestation, and around 30% at 16 to 19 weeks gestation. It has also been determined that two-thirds of malformed embryos and one-third of malformed fetuses have abnormal chromosomes (Warren & Silver, 2008).

For women with recurrent pregnancy loss, a higher rate of aneuploidy has been reported in subsequent losses when the karyotype was abnormal in the first loss, which suggests a possible reason for the losses. Awareness of factors that influence the rate of chromosomal abnormalities is an essential part of analysis in an assessment of recurrent loss etiology. These factors include gestational age, presence of malformations, a fetus that is small for the gestational age, and maternal age. Nurses who care for women with pregnancy loss or stillbirth should be familiar with this data and offer it, not only as means of providing insight, but as a means of gathering information for future pregnancies.

Identifying the genetic etiology of a pregnancy loss or stillbirth has serious implications for future pregnancies. The documentation of a cytogenetic abnormality enables the determination of a more precise recurrent risk assessment for a couple. When a common aneuploidy is identified, the recurrence risk is centered on the maternal age and specific fetal karyotype. There is no increased risk of recurrence with a 45X karyotype. With trisomies, including trisomy 21, the recurrence risk is based on the age of the mother when she delivered the initial trisomy and what her age would be at the next conception. If a woman is 30 years or older at the time of an aneuploidy birth, her risk of recurrence in a future pregnancy is only slightly greater than it was for this birth. If, however, a trisomic birth occurs in a younger woman, the recurrence risk is usually quoted as 1%; but it should be noted that women with a previous trisomic birth do have a recurrence risk for a different trisomy in another birth. If abnormalities other than trisomy are identified, an evaluation of the parental karyotype may be required if future pregnancies are desired.

Data surrounding the hospital area in which nurses work have revealed interesting potential environmental and genetic associations. Elevated risks of congenital anomalies have been found in the singleton offspring of nurses employed in particular areas of the hospital. The two areas with the highest risk include operating room nurses and the emergency department with an increase of 7.9%; however, the anomalies did vary per department. Those working in the operating room and pediatrics had the highest incidence of unspecified cardiac defects; maternal newborn nurses had a higher incidence of anomalies that involved the integument; respiratory system anomalies were higher among emergency department nurses; and alimentary tract defects were higher among nurses who worked on psychiatric floors (Dimich-Ward et al., 2011).

SECTION FIVE REVIEW

1. Chromosomal abnormalities are responsible for the majority of spontaneous abortions.
   A. True
   B. False
2. Nurses caring for women with a pregnancy loss should not offer information as to the reason for the loss.
   A. True
   B. False
3. Factors that influence the rate of chromosomal abnormalities noted in pregnancy loss include all of the following EXCEPT
   A. maternal age.
   B. gestational age.
   C. maternal weight.
   D. small for gestational age.
4. Women who experience recurrent pregnancy loss due to chromosomal abnormalities are unlikely to have another abnormality in future pregnancies.
   A. True
   B. False
5. The most common trisomy found in abortus specimens is
   A. 13.
   B. 18.
   C. 21.
   D. 16.

Answers: 1. A; 2. B; 3. C; 4. B; 5. D

POSTTEST

1. Genes are segments of DNA that code for the ___________.
   A. trait of hair color
   B. synthesis of proteins
   C. muscle contraction
   D. function of insulin
2. The result of meiosis is to produce ___________.
   A. the zygote
   B. 23 chromosomes
   C. 46 chromosomes
   D. oogonia
3. Which term is correctly used to describe all Down's persons?
   A. Aneuploidy
   B. Trisomy 21
   C. Polyploidy
   D. Translocation
4. Which of these does not contribute to genetic variability?
   A. Meiosis
   B. Crossing over
   C. Having children with a close relative
   D. Having children with someone who is not a relative
5. Several variant forms of a gene for a given trait are called ___________.
   A. autosomes
   B. alleles
   C. sex chromosomes
   D. histones
6. The genes of an individual will always be different from those of the parents.
   A. True
   B. False
7. Uniparental disomy can arise from two nondisjunction events or a trisomy and subsequent chromosome loss.
   A. True
   B. False
8. The meiotic error that causes aneuploidy is called ___________.
   A. relocation
   B. crossing over
   C. nondisjunction
   D. deletion
9. Ultrasound can be a useful tool in the evaluation of trisomic mosaicism.
   A. True
   B. False
10. The material substance of a chromosome consisting of DNA and protein that contains proteins called histones that help package DNA into a compact form to fit in the cell nucleus.
    A. Nucleic acid
    B. Cytoplasm
    C. Chromatin
    D. Genotype

Posttest answers are located in the Appendix.

CHAPTER SUMMARY

An understanding of chromosomal activity with regard to mitosis and meiosis is essential to having an understanding of the formation of trisomies and trisomy mosaicism. Mitotic and meiotic nondisjunctions are the two points at which trisomy mosaicism can begin.

- It is essential that a health care provider possesses insight into understanding the formation of trisomies in order to provide appropriate counseling for the pregnant woman.
- Trisomic mosaicism can be confined to the placenta without affecting the fetus and is believed to occur in approximately 1% to 2% of pregnancies.
- Uniparental disomy is related to trisomy by virtue of two consecutive mistakes involving either meiotic or mitotic nondisjunctions and is significant for the potential expression of autosomal recessive genes.

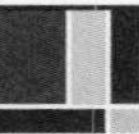

CRITICAL THINKING CHECKPOINT

Gabriella is a 25-year-old Hispanic woman who is pregnant for the second time. Her first pregnancy ended with a fetal demise at 32 weeks and unfortunately a chromosomal analysis was not done. She and her husband are concerned about this pregnancy and have requested a CVS be performed. The results come back with a diagnosis of placental mosaicism.

1. How would you explain this result to the couple?
2. What information is necessary to provide to this couple?
3. Are there any referrals you could make to help with this decision?
4. What kind of follow-up would be necessary, depending on the couple's decision?

Answers are provided in the Appendix

Pearson Nursing Student Resources

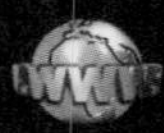

Find additional review materials at nursing.pearsonhighered.com

Prepare for success with additional NCLEX®-style practice questions, interactive assignments and activities, web links, animations, videos, and more!

ONLINE RESOURCES

PubMed Health; Mosaicism: http://www.ncbi.nlm.nih.gov/pubmedhealth/PMH0002294/

The University of British Columbia, Department of Medical Genetics: http://medgen.ubc.ca

University of Maryland Medical Center; Mosaicism Overview: http://www.umm.edu/ency/article/001317.htm

REFERENCES

Chiu, R. W. K., Akolekar, R., Zheng, Y. W. L., Leung, T. Y., Sun, H., Chan, K. C. A., et al. (2011). Noninvasive prenatal assessment of trisomy 21 by multiplexed maternal plasma DNA sequencing: Large scale validity study. *British Medical Journal, 342*, c7401. doi: 10.1136/bmj.c7401

Dimich-Ward, H., Le, N., Beking, C., Dybuncio, A., Spinelli, J., Gallagher, R., et al. (2011). Congenital anomalies in the offspring of nurses: Association with area of employment during pregnancy. *International Journal of Occupational and Environmental Health, 17*, 195–201.

Lo, Y. M. D., Chan, K. C. A., Sun, H., Chen, E. Z., Jiang, P., Lun, F. M. F., et al. (2010). Maternal plasma DNA sequencing reveals the genome-wide genetic and mutational profile of the fetus. *Science Translational Medicine, 2*(61), 61–91. doi: 10.1126/scitranslmed.3001720

National Institutes of Health. National Human Genome Research Institute. (2011). *Talking Glossary of Genetic Terms.* Retrieved February 24, 2011, from http://www.genome.gov/glossary/?id=180

Robinson W. P. (2000). Mechanisms leading to uniparental disomy and their clinical consequences. *Bioessays 22*(5), 452–459.

Robinson, W. P., & Furnival, J. (2007). *Chromosomal mosaicism.* Retrieved February 24, 2011, from http://www.medgen.ubc.ca/robinsonlab/mosaic/intro/mos_how.htm

Schuring-Blom, G. H. (2002). Chromosomal mosaicism in the placenta (in Dutch). *Ned Tijdschr Geneeskd 146*(51), 2470–2474. Retrieved January 16, 2012, from http://www.ncbi.nlm.nih.gov/pubmed/12534099

Viot, G. (2002). Confined placental mosaicism: Definition, consequences and outcome (in French). *J Gynecol Obstet Biol Reprod (Paris), 31*(1 Suppl), 2S70–74. Retrieved January 16, 2012, from http://www.ncbi.nlm.nih.gov/pubmed/11973523

Wapner, R. J. (2010). Genetics of stillbirth. *Clinical Obstetrics and Gynecology, 53*(3), 628–634.

Warren, J., & Silver, R. (2008). Genetics of pregnancy of loss. *Clinical Obstetrics and Gynecology, 51*(1), 84–95.

CHAPTER

7

Mendelian Inheritance

Cheryl Mele

LEARNING OUTCOMES

Following the completion of this chapter, the learner will be able to

1. Describe Mendelian patterns of inheritance that contribute to inherited disorders.
2. Describe the major characteristics of single gene Mendelian autosomal recessive disorders.
3. Describe the major characteristics of single gene Mendelian autosomal dominant disorders.
4. Describe the major characteristics of single gene X-linked recessive and dominant disorders.
5. Identify nontraditional Mendelian disorders such as mitochondrial disorders, genomic imprinting, uniparental disomy, and unstable triplet repeat mutations.
6. Describe the role of nurses and other health care professionals in providing information about Mendelian disease to patients and families.

This chapter presents the depiction of traditional Mendelian inheritance and nontraditional inheritance of disease. Many genetic disorders follow a **Mendelian** model of inheritance, which is often described as a single gene mutation. However, Mendelian disorders are more multifaceted, and different changes in a single gene may produce different clinical manifestations or phenotypes in individuals. The nontraditional inheritance such as **mitochondrial DNA** (mt) has become more understood. The mitochondrial disorders are from maternal inheritance and often involve deficiencies in high-energy organs.

PRETEST

1. When a set of parents has a child affected by an autosomal recessive disorder, the most likely recurrence risk is
   A. 100%.
   B. 50%.
   C. 33%.
   D. 25%.
2. New autosomal dominant disorder mutations in families in certain conditions have been associated with increased age of the father.
   A. True
   B. False
3. What is the risk for hemophilia A in the grandsons if their paternal grandfather has hemophilia A?
   A. 0%
   B. 50%
   C. 25%
   D. 100%
4. Which type of inheritance pattern occurs in a genetic disorder in which the phenotype appears in every generation, the normal family members transmit the gene to their offspring, and males and females are equally affected?
   A. Autosomal dominant
   B. Autosomal recessive
   C. X-linked dominant
   D. Mitochondrial
5. In Duchene muscular dystrophy, the median age of survival is 18 with most patients dying of
   A. cardiac arrest.
   B. ruptured aneurysms.
   C. impaired pulmonary function.
   D. malnutrition.
6. For a couple who have produced one child with cystic fibrosis, the risk for developing the disease for each subsequent child is
   A. 50%.
   B. 25%.
   C. 100%.
   D. 0%.

7. The newborn screen assesses primarily for metabolic and hemoglobinopathies disorders that are considered
   A. autosomal recessive.
   B. autosomal dominant.
   C. X-linked recessive.
   D. mitochondrial.
8. Mitochondrial disorders are inherited by
   A. maternal side.
   B. fraternal side.
   C. both maternal and fraternal.
   D. multifactorial.
9. Which of the following traits are never transmitted from the father to son?
   A. Autosomal recessive
   B. Autosomal dominant
   C. X-linked recessive
   D. Y-linked disorders
10. While genetic testing can identify the genetic composition of an individual, the ________ may not be able to accurately determine what a person actually will look like; however, the ________ can.
   A. genotype; phenotype
   B. phenotype; genotype
   C. phenotype; allele
11. Mendelian Inheritance patterns include
   A. autosomal dominate.
   B. autosomal recessive.
   C. multifactorial.
   D. Both A. and B.
12. For an autosomal dominant disease, if two affected parents have a child, what is most likely the risk of passing on the disorder?
   A. 100%
   B. 25%
   C. 50%
   D. 75%
13. Few genes are known to be located on the Y chromosome and inherited from father to son.
   A. True
   B. False
14. If an aunt has children with her nephew, which of the following terms is used to describe the relationship?
   A. Interrelatedness
   B. Recessively
   C. Inbreeding loop
   D. Consanguinity
15. A portion of individuals with a mutated gene show no signs and symptoms of the disorder.
   A. True
   B. False
16. Any tissue with mitochondria can be affected by mitochondrial disease.
   A. True
   B. False
17. Inheritance can explain conditions like baldness and gout.
   A. True
   B. False
18. An example of co-dominance is the ABO blood group.
   A. True
   B. False
19. Genetic disorders showing anticipation demonstrate increased severity with future generations.
   A. True
   B. False
20. The following are true regarding X-linked dominant disorders EXCEPT
   A. mutated gene is located on the X chromosome.
   B. X inactivation in females modifies the affect in females.
   C. affected families show excess of male offspring is 2:1.
   D. disorders are relatively uncommon.

Pretest answers are located in the Appendix.

SECTION ONE: Mendelian Inheritance

Genetic defects consist of three main categories: (1) Mendelian disorder (single gene defects), (2) chromosomal disorders (structural chromosomal errors), and (3) non-Mendelian disorders. This chapter will concentrate on Mendelian genetic disorders.

Mendelian Basics

Over 16,000 traits or disorders in humans demonstrate a single gene or Mendelian inheritance (Turnpenny & Ellard, 2012). Gregor Mendel used a series of breeding experiments in pea plants to illustrate units of inheritance. Single genes are accountable for a trait or allele, which occupies a specific **locus** on a chromosome (Skirton, Patch, & Williams, 2005). A human species inherits one allele from each parent. Mendel described in his laws of inheritance that both pairs of chromosomes separate, and genes shuffle in gametes during meiosis, leading them to be inherited in random combinations (laws of segregation and laws of independent assortment)(Lewis, 2007). Laws of segregation can be further explained according to the behavior of the chromosomes and genes during meiosis (Lewis, 2007). Mendel's second law of independent assortment follows the transmission of two or more genes on different chromosomes in maternal and paternal gametes during meiosis, which results in various combinations of genes (Lewis, 2007). That is why family members resemble one another but do not possess identical phenotypes unless identical monozygotic twins.

A gene is an elongated sequence of DNA, and it can comprise many variations. An individual who possesses identical alleles for a gene is referred to as **homozygous**. An individual who acquires two different alleles for a particular gene is referred to as **heterozygous**. The two types of alleles that may be inherited are denoted as dominant and recessive. The dominant allele uses the symbol of a capital letter and the recessive trait uses the symbol of a small letter. Two small letters (such as tt) for Mendel's short plant experiment is considered a homozygous recessive trait. Two capital letters for Mendel's tall plants (such as TT) is referred to as a homozygous dominant trait. If the tall plant mated with the short plant, another possible allele combination is one recessive allele and one dominant allele, which will result in a heterozygous combination (Tt). The *genotype* of a person is the set of alleles that make up their genetic constitution typically on genetic loci (Nussbaum, McInnes, & Willard, 2007). The *phenotype* defines the outward expression of an allele combination, or physical features of the condition. The **dominant** allele often prevails in one's phenotype.

In the human population there are numerous versions of a gene at one locus, which is defined as polymorphisms, or simply stated as many configurations of a gene (Nussbaum et al., 2007). The **wild type** gene is termed as the common phenotype found in a population. A set of alleles or traits at a certain location on a chromosome is depicted as haplotype (Nussbaum et al., 2007). A haplotype can further be defined as a combination of alleles or as a set of single nucleotide polymorphisms (SNPs) found on the same chromosome (Nussbaum et al., 2007). The disparity in a gene is due to polymorphism or mutation. A change in the DNA sequence within the gene can result in an inherited or sporadic mutation. Mutations can result from physical damage to the cell due to environmental measures such as radiation or error in DNA replication during mitosis or meiosis (Skirton, Patch, & Williams, 2005). Furthermore, when a mutation occurs, it is replicated in all daughter cells that arise from the mutated cells (Skirton, Patch, & Williams, 2005).

Principles of single gene disorders or Mendelian disorder use the same principles of inheritance of other traits such as height and eye color. Mendelian inheritance disorders or monogenic disorders are germline mutations passed onto the next generation, or they can result from a spontaneous mutation in the gametes (sperm and egg). These disorders are caused by a mutated allele or pair of mutated alleles at one genetic location on a particular chromosome (Jarvi & Chitayat, 2008). A single gene is usually defective, which is why single gene disorders are often referred to as monogenic disorders. If the defective gene is on a non-sex chromosome it is referred to as **autosomal**, and if the defective gene is on the sex chromosome it is referred to as X-linked or Y chromosomal disorder. Also, the defect is classified as either dominant or recessive. Therefore, in human genetics there are distinctive patterns of traditional inheritance named after Gregor Mendel, the "father of genetics." These common patterns of inheritance demonstrate how genetic defects pass through generation of families and are listed in the following categories:

- **Autosomal Dominant**
- **Autosomal Recessive**
- X-linked recessive
- X-linked dominant
- Y-linked

SECTION ONE REVIEW

1. Principles of single gene disorders or Mendelian disorder utilize the same principles of inheritance of other traits such as height and eye color.
   A. True
   B. False
2. Mendelian inheritance disorders or monogenic disorders are germline mutations passed onto the next generation, and they never result from spontaneous mutations.
   A. True
   B. False
3. A single gene is usually defective, which is why single gene disorders are often referred to as monogenic disorders.
   A. True
   B. False

Answers: 1. A; 2. B; 3. A

SECTION TWO: Autosomal Dominant Inheritance

Autosomal dominant inheritance occurs when a mutation in a single allele is sufficient to cause the disease or disorder in either a heterozygous or homozygous person (Nussbaum et al., 2007). Dominant disorders will acquire severe characteristics of the disease if the person inherits both mutated alleles (homozygous person) (Nussbaum et al., 2007). Only on copy of the mutated gene is required to express the trait, and the offspring have a 50% chance to pass the disorder on to a future generation. A vertical pedigree pattern is depicted with multiple generations affected. Also, offspring who do not inherit the disorder or mutations will not pass the trait onto future generations. Autosomal disorders are often caused by various disease mechanisms, and the function of genetic pathway, which sanctions the genetic alteration, will cause various clinical presentations or phenotypes (Skirton et al., 2005). Mutations also occur more often in offspring of fathers greater than 40 years of age (Turnpenny & Ellard, 2012). Over 6,000 Mendelian defects or monogenic defects have been identified and more than half are autosomal dominant (Skirton et al., 2005). Representative types of genetic disorders that respect autosomal dominant pattern are conditions such as **myotonic dystrophy**, Marfan syndrome, polycystic kidney disease, neurofibromatosis osteogenesis imperfecta, and familial hypercholesterolemia (Skirton et al., 2005). Figure 7–1 ■ illustrates autosomal dominant disorder pattern.

Myotonic dystrophy is part of a group of inherited disorders called muscular dystrophies and is the most common form of muscular dystrophy that begins in adulthood. The disorder frequently results in progressive weakness, myotonia, cardiac conduction abnormalities, feeding difficulties, somnolence, frontal

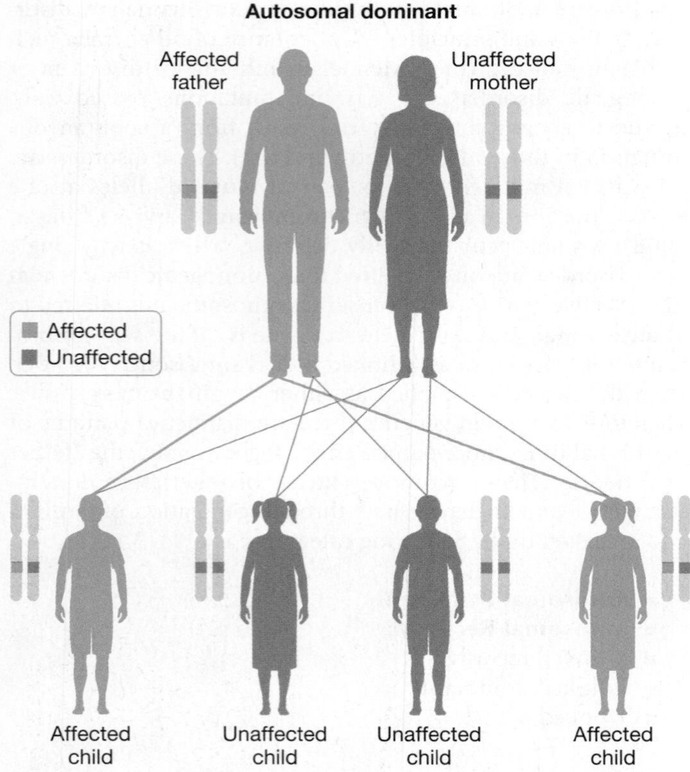

Figure 7–1 ■ Autosomal dominant disorder. In this example, a man with an autosomal dominant disorder has two affected children and two unaffected children.

Source: U.S. National Library of Medicine, 2011

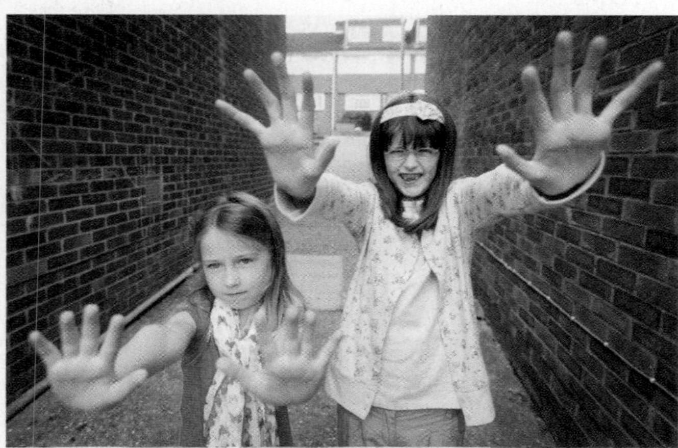

Figure 7–2 ■ Marfan syndrome in a child. A rare condition with poor prognosis. Note the phenotype consisting of pectus excavutum, narrow faces with dolichocephaly, congenital flexion contracture, and arachnodactyly (spider fingers). Prognosis depends upon severity of the cardiac malformation and congestive heart failure.

HELEN YATES/Barcroft Media /Landov

balding, and testicular atrophy (Turnpenny & Ellard, 2012). Like many autosomal dominant disorders, the age of onset is variable, and the younger the age in which the symptoms present, the more severe the case. Marfan syndrome is a disorder of the fibrous connective tissue and defect in type 1 fibrillin, a glycoprotein encoded by the FBN1 gene (Nussbaum, 2007). The affected individuals often present with Marfan stigmata: They are often extremely tall, with disproportion upper and lower body, arachnodactyl (spider fingers), pectus formation, joint laxity, myopia, mitral valve prolapse, and life-threatening aortic dissection (Turnpenny & Ellard, 2012) (Figure 7–2 ■). Consequently, due to the variability of symptoms and onset of autosomal conditions, careful history and physical assessment is key in recognition of the disorders.

Co-Dominance

In special circumstances, co-dominance occurs when the contributions of both alleles are visible in the phenotype or equally shown (Nussbaum et al., 2007). Normally, when one allele is dominant it blocks the recessive trait. However, in the case of co-dominance both alleles or variations are dominant. The ABO blood group is a prime example of co-dominance. Blood types A and B are dominant over blood type O on the red blood cells; thus the A and B blood groups are co-dominant over the O blood type (Turnpenny & Ellard, 2012). Furthermore, if a parent is blood type A and another parent is blood type B their offspring can have a phenotype of AB blood. Figure 7–3 ■ illustrates the co-dominance theory.

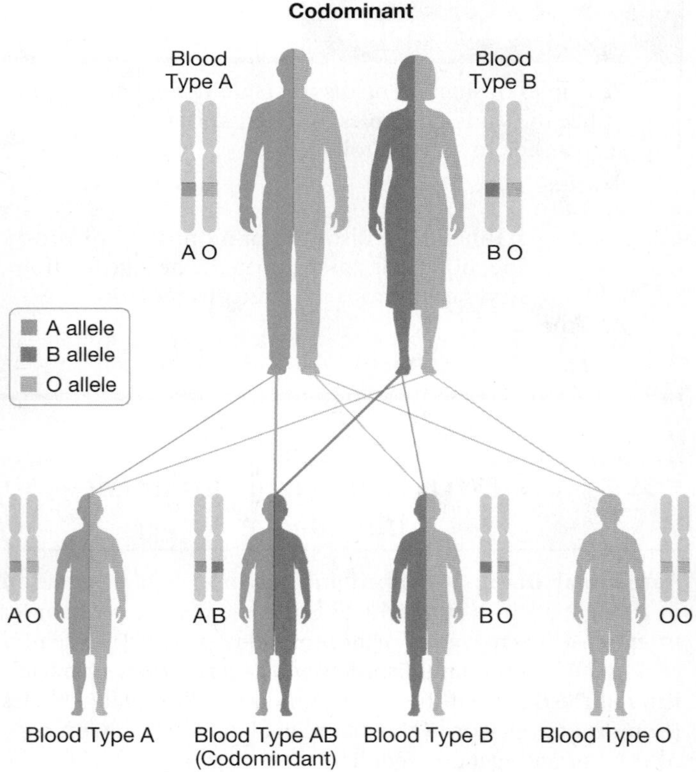

Figure 7–3 ■ Co-dominance. The ABO blood group is a major system for classifying blood types in humans. Blood type AB is inherited in a co-dominant pattern. In this example, a father with blood type A and a mother with blood type B have four children, each with a different blood type: A, AB, B, and O.

Source: U.S. National Library of Medicine, 2011

Penetrance and Expressivity

In many families genetic conditions with the abnormal phenotype can be easily distinguished from the normal one or wild type. However, clinically, individuals who carry a specific mutated allele or genotype in the same families do not express the same clinical symptoms, or severity of the disorder, and the same time in the onset of disease (Nussbaum et al., 2007). The variations can cause a challenge in diagnosis, along with pedigree interpretation. The recognized concepts **reduced penetrance** and variable **expressivity** are two ways in which such disparity in expression of a genetic condition can appear and can be explained (Nussbaum et al., 2007). *Expressivity* is defined as severity of expression of the phenotype or physical presentation of particular genetic mutation among individuals with the same disease (Nussbaum et al., 2007). *Variable expressivity* is the variation in expression of one's phenotype that can occur even if individuals in the same family have the same genotype. Phenotypic manifestations of clinical disorders are further affected by other variables, such as environment, age, and genetic location (Turnpenny & Ellard, 2012).

Neurofibromatosis (NF1) and osteogenesis imperfecta (**OI**) are classic explanations of variable expressivity (Nussbaum et al., 2007). NF1 is a mutation on the long arm of chromosome 17 that results in a loss of function of neurfibromin and involves variety of clinical disorders in the eye, nervous system, and skin (Nussbaum et al., 2007). NF1 clinical variations include café au lait spots, axillary freckling, benign fleshy tumors, Lisch nodules, life-threatening tumors in the central nervous system (CNS), and behavioral disorders (Figure 7–4 ■). OI can present with a range of classifications (I–VIII), and some are categorized as autosomal recessive inheritance. OI is a genetic mutation in the COLA1-COLA2 gene, which is a mutation in genes type 1 collagen on chromosome 7 and 17 (Turnpenny & Ellard, 2012). The mutation causes increase bone fragility and decreased bone mass. Gravity of the disorder ranges from intrauterine fractures and perinatal lethality to very mild forms without fractures. Extra-skeletal clinical symptoms include blue sclera, dentiogenesis imperfecta, hyperflexity, hearing loss, and wormian bones on skull X-rays (Leung, & Pacuad, & Lemay, 2005).

The rate of recurrence of phenotype expression in individuals who have the genotype for a certain mutation can be less than 100% (Nussbaum et al., 2007). **Penetrance** is the chance that a particular gene inherited by an individual will display a phenotypic expression or physical manifestations. Not all **carriers** of a gene mutation show clinical manifestations of the disorder. The individuals who do not express the gene in their phenotype are said to have reduced penetrance. An autosomal dominant pedigree with reduced penetrance will portray a non-typical pattern consisting of relatives who are not affected in every generation. Reduced penetrance is believed to arise due to modification of genes and their interaction with the environment (Turnpenny & Ellard, 2012).

Incomplete Dominance Inheritance

Incomplete dominance exists when one allele is expressed while the other is suppressed. In incomplete dominance, the heterozygous phenotype is intermediate between that of either homozygote (Lewis, 2007, p. 97). This results in a third phenotype or a combined phenotype, which is a blend of paternal and maternal traits. Mendel illustrated this inheritance with mating of red snapdragons with a genotype (RR) and white snapdragons with genotype (rr); the offspring resulted in pink snapdragons. A hereditary trait that displays incomplete dominance is eye color in offspring. A clinical example for Mendelian or monogenic disorder representing incomplete dominance is familial hypercholesterolemia. The phenotypes are related to the amount of receptors cells on the liver cells that take up the low-density lipoprotein form of cholesterol from the bloodstream (Lewis, 2007). The disorder can lead to premature heart disease. The rare homozygous patients (DD) possessing two mutated alleles die at a young age with coronary artery disease while the heterozygous patients with one mutated allele (Dd) suffer heart disease in early adulthood (Lewis, 2007; Nussbaum et al., 2007). Another example is achondroplasia, which is a disorder that often results in short limbs, low nasal bridge, large heads, lordosis, and normal intelligence (Lashley, 2007) (see Figure 7–5 ■). Most individuals with achondroplasia live with their disabilities and marry. However,

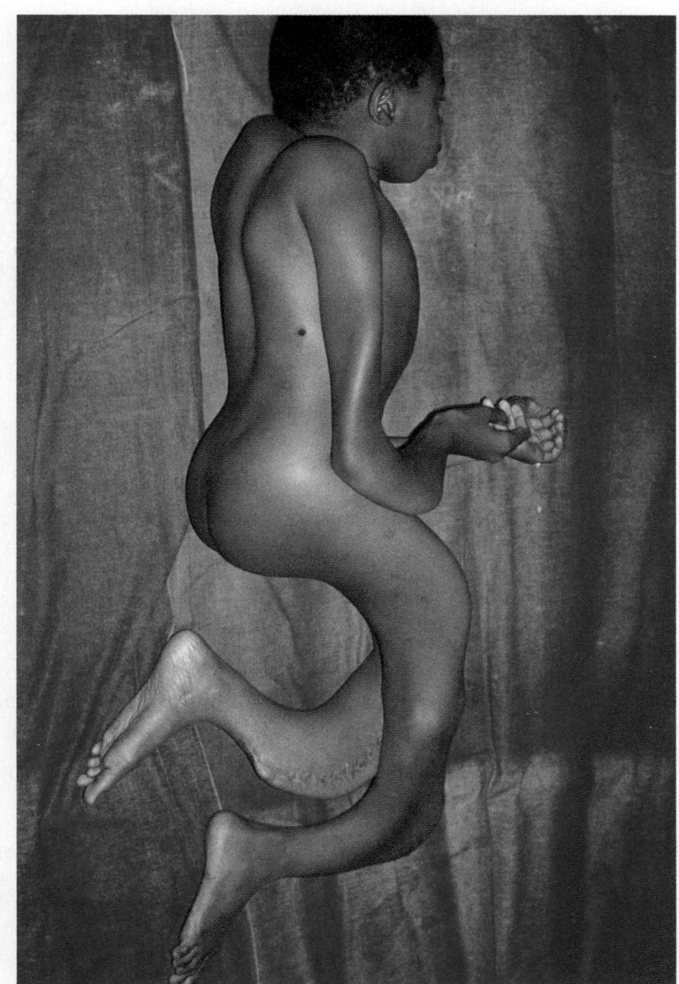

Figure 7–4 ■ Osteogenesis imperfecta type

Dr. M.A. Ansary / Photo Researchers, Inc.

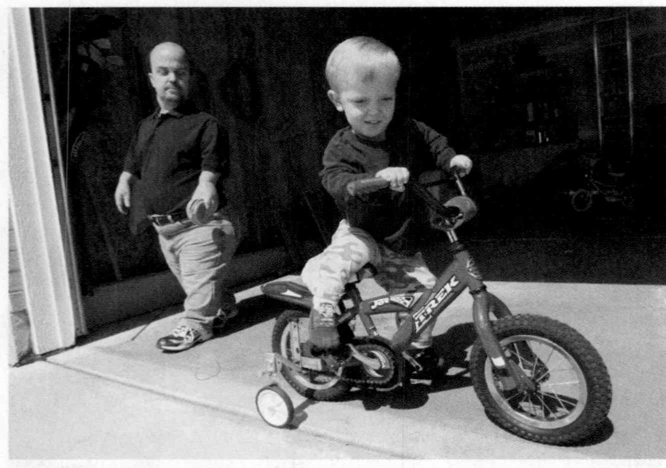

Figure 7–5 ■ Achondroplasia. The man (left) has short limbs relative to trunk length. Note also the prominent forehead, and low nasal root.
RICK WILKING/Reuters/Landov

homozygous offspring are severely affected and frequently do not survive the neonatal period (Nussbaum et al., 2007). Thus amid incomplete dominance there is a compromise or weak expression of the dominant allele over the inactive allele in a heterozygous state. The heterozygous phenotype is intermediate between the homozygous phenotype, which is often lethal.

New Mutations in Autosomal Dominant Inheritance

In autosomal dominant disorders it is common that one parent is a carrier of the mutated allele or has the genetic disorder. However, this is not always the circumstance and it is not unusual for a new spontaneous mutation or **de novo mutation** to arise in the gamete transmitted from a nonheterozygous parent (Nussbaum et al., 2007). A **new mutation** is defined as an abrupt unforeseen condition that appears due to an error occurring in transmission of gene (Turnpenny & Ellard, 2012). New dominant mutations have been allied with increased age of the father and the consequence of many mitotic divisions that male gamete stem cells undergo during a man's reproductive cycle (Turnpenny & Ellard, 2012). It has been reported that half the cases of NF1 are an end result from a new mutation rather than an inheritance (Nussbaum et al., 2007). In some conditions, such as Duchene muscular dystrophy, which is autosomal dominant, there is often a de novo mutation since those with the condition do not live long enough to reproduce.

SECTION TWO REVIEW

1. NF1 is considered a fully penetrant disorder and does not skip generations.
   A. True
   B. False
2. Myotonic dystrophy is a cause of neonatal hypertonia.
   A. True
   B. False
3. Marfan stigmata are inclusive of skeletal anomalies, myopia, and aortic valve disorders.
   A. True
   B. False
4. If a condition skips generations it may be due to reduced penetrance.
   A. True
   B. False
5. Anticipation of disease shows decrease severity of symptoms and later onset.
   A. True
   B. False

Answers: 1. A; 2. B; 3. A, 4. A; 5. B

SECTION THREE: Autosomal Recessive

Recessive disorders are expressed only when the mutated allele is present in two copies of a gene: one inherited from the mother and one from the father. In recessive disorders, if a person carries one copy of the mutated gene, then that person is labeled a carrier. Carriers normally do not have clinical manifestations of the disease. Therefore, if an offspring is born to parents who both carry an **autosomal recessive** genetic mutation, each offspring has a 1 in 4 chance of getting the malfunctioning genes from both parents and developing the disease. The offspring will have a 50% chance of inheriting one genetic mutation (a carrier of the disorder). If an individual who is homozygous for an autosomal recessive disorder has offspring, they will have a 50% chance of being affected. Such a pedigree is understood to display pseudodominance (Turnpenny & Ellard, 2012). Furthermore, most individuals affected by autosomal recessive disorders are probably compound heterozygotes, which means there are a variety of mutations identified for the same locus (Turnpenny & Ellard, 2012). This explains the variations in clinical manifestations for **hemoglobinopathy**, β thalassemia, and cystic fibrosis.

A depiction of autosomal recessive disorder can be demonstrated with sickle cell disease (**SCD**). For a child to have SCD he or she will have inherited two copies of the mutation (homozygous genotype) and both parents most often are carriers of the disorder (heterozygous genotype). SCD is one of a group of hereditary hemoglobinopathies that are caused by mutations in the genes for globin that construct hemoglobin (Skirton et al., 2004). Normal structure of hemoglobin is important to absorb and release oxygen to the tissues. SCD causes abnormal construction of a hemoglobin molecule (crescent shape) under low oxygen conditions and stress. The clinical result is a sickle cell crisis in which a crescent-shaped hemoglobin molecule is inefficient in carrying oxygen, causing obstruction to blood flow and ischemia, or tissue infarction (Skirton et al., 2004). Possible complications of SCD disorder are anemia, immunosuppression, gallstones, delayed growth, aplastic crisis, ulcers, retinopathy, and stroke. Figure 7–6 ■ provides an illustration of the autosomal recessive mode of inheritance.

Cystic fibrosis (CF) is another common autosomal recessive disorder in those with western European ancestry. It is less common in those with African or Asian ancestry. CF has been isolated and mapped on chromosome 7q31 and involves CFTR gene (Genetic Home Reference, 2007). More than 1,500 mutations of the CFTR gene have been identified (Turnpenny & Ellard, 2012). Mutations in the CFTR gene interrupt the role of the chloride channels by adjusting the movement of chloride ions and water across cell membranes (Genetic Home Reference, 2007). Levels of mutations correlate with a clinical phenotype; the greater the dysfunction in the CFTR gene, the more severe the manifestations of the disease. As a consequence, cells that contour the passageways of the lungs, pancreas, and other organs create mucus that is copious and gluey. The thick mucus clogs the airways and other organs, causing the characteristic signs and symptoms of cystic fibrosis such as recurrent episodes of pneumonia, constipation, weight loss, pale, foul-smelling stools, and diabetes. Infertility is also an issue with both sexes with congenital bilateral absence of vas deferens, and thick secretions of cervix and fallopian tubes (Read & Donnai, 2007).

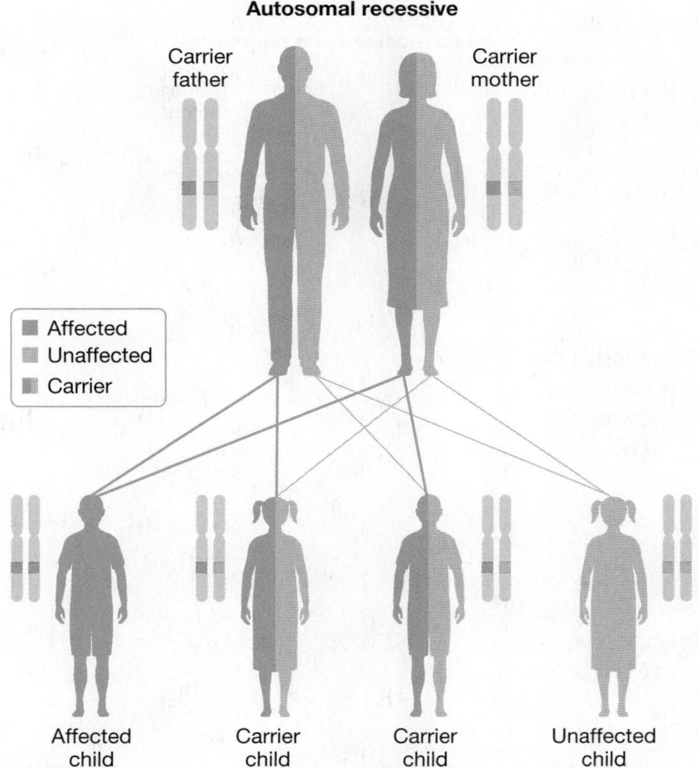

Figure 7–6 ■ Autosomal recessive. Two unaffected parents each carry one copy of a gene mutation for an autosomal recessive disorder. They have one affected child and three unaffected children, two of which carry one copy of the gene.

Source: U.S. National Library of Medicine, 2011

Children often present in the newborn period, with failure to thrive, and/or frequent respiratory infections. Chronic lung disease caused by recurrent infection eventually leads to fibrotic change in the lungs with secondary pulmonary hypertension or cor pulmonale (Turnpenny & Ellard, 2012). Population screening is provided in the newborn screen and genetic testing provides confirmation of the disease. The outlook for CF has improved over the years, but children with the disorder require frequent hospitalizations, chest physical therapy, bronchodilators, pancreatic enzymes, and increased calorie requirements. The disorder is frequently fatal but promise of gene therapy is being investigated due to the obtainability of target organs (Turnpenny & Ellard, 2012).

A majority of the autosomal recessive disorders are due to loss of a genetic function or deficiency of an enzyme in the metabolic pathway or proteins in signaling cascade (Nussbaum et al., 2007; Skirton et al., 2004). Many of these disorders are included in newborn screening panels because devastating clinical manifestations are frequently present early in life. Autosomal recessive metabolic disorders, if left untreated, may result in seizures, mental retardation, or death. The federal government only mandates screening for hypothyroidism and **phenylketonuria (PKU)** in all 50 states. Newborns with PKU disorder are defective of an enzyme called phenylalanine hydroxylase, which is needed to break down an essential amino acid called phenylalanine. Early detection is essential for prevention of neurologic complications. Treatment requires specialized formula and lifelong restriction of protein and artificial sweeteners (aspartame) in their diet. Other examples of autosomal recessive disorders include maple syrup urine disease, **ataxia telangiectasia**, and lysomal storage disease (Hurler syndrome).

Consanguinity

Inquiries into one's family history might reveal the risk of consanguinity, or the relatedness of individuals who marry each other. Consanguinity promotes a higher risk for rare alleles and more likely an increased risk for autosomal recessive disorders in offspring (Turnpenny & Ellard, 2012). The rarer a recessive disorder, the greater the prevalence of consanguinity among the parents of the affected offspring. Alkaptonuria is a prime example. It is a disorder in which the body fails to properly break down certain amino acids (tyrosine and phenylalanine). It is a defect in the HGD gene and results in brown-black-colored urine when it hits the air as well as other symptoms like arthritis in the spine later in life (Lewis, 2007). This disorder was scrutinized and found in more than one-fourth of cases in which most of the parents were first cousins (Turnpenny & Ellard, 2012).

SECTION THREE REVIEW

1. PKU is a condition that can impact the neurologic function of a child.
   A. True
   B. False
2. Most autosomal recessive disorders present in adulthood.
   A. True
   B. False
3. The newborn screen only tests for PKU and congenital hypothyroidism.
   A. True
   B. False

Answers: 1. A; 2. B; 3. A

SECTION FOUR: X-Linked Disorders

X-Linked Recessive

X-linked inheritance is determined by a genetic mutation on the X chromosome. The majority of X-linked inheritances are recessive disorders. The X-linked disorders are mutations on the X chromosome and are almost exclusively seen in males. A male with a mutated allele on the X chromosome is described as hemizygous because he only has one X chromosome (Turnpenny & Ellard, 2012). The affected males inherit the disorder from their mothers. Females who possess one mutated allele are carriers because they have two X chromosomes, and they will need two mutated alleles on their X chromosomes to exhibit the disorder. Therefore, the disorder is frequently passed from an affected male through his carrier daughters, who pass the mutation onto their sons, since no X chromosome is transmitted from father to son (Jarvi & Chitayat, 2008). Statistically speaking, if a woman is a carrier, there is a 1 in 2 chance that her son will be affected with the disorder and a 1 in 2 chance that her daughter will be a carrier. Figure 7–7 ■ illustrates the mode of inheritance of X-linked recessive disorder.

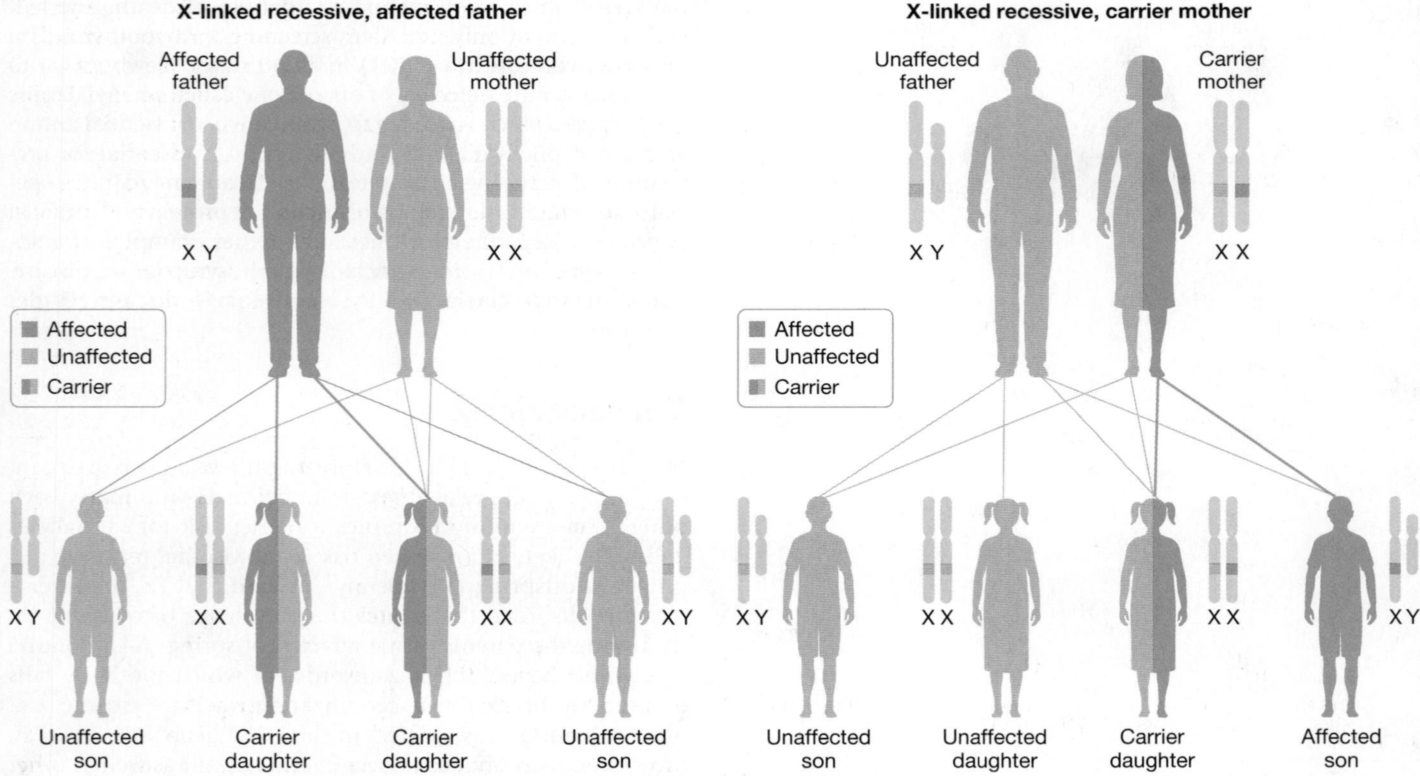

Figure 7–7 ■ X-linked recessive. A man with an X-linked recessive condition has two unaffected daughters who each carry one copy of the gene mutation, and two unaffected sons who do not have the mutation. A woman with an X-linked dominant condition has an affected daughter, an affected son, an unaffected daughter, and an unaffected son.

Source: U.S. National Library of Medicine, 2011

Examples of X-linked recessive disorders include hemophilia, Kallmann syndrome, and Duchenne Muscular Dystrophy (**DMD**). Male patients with Kallmann syndrome have hypogonadism secondary to defect of hypothalamic gonadotropin-releasing hormone, and clinical features such as craniofacial abnormalities, anosmia (reduced smell), underdeveloped genitalia, infertility, brittle bones, hearing loss, and renal abnormalities (Jarvi & Chitayat, 2008).

Hemophilia is a bleeding disorder; those individuals with the disorder can have prolonged bleeding after trauma or surgery. The major types of hemophilia are Hemophilia A (classic) and Hemophilia B (Christmas disease). Hemophilia A is caused by an abnormality in the F8 gene, which causes an dysfunction in the protein named Factor VIII, which is involved in the coagulation cascade (Turnpenny & Ellard, 2012). Hemophilia B is a mutation in the F9 gene and causes a dysfunction in the protein that causes abnormalities in Factor IX (Turnpenny & Ellard, 2012).

Hemophilia results in altered blood clotting that can cause excessive bleeding. Treatment often results in administration of the deficient factor v. Hemophilia A and B are excellent candidates for gene therapy because only a small surge in the deficient plasma factor will be a major clinical advantage; in animal models severe forms reverted to mild after treatment (Turnpenny & Ellard, 2012).

Duchenne muscular dystrophy (DMD) represents one of the most common neuromuscular disorders in children, and often causes early demise. The gene mutation associated with the disorder involves absence of dystrophin, a protein critical for maintenance of the muscle (Zak & Chan, 2010). Absence of dystrophin will result in generalized muscle weakness that progresses over time. Clinical manifestations usually exist prior to the age of 6 and can emerge early in infancy. Some of the manifestations include fatigue, delayed walking, difficulty climbing stairs and running, clumsy, enlarged appearance of calves (pseudohypertrophy), and fatigue (Zak & Chan, 2010). The Gower sign during the toddler years, which involves the child's inability to rise from the floor in a normal fashion, is a red flag for the disorder. In order to stand, the child will roll over onto his hands, uses his hands for support, and get up by bracing his arms on his legs. The disorder is progressive and in the teenage years the child will lose his ability to ambulate, and it will impact cardiac–respiratory muscles. DMD diagnosis is made through evaluation of clinical symptoms, muscle biopsy (absence of dystrophin), elevated creatine levels (muscle wasting), electromyography (**EMG**), and DNA testing for presence of the gene (Palmiera & Sbelendorio,2007). The child's death typically occurs due to pulmonary complications, and/or congestive heart failure in the late teenage years or early 20s. Treatment involves maximizing quality of life with corticosteroids (which protect muscle fibers from damage), promoting mobility with equipment and therapies, and emotional support for the child and family (Palmiera & Sbelendorio, 2007).

A summary of X-linked recessive disorder include the following criteria:

- The condition is apparent almost exclusively in males.
- The trait is passed from an affected male to his daughters and then to 50% of his daughters' sons.
- The trait is never directly transferred from father to son.
- The trait is transferred from a series of female carriers; the affected males are directly related to another through the females (Gunder & Martin, 2011).

X-Linked Dominant

X-linked dominant disorders are rare. There are differences in gene expression between affected males and females. A male who inherits the X-linked dominant allele is more severely affected than the heterozygous female because the male has no other allele to offset the dominant mutation (Lewis, 2007). Thus, the X-linked dominant disorders are frequently lethal in males. X-linked dominant inheritance resembles autosomal dominant inheritance where both the daughters and males of an affected female have a 50% chance of being affected (Turnpenny & Ellard, 2012). However, an affected male only transfers the trait on to his daughters and not his sons. Therefore, direct male-to-male transmission cannot happen. Examples of X-linked dominant traits are hypophosphatemia (Vitamin D resistant rickets), Charcot-Marie-Toothe disease (motor and sensory neuropathy), some types of OI (brittle bone disease, hearing loss, and blue sclera) and Incontinentia Pigmenti (skin disorder) (Turnpenny & Ellard, 2012). X-linked dominant is illustrated in Figure 7–8 ■.

The disorder of Incontinentia Pigmenti (**IP**) demonstrates the difference in the severity of X-linked dominance disorders between male and female inheritance. Incontinentia Pigmenti is a defect in the **NEMO** gene on the X chromosome (Lewis, 2007). Affected females with Incontinentia Pigmenti at birth have blisters, hyperpigmentation within the first few weeks, and **CNS** abnormalities (Jones, 2006). In contrast males affected with the disorder do not survive and women with the disorder have a high rate of spontaneous abortion (Lewis, 2007). Rett syndrome is another disorder that exclusively occurs in females and lethal in hemizygous males (Nussbaum et al., 2007). Rett syndrome results originally with normal growth and development in the first year of life, followed by a rapid neurologic deterioration and loss of developmental milestones. The infant often develops autistic features, seizures, irritable behaviors, ataxia, and typical wringing and flapping arms/hands. The deterioration may halt and the individual can survive for decades with the severe neurologic deficiency (Nussbaum, et al., 2007).

A summary of X-linked dominant inheritance criteria include the following:

- Expressed in the female in one copy.
- Males have more severe effects than females.
- Transmission from male to all daughters but not to sons.
- High rates of miscarriages in females and lethality in males.
- Affected females are more common than males and a milder expression of the phenotype.

(Gunder & Martin, 2011)

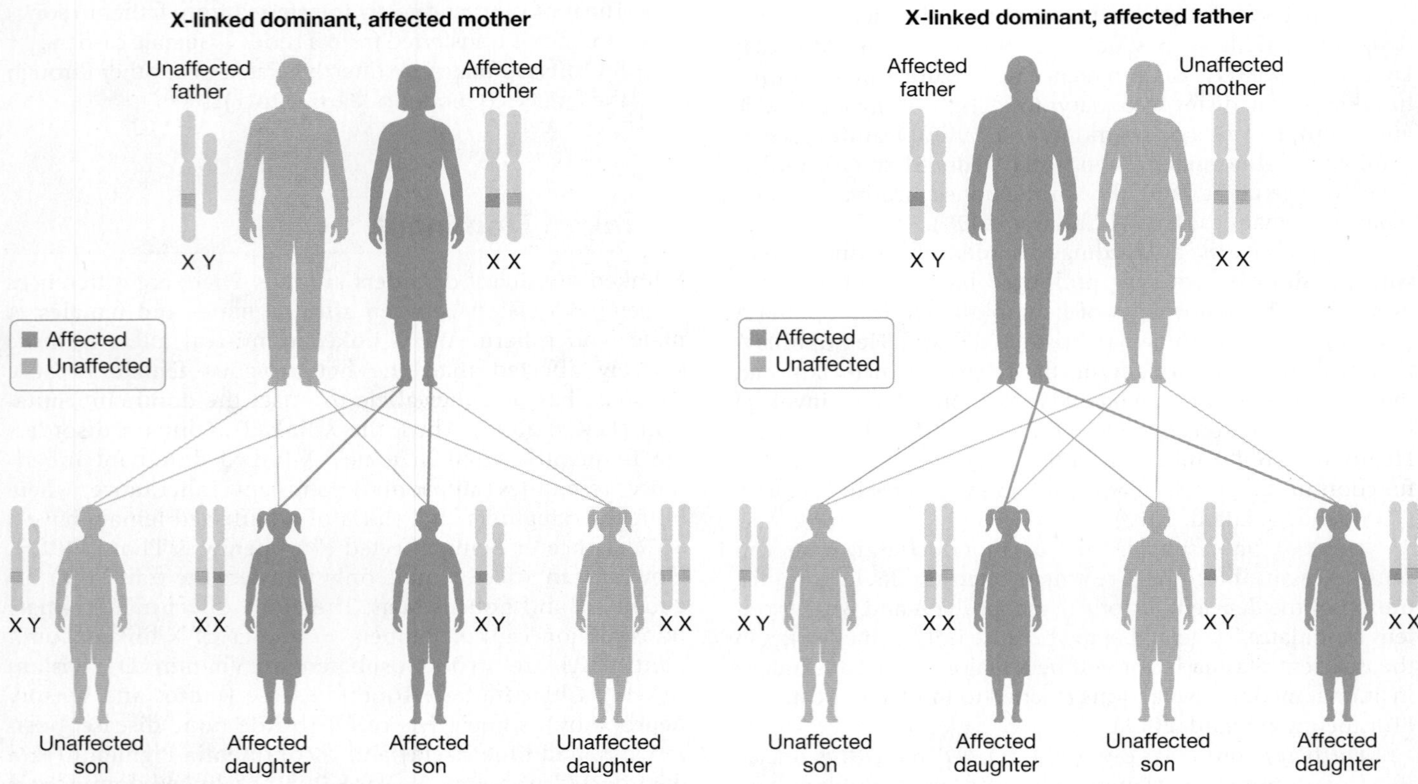

Figure 7–8 ■ X-linked dominant. A woman with an X-linked dominant condition has an affected daughter, an affected son, an unaffected daughter, and an unaffected son. A man with an X-linked dominant condition has two affected daughters and two unaffected sons.

Source: U.S. National Library of Medicine, 2011

X-Inactivation

Females have two alleles for every gene on the X chromosome; in contrast males have only one. A mechanism called X inactivation equalizes this disparity (Lewis, 2007). The clinical significance of X inactivation is insightful and leads the females to have two cell populations (Nussbaum et al., 2007). During embryonic development, 75% of the genes on the X chromosome in each cell is inactivated and the remaining is expressed differently (Lewis, 2007). The selected genes, which are assigned as active versus nonactive in the offspring, are randomly inherited. How does this phenomenon affect X-linked genetic disorders? Depending upon what genes are active in the two chromosomes, X-linked disease could have diverse presentations of the disorder in females due to the proportion of the cells that acquire the mutated allele on the active X chromosome (Nussbaum et al., 2007).

Y-Linked Disorders or Holandric Inheritance

The Y chromosome is the smallest chromosome and few genes are known to be located it. Some of the genes that are well known on the Y chromosome have been associated with skin abnormalities (porcupine skin), hairy ears, webbed toes, height determination, and tooth enamel anomalies, but evidence is debatable (Turnpenny & Ellard, 2012). Most Y-linked genes have to do with male sex determination. H-Y histocompatibility antigen and genes involved in spermatogenesis are carried on the Y chromosome, and therefore manifest holandric inheritance (Turnpenny & Ellard, 2012, p. 117). Y-linked inheritance occurs exclusively in males and male-to-male transmission. None of the affected males' daughters will inherit the trait.

Here is a summary of criteria for Y-linked disorders:

- It only affects males.
- Affected males must transmit the disorder to their sons.

SECTION FOUR REVIEW

1. Y-linked disorders have severe clinical significance and are fatal.
   A. True
   B. False
2. Because of X-inactivation in females, X-linked disorders can have a diverse presentation.
   A. True
   B. False
3. Hemophilia A and B will not benefit from gene therapy because a large amount of factor in the plasma is required to have beneficial results.
   A. True
   B. False
4. X-linked dominant disorders in males are often lethal.
   A. True
   B. False

Answers: 1. B; 2. A; 3. B; 4. A

SECTION FIVE: Nontraditional Inheritance Patterns

Mitochondrial Inheritance

The mitochondria of the cells contain 37 genes and there are approximately 1,000 mitochondrial DNA (**mtDNA**) molecules per cell (Nussbaum et al., 2007). Mitochondria are the "powerhouse of the cell" and the organelles that use oxygen in process of energy production. The genes found within the mitochondria are key in the production of several of the enzymes that initiate the biochemical process to generate the body's source of energy, a chemical named ATP (adenosine triphosphate) (Nussbaum et al., 2007; Turnpenny & Ellard, 2012). The cells in the body, especially in organs such as the brain, heart, retina, skeletal muscle, kidneys and liver, cannot function normally unless they are receiving a continual supply of energy (Nussbaum et al., 2007; Turnpenny & Ellard, 2012).

Diseases involving mitochondrial disorders are associated with faulty genes with a reduction of ATP or deficient energy in the cells of the aforementioned high-energy organs (Skirton et al., 2005). The cells of different tissues or organs can vary with faulty mutations and are created by deletions or other genetic abnormalities that frequently involve one or more organs like the brain, eyes, and heart (Lashley, 2007).

Mitochondrial inheritance is passed through maternal lines where they are abundant (Lashley, 2007). Paternal mitochondria could be transferred, except it is lost early in embryogenesis because the mitochondriaare located in the sperm's tail, which is lost during fertilization (Lashley, 2007; Skirton, et al., 2005) (see Figure 7–9 ■). The mitochondria independently replicate and then segregate randomly into daughter cells (Nussbaum et al., 2007). A mutation in the mitochondrial DNA can be present in all maternal DNA copies, which is termed as *homoplasmy* (identical mutated genome), or in some of the DNA copies, termed *heteroplasmy* (assorted population of mutated and normal genome) (Lashley, 2007; Skirton, et al., 2005). Thus, the percentage of mitochondrial genes with a mutation varies between cells and tissues, and explains the assorted phenotypes or variability of clinical manifestations observed in patients with the disorder (Turnpenny & Ellard, 2012). Whether symptoms of the disorder ensue will be contingent upon whether the quantities of deficient genes in the mitochondria are above the critical threshold and impede energy production in certain organs (Nussbaum et al., 2007).

Mitochondrial disorders tend to be progressive, and the age of onset fluctuates in families and individuals. Unexplained hearing loss, exercise intolerance, and generalized fatigue may be early symptoms and can prompt genetic investigation (Lashley, 2007). Also, a high incidence of mid- and late pregnancy loss is a common occurrence that often goes unrecognized (Chinnery, 2000). Laboratory investigations will find abnormalities in serum lactate, pyruvate after exercise, and ragged red fibers in a muscle biopsy in myoclonic epilepsy (Lashley, 2007). For example, a mother could have a child born that develops severe encephalopathy and suffers demise; subsequent genetic testing on blood and muscle discover a mitochondrial mutation. The mother is then tested and found to have the mutation in small levels solely in her muscle. Counseling on the advisability of future pregnancies is suggested because it is certain that the mutation will be passed on but the severity to future offspring is unknown.

Known conditions of mitochondrial inheritance disorders include Leber hereditary optic neuropathy (progressive visual impairment), myoclonic epilepsy, Kearns-Sayre syndrome (a neuromuscular disorder), and cardiomyopathies (Lashley, 2007). Genetic diagnosis and counseling can be difficult due to the complexities of the disorder, variability of symptoms, and the inability to give precise risk of passing the responsible gene on to the offspring (Skirton et al., 2005).

Mitochondrial inheritance criteria include the following:

- The mutated gene is located in the mitochondrial DNA.
- Inheritance is through maternal transmission and lost in paternal transmission.
- Males and females are affected in equal numbers.
- Variability in expression of the disorder is common; there is a wide spectrum of the disorders.
- Normal and mutated mitochondrial DNA for the same allele can be in the same cell (heteroplasmy).

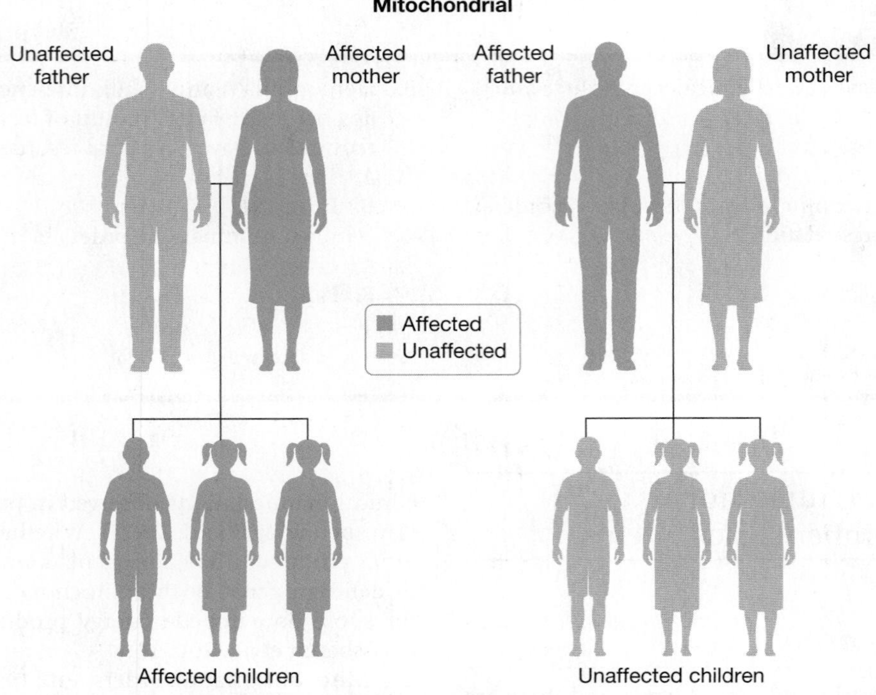

Figure 7–9 ■ Mitochondrial. In one family, a woman with a disorder caused by a mutation in mitochondrial DNA and her unaffected husband has only affected children. In another family, a man with a condition resulting from a mutation in mitochondrial DNA and his unaffected wife have no affected children.
Source: U.S. National Library of Medicine, 2011

- All children of homoplasmy mutations will inherit the mutation.
- Males will not pass on the mitochondrial disorder to their children.
(Lashley, 2007)

Mitochondrial disorders are triggered by mutations of mtDNA and maternally inherited. Some mitochondrial disorders affect only a single organ (e.g., the vision in Leber hereditary optic neuropathy), but many involve various high-energy organ systems and regularly present with obvious neurologic and myopathic characteristics (Chinnery, 2000). Mitochondrial disorders may present at any age, and variable clinical manifestations can appear in a family. Nonetheless, significant clinical inconsistency occurs and various persons do not precisely fit into single certain classifications. Common clinical features of mitochondrial disease involve dysfunction in high-energy organs and neurologic findings. An individual may present with exercise intolerance, cardiomyopathy, sensor neural deafness, optic atrophy, pigmentary retinopathy, diabetes mellitus, seizures, dementia, migraine, ataxia, and spasticity (Chinnery, 2000; Turnpenny & Ellard, 2012).

Mosaicism

The majority of the time when an individual has a chromosomal error it exists in every cell of the body. However, an individual may have different cell lines in a particular tissue of the body, through an error occurring during mitosis after fertilization of the zygote (Liang, & Schaffer, 2008). Mosaicism depicts the existence of cells that differ in their genetic constituent from other cells in the body. This occurrence would result in a person composed of two or more different cell lines. Mosaicism can occur in somatic tissue (affecting cells other than the gametes) or germ cells (affecting egg and sperm cells). Peculiar patterns of inheritance or phenotypic characteristics in an affected individual are accounted for by the phenomenon of mosaicism. (Turnpenny & Ellard, 2012). It has shown to have clinical implications in many disorders and plays a role in autosomal single gene defect disorders (Nussbaum et al., 2007).

A person who has a somatic mosaicism may or may not be affected by the disorder or have a milder phenotype. Only a minor proportion of the cells encompass the mutation, or the mutation is limited to a fixed segment of the body. Several genetic conditions have demonstrated somatic mosaicism such as NF1, cancer, and trisomy 21. Neurofibromatosis is a cutaneous genetic disorder that disrupts cell growth in nervous system and is characterized by high penetrance with a variable expression of the disorder. NF1 is sometimes segmented to one part of the body and may be caused by mosaicism (Turnpenny & Ellard, 2012). For example, an individual could present with multiple café au lait macules on the abdomen and Lisch nodules on the iris without systemic involvement. In such cases it is hypothesized that mosaicism results from somatic mutation occurring late in embryological development in contrast to an earlier mutation that caused widespread disease (Liang & Schaffer, 2008). When a mutation occurs very early in development, then it may be present in both somatic and germline cells and is called gonosomal mosaics.

Germline mosaicism can be detected with any inheritance pattern. However, it is typically appreciated with autosomal dominant and X-linked disorders, such as NF1, OI, hemophilia, and DMD (Nussbaum et al., 2007). Most parents are unaware they have a germline mutation until they have offspring that are affected. There is documented evidence of low-level germline mutations in OI and NF1 in the sperm of a percentage of clinically normal fathers that resulted in affected children with different mothers (Turnpenny & Ellard, 2012). The mutation is thought to be present in the parents' gametes (ovaries and testes) and will exist in every cell line of the developing fetus (Nussbaum et al., 2007). Therefore, the offspring will be affected with clinical manifestations and not be mosaic like the parent. The recurrence risk for parents with germline mosaicism for an inherited disorder can be challenging to predict due to the difficulty in testing the proportion of mutation in the germline cells (Liang & Schaffer, 2008). Thus, phenotypically normal parents of a child whose disorder is considered to be a new mutation ought to be counseled that the risk of reoccurrence is not negligible because they may carry the mutation in their germline (Turnpenny & Ellard, 2012). Furthermore, patients with mosaic forms of disorders or diseases should undergo a thorough physical exam of first-degree relatives, and appropriate genetic evaluation (Liang & Schaffer, 2008).

Genomic Imprinting

Genomic is an epigenetic phenomenon and defied the principles that genes on homologous chromosome were expressed uniformly (Turnpenny & Ellard, 2012). It is now recognized that genes inherited either from the mother or the father can result in diverse clinical distinctions; this is signified as genomic imprinting. Several disorders are associated with imprinting such as **Prader-Willi syndrome** and **Angelman syndrome** (see Figure 7–10a ■ and 7–10b ■). Both are caused by the deletion/impairment of the region on chromosome 15q11–13 (Jarvi & Chitayat, 2008). Prader-Willi syndrome is a deletion in paternal gene on chromosome 15 and is characterized by hypotonia, hypogonadism, childhood obesity, hyperphagia, aggressive behavioral issues, and failure to thrive in infancy. In contrast, Angelman syndrome is a deletion on chromosome 15q11–13 on the maternal side, which has entirely dissimilar clinical manifestations or phenotype. Children with Angelman syndrome are often autistic with a happy demeanor. They have other neurologic disorders such as seizures, speech, and gait abnormalities.

Unstable Repeat Expansions

An entire new category of genetic disorders has been studied, named unstable repeat **expansions** and present in everyone's genome. The most common repeats associated with disorders include the three nucleotides, which are cytosine (C), guanine (G), and thymine (T), and which have a customary number of permissible repeats. Normally, there are fewer than 20–40 repeats in the nucleotides in a given genome before abnormalities result (Lashley, 2007). The molecular device by which such expansion can result is not clearly comprehended but most likely owed to a type of DNA replication error known as slipped mis-pairing (Lashley, 2007; Nussbaum et al., 2007). The differences in the number of unstable repeats are due to the length, number, and degree, to which the nucleotides are unbalanced during meiosis or mitosis (Nussbaum et al., 2007). This number of repeats or errors in the genetic code of nucleotides explains if the patient is rendered normal, presymptomatic, or fully affected (Nussbaum et al., 2007; Lashley, 2007). Normally an individual can have up to 54 repeats of the CGG codon in the case of Fragile X syndrome. Premutation or presymptomatic would be considered a repeat codon number of 54–230 in Fragile X (Genetic Home

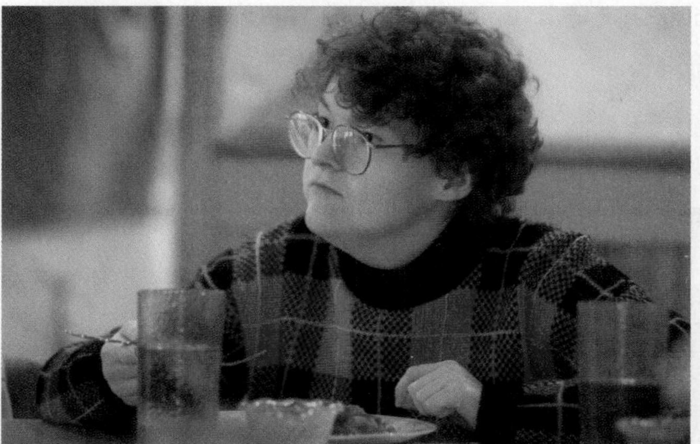

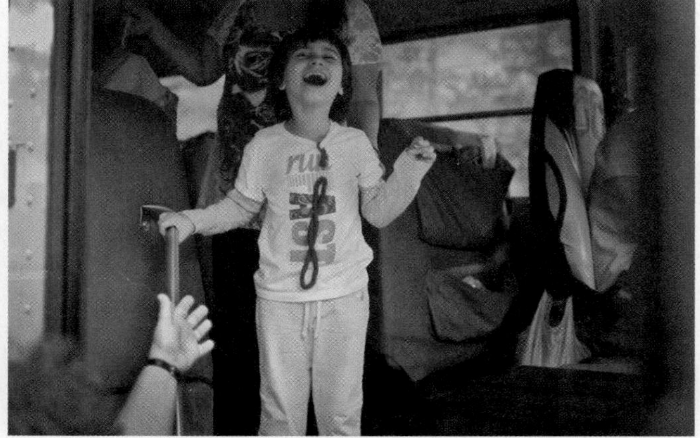

Figure 7–10 ■ Prader-Willi and Angelman syndrome are characterized by deletion of chromosome 15 with demonstration of imprinting. (a) In Prader-Willi, note the hypotonia and upslanting palpebral fissure; it is known for obesity, hypogondanism, and small feet and hands. (b) Angelman syndrome, or "puppet-like," is shown by abnormal gait, large wide mouth, and deep-set eyes.

RICH SUGG KRT/Newscom; The Washington Post/Getty Images

Reference, 2007; Read & Donnai, 2007). An affected individual would be an individual with > 230 repeats of the genetic codon (Genetic Home Reference, 2007; Read & Donnai, 2007). As the abnormal genetic codon is passed on from generation to generation, it can undergo **anticipation**; consequently, more severe symptoms of the disorder will arise (Read & Donnai, 2007). The majority of unstable repeat expansions disorders comprise neurologic conditions that possess a dominant pattern (Nussbaum et al., 2007). Certain well-known unstable repeat expansion disorders and the affected sites are Fragile X (CCG), congenital myotonic dystrophy (CTG), and Huntington disease (CAG) (Turnpenny & Ellard, 2012).

Fragile X syndrome is the most common hereditary disorder for mental retardation and is also associated with autism and hyperactivity. Fragile X is a mutation in the Fragile X Mutation Protein (FMRP gene). Fragile X syndrome occurs due to the unusual CGG repeats in the FMRP gene, with the major instability occurring during maternal meiosis (Turnpenny & Ellard, 2012). These abnormal numbers of repeats cause less FMRP production; the more repeats that occur, the worse the symptoms of the disorder. Fragile X has a classic phenotype, with a long face, high arch, macro-orchidism, prominent jaw, connective tissue weakness (mitral valve prolapse), striae, and hyperextensibility of joints. Female carriers can present with mild phenotype characteristics, and 50% with full mutation will show mild to moderate learning disabilities (Turnpenny & Ellard 2012). Fragile X is depicted in Figure 7–11 ■.

Huntington disease (HD) is characterized by a slowly progressive movement disorder and impairment of intellectual capacity or dementia during mid-life. HD has a variable age of onset, known anticipation in the CAG repeats, often complete penetrance, and small mutation rate (Turnpenny & Ellard, 2012). If symptoms present in early childhood or adolescence (juvenile HD), inheritance is often passed from the paternal side (Nussbaum et al., 2007). Interesting to note, HD was the first disorder mapped by linkage analysis using polymorphic DNA markers, and HD homozygous individuals are no more severely affected than heterozygous individuals (Turnpenny & Ellard, 2012). This phenomenon contradicts with other dominant single gene defects.

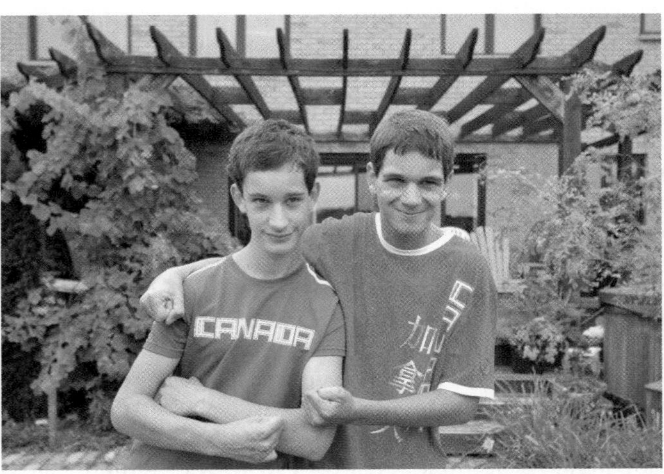

Figure 7–11 ■ Fragile X syndrome. Note the characteristic features: a long face, forehead bossing, and macrocephaly.
ZUMA Press/Newscom

Uniparental Disomy

In the case of uniparental disomy the child inherits both copies of a chromosome pair or chromosome region from the same parent instead of one copy of a chromosome inherited from both parents (Nussbaum et al., 2007). Thus, the child acquires both chromosomes from the mother or father. If no altered gene is inherited this might not be problematic. This can convert into a grave concern, especially if the parent is a carrier of a recessive disorder like PKU. The child would have inherited both mutated alleles from one parent and developed the disease even though the other parent is not a carrier of the disorder. Remarkably, many individuals who develop Prader-Willi syndrome and Angleman syndrome inherit the disorder owing to uniparental disomy (Nussbaum et al., 2007). It is also possible to have uniparental disomy for areas of chromosomes responsible for structural anomalies (Skirton et al., 2005).

SECTION FIVE REVIEW

1. Homoplasmy refers to the presence of more than one mutation in the mitochondria.
   A. True
   B. False
2. Most of the human genome is subject to imprinting.
   A. True
   B. False
3. In X-linked inheritance, germline mosaicism does not need to be considered.
   A. True
   B. False
4. In uniparental disomy, the child inherits both copies of a chromosome pair or chromosome region from the same parent instead of one copy of a chromosome pair.
   A. True
   B. False
5. Fragile X is the most common hereditary disorder that is associated with mental retardation.
   A. True
   B. False

Answers: 1. B; 2. A; 3. B; 4. A; 5. A

SECTION SIX: Implications for Nursing Practice

Genetic disease affects 5%–10% of children and 3% of the newborn population (Elias, 2003; Toomey, 1996). One-third to one-half of pediatric hospital admissions are due to a disease with genetic origins (Toomey, 1996). Achievement of the Human Genome Project in 2003 presaged the genomic era of health care (Elias, 2003). Research associated with the Human Genome Project has revealed that essentially the majority of diseases contain a genetic and environmental component, both of which contribute to a patient's well-being. It is acknowledged that some diseases transpire because of a specific or single gene mutation and hence are often inherited, such as the Mendelian single genetic disorders. Families are becoming acquainted with inherited genetic risks with certain disorders and pursuing guidance. Genetics is impacting every aspect of medical care with the advances in knowledge of the disease in relation to one's genetic contribution.

History and Physical Exam

Nurses need to be prepared to convey genetically proficient care in various health care delivery systems to individuals, families, and communities. Nurses in maternal–child health surroundings may be the initial health care provider to suspect a pediatric patient may have a genetic condition. Nurses are the main health care professionals at the patient's bedside and are often the first to obtain a comprehensive patient history and physical exam. The comprehensive history includes maternal pregnancy, neonatal period, family history, and history of current illness. By performing a thorough assessment, nurses may identify a genetic hereditary disease that requires further genetic testing and evaluation. Clues in the history and physical exam that may suggest a Mendelian genetic disorder but that are not inclusive would be consanguinity, abnormal fetal ultrasound, cutaneous disorders, hyptonia, seizure, growth abnormalities, developmental delays, and abnormal newborn screens. Nurses should also be able to complete and interpret a basic pedigree as part of a genetic history. This would enable nurses to have a better understanding of the pattern of Mendelian inheritance, so they can teach and counsel parents' further risks to their offspring.

Diagnostic Testing

Common laboratory and diagnostic testing are employed to detect Mendelian disorders, although diagnosis of genetic disorders is based upon both clinical manifestations and confirmation by genetic testing. Conventional newborn screening is performed in the perinatal setting. Parents who employ direct-to-consumer genetic tests may ask questions about test outcomes to nurses. Researchers recently developed new tests designed to simultaneously detect genetic mutations involved in more than 400 rare hereditary disorders (like Mendelian disorders) and screen prospective parents for mutations (Singer, 2011). In either instance, nurses must have knowledge of the procedure for testing, what the test is evaluating, and the ability to educate the family.

Genetic Competencies in Hereditary Disorders and Patient Advocacy

Pediatric nurses often care for children with genetic conditions, such as SCD and CF, who require repeated hospitalization. Nurses perform a critical role in the genetic referral, consultation process, and teaching. Countless times the nurse is the original contact with patients and families, as well as being the provider who delivers follow-up care. Nurses in maternal–child health settings and specialty clinics require genetic preparation to assist asymptomatic or symptomatic individuals and families who are progressively pursuing communication about their possibility for an inherited disease. For the aforementioned reason, nurses should undertake genetic literacy to acquire proficiency in the current genomic age. The American Nurses Association (ANA) and International Society of International Genetic Nurses (ISONG) have established genetic competency for the professional and advanced practice nurses. The ANA/ISONG statement on the scope and standards of genetics and genomic nursing practice is as follows:

> All licensed registered nurses, regardless of their practice setting, have a role in the delivery of genetics services and the management of genetic information. Nurses require genetics and genomics knowledge to identify, refer, support, and care for persons affected by, or at risk for manifesting or transmitting conditions or diseases with a genetic component. As the public becomes more aware of the genetic contribution to health and disease, nurses in all areas of practice are being asked to address basic genetics- and genomics-related questions and service needs.

These competencies are pertinent to the preparation and practice of all registered nurses, regardless of the clinical setting, professional role, or specialization. The proficiencies are defined by both organizations and are related to professionalism, clinical practice, family education, and support. By purely assimilating genetics into the nursing process, the

Emerging Evidence

As exhibited with these examples of the Mendelian disorders, understanding the genetic transmission of a disorder plays a critical function in diagnosing and managing the disorders. Persons with a solid family history of autosomal dominant disorders such as cardiovascular disease should be assessed with a distinctive approach in contrast to individuals with sporadic diseases (Kim, Devereux, & Basson, 2011). Significant clinical heterogeneity exists with all of the previously mentioned Mendelian disorders, and the manifestation of a strong family history is usually a foremost diagnostic benchmark (Kim et al., 2011). Recognition of the different patterns of diseases within a pedigree, comprising mode of inheritance and heritable disease risk factors, assists diagnosis of these Mendelian disorders. Genetic testing is obtainable for many disorders, which can explain the genetic risk; direction for management and prevention are available for individuals/families (Scheuner, Yoon, & Khoury, 2004). However, evidence-based guidelines need further exploration.

maternal–child nurse can advance the standard of care with the pediatric family. The maternal–child nurse should know specific genetic resources in order to provide education and health promotion to children and families with hereditary genetic disorders. Also, apprising families of what to anticipate from a genetic evaluation and reinforcing information attained during a genetic counseling and testing is noteworthy.

The nurse needs to be a supportive and patient advocate. A known offspring with a hereditary genetic disorder can produce an array of emotions. The parents may experience a sense of loss of a normal child. The family often feels emotions such as shock, anger, anxiety, self-blame, denial, and confusion. Certainly other family members may need to be involved in the genetic evaluation process, which can heighten emotions and family discourse. One of the important roles of the maternal–child nurse caring for the family is keeping the family abreast of consults being arranged, tests being performed, and clarifications of findings. The maternal–child nurse does not need to be a genetic expert. However, a baseline understanding of genetic hereditary disorders and genetic testing will support a family through this stressful endeavor. Ultimately, increased cognizance for genetic disorders by the maternal–child nurse will promote patient advocacy and family wherewithal.

SECTION SIX REVIEW

1. Nurses in maternal–child surroundings may be the initial health care provider to suspect a pediatric patient with a genetic condition.
   A. True
   B. False
2. Parents who have a child diagnosed with a hereditary disorder may feel symptoms of grief and loss.
   A. True
   B. False
3. Name some clues in a nurse's assessment and physical exam of patients that may alert to a hereditary genetic disorder.

Answers: 1. A; 2. A; 3. Mendelian genetic disorder, but not inclusive would be consanguinity, abnormal fetal ultrasound, cutaneous disorders, hypotonia, seizure, growth abnormalities, developmental delays, and abnormal newborn screens.

POSTTEST

1. Which one of the following genetic disorders is an example of imprinting?
   A. Duchene Muscular Dystrophy
   B. Factor V Leiden
   C. Prader-Willi syndrome paternal
   D. Tay-Sachs
2. Which one of the following symptoms is associated with Fragile X?
   A. Autism
   B. Obesity
   C. Short stature
   D. Delayed puberty
3. The newborn screen assesses primarily for metabolic and hemoglobinopathies disorders that are considered
   A. autosomal recessive.
   B. autosomal dominant.
   C. X-linked recessive.
   D. mitochondrial.
4. All of the following describes mosaicism EXCEPT
   A. Somatic mosaicism can result in less severe clinical manifestation of a single gene defect
   B. Disorders like Duchene muscular dystrophy , osteogenesis imperfecta and hemophilia have been associated with mosaicism
   C. The mutation is present in all of the germline cells
   D. The mutation is present in proportion of the gonadal cells
5. What single gene disorders can cause mental retardation? (Select all that apply.)
   A. Phenylketonuria
   B. Congenital hypothyroidism
   C. Sickle cell disease
   D. Achondroplasia
6. Consanguinity is an important issue in which inheritance pattern?
   A. Autosomal dominant
   B. Autosomal recessive
   C. X-linked recessive
   D. X-linked dominant
7. Which type of Mendelian inheritance is never transmitted from father to son? (Select all that apply.)
   A. Autosomal dominant
   B. Autosomal recessive
   C. X-linked recessive
   D. Mitochondrial inheritance
8. All of the following characteristics describe osteogenesis imperfect EXCEPT
   A. the majority of the types are autosomal dominant.

B. deafness is common.
C. frequent fractures.
D. mental retardation.

9. Maple syrup urine disorder and PKU are inborn errors of metabolism, and if undiagnosed can cause all of the following EXCEPT
A. mental retardation and seizures.
B. anemia.
C. hyptonia.
D. death.

10. What are the 2 autosomal recessive disorders mandated in 50 states to screen in the newborn screen at 48 hours of life?
A. Congenital hypothyroidism and PKU
B. PKU and sickle cell disease
C. Cystic fibrosis and congenital hypothyroidism
D. Turner syndrome and Fragile X

11. Which of the following symptoms are found in Marfan syndrome?
A. Brushfield spots
B. Shield chest with wide space nipples
C. Six or more café au lait macules
D. Pectus excavatum in the sternum

12. A mom discovered that she is pregnant with a male child. There is a maternal family history of factor VIII hemophilia (X-linked recessive disorder). What will you tell this patient regarding genetic transmission?
A. There is 25% chance of transmission.
B. There is 50% chance of transmission.
C. There is 0% of chance of transmission.
D. There is 100% chance of transmission.

13. Which of the following characteristics of Fragile X is true?
A. It only affects males.
B. It is the most common hereditary cause of mental retardation.
C. Most individuals die in infancy.
D. Physical disabilities are common.

14. The physical exam of a 6-year-old identifies seven smooth-bordered, light brown lesions measuring > 0.5 cm and irregular. To confirm neurofibromatosis, what other physical findings should be present?
A. Cataracts and axillary freckling
B. Dysmorphic facial features and low set ears
C. Errors of metabolism
D. Gait anomaly and paralysis

15. Which of the following is an X-linked dominant condition?
A. Cystic fibrosis
B. Hemophilia
C. Rett syndrome
D. Alkaptonuria

16. Which of the following terms refers to the fact that different people with the same genotype can have variety in phenotype?
A. Reduced penetrance
B. Variable expressivity
C. Incomplete dominance
D. Co-dominance

17. What is the most likely explanation for a set of unaffected parents having two children with a highly penetrant, autosomal dominant disorder? (Select all that apply.)
A. Variable expressivity
B. Co-dominance
C. Germline mosaicism in one of the parents
D. Reduced penetrance

18. Autosomal dominant conditions are due to loss of a genetic function or deficiency of an enzyme in the metabolic pathway, which often presents early on in the newborn period.
A. True
B. False

19. Anticipation is a finding in a genetic disorder in which the severity of a phenotype increases and age of onset decreases as some genetic disorders are passed through families.
A. True
B. False

20. Which of the following is true about mitochondrial inheritance?
A. There is heteroplasmy or homoplasmy.
B. The mitochondria segregate randomly as cells divide.
C. Mitochondria are maternally inherited.
D. The disorder occurs in high energy organs like the heart and kidney.
E. All of the above

21. A process that can greatly affect the presentation of an X-linked phenotype in carrier females is
A. interfering mutations.
B. X-inactivation.
C. mitochondrial disorders.
D. recombination.

Posttest answers are located in the Appendix.

CHAPTER SUMMARY

Only a single mutated copy of the gene will be needed for a person to be affected by an autosomal dominant disorder. Every affected person generally has one affected parent and both sexes are equally affected. Unaffected individuals do not transmit mutated alleles to their future offspring. Ailments that are autosomal dominant occasionally have reduced penetrance and variable expressivity, which means that although only one mutated copy is required, not all individuals who inherit that mutation go on to develop the disorder and there is variation of the disease in families (Turnpenny & Ellard, 2012). Autosomal dominant disorders are associated with advanced paternal age and with distinct malformations and physical features, and they involve a particular structural protein defect (Lashley, 2007).

Autosomal dominant inheritance criteria include the following:

- On a pedigree, a vertical pattern is displayed and often does not skip generations.
- Each person inheriting the disorder has one affected parent.
- Each offspring of an affected parent has a 50% chance of inheriting the disorder.
- Males and females are equally affected.
- Unaffected individuals will not pass onto future generations.
- Autosomal disorders phenotypes are often age dependent and less severe than autosomal recessive phenotypes and are associated with malformations and physical dysmorphisms.

(Gunder & Martin, 2011)

In autosomal recessive inheritance the disorder often skips generations and presents in offspring and siblings. The parents of the affected children commonly do not exhibit the disorder but are carriers of the mutated allele (heterozygous). Two copies of the mutated gene (homozygous) are needed for phenotypic manifestations and to develop the clinical disease. Each offspring often has parents who are carriers of the mutated allele. If both parents are carriers then their offspring have a 25% chance to inherit the disorder, a 50% chance to be carriers of the mutated allele, and a 25% chance to be disease free (noncarriers) (Jarvi & Chitayat, 2008). Unlike autosomal dominant disorders, the typical age of presentation is newborn or early childhood (Turnpenny & Ellard, 2012). Spontaneous mutation is rare and consanguinity more commonly presents than in other hereditary conditions (Lashley, 2007). Typical examples of autosomal disorders are many metabolic disorders and inborn errors of metabolism, cystic fibrosis, and hemoglobinopathies.

Autosomal recessive inheritance criteria include the following:

- Parents of affected children are often carriers and unaffected by the disorder.
- Autosomal recessive disorders skip generations.
- If two parents carry at least one mutation then each child has a 25% risk of having the disorder.
- If two parents carry at least one mutation then each child has a 25% chance of being unaffected.
- If two parents carry at least one mutation then each child has a 50% risk being a carrier of the disease.
- Autosomal recessive disorders affect males and females equally.

(Gunder & Martin, 2011)

Unlike the autosomal dominant or autosomal recessive mutations, which affect men and women equally, X-linked disorders affect more men than women. Women who present with the disorder inherit two mutated copies of the X-linked mutation (Jarvi & Chitayat, 2008). The majority of the transmission of the disease is from an affected man through his carrier daughters to his grandsons (Jarvi & Chitayat, 2008).

Y-linked or holandric disorders have little clinical significance and are male sex limited (Lashley, 2007). Y chromosome interstitial deletions have been associated with male reproductive disorders such as nonobstructive azoospermia (Nussbaum et al., 2007). Thus, all sons of an affected father will inherit the disorder, and the age of presentation varies (Read & Donnai, 2007).

Mitochondrial disorders are triggered by mutations of mtDNA and maternally inherited. Some mitochondrial disorders only affect a single organ (e.g., the vision in Leber hereditary optic neuropathy), but many involve various high-energy organ systems and regularly present with obvious neurologic and myopathic characteristics (Chinnery, 2000). Mitochondrial disorders may present at any age, and there are variable clinical manifestations in a family. Nonetheless, significant clinical inconsistency occurs and various persons do not precisely fit into a single certain classification. Common clinical features of mitochondrial disease involve dysfunction in high-energy organs and neurologic findings. An individual may present with exercise intolerance, cardiomyopathy, sensor neural deafness, optic atrophy, pigmentary retinopathy, diabetes mellitus, seizures, dementia, migraine, ataxia, and spasticity (Chinnery, 2000; Turnpenny & Ellard, 2012).

A variety of inheritance patterns has been presented. While some of the traditional patterns are predictable in a bulk of hereditary conditions there are exceptions to the rules. Other single genes disorders have established newly definitive inheritance patterns contrary to nontraditional inheritance patterns, such as mitochondrial inheritance, imprinting, mosaicism, and uniparental disomy. Genetic expression is diverse for some chromosomal regions and also contingent upon inheritance from the maternal or paternal origin. The complexity and discovery of genetic information is likely to continue. This will provide challenges to the health care providers in the role of interpreting family history and counseling with recurrence or probabilities.

CHAPTER SUMMARY (Continued)

Despite the sophistication of genetics studies and health care delivery, an accurate family history and exam remains the fundamental instrument for nurses to employ in patient care. A thorough nursing assessment and examination can provide clues to genetic disorders, like Mendelian or monogenic disorders. Other atypical or complex inheritance patterns should not be ignored and nurses should be familiar with mitochondrial mutations and germline mosaicism presentations. A family pedigree is an important tool the nurse should incorporate in the family history and assessment. The determination of the inheritance pattern can be identified in a pedigree and aid in the diagnosis of a Mendelian genetic disorder.

Nurses play an important role in genetic referral, consultation process, and teaching. Families coping with hereditary genetic disclosures require a formulation of choices, especially with a concern towards reproduction. The maternal–child nurse must keep in mind that families will need resources and help in gathering information to make knowledgeable decisions. Furthermore, understanding genetic inheritance maybe the first step in finding ways to improve health and provide innovative treatments and a possible cure. Thus, baseline genetic knowledge regarding hereditary patterns is a vital component for the maternal–child nurse.

CRITICAL THINKING CHECKPOINT

Case 1

Carol is a second child of Donald and Pam Green. Carol's older brother George is now 3 years of age and without any health problems. Carol however is a different matter. Her parents have been concerned from birth. She had a delayed meconium stool at birth. She was also very slow to gain weight and had frequent respiratory infections and cough the first few months of life. The pediatrician at first thought this was due to George being in daycare and developing frequent upper respiratory infections. At 6 months of age Carol was admitted to the hospital with respiratory distress and pneumonia. She had never doubled her birth weight despite adequate fluid intake and she was below the 5% in height and weight on the growth chart. Her bowel movements were also bulky and foul smelling. The physicians suspected cystic fibrosis and ordered a sweat test. The result was Na+ level 85 mmol/l, which is reflective of CF. The diagnosis was a shocking revelation to the family. The family requested to speak to a geneticist for guidance. Like most cases of CF, the clinical history and physical exam along with positive sweat test made the diagnosis secure. CF is an autosomal recessive disorder and caused by a mutation on chromosome 7 with the CFTR gene.

1. What further data should the nurse gather from Donald and Pam before referring the family to a genetic specialist?
2. What are the signs and symptoms of CF? The prognosis? Is it linked to any ethnic group?
3. Donald and Pam ask the nurse how CF can be genetic if no one in their family ever had the disorder. What is the correct response?
4. Donald and Pam ask if other family members should know and be tested. What is the nurse's advice? What type of genetic testing should the nurse suggest?
5. The family have inquires about new genetic treatments for CF. Search websites and other literature to learn more about CF and new genetic treatments or research.

Case 2

Ellen and Allen wanted to have children right after they were married. The couple was of Jamaican descent. Ellen became pregnant quickly but suffered a miscarriage at 10 weeks. The next pregnancy was 6 months later but the ultrasound scan at 30 weeks showed the baby was very small. The couple was not concerned since they were both of short stature and petite. However, when their daughter Helen was born at 37 weeks gestation, the couple knew something was troublesome. The neonate's length, head circumference, and weight were well below the third percentile. On physical exam, the infant also had a heart murmur and dysmorphic facial features. The child was diagnosed with complex heart defect and critical aortic stenosis and was referred for a genetic evaluation. The nurse inquired further into the family history and discovered that Ellen's sister also had several miscarriages. Her aunt also had a child who died from a heart problem and stillbirth before she had a healthy child.

1. Based on the history, what kind of Mendelian disorder could this suggest?
2. What type of genetic testing would be part of the genetic evaluation?
3. What type of response or emotions might the family experience after a birth of a child with malformations and suspected hereditary genetic disorder? How can the nurse provide support for this family situation?

Case 3

Matt is the first son of June and Ryan. They have one daughter named Kyra. Kyra was quick with her developmental milestones and walked at 9 months of age. Matt seems slower in achieving his fine and gross motor developmental milestones compared to his sister. June associated it with being a boy. June took Matt to see the nurse practitioner during his 24-month-old visit. When comprising a history, June said that

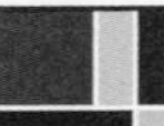

CRITICAL THINKING CHECKPOINT *(Continued)*

Matt did not walk until he was 20 months old. On observation, the nurse practitioner noted the toddler was clumsy, had enlarged calves, and when he got up from the floor, he rolled onto his hands and knees, using the chair to support some of his weight; and then he braced his arms against his legs (Gower's sign). Both the nurse practitioner and June were concerned about Matt's development. With further probing into the family history, the nurse learned June's uncle had died during his teenage years with DMD. The nurse practitioner referred Matt to a neurologist and geneticist.

1. What clues in this scenario suggest Matt has DMD?
2. What type of inheritance pattern is DMD?
3. What type of diagnostic testing confirms the disorder?

Case 4

Fred is 18-year-old high school student who is graduating and plans to attend college at the University of the Arts. He enjoys painting, sculpting, and going out with his friends. He admits to drinking alcohol at parties on the weekend. He always had good eyesight but within the last week he has noticed that his vision was blurred and the colors of the paints paler than usual. These symptoms cause his mother to bring him to see the nurse practitioner at the family health center. The nurse practitioner performed a complete history and physical exam. The family history is significant. His mother, Francis, is a healthy woman, but her brother has been blind since age of 27 years of age with optic atrophy. His mother's sister, Doris, also has serious visual problems, which first occurred when she was 45 years of age, and heart rhythm problems. Based on the presentation and history the nurse practitioner sent Fred to the eye hospital for ophthalmologist referral. At the hospital, the nurse read the report and found disk swelling (pseudoedema of the nerve fiber layer) and increased tortuosity of the retinal vessels. This combined with the history represents Leber hereditary optic neuropathy (Donnai & Reed, 2007). The ophthalmologist referred Fred to a geneticist due to his family history and clinical exam. Gradually over the next several months he has lost his vision, unable to paint and refocus his career.

1. What type of inheritance is Leber hereditary optic neuropathy? Will Fred's children be affected with the disorder?
2. What clues in history and physical exam suggest a hereditary disorder?
3. What would be an essential nursing intervention for Fred and his family?

Answers are provided in the Appendix

ONLINE RESOURCES

Cincinnati's Children's Hospital Genetic Education Program (1999–2011): http://www.cincinnatichildrens.org/education/clinical/nursing/genetics/default/

Genetic Home Reference: Your Guide in Understanding Genetic Conditions (2012): http://ghr.nlm.nih.gov

National Coalition for Health Professionals Education in Genetics (2012): http://www.nchpeg.org

Online Mendelian Inheritance in Man, OMIM (2012): http://www.ncbi.nlm.nih.gov/sites/entrez?db=OMIM

REFERENCES

American Nurses Association (ANA) & International Society of Nurses in Genetics. (ISONG). (2007). *Genetics/genomics nursing: Scope and standards of practice.* Silver Spring: MD.

Chinnery, F. P. (2000). Mitochondrial disorder reviews. In Pagon, R. A., Bird, T. D., Dolan, C. R., et al. (Eds.), *Gene Reviews*. Seattle, WA: University of Washington, Seattle.

Elias, E. R. (2003). Genetic evaluation in the newborn. *Neoreviews, 4*, 10, 277–282.

Genetic Home Reference (2007). *Cystic fibrosis.* Retrieved March 9, 2012, from http://www.ncbi.nlm.nih.gov/condition/cystic-fibrosis

Genetic Home Reference (2007). *Fragile X syndrome*. Retrieved February, 14, 2012, from http://www.ncbi.nlm.nih.gov/condition/fragile-x-syndrome

Gunder, L., & Martin S. (2011). *Essentials of medical genetics for health professionals.* Sudbury, MA: Jones and Bartlett.

Jarvi, K., & Chitayat, D. (2008). The genetics you never knew: A genetics primer. *Urologic Clinics,* 35, 243–256.

Jones, K. L. (2006). *Smith's recognizable patterns of human malformation* (6th ed.). Philadelphia, PA: Elsevier.

Jordie, L., Carey, J. C., Bamshad, M. J., & White, R. L. (2001). *Medical genetics* (2nd ed.). Mosby. Retrieved August 11, 2011, from http://medgen.genetics.utah.edu/index.htm

Kim, L., Devereux, R., & Basson, C. (2011). Impact of genetic insights into mendelain disease on cardiovascular clinical practice. *Circulation, 143,* 544–550.

Lashley, F. R. (2007). *Essentials of medical genetics in nursing practice.* New York, NY: Springer.

Leung, A., Pacuad, D., & Lemay, F. (2005). Boy with blue sclerae: What is your diagnosis? *Consultant for Pediatricians, 4*(7), 331–335.

Lewis, R. (2007). *Human genetics: concepts and applications* (7th ed.). New York, NY: McGraw Hill, pp. 75–85.

Liang, C., & Schaffer, J. (2008). Mosiac neurofibromatosis type 1. Dermatology Online Journal, 14(5), 6. Retrieved January 12, 2012, from http://dermatology-s10.cdlib.org/145/nyu/cases/041707-2html

Nussbaum, R. L., McInnes, R. R., & Willard, H. F. (2007). *Thompson & Thompson genetics in medicine* (7th ed.). Philadelphia, Pa: Elsevier, pp. 115–146.

Palmiera, B., & Sbelendorio, V. (2007). Duchenne muscular dystrophy: An update part II. *Journal of Clinical Neuromuscular Disease, 8* (3), 122–151.

Read, A., & Donnai, D. (2007). *New clinical genetics* (1st ed.). Oxfordshire, UK: Scion Publishers, pp. 220–248.

Scheuner, M., Yoon, P., &, Khoury, M. (2004). Contribution of mendelian disorders to chronic disease: opportunities for recognition, intervention and prevention. *American Journal of Medical Genetics: Seminars in Medical Genetics, 125C*(1), 50–65.

Simon, E. (2011). January 14. A test for 400 inherited disease. *Technology Review*. Retrieved March 1, 2012, from http://www.technologyreview.com/biomedicine/27054/page1/

Skirton, H., Patch, C., & Williams, J. (2005). *Applied genetics in healthcare*. New York, NY: Taylor and Francis Group.

Toomey, K. (1996). Medical genetics for the practitioner. *Pediatrics in Review, 17,* 163–174.

Turnpenny, P., & Ellard, S. (2012). *Emery's elements of medical genetics* (14th ed.). Philadelphia, Pa: Elsevier.

U.S. National Library of Medicine. (2011, August 22). *Your guide to understanding genetics*. Retrieved August 24, 2011, from Genetic Home Reference, http://ghr.nlm.nih.gov/handbook/illustrations

Zak, M., & Chan, V. W. (2010). Pediatric neurologic disorders. In S. M. Nettina (Ed.), *Lippincott manual of nursing practice* (9th ed.). Philadelphia: Lippincott Williams & Wilkins, pp. 1543–1573.

CHAPTER

8 Genetics and Fetal Development

Cindy M. Little

LEARNING OUTCOMES

Following the completion of this chapter, the learner will be able to

1. Summarize the development of the different key organ systems during pregnancy.
2. Differentiate between the changes in development during gestation weeks 3 through 38.
3. Discuss the development and function of the placenta during fetal development.
4. Describe the various factors that can influence or interfere with fetal development.
5. Identify the process and genetics in the development of fraternal (dizygotic) and identical (monozygotic) twins.
6. Discuss the chromosomal abnormalities that can occur in autosomes or sex chromosomes that may result in congenital anomalies or birth defects.

This chapter presents the process of pre-embryonic, embryonic, and fetal development and the genetic influences on prenatal development. The chapter covers **fertilization**, implantation, and pre-embryonic development that occur in the first two weeks of pregnancy. This includes development of the major components of pregnancy: the placenta and umbilical cord, the yolk sac, amnionic fluid, and fetal circulation. In addition, this chapter discusses the embryonic stage, which is between 2 and 8 weeks gestation and includes multiple gestation, as well as fetal development from weeks 9 through 38. It also includes both environmental and genetic factors that influence fetal development. This chapter provides information on how prenatal care maximizes the health benefits during pregnancy as well, and discusses fetal loss and nursing care for families who have experienced the loss of a baby.

PRETEST

1. Based on the last menstrual period, a full-term pregnancy lasts how many weeks?
   A. 28
   B. 38
   C. 40
   D. 42
2. Ovulation occurs
   A. 14 days after the start of the menstrual cycle.
   B. 14 days before the start of the menstrual cycle.
   C. midway between two menstrual periods.
   D. every other month.
3. The functions of the placenta include all of the following EXCEPT
   A. it provides a passage of essential nutrients for the fetus.
   B. it provides the exchange of metabolic and gaseous products.
   C. it produces hormones necessary for fetal development.
   D. it forms a barrier to microorganisms such as bacteria and viruses.
4. Identical twins are called
   A. monozygotic.
   B. dizygotic.
   C. conjoined.
   D. vanishing.
5. Based on the last monthly period, the ninth week marks the beginning of the fetal period.
   A. True
   B. False
6. Fetal movement felt by the mother around 16 to 20 weeks is called
   A. lightening.
   B. induction.
   C. quickening.
   D. dropping.

7. A congenital anomaly called a malformation is a(n)
   A. interruption of normal development process.
   B. alteration in form or shape resulting from mechanical forces.
   C. subnormal development of tissue that often affects several organs.
   D. a structural defect of an organ or larger body region.
8. An example of a numerical autosomal chromosomal abnormality such as a trisomy is
   A. Turner syndrome.
   B. Jacob's syndrome.
   C. Down syndrome.
   D. Klinefelter syndrome.
9. The purpose of preconception counseling includes all of the following EXCEPT to
   A. identify risk factors for complications in pregnancy.
   B. determine the best methods of contraception.
   C. assess nutritional status.
   D. screen for diseases that may be genetically transmitted.
10. A cause of fetal loss or demise is
   A. morphologic abnormalities.
   B. immunologic disorders.
   C. infection.
   D. All of the above

Pretest answers are located in the Appendix.

SECTION ONE: Fertilization, Implantation, and Pre-Embryonic Stage

Pre-embryonic development begins with the female reproductive cycle, which consists of an ovarian cycle and a uterine cycle. These cycles work simultaneously in a cause-and-effect manner. The ovarian cycle has two phases: the **follicular phase** and the **luteal phase**. The uterine cycle consists of four phases: the **menstrual phase**, the **proliferative phase**, the **secretory phase**, and the **ischemic phase**. **Ovulation** occurs approximately 14 days prior to the expected menstrual cycle. If fertilization does not occur, the cycle begins again on the first day of menses. During the follicular phase (days 1–14), **follicle stimulating hormone (FSH)** is released by the anterior pituitary in response to **gonadotropin releasing hormone (GnRH)**. FSH is responsible for causing the primary ovarian follicle to mature. During this time the follicle secretes estrogen, which augments the follicle's development in preparation for ovulation and contributes to the proliferation phase of the uterus.

The luteal phase (days 14–28) begins on about the 14th day of the cycle (in a 28-day cycle) and the mature **graafian follicle** appears. **Luteinizing hormone (LH)** contributes to the final maturation of the graafian follicle and ovulation occurs. The ovum is released near the **fimbria** of the fallopian tube and begins its journey through the tube to the uterus. Some women experience lower abdominal midcycle pain, known as **mittelschmerz**, during ovulation.

The ruptured follicle undergoes changes and becomes the **corpus luteum** and secretes large amounts of progesterone to maintain a pregnancy if fertilization has occurred. Approximately 7 days after ovulation, if fertilization has not occurred, the corpus luteum loses its secretory function, estrogen and progesterone levels drop, and the cycle starts again with a surge in FSH.

The uterus also responds to the hormonal fluctuations and coincides with the ovarian phases. Approximately a week after the onset of menses, based on a 28-day menstrual cycle, the vaginal bleeding subsides and the uterine lining known as the **endometrium** begins the proliferative phase (days 7–14) to prepare for a pregnancy. The endometrial glands become distended, blood vessels become dilated and engorged, and the lining thickens in response to increasing amounts of estrogen. During this time the cervical mucus becomes, thin, watery, and more alkaline and becomes more favorable to allow sperm to enter the uterus. The cervical mucus shows increased elasticity known as **spinnbarkeit**, which is measured in centimeters when stretched and is a sign that ovulation is occurring. Following ovulation, the secretory phase (days 15–26) begins and the secretory glands of the endometrium become thicker and more convoluted, endometrial cells accumulate glycogen, proteins, and sugars, vascularity increases greatly, and small amounts of endometrial fluid are secreted in preparation for implantation. The ischemic phase (days 27–28) begins a few days before menses if fertilization does not occur. During this phase vascular changes occur in the endometrium and areas of the lining become necrotic. Eventually the menstrual phase (days 1–6) begins with the shedding of the endometrial lining; however, the basal layer remains intact so the endometrial lining can regenerate and the cycle begins again (see Figure 8–1 ■).

Fertilization

Two to three hundred million sperm enter the female genital tract during a single ejaculation; however, only about 200 actually reach the ovum. The 3–4 cm of semen help buffer the acidic vaginal secretions. The sperm remain viable in the female genital tract for 2 to 3 days but are thought to be healthy and fertile for 24 hours. The ovum remains viable for 6 to 24 hours. Thinning of the cervical mucus caused by the high levels of estrogen allows sperm to move easily through the cervix and into the uterus. Transit time for the sperm to reach the ovum takes an average of 5–7 hours. Fertilization usually takes place in the **ampulla**, which is the outer third of the fallopian tube. Peristalsis, which occurs in the fallopian tubes, is also caused by high levels of estrogen that propel the fertilized ovum toward the uterus. This takes about 72 to 96 hours (Figure 8–2 ■).

The ovum is surrounded by a clear, thick, transparent, noncellular glycoprotein membrane called the **zona pellucid**, whose thickness can influence the fertilization rate. Elongated follicular cells called the **corona radiata** radiate from the

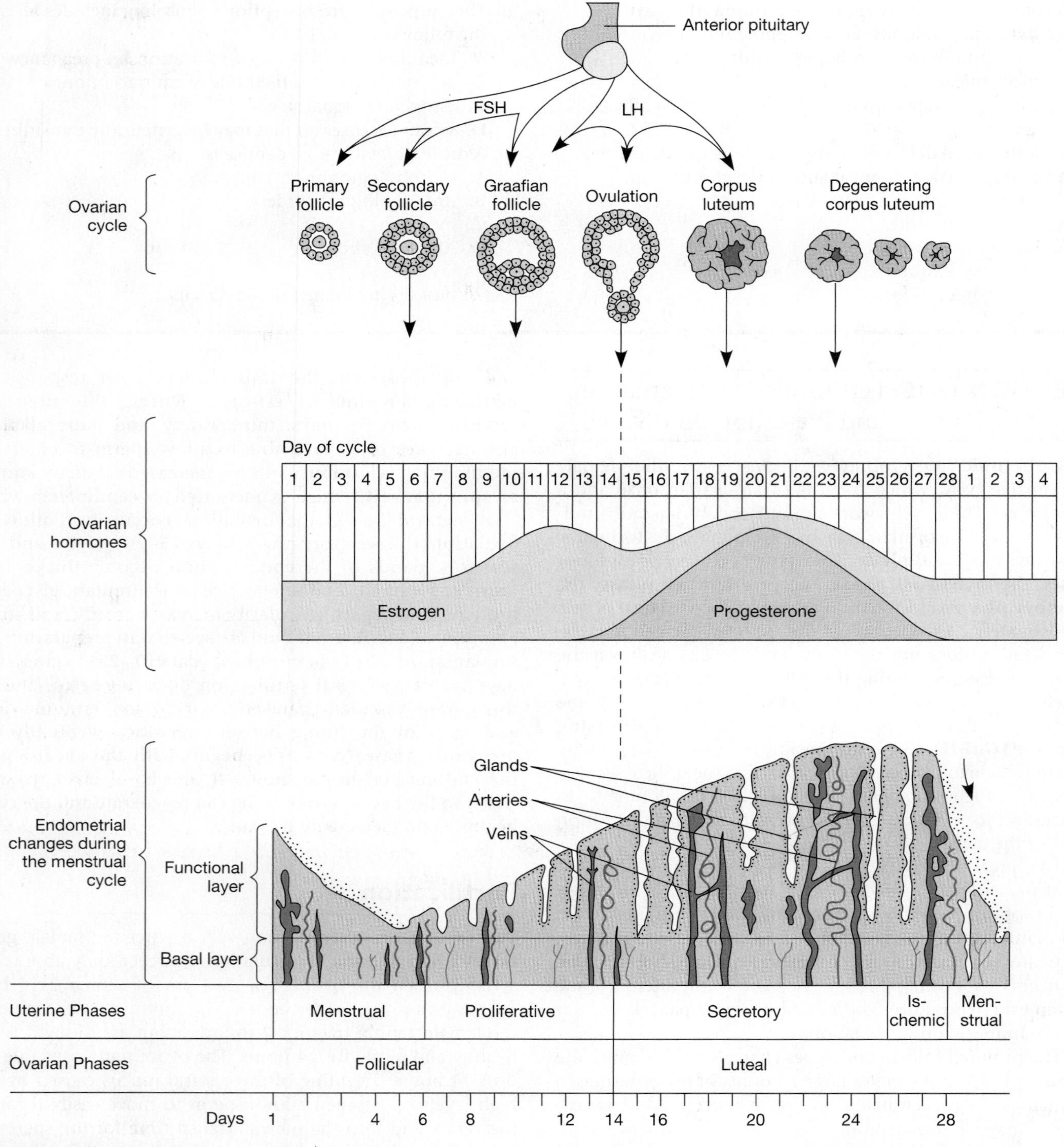

Figure 8–1 ■ The female reproductive cycle

ovum and surround the zona pellucid, and supply protein to the cell. Sperm must undergo the process of **capacitation**, which is the removal of the sperm head plasma membrane (**acrosome**), eventually causing a chemical reaction. Following capacitation is the **acrosomal reaction**, in which the acrosomes in the head of the sperm release an enzyme as they approach the ovum. Once this occurs, the sperm become *hyperactivated*. This process allows the sperm to break down the corona radiate, making it possible for only one sperm to penetrate the ovum. Once the sperm penetrates the zona pellucid, another chemical reaction occurs, causing hardening of the zona pellucid and preventing other sperm from entering the ovum. This is known as a **block to polyspermy** (Moore & Persaud, 2008).

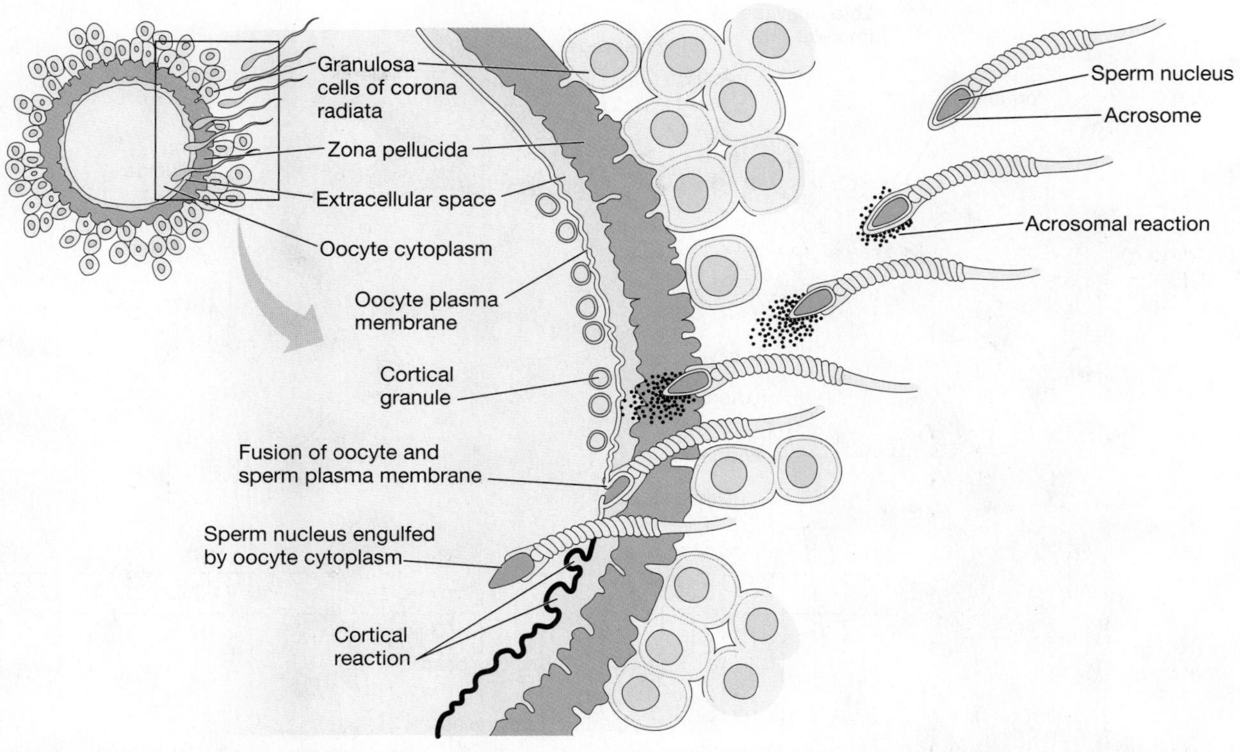

Figure 8–2 ■ Sperm penetration of an ovum

As soon as the head of the sperm enters the ovum, the tail and **mitochondria** degenerate. (This is why all mitochondria in humans are of maternal origin.) The nucleus of the sperm eventually fuses with the nucleus of the ovum, which at that moment produces a new single-celled individual, or **zygote**. The nucleus from each gamete (the ovum and sperm) contain a haploid number of chromosomes (23) and they join creating a diploid (46) zygote, which earns half of its chromosomes from the father (sperm) and half from the mother (ovum) (see Figure 8–3 ■).

The sex (gender) of the zygote is also determined immediately at fertilization. Females have two X chromosomes and males have one X and one Y chromosome. The gametes from a female contain only an X; however, the gametes from the male can be a Y or an X. If the ovum contributes an X and the sperm contains a Y chromosome, the resulting zygote is a male. The SRY gene (sex-determining region of the Y) located on the Y chromosome determines maleness (Lewis, 2010). The ovum contributes only an X; when the sperm contains an X chromosome, the resulting zygote is a female. Because X chromosomes are larger and contain more genes than the Y chromosome there are more X-linked traits.

The pre-embryonic stage begins once the ovum is fertilized and lasts for 14 days. As the zygote travels down the fallopian tube to the uterine cavity, cellular multiplication begins. This rapid mitotic division is called **cleavage** and the cells continuously double, forming new cells called **blastomeres**, within the zona pellucida. When cleavage has produced 16 cells it forms a solid ball called the **morula**. The morula continues to develop for approximately 24 hours until it contains 16–32 cells. The formation of a cavity caused by an increase in intracellular fluid begins to transform the cells to a solid mass of cells creating a blastocyst. Some of the cells differentiate to form the **trophoblast**, which replaces the zona pellucid and eventually develops into one of the embryonic membranes, the **chorion**. The blastocyst develops into an embryonic disc, which will continue developing into the fetus and the **amnionic membrane** (Moore & Persaud, 2008).

Implantation

The blastocyst partially imbeds itself into the endometrium by the beginning of the second week. During this time the exchange of oxygen and carbon dioxide occurs by diffusion. By the second week, the blastocyst continues to penetrate into the endometrial capillaries until it is completely covered and the trophoblast connects with the endometrium for more nourishment while preparing for the development of what will become the **chorionic villi**.

The endometrium increases in thickness and vascularity starting in the proliferative phase of the menstrual cycle and continues under the influence of progesterone from the corpus luteum now that fertilization has occurred. Once implantation takes place the endometrium is called the **decidua** and consists of three layers: the **decidua capsularis**, the part that covers the blastocyst; the **decidua basalis**, the part under the implanted blastocyst that becomes the maternal part of the placenta; and the **decidua vera**, the part that lines the uterine cavity. The chorionic villi will connect with the deciduas basalis to form the fetal part of the placenta.

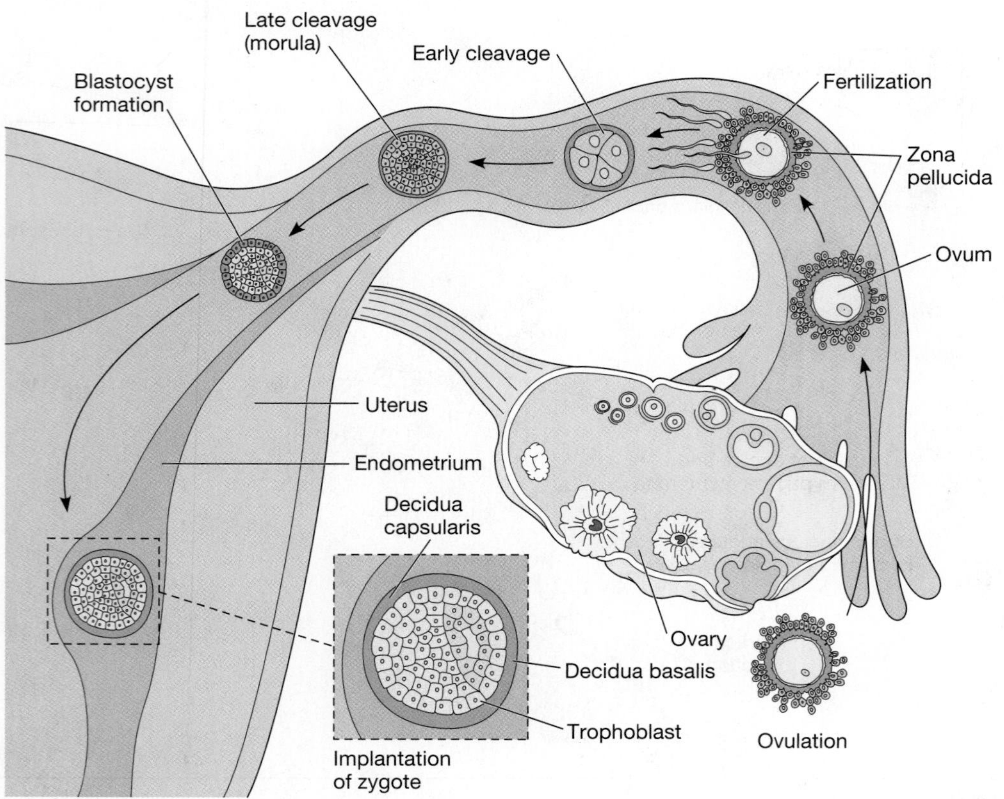

Figure 8–3 ■ During ovulation, the ovum leaves the ovary and enters the fallopian tube

After implantation, the embryo releases **human chorionic gonadotropins (hCG)**. hCG rapidly increases within the first 4 weeks of pregnancy. The hCG signals the corpus luteum to continue secreting progesterone thereby supporting a thick endometrium for the zygote and maintaining the pregnancy until the placenta is large enough to secrete progesterone.

Multifetal Pregnancy

A multifetal pregnancy has a higher risk of fetal morbidity and mortality than does a single pregnancy. The incidence of multiple gestation has increased in the past three decades, partly because of assisted reproductive technologies (**ART**) and the use of ovulation induction (OI) to treat infertility. The natural development of twins occurs in about 1 in 81 pregnancies (Lewis, 2008). Triplets or higher order multiple births increased more than 400% during the 1980s and 1990s. One factor thought to be responsible for this rise is delayed childbearing. Fertility starts to decline around age 32 and older women are seeking ART for help in getting pregnant (Little, 2010).

Multiples occur early in embryonic development. Twins that originate from two zygotes are fraternal or **dizygotic (DZ)** and are the result of two oocytes fertilized by two different sperm. This can be the result of both ovaries ovulating in the same month or two oocytes being released from the same ovary and fertilized by two separate sperm. DZ twins can be the same gender or opposite gender, do not share the same phenotypes, and are no more alike than any two siblings born at different times. DZ twins always have two placentas, two amnions, and two chorions; however, the chorions and placentas may be fused. DZ twinning shows a familial pattern possibly because of the mother's genotype. Some women ovulate two oocytes in a month (double ovulation) (Lewis, 2008).

Identical or **monozygotic** twins (**MZ**) develop from a single fertilized oocyte and develop from one zygote. They are genetically identical, are of the same gender, and have the same phenotype (appearance). MZ twinning originates in one of three points of development. About one-third experience early division of the embryonic blastomeres during the first three days of development. These twins have separate amnions (**diamniotic**), separate chorions (**dichorionic**), and possibly two separate placentas (although the placentas may be fused). If the division of the inner cell mass of the blastocyst occurs after day 5 but before day 9 when the chorionic cells have differentiated but the amnion cells have not,

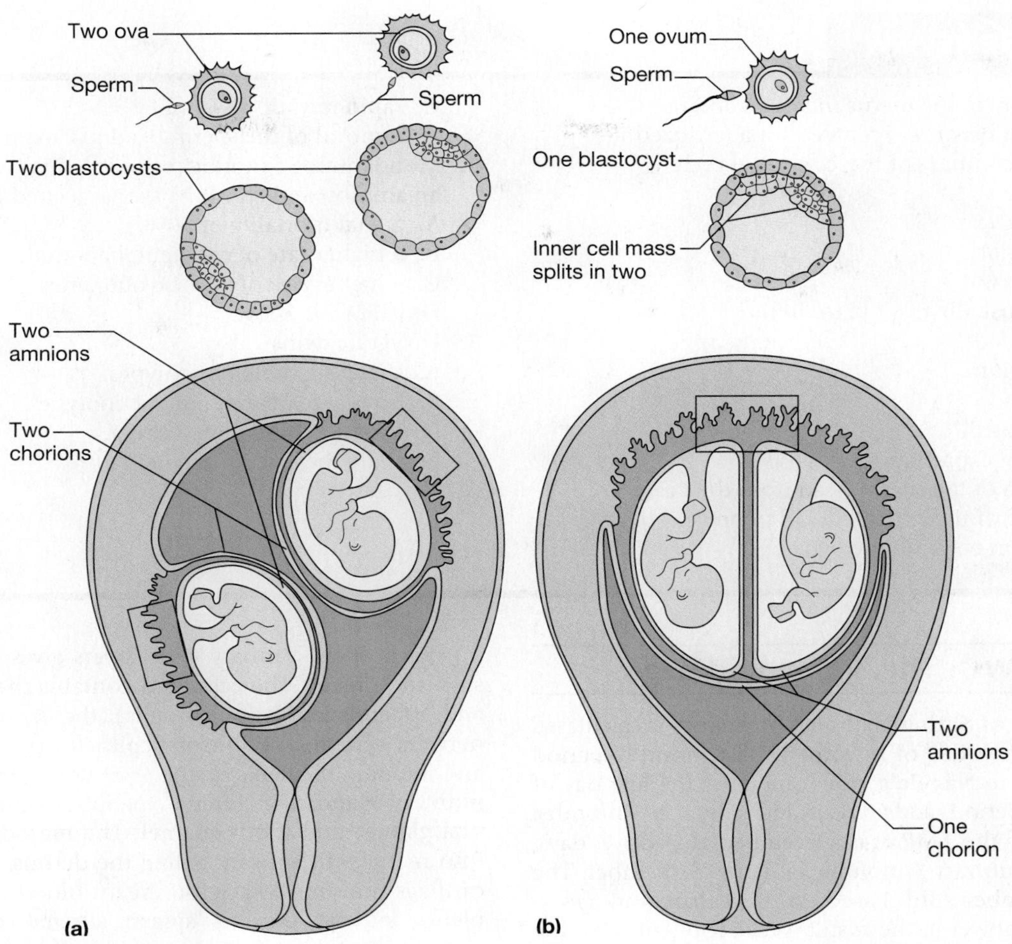

Figure 8–4 ■ (a) Formation of fraternal twins (b) Formation of identical twins

these twins will share a chorion (**monochorionic**) but have separate amnions (diamniotic). This occurs in about two-thirds of MZ twins. Rarely, the embryonic disc will divide into two after the amnion and the chorion have formed on approximately day 7 to 13 following fertilization. This results in a shared amnion (**monoamniotic**) and a shared chorion (monochorionic).

A monoamniotic–monochorionic twin pregnancy is associated with a fetal mortality of 50% (Beckman et al., 2010). MZ twins have the potential for multiple complications. The umbilical cord can become entangled to the point where the circulation is interrupted and one or both fetuses can die. MZ twins have a higher rate of congenital anomalies and both twins may have the same birth defects. Other complications such as twin-to-twin transfusion syndrome and twin-reversed arterial perfusion put both fetuses at high mortality risk. Abnormalities within the placenta may cause intrauterine growth restriction or discordant fetal size. Occasionally a pregnancy is complicated by one twin who is acardiac and anencephalic or one with severely discordant structural anomalies in which the treatment is selective termination. Monochorionic twin pregnancies have a high risk for adverse outcomes, which may result in demise of one or both twins (Rand & Lee, 2009). Spontaneous loss of one fetus in a twin pregnancy is common and occurs in approximately 30% of twin pregnancies (Little, 2010). This phenomenon is known as **vanishing twin** and usually occurs in the first trimester (see Figure 8–4 ■).

Other multifetal pregnancies such as spontaneous triplet gestation can occur from one zygote and can be identical, or from two zygotes and develop into a set of identical twins and one singleton, or from three zygotes and be three separate (fraternal) individuals of the same gender or of a different gender. In rare cases, if the embryonic disc does not divide completely after the group of cells develops into two fetuses around days 13–15, the result is a **conjoined twin**. Most conjoined twins cannot be separated as they share major organs or other structures; however, some are connected by skin or other tissue and can be surgically separated successfully.

SECTION ONE REVIEW

1. The vascularity of the uterus increases and the endometrium becomes prepared for a fertilized ovum in which phase of the menstrual cycle?
   A. Menstrual
   B. Proliferative
   C. Endometrial
   D. Luteal phase
2. Fertilization usually takes place in the
   A. ovary.
   B. endometrium.
   C. ampulla.
   D. zona pellucid.
3. The process of capacitation involves
   A. separation of the sperm head from the tail.
   B. hardening of the zona pellucid to prevent other sperm from entering the ovum.
   C. rapid mitotic division.
   D. removal of the sperm head plasma membrane.
4. Monoamniotic-monochorionic twins (twins that share an amnion and chorion) are associated with
   A. a fetal mortality of 50%.
   B. a higher rate of congenital anomalies.
   C. a higher risk of adverse outcomes.
   D. All of the above
5. Dizygotic twins
   A. share the same phenotypes.
   B. do not share the same phenotypes.
   C. are always the same gender.
   D. share the same placenta.

Answers: 1. B; 2. C; 3. D; 4. D; 5. B

SECTION TWO: The Embryonic Stage

The expectant date of birth in a human pregnancy is calculated according to the first day of a woman's last monthly period (**LMP**). According to **Nägele's rule**, one takes the first day of the last monthly period, adds 7 days and subtracts 3 months. If the first day of the LMP was December 16, add 7 days, which is 23 and subtract 3 months, which is September. The due date is September 23rd. Based on this calculation, gestation is 40 weeks; however, the first 2 weeks correlate with the woman's menstrual cycle and development of the ovum, and fertilization and implantation actually take place after the first 2 weeks. The field of embryology considers fertilization of the ovum and formation of the zygote as the beginning of gestation, which calculates to 38 weeks. This chapter will use the embryology standard of calculation as 38 weeks gestation. The embryonic stages of development begin in the third week through the eighth week, during which time the human conception is considered an **embryo**. From the beginning of week 9 through week 38 it is called a **fetus**.

Organogenesis (2–8 Weeks)

Rapid development of the embryo from the embryonic disc takes place during week 3. During formation of the two-layered embryonic disc, a primary structure forms along the longitudinal midline of the disc that is known as the **primitive streak**, a longitudinal thickening of the epiblast that establishes bilateral symmetry and initiates the germ layer formation of the **ectoderm** and the **endoderm**. A third layer forms in the middle that is known as the **mesoderm**. This three-layered formation is called the primordial embryo and is also referred to as the gastrula. **Gastrulation** is the process of the two-layer (bilaminar) disc becoming a three-layer (trilaminar) embryonic disc. It is the beginning of morphogenesis, the development of the body form. Cells from each of these layers are destined to become a specific cell type (Moore & Persaud, 2008).

Each of the primary germ layers gives rise to certain tissues and organs. The ectoderm contains the epidermis (skin) and appendages (hair and nails), the central and peripheral nervous system, the sensory epithelia of the eye, ear, nose, and mouth, the lens of the eye, the mammary gland, the pituitary gland, the adrenal medulla, subcutaneous glands, oral glands, and tooth enamel. The mesoderm differentiates into many structures including the dermis, connective tissue, cartilage and bone, skeleton, heart, blood, lymphatic tissues, pleura, kidneys, muscles, spleen, adrenal cortex, ovaries and testes, genital ducts (which turn into the internal and external genitals), and the serous membrane lining the body cavities. The endoderm gives rise to the epithelial lining of the respiratory and gastrointestinal tracts; the primary tissue of the liver

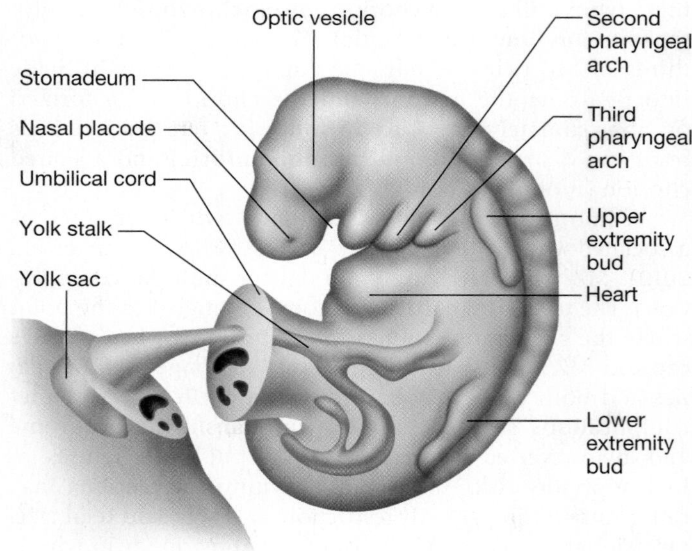

Figure 8–5 ■ The primordial embryo

and pancreas; urinary bladder; urethra and associated glands; vagina; parenchyma of the tonsils, thyroid, and parathyroid glands; the thymus; and the epithelial lining of the tympanic cavity, tympanic antrum, and auditory tube (Moore & Persaud, 2008) (see Figure 8–5 ■).

Development of the embryo depends on a coordinated interaction of genetics and environmental factors. Mechanisms that guide differentiation and control synchronized development include interaction between the tissues, controlled proliferation, regulated migration of the cells, and programmed cell death. Each system has its own developmental pattern. Cells, also known as stem cells, which make up early embryonic tissue, are **pluripotent**, meaning they have the potential to become any type of cell. Development of tissue from the cells occurs in response to cues from the surrounding and adjacent tissue, which is known as **induction**. This interaction between the tissue and cells is required for development and normal functioning of each organ (Lewis, 2008; Moore & Persaud, 2008).

Normal Development – Embryo

The embryonic stage starts at the beginning of the third week following conception and continues through the eighth week. During the third week, **organogenesis** begins, as stated previously, and the development of the body form begins with gastrulation, which gives rise to specific tissues and organs. The neural tube, notochord, coelomic spaces, and a primitive cardiovascular system and blood cells develop during this time. The neural folds fuse to form the neural tube. The notochord is a flexible, rod-shaped body that defines the primordial axis of the embryo and serves as the basis for development of the bones of the head and vertebral column. It eventually develops into the nucleus pulposus of each intervertebral disc. The coelomic space is a primitive cavity that will form three body cavities: the pericardial cavity, the pleural cavity, and the peritoneal cavity (Moore & Persaud, 2008).

At the beginning of the third week the blood vessels begin to form. The development of the cardiovascular system correlates with a decrease of yolk in the ovum and **yolk sac** and the urgent need for nourishment for the embryo. There is an urgent need for nourishment because the yolk sac cannot sufficiently supply it, so the placenta has to develop and kick in. The yolk sac produces primitive red blood cells between the 3rd and 6th weeks, when the liver begins making blood cells. (The yolk sac incorporates itself into the umbilical cord by week 10.) Blood vessel formation begins in the third week and blood cells develop from the endothelial cells. A primitive heart tube gives rise to the embryo's heart. This tube joins with blood vessels in the embryo to form a primordial cardiovascular system and is the first organ to actually function. The heart and cardiovascular system requires energy so the placenta has to grow and take over from the yolk sac that is decreasing in size. The heart begins to beat and the blood begins to circulate by the end of the third week. Finally, there is rapid development of the chorionic villi during this time, which greatly increases the surface area of the placenta and allows for the exchange of nutrients and oxygen between the mother and embryo.

In week four, rapid growth produces major changes in the body form. Longitudinal folding of the embryonic disc changes the straight form to a C-shaped curved form. Transverse folding occurs also as the right and left folds come toward the midline, changing the flat form to a cylindrical form. Upper and lower limb buds appear, and four pairs of branchial arches that will form the face and neck structures are visible. The embryo now has the rudiments of the ears (otic pit) and the lens of the eye. The lungs and kidneys begin to develop.

During the fifth week the extensive growth of the head exceeds the rest of the body, as shown in Figure 8–6 ■. This enlargement is caused by the rapid growth of the brain and facial structures. The structures for the face and eyes are beginning. Lower limb buds appear and upper limbs are paddle shaped. Development is cephalocaudal, meaning development proceeds from top to bottom or head to toe. The circulatory system and the heart show rapid development at this time.

The nose, mouth, and palate begin to take form, and the eye is now visible, as retinal pigment forms during the sixth week. The upper limbs begin to show differentiation at the elbows and hand plates. Digital rays, which eventually become fingers, begin to develop in the hand plates. The head is larger than the trunk and is curved over the large heart. Fetal circulation begins to be established. The lungs and the primitive skeleton have begun to form. It has been reported that in the sixth week, embryos have shown spontaneous movements.

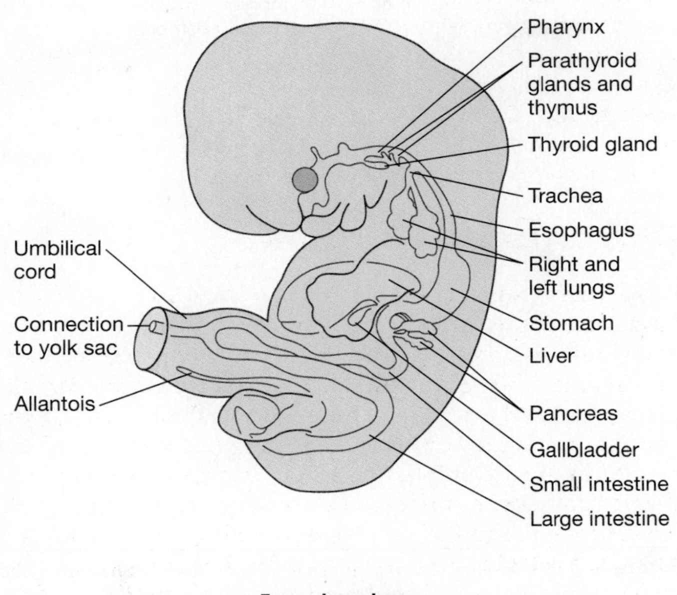

Figure 8–6 ■ The embryo at 5 weeks

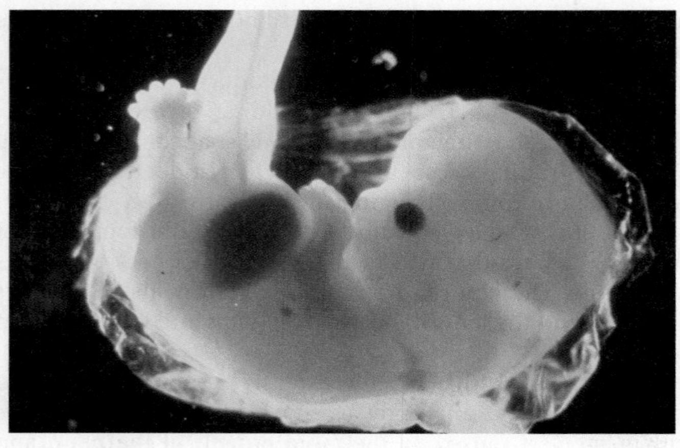

Figure 8–7 ■ The embryo at 7 weeks
Petit Format / Photo Researchers, Inc.

At seven weeks the embryo shows straightening of the trunk and the head is nearly erect. Although the abdomen is less protuberant, the gastrointestinal tract is experiencing many changes. The urogenital development is beginning. The eyelids are beginning to form, the external ears are evident, the tongue is developing, and early tooth buds are present. By the end of the seventh week the embryo resembles a human being, as depicted in Figure 8–7 ■.

In the final and eighth week of organ development, all essential internal and external structures are present. The head is more rounded and shows human characteristics. The facial features begin to develop, and the eyes and external ears assume their final shape. External genitals are visible, but gender of the embryo is not identifiable. Ossification of the long bones continues during this time. Maternal–fetal circulation is well established, as shown in Figure 8–8 ■.

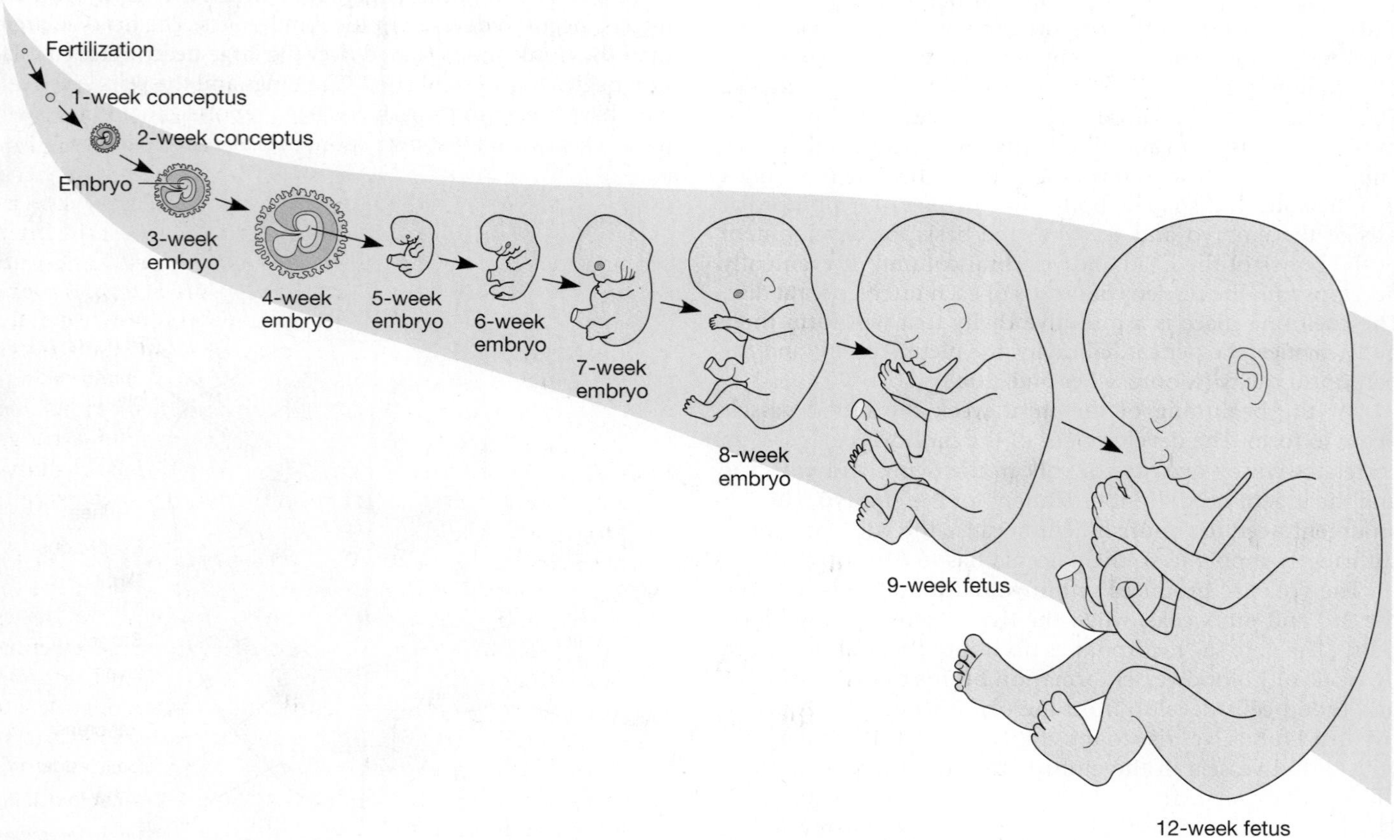

Fertilization
1-week conceptus
2-week conceptus
Embryo
3-week embryo
4-week embryo
5-week embryo
6-week embryo
7-week embryo
8-week embryo
9-week fetus
12-week fetus

Figure 8–8 ■ The actual size of a human conceptus, from fertilization to the early fetal stage

SECTION TWO REVIEW

1. Based on when fertilization occurs, the developmental stage that takes place between gestation week 9 through week 38 is called the _________ stage.
   A. embryonic
   B. fetal
   C. organogenesis
   D. primordial
2. The three germ layers from which all tissues and organs develop are all of the following EXCEPT
   A. the primary germ.
   B. the ectoderm.
   C. the endoderm.
   D. the mesoderm.
3. The fetal heart begins to beat in which gestational week (following fertilization)?
   A. 2
   B. 3
   C. 4
   D. 6
4. All internal and external structures are present in the fetus by which week?
   A. 6
   B. 8
   C. 12
   D. 18
5. During week 5 the extensive growth of the head exceeds the rest of the body. This is caused by
   A. enlargement of the bones.
   B. an increase in maternal hormones.
   C. the rapid growth of the brain and facial structures.
   D. an increase in the size of the placenta.

Answers: 1. B; 2. A; 3. B; 4. C; 5. D

SECTION THREE: Fetal Development

For clinical purposes, pregnancy is divided into three trimesters. The entire embryonic period and the first two weeks of the fetal period make up the first trimester. Each trimester is approximately 13 weeks. The 10th week postfertilization is the 12th gestational week, based on the date of the last monthly period (LMP) and the total pregnancy lasting 40 weeks. The ninth week marks the beginning of the *fetal period*. From this point on gestation is based on the LMP.

Structural Development

Placenta

As the trophoblast imbeds into the endometrium, it differentiates into two layers: the **cytotrophoblast**, or the inner layer; and the **syncytiotrophoblast**, or the outer layer. As the syncytiotrophoblast invades the endometrial **stroma**, hollow spaces called **lacunae** (the forerunners of the **intervillous space**) fill with embryotroph, a mixture of maternal blood and secretions that provides nutrition to the embryo. The cytotrophoblast cells proliferate, forming secondary and tertiary villi that completely infiltrate the decidua. As this is occurring, remnants of the decidua covered with trophoblast form the placental septa. The placental septa divide the placenta into 15–30 segments called **cotyledons**. The septa allows compartmentalization of the uteroplacental circulation; therefore, if an infarction or other pathology occurs in one cotyledon it is restricted to that space and remains localized.

Exchange of nutrients and gases across the placenta are minimal during the first 3 to 5 months of fetal development. Placental circulation consists of two separate circulations: maternal and fetal, as shown in Figure 8–9 ■. The placental membrane is made up of trophoblast, connective tissue in the chorionic villi between circulating fetal and maternal blood. Placental transfer, the transfer of nutrients and gases between the fetal and maternal circulation, takes place across the placental membrane. Maternal placental circulation takes place outside the maternal circulatory system. Maternal blood rich in oxygen and nutrients enters the intervillous space through the spiral arteries of the endometrium under great pressure that is produced by the maternal blood pressure. The blood is dispersed laterally and flows over the chorionic villi, allowing the exchange of materials between the maternal and fetal circulations. Waste products and deoxygenated maternal blood exits through the venous outlet. Placental perfusion can be altered by many physiologic changes in the mother or fetus, such as a drop in maternal blood pressure, tetanic labor contractions, or an increase in the fetal heart rate.

The placenta is designed to provide for and protect the fetus. The placenta is fetal in origin but relies entirely on the maternal blood to sustain life. Its main functions are to provide the fetus with oxygen, to provide passage of essential nutrients, to provide metabolic substances such as hormones for fetal use, and to allow for excretion of carbon dioxide and other metabolic wastes. The fetus acquires passive immunity from the maternal antibodies that cross the placenta; however, protozoal, bacterial, and viral infections can cross the placental membrane and infect the fetus.

Placental Transport Function. The placenta serves three primary functions: 1) It provides the fetus with exchange of metabolic and gaseous products, 2) it acts as an organ of transfer, and 3) it produces the hormones necessary for fetal development and maintenance of pregnancy. The methods by

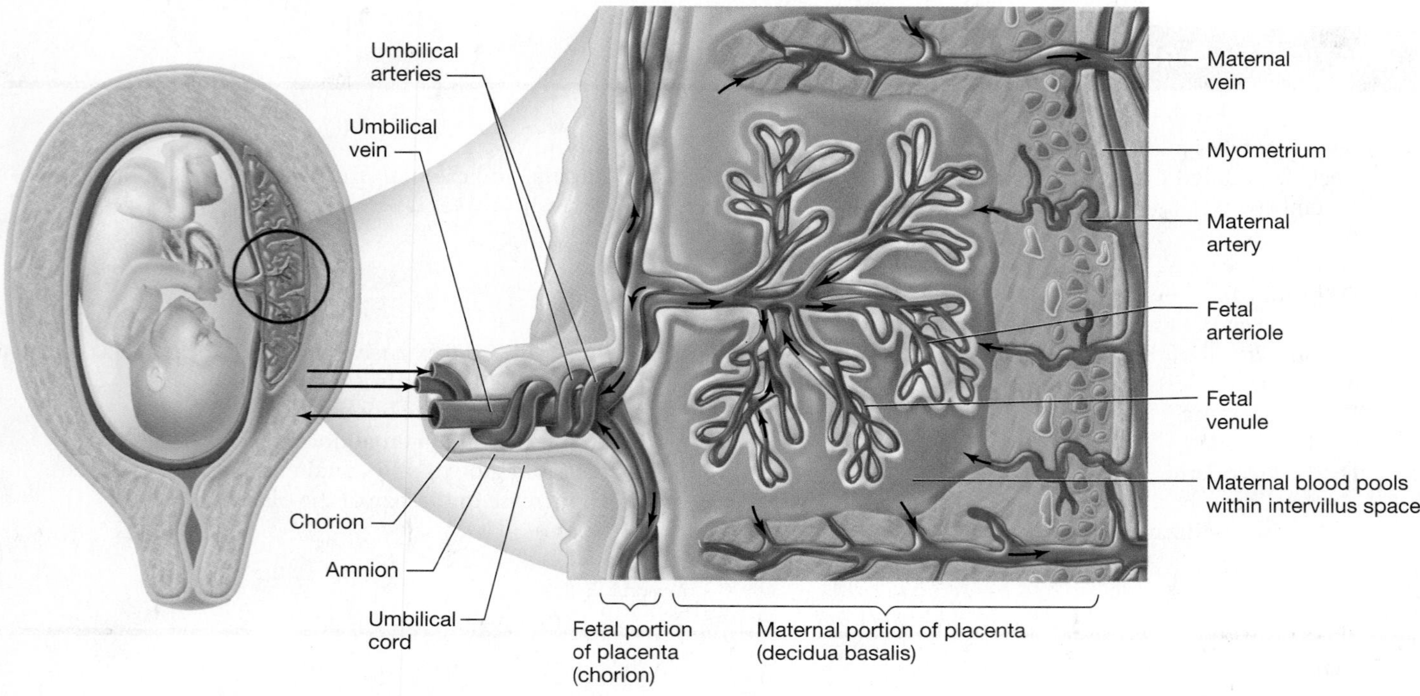

Figure 8–9 ■ Vascular arrangement of the placenta

which the placenta can transfer materials across the placental membrane occur by the following mechanisms:

- *Simple diffusion*: the passive transfer of materials from a higher concentration to a lower concentration. This mechanism is used in the transfer of oxygen, carbon dioxide, water, electrolytes, and drugs (both legal and illegal).
- *Facilitated transport*: the movement of molecules from an area of greater concentration to an area of lower concentration, which is facilitated across the placental membrane for more rapid or direct transfer. Glucose, galactose, and some oxygen molecules are transported by this method.
- *Active transport*: the transfer of molecules from an area of greater concentration to an area of lower concentration and back to areas of higher concentration against an electrochemical gradient. The placenta facilitates diffusion by active transport. Substances that are essential for rapid fetal growth but are low in concentration (including calcium, iron, amino acids, free fatty acids, carbohydrates, and vitamins) are actively transported across the placenta.
- *Pinocytosis*: the movement of molecules across the fetal membrane to become part of fetal circulation. The molecules are engulfed by amoeba-like cells, forming plasma droplets. This mechanism is used to transfer large protein molecules with a high molecular weight (such as albumin) and maternal antibodies (such as immune gamma globulin G).
- *Leakage (breaks between cells)*: the gross breaks in the chorionic villi that allow for passage of intact cells. The hydrostatic pressure gradient is typically from fetus to mother; however, red and white blood cells have been found to travel in either direction. An example is the sensitization of an Rh-negative woman who is exposed the blood cells of her Rh-positive fetus. Breaks are occasional and probably occur during labor or with placental disruption (Knuppel, 2007).

Placental Endocrine Function. The placenta synthesizes, produces, and secretes hormones that are vital to the survival of the fetus. These hormones include human chorionic gonadotropins (hCG), **human placental lactogen (hPL)** (which is also known as human chorionic somatomammotropin), progesterone, and estrogen. Following conception and throughout the first trimester, progesterone, which is provided by the corpus luteum of pregnancy, is the principal source of gestational steroids. Human chorionic gonadotropin is a glucoprotein that is produced by the syncytiotrophoblast of the placenta and signals to the corpus luteum to continue producing progesterone. After the 11th week the placenta provides enough progesterone and estrogen to maintain the pregnancy. Doubling values of hCG in early pregnancy is a reassuring sign that the pregnancy is viable. Conversely, abnormally slow doubling times could mean a bad prognosis indicating an impending spontaneous abortion or ectopic pregnancy. Human chorionic gonadotropin is thought to have immunologic capabilities to protect the placenta and embryo from being rejected by the mother. Concentrations of hCG peak at 2–3 months and decrease to a plateau that is maintained until delivery (Knupple, 2007).

Human placental lactogen (hPL) is also produced by the placenta and synthesized by the placenta's syncytiotrophoblastic layer. It is biologically similar to pituitary growth hormone—it is known as the "growth hormone of pregnancy." Human placental lactogen stimulates metabolic and lactogenic activity in the mother to assure that more protein, glucose, and minerals are available to the fetus.

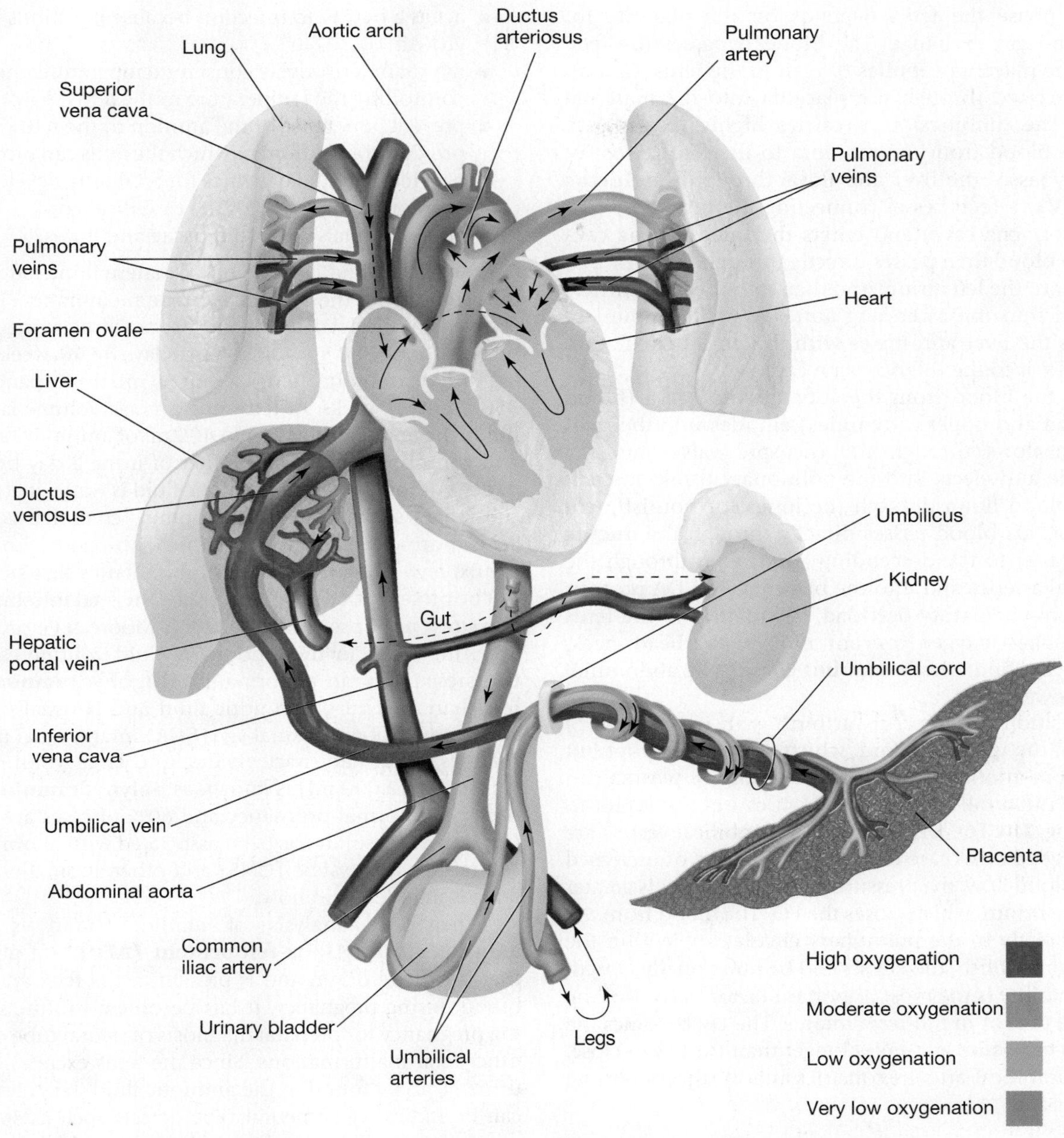

Figure 8–10 ■ Fetal circulation

Umbilical Cord

The thick embryonic body stalk attaches the embryo to the yolk sac and contains blood vessels—two arteries that carry blood from the embryo to the chorionic villi and a vein that returns blood to the embryo. The stalk becomes the umbilical cord that attaches the fetus to the placenta. An umbilical cord with only two vessels (absence of one artery) has been associated with chromosomal and fetal abnormalities, most commonly of the cardiovascular system.

Surrounding the blood vessels is a connective tissue called **Wharton's jelly**. This tissue helps to protect the umbilical cord from compression and kinking. The cord grows longer as the baby grows; at birth, it is about 50–60 cm in length and 1–2 cm in diameter. Occasionally a cord may be twisted or knotted, but in most cases this is not clinically significant as long as there was no damage to the blood vessels within the cord. Umbilical cord sampling under guided ultrasound can be used for prenatal genetic testing and other screenings and as a means to correct Rh isoimmunization in the fetus.

Fetal Circulation

The fetal cardiovascular system is designed to serve the fetus in utero and allows transformation to extrauterine circulation at birth (see Figure 8–10 ■). Fetal circulation has three phases: intrauterine, transition, and post-birth. During the intrauterine phase the fetus depends on the placenta for metabolic and gas exchange. The blood bypasses the fetal lungs, and the placenta supplies oxygen to the fetus. Carbon dioxide is excreted through the placenta into the maternal circulation. The umbilical vein carries highly oxygenated, nutrient-rich blood from the placenta to the fetus. Most of the blood bypasses the liver and flows through the **ductus venosus (DV)** (a fetal vessel connecting the umbilical vein to the inferior vena cava) and enters the inferior vena cava directly. This blood then passes directly through the **foramen ovale (FO)** into the left atrium and then into the left ventricle to be ejected into the ascending aorta. A small amount of blood enters the liver and mixes with the portal circulation and then flows into the inferior vena cava.

Most of the blood from the superior vena cava (blood from the head and upper extremities) empties into the right atrium, then flows through the tricuspid valve into the right ventricle and ejects into the pulmonary trunk. A small amount of blood flows through the lungs for nourishment only. Most of this blood passes directly through the **ductus arteriosus (DA)** to the descending aorta, then through the two umbilical arteries and into the placenta. The DA protects the lungs from circulatory overload. Circulation in the fetus carries the highest oxygen concentration to the head, neck, brain, and heart, and a lesser amount goes to the abdominal organs and lower body.

The transition phase occurs at birth with two events: 1) the cutting of the umbilical cord, which causes an abrupt but transient rise in arterial pressure, and 2) a rise in plasma carbon dioxide and a fall in oxygen, which causes the infant to start breathing. The FO, DA, DV, and the umbilical vessels are no longer needed and cease to function. Because of increased pulmonary blood flow, the pressure in the left atrium is greater than the right atrium, which closes the FO. The blood from the right flows directly to the pulmonary circulation. Within the first few days after birth, the DA should be functionally closed. Oxygen availability is the most important factor in controlling the closure of the DA in full-term infants. The DV becomes the **ligamentum venosum** and takes longer than the DA to close. Finally, the umbilical arteries constrict after birth, preventing loss of fetal blood.

Amniotic Membrane/Fluid

During implantation the embryonic membranes begin to form and surround the embryo and fetus. The thick, outermost membrane that forms from the trophoblast is the chorion. Between 7 and 12 weeks gestation, the amniotic fluid increases, causing the amnion to enlarge and bringing the amnion and chorion together. The amnion is a thin membrane containing amniotic fluid. As the two layers come together they form the amniotic sac, which is filled with amniotic fluid that protects the embryo.

Amniotic fluid contributes several critical functions in the development of the fetus. The primary functions of the amniotic fluid are to

- act as a shock absorber and cushion the fetus against severe injury.
- act as a barrier to infection because it inhibits bacterial growth.
- maintain a relatively constant temperature, thereby controlling the temperature of the fetus.
- prevent adherence of the amnion to the fetus, thereby providing a medium in which the fetus can move freely.
- provide essential enzymes for fetal lung development.
- prevent compression of the umbilical cord.
- allow for analysis of fetal tissue and fluids.

Amniotic fluid is made up of maternal interstitial fluid by diffusion across the amniochorionic membrane. Fluid is also secreted by the fetal lungs and by expelling urine. The lungs secrete about 300 to 400 ml per day. By 10 weeks the total amount of amniotic fluid is about 30 ml; this expands to about 350 ml at 20 weeks. At term, the average volume is 800 ml of fluid. The fetus swallows up to 400 ml of amniotic fluid per day and contributes about half a liter of urine a day by late pregnancy. Although 99% of amniotic fluid is water, it also contains substances such as sodium, albumin, epithelial cells, amino acids, hormones, enzymes, lecithin, sphingomyelin, bilirubin, vernix, and lanugo. Meconium, the infant's first stool, should not be present but can be excreted by the fetal intestines because of a stress response (Knuppel, 2007; Moore & Persaud, 2008).

Alterations in the amount of fluid volume can indicate the presence of an abnormality. **Oligohydramnios** refers to less than 400 ml of amniotic fluid and is usually associated with a small-of-gestational age (**SGA**) infant, renal tract abnormalities, or urinary tract obstruction. High volumes of fluid (more than 2,000 ml) is known as **polyhydramnios**. This can occur in a normal pregnancy and 60% of cases are idiopathic (unknown cause). It has been associated with anomalies of the central nervous system (CNS) and other anomalies where the fetus is unable to swallow.

Diagnostic analysis of amniotic fluid is done by **amniocentesis**. **Alpha-fetoprotein (AFP)** is a glycoprotein that is of fetal origin and is present in the fetal and maternal blood during pregnancy. It has become a routine screen during pregnancy for prenatal diagnosis of neural tube defects and other fetal malformations. Since the fetus excretes AFP in the urine it can be found in the amniotic fluid. High levels of AFP can be indicative of neural tube defects such as spina bifida, omphalocele, and gastroschisis. It also runs high in a multiple gestation. Low levels of AFP have been predictive for Down syndrome. AFP can also be used to screen for morphologic chromosomal abnormalities and inborn errors of metabolism. Cells from the skin, the gastrointestinal and genitourinary tracts, and the amnion are present in the amnionic fluid by 16 weeks. By the 11th week, karyotyping from the amniotic fluid can be performed.

Normal Growth and Development

Nine to Twelve Weeks

By the 12th week the fetus weighs about 45 grams (1.6 oz) with a crown rump length of 8 cm (3.2 inches). The fetal head is disproportionately large in relation to the body. The ears are low-set and the eyelids are closed. The face is well formed but broad and the eyes are widely separated. Tooth buds appear for the baby teeth. The fetus can swallow and make respiratory movement. The legs are not as developed as the arms and are not as long as their final relative length. The intestines have returned to the abdomen from the proximal end of the umbilical cord and the external genitalia are now easily distinguishable. Fingernails are present and the fetus can curl his fingers to make a fist. Red blood cells are produced by the liver. The kidneys begin producing urine and the fetus discharges urine into the amniotic fluid. The heartbeat can be heard; the normal fetal heart rate is 120 to 160 beats per minute (see Figure 8–11 ■).

Thirteen to Sixteen Weeks

During this period, rapid growth and development occur. The head is relatively small compared to that of a 12-week fetus and scalp hair patterning occurs during this time. Fine hair called **lanugo** begins to grow on the head. The external ears are close to their normal positions on the head. Ossification of the fetal skeleton is active during this time. The lower limbs have lengthened and limb movements become more coordinated and intentional; however, they are not yet felt by the mother. Reflex response and muscular activity begin. Fingerprints are now developed. The fetus opens her mouth, makes a sucking motion, and swallows amniotic fluid. The fetus begins producing meconium in the intestines. In females, the ovaries differentiate and contain primordial follicles. By 16 weeks, the fetus weighs 200 g (7 oz) and has a crown rump length (**C-H**) of 13.5 cm (5.4 inches) (see Figure 8–12 ■).

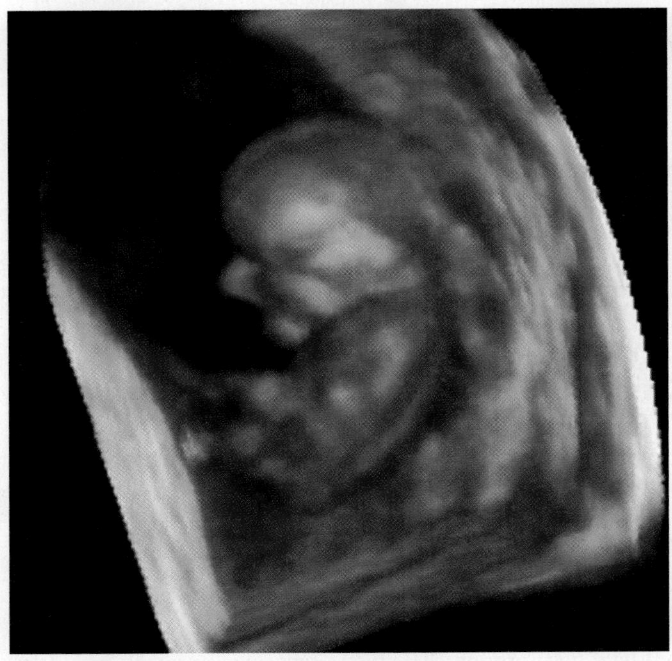

Figure 8–11 ■ The fetus at 9 weeks

Dr. Najeeb Layyous/Photo Researchers, Inc.

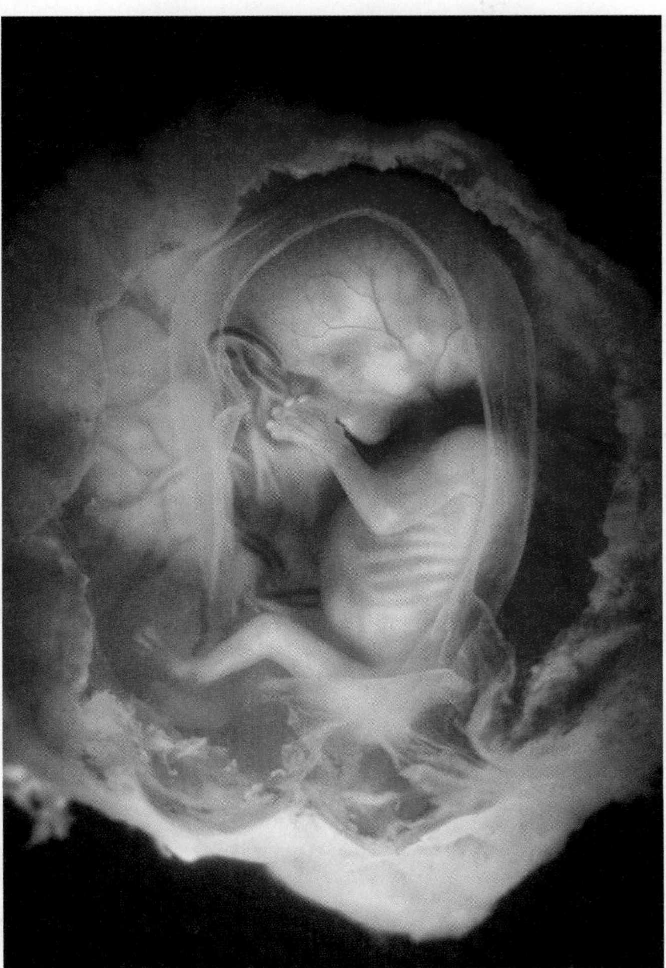

Figure 8–12 ■ The fetus at 14 weeks

Petit Format / Photo Researchers, Inc.

Seventeen to Twenty Weeks

This is a period of slower growth. The limbs are now in proportion to the rest of the body and the muscles are well developed. Fetal movement can now be felt by the mother—this is known as **quickening**. The skin is covered in a cream cheese-like coating called **vernix caseosa**, which is made up of fatty secretions from sebaceous glands and epithelial cells and protects the fragile skin from abrasions and chapping. Lanugo, the fine, downy hair found on the head, is now present all over the body and helps to hold the vernix caseosa on the skin. Brown fat, which forms in the base of the neck, posterior to the sternum, and the perineal area, is a source of heat production for the newborn. Toenails are now present and eyebrows and eyelashes are beginning to form. At 18 weeks the uterus is formed in the female fetus. At 20 weeks, myelination of the spinal cord begins. Also at this point, the testes begin to descend in the male fetus. IgG fetal antibodies can be detected. At 20 weeks the fetus has a crown to heel (C-H) length of 25 cm (10 inches) and a weight of 435 g (15 oz), as depicted in Figure 8–13 ■.

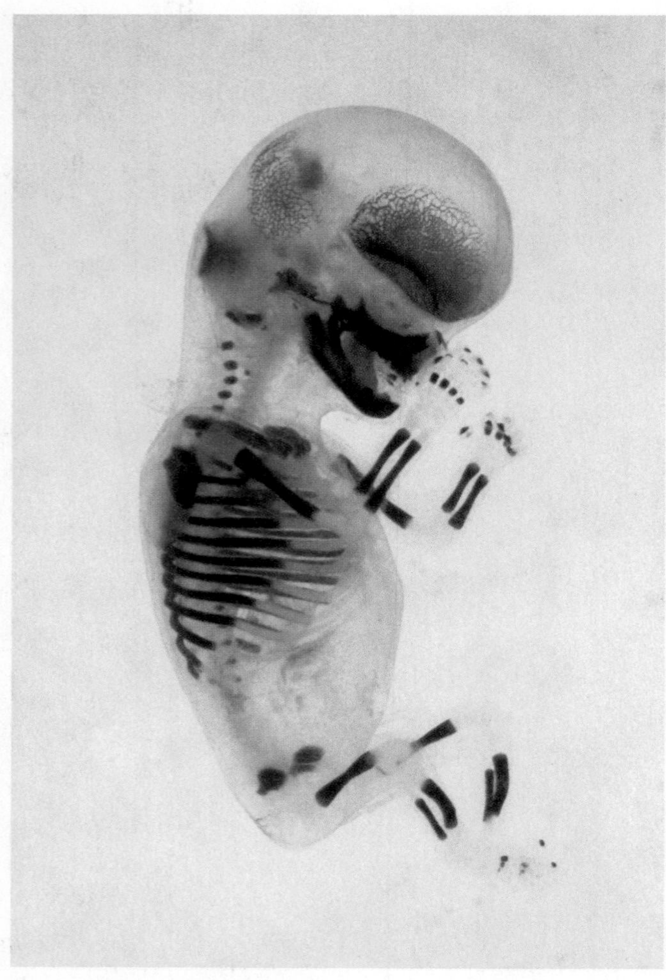

Figure 8–13 ■ The fetus at 20 weeks
Biophoto Associates/Photo Researchers, Inc.

Twenty-One to Twenty-Five Weeks

During this period there is a substantial weight gain. The skin is wrinkled and a translucent pink-red because the blood is visible through the capillaries. There is little subcutaneous fat. Bone marrow begins to make red blood cells. The fetus has a hand grasp and a startle reflex. At 21 weeks rapid eye movements begin. Eyebrows and eyelashes are fully formed. Teeth in the form of hard tissue are forming, which will become the second molars. IgG levels reach maternal levels. At 24 weeks, the interalveolar walls of the lungs begin to secrete surfactant. The fetus has a C-H length of 28 cm (11.2 inches) and a weight of 780 g (1 lb, 11 ½ oz) at 24 weeks gestation.

Twenty-Six to Twenty-Nine Weeks

The fetus now has vasculature of the lungs that are developed enough to provide gas exchange if he were to be born at this time. The CNS is mature enough that it can direct breathing movements and control body temp. There is considerable subcutaneous fat under the skin to help maintain body temperature. The eyelids begin to open and close. In males, the testes descend into the inguinal canal and upper scrotum. A fetus at 28 weeks has a C-H length of 35 cm (14 inches) and a weight of 1,200–1,250 g (2 lb, 12 oz).

Thirty to Thirty-Four Weeks

During this time there is a rapid increase in body fat and muscle. White fat makes up about 8% of the body weight and the fetus actually looks plump. The bones are fully developed but are soft and pliable. The CNS is developed enough to maintain body temperature if she were to be born now; however, the lungs are still not fully mature. The papillary light reflex of the eye is present at 30 weeks. More reflexes are present. The fetus begins storing calcium, iron, and phosphorous. At 32 weeks the fetus is 38–43 cm long (C-H) (15.2–17.2 inches) and weighs 2,000 g (4 lb, 7 oz).

Thirty-Five to Thirty-Six Weeks

The fetus starts to fill out and look "plump" and the skin is less wrinkled. He exhibits a spontaneous orientation to light and has a strong grasp reflex. At 36 weeks the fetus has a C-H length of 42–48 cm (16.8–17.2 inches) and weighs 2,500–2,750 g (5 lb, 8 oz to 6 lb, 1 oz).

Thirty-Seven to Forty Weeks

In the last few weeks, the fetus gains 14 grams of fat per day, and white fat makes up 16% of his total weight. As the fetus fills the uterine cavity, the amniotic fluid decreases to about 500 ml or less. The fetus is considered full term between 38 and 40 weeks. The skin is normally bluish-pink and the lanugo disappears. The chest is prominent, and mammary glands protrude slightly in both males and females. In a full-term male the testes are in the scrotum, and in females the labia majora is well developed. The earlobes are firm and the fingernails extend beyond the fingertips. There is a slowing of growth as birth approaches. The CNS is developed enough to carry out some integrative functions. The lecithin–sphingomyelin (**L/S**) ratio approaches 2:1 indicating lung maturity. At term, the fetus weights 3,200 g or more, and is 48–52 cm (19–21 inches) long.

Genetic Factors that Influence Fetal Development

Genetic abnormalities as well as exposures to certain toxins, radiation, and infections can cause congenital anomalies in the embryo or fetus. The time in which an embryo is most vulnerable to malformations caused by **teratogens** is during the first eight weeks of development. This is called the **critical period**; however, some organs, such as the brain, are sensitive throughout fetal development. The terms *congenital anomaly, birth defect,* and *congenital malformation* are used synonymously to describe structural abnormalities in an infant; however, there are four classifications of congenital anomalies: **malformation**, **disruption**, **deformation**, and **dysplasia**.

- A malformation is a structural defect of an organ or larger body region. It can result from abnormal embryonic development such as a chromosomal abnormality of the gamete at fertilization.
- A disruption is an interruption of a normal developmental process. A disruption cannot be inherited.
- A deformation is an alteration in form or shape resulting from mechanical forces and occurs in otherwise healthy tissue.
- Dysplasia is abnormal development of tissue that often affects several organs.

Birth defects are the leading cause of infant death, causing more than 20% of all infant deaths. Approximately 1 in every 33 babies (about 3%) is born with a birth defect (Heron et al., 2009). The causes of congenital anomalies are genetic or environmental factors or a combination of both, known as **multifactorial inheritance** (Lewis, 2008; Moore & Persaud, 2007).

Genetic Factors

Presently, a small number of genetic anomalies can be diagnosed early in pregnancy because of the availability of ultrasound and prenatal genetic testing. Genetic factors cause about one-third of all birth defects, and at least half of all spontaneous abortions are the result of chromosomal abnormalities. Chromosomal abnormalities are present in 6% to 7% of zygotes and many never reach the stage of cleavage. Abnormalities in chromosomes can be found in the autosomes and/or the sex chromosomes and are divided into two types of changes: numerical abnormalities or structural abnormalities.

Numerical Chromosomal Abnormalities

The most common chromosomal abnormalities are aneuploids, meaning there is an extra single or a missing single chromosome. These include trisomies and monosomies and are most often caused by nondysjunction, the failure of the paired chromosomes to separate during meiotic division resulting in an unequal distribution of a pair of chromosomes. The zygote will have either 45 or 47 chromosomes instead of the normal 46. The most common aneuploids are trisomy 13, 18, and 21. The occurrence of trisomies becomes more frequent as maternal age increases. Monosomies occur when one of the gametes is missing a chromosome and most are so severe that they cease to develop and die. An individual with mosaicism, having two or more distinct cell types containing a different number of chromosomes, may have a less severe phenotype or milder version of the condition (see Chapter 6). In some individuals, health may not be affected depending on which cells have the extra chromosome.

Down syndrome, or trisomy 21, was first described by British physician Dr. John Langdon Haydon Down in 1866. Clinical features can vary depending on the genotype. If it is caused by a mosaicism, the infant may not be severely affected. Typically, an individual with Down syndrome has dysmorphic features such as tongue protruding through the lips, small jaw and very small airway, high, arched palate, low-set ears, broad, short fingers, abnormal pattern of creases of the hands, loose joints, poor reflexes, epicanthal folds, and straight, sparse hair, as depicted in Figure 8–14 ■. Developmentally, people with Down syndrome are challenged, with varied degrees of mental retardation. Many experience medical problems including heart and kidney defects, hearing and vision loss, gastrointestinal problems, and a suppressed immune system. They are 15 times more likely to develop leukemia than a child without Down syndrome and are 25% more likely than the general public to develop Alzheimer disease after age 40. Currently, the average life expectancy is in the 50s.

Trisomy 18 is also known as Edwards syndrome and was first described by John Hall-Edwards, a British geneticist, in 1960. Trisomy 18 has three copies of chromosome 18 and most cases are caused by nondisjunction in meiosis

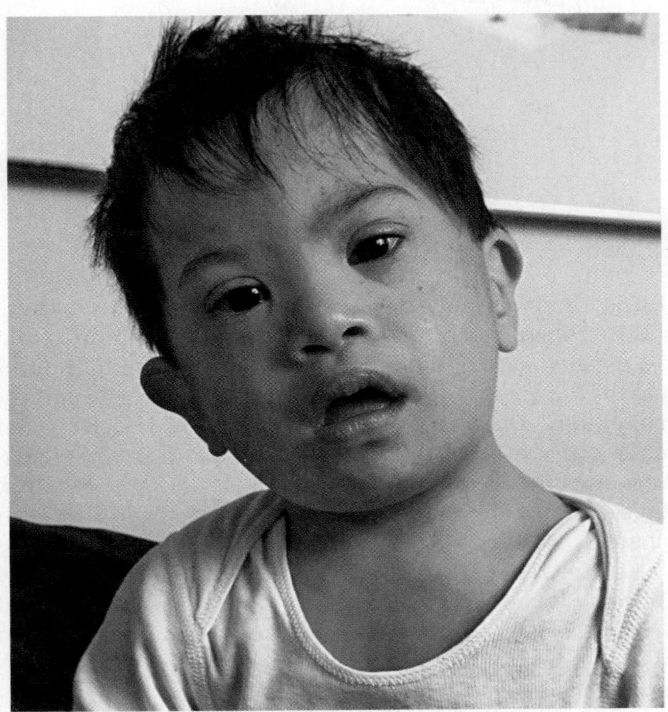

Figure 8–14 ■ Picture of a child with Down syndrome
George Dodson/Pearson Education/PH College

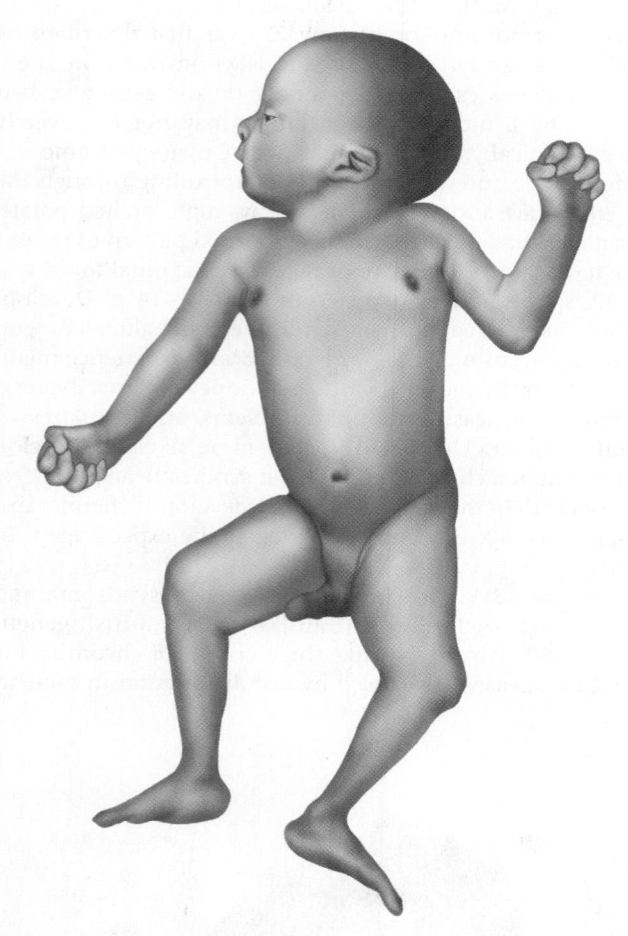

Figure 8–15 ■ Picture of a child with trisomy 18

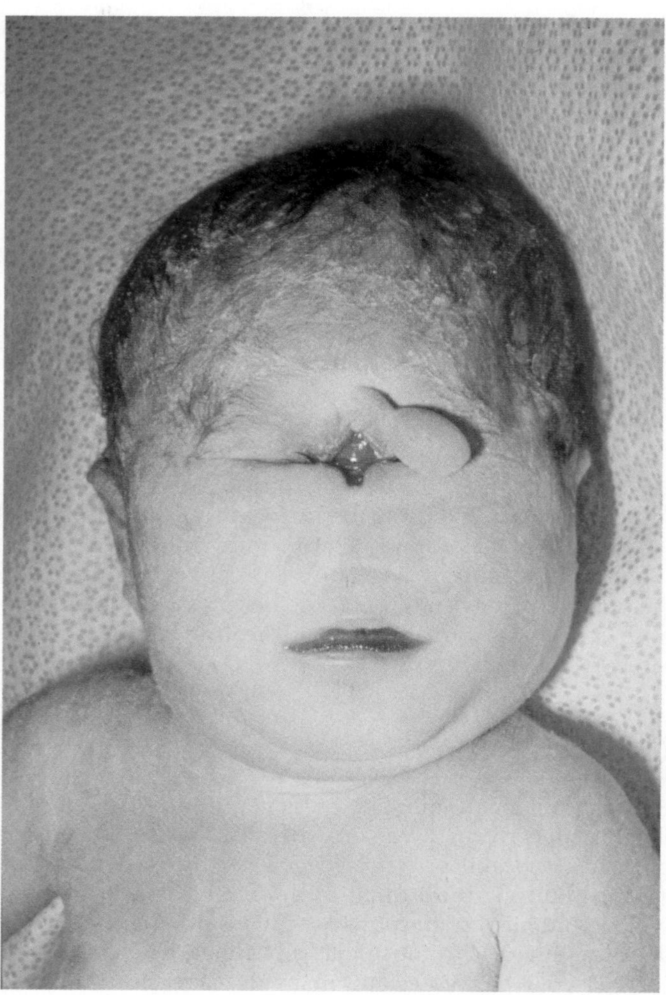

Figure 8–16 ■ Picture of a child with trisomy 13
Ralph C. Eagle, Jr./Photo Researchers, Inc.

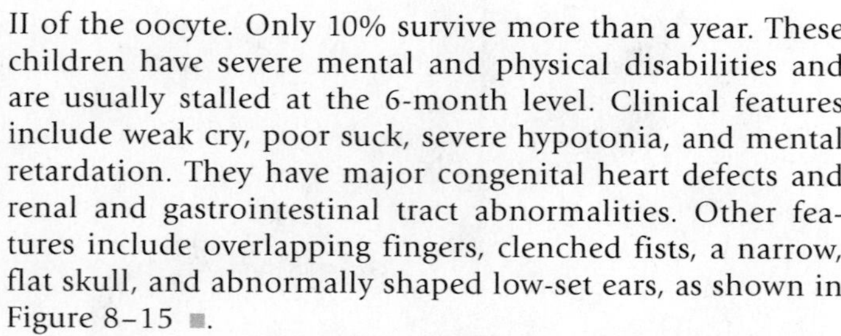

II of the oocyte. Only 10% survive more than a year. These children have severe mental and physical disabilities and are usually stalled at the 6-month level. Clinical features include weak cry, poor suck, severe hypotonia, and mental retardation. They have major congenital heart defects and renal and gastrointestinal tract abnormalities. Other features include overlapping fingers, clenched fists, a narrow, flat skull, and abnormally shaped low-set ears, as shown in Figure 8–15 ■.

Trisomy 13, or Patau syndrome, was first observed by Thomas Bartholin in 1657 but was later genetically identified by Klaus Pautau in 1960. Severe malformations include fusion or absence of the eyes, microcephaly, microphthalmia, malformed ears, micrognathia, cleft lip and palate, and polydactyly, as depicted in Figure 8–16 ■. Severe anomalies include the heart and gastrointestinal tract. Most do not survive the first year and do not progress developmentally past 6 months. The exception is if they are mosaic.

Numerical Sex Chromosomal Abnormalities

Trisomy of the sex chromosomes is more common; because there are no physical symptoms or characteristics in childhood, these may go undiagnosed until puberty. Most sex chromosomal abnormalities are the result of nondisjunction and are the type with an extra or missing Y or X chromosome. Disorders that have more X or Y chromosomes are extremely rare. Those with mosaic sex chromosome abnormalities have fewer and milder symptoms and fertility may not be impaired. The most well-known disorder of sex chromosome mosaicism is associated with women who took diethylstilbesterol (DES) during pregnancy. Uterine malformation, hormonal problems, and miscarriage are associated with daughters of women who took DES.

One of the most common sex chromosomal aneuploidy is Turner syndrome, also known as XO syndrome. In 1938, Dr. Henry Turner, an American endocrinologist, described several young women with short stature, broad chests, skin folds on the back of their "webbed" necks, low hairline, and malformed elbows who were sexually underdeveloped. It was later discovered that cells from women with the syndrome lacked a **Barr body**, a dark spot on the inactivated X chromosome indicating a second activated X chromosome. In Turner syndrome, one of the sex chromosomes (X) is missing or has some abnormality. Because two X chromosomes are required for normal sexual maturation, secondary sex characteristics do not develop. Occasionally one X chromosome is missing in some but not all of the cells. This is known as mosaicism. Women who have this mosaicism may have children but with a high risk of an abnormal number of chromosomes. Prenatal diagnosis is currently available by ultrasound or by karyotype with amniocentesis.

Sex chromosomal aneuploidys in males include Klinefelter Syndrome (XXY) and Jacob's syndrome (XYY). In males with Klinefelter syndrome, the most noted symptoms do not appear until puberty. They include tall stature with long arms and legs, large hands and feet, obesity with fat distribution of a female, development of breast tissue, speech and language delays, and reading problems. There is incomplete development of secondary sex characteristics and many are infertile. In Jacobs's syndrome the karyotype is XYY and can occur from nondisjunction in the male. In most cases the male is normal but may have some symptoms as tall stature, acne, and speech and reading problems.

Structural Chromosomal Abnormalities

Abnormalities in the structure of a chromosome results from breakage of the chromosome that is repaired incorrectly or rearranged (see Figure 8–17 ■). These abnormalities can occur as translocations, inversions, deletions, or duplications. (These are explained in detail in Chapter 5). Translocations occur when the genetic information stays the same but is rearranged or exchanged and does not necessarily result in abnormal development. Inversion occurs when a segment of the chromosome is reversed. Deletions occur when genetic material in the chromosome and a portion of the chromosome is lost. The consequences in the phenotype depend on the size of the deletion and the material that was deleted. An example of a deletion is **cri du chat syndrome** in which an infant has a characteristic cry sounding like the meow of a kitten. The symptoms are low birth weight, microcephaly, growth restriction, and severe mental retardation due to a missing part of chromosome 5. A duplication can involve all or part of a gene but there is no loss of genetic material; rather, part of the chromosome is duplicated. Duplications are less harmful since no genetic material is lost and they are more common than deletions.

A microdeletion occurs de novo (for no apparent reason) when a tiny piece of chromosomal material is missing and cannot be seen by routine chromosomal analysis; rather a special technique called fluorescent in situ hybridization (**FISH**) must be used. Microdeletions are a cause of congenital anomalies.

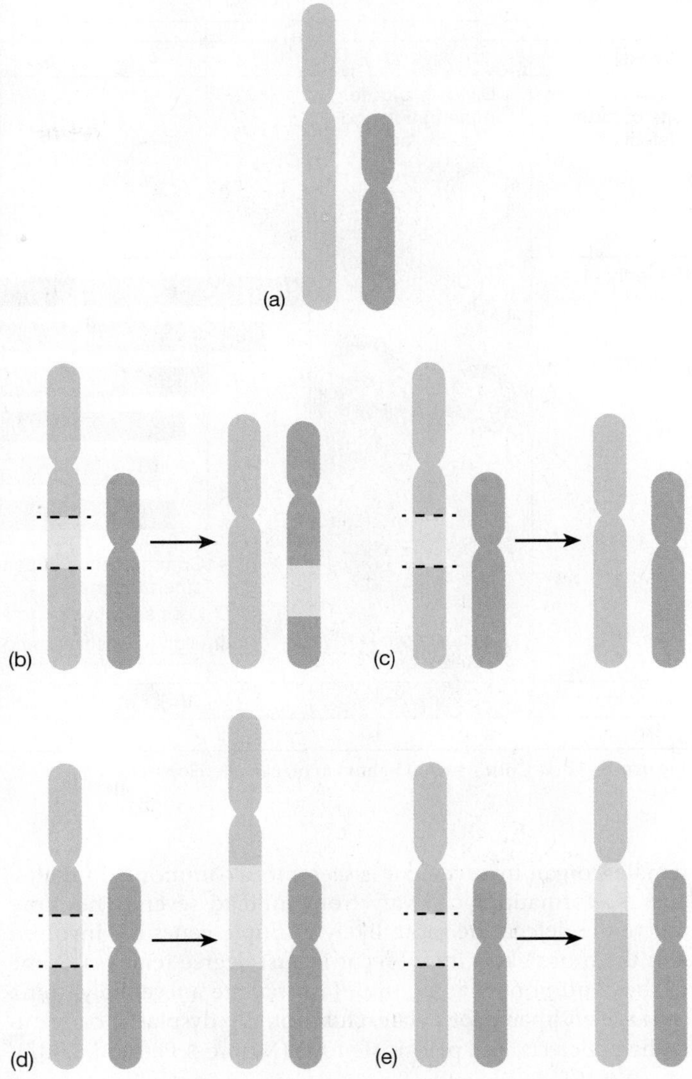

Figure 8–17 ■ Chromosome abnormalities

Babies with microdeletions are often "floppy" and weak, with a weak suck. They cannot breastfeed and have difficulty taking a bottle. They have delayed speech and learning disabilities but are friendly and pleasant. They have more serious symptoms involving multiple organs later in life (see Figure 8–18 ■) (Moore & Persaud, 2007).

Multifactorial Causation

There are several conditions that are inherited because of a combination of environmental and genetic factors. Multifactorial traits occur with greater frequency in individuals in a particular family than they do in the general public. The more affected family members there are, the more likely it is to occur in other members. Tissue anomalies are expressed more frequently in

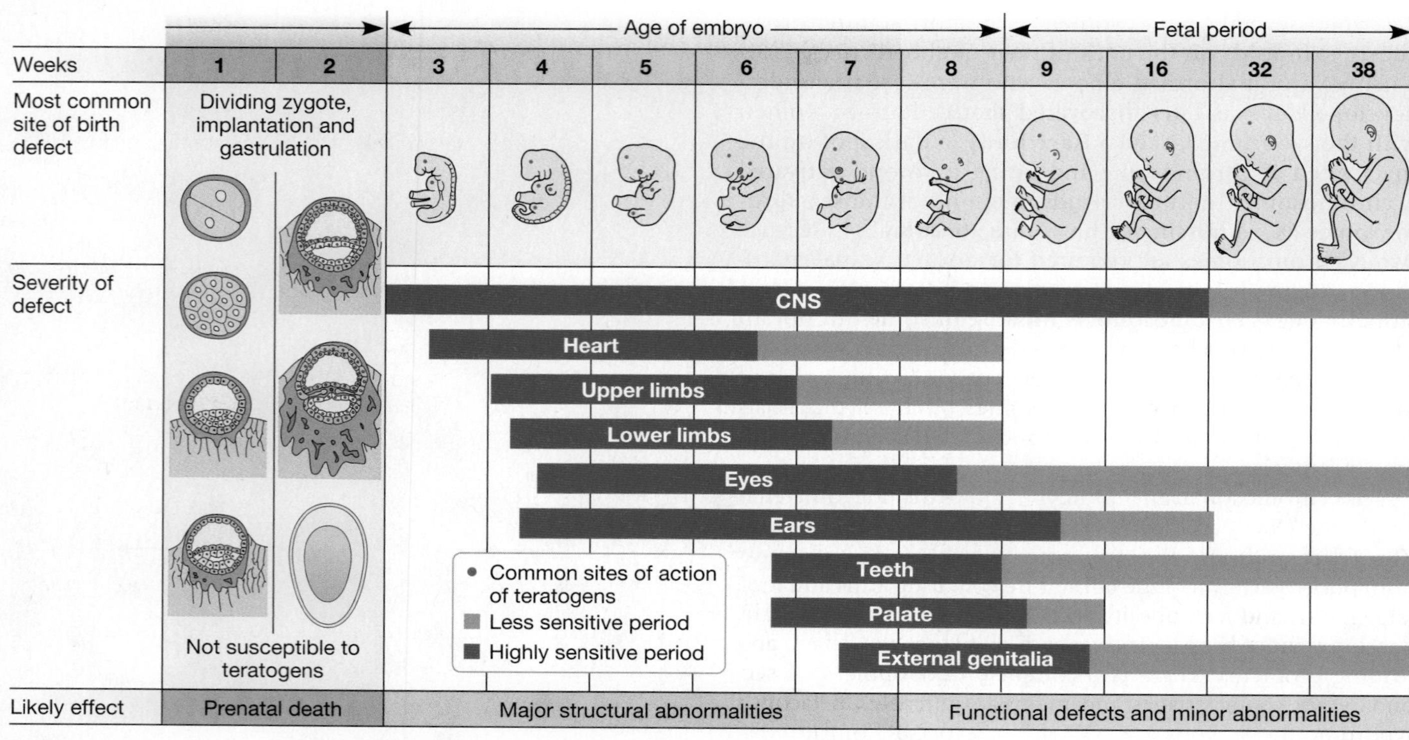

Figure 8–18 ■ Critical period in human prenatal development

females, organ involvement is seen more commonly in males, and malformations can vary from mild to severe. The more severe the defect, the more likely multiple genes are involved and the more likely it will recur in first-degree relatives. Some of the conditions that are multifactorial are anecephaly, spina bifida, cleft lip and/or palate, clubfoot, hip dysplasia, congenital heart defects, and pyloric stenosis (Moore & Persaud, 2007).

Environmental Factors

Seven to ten percent of congenital anomalies are caused by environmental factors (Moore & Persaud, 2007); however, most birth defects whose causes are unknown are believed to be a combination of both genetics and environment (Wlodarczyk et al., 2011). The most vulnerable or critical period during which structures are sensitive to environmental agents, known as teratogens, is during the first eight weeks of pregnancy (based on fertilization) when cell division, cell differentiation, and morphogenesis takes place. Each organ or structure has its own critical period in which exposure to teratogens can cause malformations or functional disturbances in varying severity depending on the timing and the teratogens. The critical period for development of the brain is between 3 to 16 weeks gestation. A disturbance during this period causes approximately two-thirds of all birth defects. Unfortunately, a woman may not know she is pregnant during the critical period and may be exposed to teratogens during that time (see Table 8–1). Whether or not the exposure will cause birth defects may depend on the mother's genes. For example, valproic acid taken for seizures may cause birth defects in fetuses of women who have a certain gene variant (MTHFR C677T, MIM 607093). Women who test positive for this variant can switch medications before conceiving (Lewis, 2008). Teratogens are agents such as chemicals, viruses, drugs, radiation, maternal disease, and other environmental factors that cause birth defects. The use of hot tubs or saunas is also included in this definition as they can cause hypothermia in the pregnant woman, which can lead to neural tube defects or pregnancy loss.

Infectious Agents

Rubella. Rubella (German measles) is a viral infection that is spread through the air or by close contact and usually causes a fever, headache and general malaise. An individual is contagious one week before the rash appears to two weeks after the rash disappears. The virus crossed the placenta and can infect the embryo/fetus. Exposure to rubella in the first trimester can cause cataracts, permanent hearing loss, cardiac malformations (especially patent ductus arteriosus and pulmonary stenosis), and congenital rubella syndrome. A fetus that is exposed in the second or third trimester has a lower risk of anomalies; however, he can develop learning disabilities and speech and hearing problems. Prevention of infection with rubella is the primary goal, and women should be serologically tested to determine if the rubella antibody is present. If a woman is not immune, she should be vaccinated as long as she is not pregnant and is certain to avoid pregnancy for at least 6 months.

TABLE 8–1: Microdeletion and Microduplication syndromes

Syndrome name	Clinical features	Chromosome findings	Origin
Angelman's	Microcephaly, macrosomia, ataxia, excessive laughter (happy and excitable demeanor), seizures, delayed development, intellectual disability, severe speech impairment	Del 15 q12 (most cases)	Maternal
Beckwith-Wiedemann	Macrosomia, macroglossia, some cases of omphalocele, hypoglycemia, hemihypertrophy, transverse ear lobes	Dup 11 q15 (some cases)	Paternal
DiGeorge	Thymic hypoplasia, parathyroid hypoplasia, conotruncal cardiac defects, facial dysmorphism	Del 22 q11 (some cases)	Either parent
Miller-Dieker	Type 1 lissencephaly, facial dysmorphism including mid-face hypoplasia, low set, abnormally shaped ears and small jaw, seizures, sever developmental delay cardiac anomalies, spasticity	Del 17 q13.3 (most cases)	Either parent
Prader-Willi	Hypertonia, hypogonadism, obesity with hyperphagia, narrow bifrontal skull, almond eyes, short stature, small hands and feet, mild developmental delay	Del 15 q12 (most cases)	Paternal
Smith-Magenis	Bracycepahaly, broad nasal bridge, prominent jaw, broad hands, sleep disturbance, delayed speech, mild to moderate intellectual disability	Del 17 q11 .2	Either parent
22q11.2 deletion syndrome Also called Velocardiofacial (or Shprintzen's)	Symptoms vary widely: Palatal defects, hypoplastic alae nasi, long nose, conotruncal cardiac defects, facial dysmorphism, learning disabilities	Del 22 q11 (most cases)	Either parent
Williams	Short stature, hypercalcemia, cardiac anomalies (esp. supravalvular aortic stenosis), elfin-like facial characteristics, mild to moderate intellectual disability	Del 15 q12 (most cases)	Either parent

Cytomegalovirus. **CMV** is a virus belonging to the herpes family. It is passed from infected individuals by direct contact of body fluids (urine, saliva, breast milk, blood, and semen). Approximately 30% to 50% of women have never been infected with CMV. One-third of women who have a primary infection during pregnancy will pass it on to their fetus as the virus crosses the placenta (CDC, 2010). Children, especially those in daycare settings, can transmit the virus to their mothers. Among infants who are infected, one in five will have permanent disabilities, including microcephaly, meningoencephalitis (which causes mental retardation), hearing and vision loss, and seizures. There is no cure; therefore, it is necessary to reduce the risk of transmission through hand washing and avoiding sharing food, drink, and eating utensils with children.

Toxoplasmosis. Toxoplasmosis is caused by a protozoan, Toxoplasma gondii. Infection is transmitted by eating raw or undercooked meat, handling soil or cat litter contaminated with feces of infected cats, or cleaning bird cages. A primary infection in pregnancy may produce no symptoms for the mother but can cause congenital toxoplasmosis. Headache, mild fever, enlarged lymph nodes, or sore throat may be present in the mother; however, infection in the fetus can cause severe problems. A woman has a 30% chance of passing the infection on to her fetus, but the risk and the severity depends on the timing of the exposure in the pregnancy. Congenital toxoplasmosis can include changes in the brain (intracranial calcifications), chorioretinitis, microcephaly, micropthalmia, hydrocephalus, and seizures. Treatment started early and throughout the first year of life with pyrimethamine and sulfadizine is extremely effective, even for babies with severe symptoms.

Herpes Simplex Virus (HSV). **HSV** is the most common sexually transmitted disease among adult women and is transmitted across broken skin and mucus membrane by direct exposure to the virus. Primary onset of HSV during late pregnancy carries a 30% to 50% risk of neonatal infection. During this time the mother does not have time to develop antibodies. Infection to the fetus is transmitted during birth 85% of the time. Neonatal infection has a mortality rate of 50%. Sequela of those who survive include significant neurologic defects, blindness, and seizures. Women with an active outbreak are usually scheduled for a Cesarean delivery to prevent exposure of the virus to the infant.

Human Immunodeficiency Virus (HIV). **HIV** is a virus and the cause of acquired immunodeficiency syndrome (**AIDS**). HIV is transmitted through body fluids, such as blood, semen, genital fluids, and breast milk. HIV can be transmitted during pregnancy, labor, or delivery, and through breastfeeding. Breastfeeding is not recommended for women infected with HIV. Treating a woman prophylactically with antiretroviral drugs during pregnancy and labor decreases the viral load of HIV in a woman's body and therefore reduces the risk of maternal–fetal transmission. Anomalies associated with HIV are microcephaly, growth failure, and craniofacial features.

Syphilis. Syphilis is caused by a spirochete called Treponema pallidum and can cross the placenta as early as 9 to 10 weeks gestation. It is usually transmitted through sexual contact but can also be transmitted by contaminated needles, especially with drug users, or through nonsexual contact with an infected lesion. A first-time infection acquired during pregnancy (primary infection) can cause serious congenital anomalies or stillbirth. Untreated primary or secondary syphilis in the mother is usually transmitted, and latent or tertiary syphilis is not. Congenital syphilis is classified as early or late. Early congenital syphilis manifests during the first three months of life and symptoms include vesiculobullous lesions, rash, lymphadenopathy, hepatospleenomegaly, and a mucopurulent nasal discharge known as "snuffles." Late congenital syphilis occurs about or after age 2 and symptoms include gummatous ulcers on the nose, septum, and palate; bossing of frontal and parietal bone; optic atrophy leading to blindness; interstitial keratitis; corneal scarring; and sensorineural deafness. Neurosyphilis is usually asymptomatic. Screening for syphilis during pregnancy should be done early at the first prenatal visit and again later in high-risk women. Treatment as soon as possible can prevent complications and transmission of the infection to the fetus. Teratogens known to cause human congenital anatomical anomalies or birth defects are shown in Table 8–2.

Drugs/Medications

In the late 1950s to early 1960s, thalidomide, a mild tranquilizer, was given to women to relieve nausea in early pregnancy. The drug was taken around the sixth to eighth week of pregnancy, when the limbs were beginning to form. Many of these babies were born with major birth defects, and missing arms and legs. Some had radial aplasia, the lack of the thumb and adjoining bones in the lower arm. Other malformations included the eyes, ears, heart, kidneys, genitals, GI tract, and CNS. Thalidomide is still used today for treatment of leprosy, multiple myeloma, and AIDS; however, women should be on strict birth control when taking the drug to avoid pregnancy with fetal exposure to thalidomide, (Thalidomide, 2010).

Diethylstilbestrol (**DES**) a synthetic, nonsteroidal estrogen, was prescribed between 1938 and 1971 for women who experienced bleeding and risk of premature birth. In the 1970s it was observed that daughters of women who took DES,were born with uterine abnormalities (T-shaped uterus), an increased risk of clear cell adenocarcinoma of the vagina and cervix and breast cancer, reproductive tract anomalies, and an increased incidence of infertility and adverse pregnancy outcomes. Sons born to women who took DES in pregnancy had an increased risk of genitourinary abnormalities including epididymal cysts.

Antiepileptic drugs are known to have teratogenic potential, and women who take these medications during pregnancy have a two- to three-fold higher incidence of having a baby with a birth defect than the general population; however, not all exposed fetuses have been born with birth defects. It is now believed that either maternal or fetal genetics predispose the fetus to an abnormal phenotype (Wlodarczyk et al., 2011). Drug safety is a primary concern during pregnancy, especially in women with pregestational diseases or conditions. Most medications are relatively safe in pregnancy and have no effect on embryo/fetal development. However, just because a medication is considered to *not* be a teratogen does not mean it is safe in pregnancy. Safety of a medication is usually not tested in pregnant women and rightly so, as it would be unethical to expose a fetus to a possible teratogen.

The Food and Drug Administration (**FDA**) has established five categories of medications for pregnancy, discussed in Table 8–3.

Drugs that are known teratogens that can cause birth defects include antibiotics (streptomycin, tetracycline), antineoplastic agents (amniopterin, methotrexate), anticoagulants (Coumadin), anticonvulsants (phenytoin, valproic acid), hormones (adrenocorticoids, diethylstilbestrol [DES]), antithyroid drugs, psychotropics, and retinoic acid (Vitamin A).

Alcohol

Women who consume alcohol during their pregnancy risk having a child with fetal alcohol syndrome (**FAS**). A major factor in development of FAS is the timing, amount and frequency of alcohol consumption during pregnancy. Children born to alcoholic mothers exhibit a characteristic pattern of development that includes craniofacial abnormalities: microcephaly, smooth philtrum, thin upper lip, small palpebral fissures and short nose. Central nervous system abnormalities are expressed as

TABLE 8–2: Common Tetrogens (Agents) Known to Cause Congenital Anatomical Anomalies or Birth Defects in Humans

	Agent Common Congenital Anatomical Anomalies or defects
Chemical	
Methyl mercury	Complex of neurological symptoms, including cerebral palsy, ataxia, disturbed psychomotor development and mental retardation sometimes accompanied by microcephaly
Polychlorinated biphenyls (PCBs)	Low birth weights, skin pigmentation of gums, nails and groin, calcification of the skull, rocker bottom heal, conjunctivitis
Drug	
Alcohol	Fetal alcohol syndrome (developmental and mental retardation), intrauterine growth restriction, microcephaly, ocular anomalies and joint abnormalities, short palpebral fissures
Aminopterin	Skeletal defects, growth retardation, malformation of the CNS, meroencephaly (most of the brain is absent)
Androgens and high doses of progestogens	Masculinization of female external genitalia, ambiguous external genitalia, Fusion of the labia minora, clitoral hypertrophy
Cocaine	Cerebral infarction, prematurity, microcephaly, urogenital anomalies, neurobehavioral disturbance
diethstilbestrol	Abnormalities of uterus and vagina, clitoromomegaly, vaginal adenocarcinomas
Isotrentinoin (13-cis-retinoic-acid)	Absent or defective ears, absent or small jaws, cleft palate, aortic arch abnormalities, thymic deficiencies, CNS abnormalities
Lithium carbonate	Heart and large vessel anomalies, Ebstein's anomaly, neural tube defects, talipes, microtia, and thyroid anomalies
Methotrexate	Multiple anomalies, skeletal and facial including cranium, face, limbs, vertebral column.
Phenytoin (Dilantin)	Fetal hydantoin syndrome manifested by intrauterine growth restriction and microcephaly, risk of cleft palate and congenital heart disease, inner epicanthal folds, eye lid ptosis, depressed nasal bridge, phalangeal hypoplasia
Tetracycline	Affects bone growth, stained teeth, hypoplasia of tooth enamel.
Thalidomide	Variable degree of deformities of the limbs, meromelia, amelia, facial anomalies, malformations of the ear, deafness, phocomelia, Fallot tetralogy, inguinal hernia, recto-vaginal fistula, cryptorchid testes, ectopic kidneys, absent or hypoplastic humerus, absent digits cardiac and kidney defects
Valoproc Acid	Craniofacial anomalies, NTDs, hydrocephalus, heart and skeletal defects
Warfarin	Nasal hypoplasia, stippled epiphysis, hypoplastic phalanges, eye anomalies, mental retardation
Infection	
Cytomegalovirus	Microcephaly, chorioretinitis, sensorineural hearing loss, delayed psychomotor/mental development, hydrocephaly, cerebral palsy, brain (periventricular) calcification
Herpes simplex virus	Skin vesicles and scarring, chorioretinitis, hepatomegaly, thrombocytopenia, petechiae, hemolytic anemia, hydrnagencephaly
Human parvovirus B 19	Eye defect, changes in fetal tissue
Rubella virus	Sensorineural deafness, Eye abnormalities retinopathy, cataract and microphthalmia, Congenital heart disease—especially patent ductus arteriosusm, Spleen, liver or bone marrow problems, Mental retardation, (microcephaly), Eye defects, Low birth weight, Thrombocytopenic purpura, Hepatomegaly, Micrognathia
Toxoplasma gondii	Encephalitis, necrotizing retinochoroiditis, nasal malformations,
Treponema pallidum	Hydrocephalus, congenital deafness, mental retardation, abnormal teeth and bones.
Venezuelan equine encephalitis virus	Microcephaly, microphthalmia, cerebral agenesis, CNS necrosis, hydrocephalus
Varicella virus	Cutaneous scars, defects of muscle and bone, malformed and paralyzed limbs, Microcephaly, blindness, seizures, and mental retardation
Radiation	
High levels of ionizing radiation	Small skull size (microcephaly), blindness, spina bifida, and cleft palate.

TABLE 8–3: FDA Classification of Drugs in Pregnancy

Risk Factor Category	FDA Classification/Medications in Pregnancy
A	Adequate, well-controlled studies have failed to demonstrate a risk to the fetus.
B	Animal studies have demonstrated no risk to the fetus; however, there are no adequate or well-controlled studies in pregnant women OR animal studies have shown an adverse effect but adequate studies in pregnant women have failed to demonstrate a risk.
C	Animal studies have shown an adverse effect on the fetus but there are no adequate studies on humans. Benefits to mother may outweigh potential risks to fetus.
D	There is positive evidence of human fetal risk; however, potential benefits may outweigh the potential risks in a life-threatening situation or with a serious disease in which safer drugs cannot be used or are ineffective.
X	Contraindicated in pregnancy. Adequate, well-controlled studies in animals or pregnant women have demonstrated positive evidence of fetal anomalies or risks that clearly outweigh any possible benefit in pregnant women.

cognitive impairment, impaired fine motor skills, developmental disabilities, impulse control, attention deficit hyperactive disorder, or seizure disorder. Physical growth is often restricted. Since the brain develops throughout pregnancy it is especially vulnerable to teratogenic effects during any stage of pregnancy.

Fetal alcohol spectrum disorder (**FASD**) is a modern term that describes a range of permanent effects of fetal alcohol exposure during pregnancy as depicted in Figure 8–19 ■. It includes FAS, and features vary in severity depending on the timing of the exposure in pregnancy and the amount of alcohol consumed. Alcohol is considered a category D drug by the FDA and therefore is contraindicated in pregnancy. Women need to be advised that the amount of alcohol that causes FAS is unknown and abstinence during pregnancy is the best practice.

Tobacco

The dangers of smoking cigarettes have been well documented especially for pregnancy. Smoking during pregnancy has an increased risk of preterm birth (**PTB**), low birth weight (**LBW**), premature rupture of membranes (**PROM**), placenta previa, placental abruption, and stillbirth (Murin, Rafii, & Bilello, 2011). Nicotine has neuro-teratogenic effects during pregnancy and can cause DNA and chromosomal damage to human germinal cells, oocytes, and sperm. Nicotine is a vasoconstrictor and causes a decrease in oxygenated blood to the fetus resulting in growth restriction. Paternal smoking and to a greater degree maternal smoking is associated with LBW (< 2500 gm). Adverse effects in development can be seen in children and adolescents, and they include mood and conduct disorders, an increased rate of behavioral problems, anxiety, depression, antisocial behavior, and childhood obesity (Murin, Rafii, & Bilello, 2011).

Multiple genes responsible for angiogenesis, blood vessel integrity, and inflammation have been implicated in pregnant women who smoke while pregnant. Some of these genes have shown a strong interaction with smoking. Women who smoke and have one or two of the gene variants have a higher risk of having an infant with gastroschisis compared to women with "wildtype alleles" who smoke. Women with certain genotypes and who smoke are at a high risk for having babies with structural defects such as cleft lip and palate (Wlodarczyk et al., 2011).

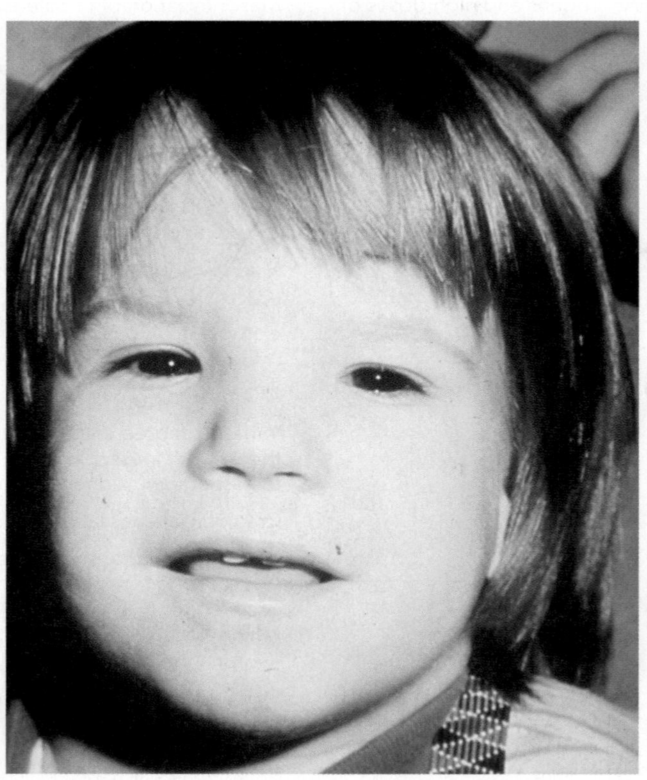

Figure 8–19 ■ Picture of a child with fetal alcohol syndrome

Source: Streissguth, A.P, Clarren, S.K., & Jones, K.L. Natural history of the Fetal Alcohol Syndrome: A ten - year follow-up of eleven patients. The Lancet,(13 July, 1985), 85-91.

Ionizing Radiation

Exposure to large amounts of radiation during pregnancy can be detrimental to the fetus; however, exposure during pregnancy is rare. High levels can cause injury to fetal cells and chromosomes. High levels of exposure have been known to cause growth retardation, microcephaly, spina bifida cystic, retinal changes, cataracts, skeletal and visceral abnormalities, and cleft palate. The brain is more vulnerable to exposure during weeks 8 to 16 after fertilization and can result in severe mental retardation. All women should avoid radiation exposure during pregnancy if possible; however, if an X-ray is absolutely needed, the abdomen should be effectively shielded from the exposure.

Illicit Drugs

Cocaine, one of the most widely used street drugs by women of childbearing age, has been associated with PTB, LBW, PROM, and placental abruption. Cocaine slows prenatal growth, especially head growth. If used in early pregnancy there is an increased risk of spontaneous abortion (miscarriage). Children born of women who use cocaine have a higher risk of PTB and LBW, have difficulty eating, and are more likely to be ill in the first year. Significant CNS problems are not always observed until the child is older. These include attention and behavioral problems and language and learning disabilities. Babies whose mothers use cocaine during pregnancy also have an increased risk of **sudden infant death syndrome (SIDS)**.

There have been no observed teratogenic effects of marijuana to date. Because marijuana is an illegal drug, research studies have been hindered. Individuals are not always forthcoming or reliable about their drug use, and strength or dose of any street drug is usually unknown. Researchers continue to follow drug use in pregnancy to determine its teratogenicity.

Maternal Disease

Poorly controlled carbohydrate metabolism in the diabetic woman is associated with major congenital anomalies in the fetus. The incidence of birth defects in these women is three to four times higher than in the general population (Sadler, 2010). Abnormalities, which usually occur in weeks 5 to 8 of organogenesis, include brain anomalies, skeletal defects, neurodevelopmental abnormalities, and congenital heart defects. Hyperglycemia at the time of conception and early fetal development is a determinant of the risk and severity of congenital anomalies. Ideally, strict control of blood sugar should be initiated prior to conception and women who have diabetes should be followed by a perinatologist to achieve the best pregnancy outcome.

Women with phenylalanine hydroxylase deficiency (phenylketonuria [PKU]) and hyperphenylalaninemia have an increased risk of having a baby with congenital anomalies if their phenylalanine levels are high when they become pregnant. Most babies will have microcephaly and mental retardation. Other defects include congenital heart disease and low birth weight. A study to determine the effects of a phenylalanine-free diet during pregnancy found that women whose blood phenylalanine levels were under control at the time of conception were likely to have healthy babies (Koch et al., 2003).

Heavy Metals

Prenatal exposure to lead is clearly linked to neurologic deficits in children. Lead exposure has been associated with spontaneous abortion, PTB, LBW, and development delays. Lead can be found in lead crystal glassware, arts and crafts supplies, old and some new painted toys, lead solder in some canned foods, cigarette smoke, and cosmetics.

Eating fish is the major cause of methylmercury exposure. Mercury can cause severe neurologic symptoms including behavioral disturbances resembling cerebral palsy. Other sequelae from high levels of mercury include severe brain damage, mental retardation, seizures, and blindness. Pregnant women should avoid eating swordfish, shark, king mackerel, and tilefish, the fish with the highest levels of methylmercury. Albacore tuna should be limited to 6 ounces or less per week.

Bisphenol-A

Bisphenol-A (**BPA**) is an organic compound used to make polycarbonate plastic, epoxy resins, and dental sealants. Plastics with a recycle code of 1, 2, 4, 5, and 6 are not likely to contain BPA. BPA can be found in the plastic lining of canned goods, plastic baby bottles, and polycarbonate plastic containers. The chemical structure of BPA is similar to that of estrogen and can have the same effect on the body. Some studies have suggested a relationship between BPA and meiotic aneuploidy. High serum levels of BPA have been associated with recurrent first trimester miscarriages, changes in breast tissue, preeclampsia, **IUGR**, and PTB. In men, BPA has been linked to male reproductive function including erectile function. Women who are trying to conceive or who are pregnant should avoid the use of plastic that contains BPA (Stillerman, Mattison, Giudice, & Woodruff, 2008). In 2010, Maine's Board of Environmental Protection voted unanimously to ban the sale of baby bottles and other food and beverage containers that contained BPA.

Obesity

Sixty percent of women in the United States are considered obese or overweight. Obesity is classified as having a Body Mass Index of >30 kg/m^2. More than 40% of pregnant women are overweight or obese (Gunatilake & Perlow, 2011). Women who are obese during pregnancy have a higher risk than normal weight women of having multiple adverse maternal, fetal, and neonatal outcomes, probably due to nutritional deficiencies, poor metabolic control, and coexisting medical complications that interfere with organogenesis. Miscarriage and congenital anomalies occur more frequently in obese women compared to the general population. Congenital anomalies include microcephaly, neural tube defects, cardiac anomalies, cleft lip and palate, anorectal atresia, diaphragmatic hernia, hydrocephalus, hypospadius, and limb reduction. Ideally, preconception counseling and weight loss would be achieved for the best perinatal outcome (Gunatilake & Perlow).

Other

Chromosomal abnormalities and DNA mutations have been associated with advanced paternal age. Older men have an increased risk of fathering a child with an autosomal dominant genetic disorder such as Marfan syndrome or achondroplasia. Other anomalies associated with advanced paternal age are orofacial clefts, hydrocephalus, neural tube defects, hypospadius, malformation of extremities and limb reduction defects, tracheoesophageal fistula or atresia, and congenital heart defects. Men younger than 20 years old are also considered high risk for fathering a child with a birth defect (Green et al., 2010).

An increased risk of new gene mutations is associated with advanced paternal age. There is also evidence that an increase in complex disorders such as some types of cancer, congenital anomalies, schizophrenia, and autism spectrum disorders are associated with advanced paternal age (Toriello & Meck, 2008).

SECTION THREE REVIEW

1. The time in which a fetus is most vulnerable to malformations during the first 8 weeks of pregnancy is called the
   A. malformation period.
   B. pre-embryonic period.
   C. significant period.
   D. critical period.
2. The skin covering on the fetus, which is made up of fatty secretions from sebaceous glands and epithelial cells, is called
   A. vernix caseosa.
   B. lanugo.
   C. meconium.
   D. amnion.
3. Genetic and environmental causes of congenital anomalies are called
   A. environ-genetic inheritance.
   B. multifactorial inheritance.
   C. chromosomal inheritance.
   D. multiple gene inheritance.
4. A teratogen can be all of the following EXCEPT
   A. prenatal vitamins.
   B. maternal disease.
   C. medications.
   D. infection.
5. Chromosomal abnormalities and DNA mutations have been associated with advanced paternal age.
   A. True
   B. False

Answers: 1. D; 2. A; 3. B; 4. A; 5. A

SECTION FOUR: Prenatal Care

Ideally, women would seek counseling prior to becoming pregnant to identify risk factors for complications in pregnancy, screen for diseases that may be genetically transmitted, assess nutritional status, discuss potential teratogens, and promote a healthy lifestyle. The American College of Obstetricians and Gynecologists (ACOG; 2005) recommends ongoing education and screening on all women of reproductive age in order to identify potential risks to a woman and her fetus prior to a pregnancy and between each pregnancy. The purpose of preconception counseling is to optimize healthy perinatal outcomes.

Emerging Evidence

Several studies have confirmed that folic acid or folic acid–containing multivitamin supplementation taken in the preconception period can prevent neural tube defects, congenital cardiovascular abnormalities, and possibly other defects (Czeizel & Banhidy, 2011).

- Maternal opioid treatment 1 month prior to pregnancy and during the first trimester (within 3 months after conception) showed an association with certain types of birth defects including several types of congenital heart defects (Broussard et al., 2011).
- In the past two decades it has been recognized that adult diseases can be influenced by prenatal and environmental exposures; this is known as fetal programming. Conditions during pregnancy can change gene expression during development and may lead to permanent programming of tissue function (Lau, Rogers, Desai, & Ross, 2011).

Preconception Counseling

During the preconception assessment the provider should obtain a comprehensive medical, surgical, reproductive, psychological, social, and family/genetic history followed by a complete physical examination. Equally important is the potential father's medical, family, and reproductive history. This information is valuable in identifying preexisting conditions that may affect pregnancy or inherited disorders that could be passed on to the fetus. Risks can be reduced in diseases such as diabetes if strict metabolic control can be established prior to pregnancy. A three-generation family pedigree and carrier testing should be done for common genetic disorders. Women at risk for passing on a genetic anomaly or birth defect can be counseled about options with assisted reproductive technologies such as preimplantation diagnosis.

Establishing healthy eating habits is essential to a healthy pregnancy. A nutritional assessment should be made and referral to a dietitian may be necessary. Women should be instructed to take preconception or prenatal vitamins that contain 0.4 mg of folic acid at least 1 month prior to conception in order to prevent neural tube defects in the fetus. It is recommended that all women of childbearing age regularly take 0.4 mg of folic acid because of the high incidence of unintended pregnancy. Women need to be encouraged to continue an established exercise routine during pregnancy or to start an exercise program before becoming pregnant (ACOG; 2009).

Other important items that should be assessed are (a) potential teratogenic exposures in the workplace or in the home; (b) the use of alcohol, cigarettes, and/or recreational drugs; (c) risk measures to avoid or prevent exposure to infections; (d) up-to-date vaccinations; (e) mental health issues; and (f) *all* medications and dietary supplements. The provider should discuss the need for any prescribed medications. Medications that the woman may be taking for a chronic medical condition such as asthma, diabetes, or hypertension may need to be changed during the pregnancy. Finally, a preconception visit is an ideal time to begin educating women about what to expect with routine prenatal care and to answer any questions they may have about any aspect of pregnancy.

Prenatal Care

The ultimate goal in pregnancy is to have a healthy mother who gives birth to a healthy infant. Women who seek early and regular prenatal care are more likely to have healthier babies (Gabbe, Niebyl, & Simpson, 2007). Prenatal care is more than just health care; it also includes screening, counseling, and education. Medical care includes diagnosing the pregnancy and monitoring its progress. Should a complication develop, it can be identified early and a management plan can be initiated. The prenatal visits provide an opportunity for educating the patient on aspects surrounding the pregnancy and the prenatal care. Women should seek prenatal care as soon as possible after the first missed menstrual period.

Once the pregnancy is confirmed, a complete assessment of the pregnant woman is needed. During the initial prenatal visit the woman is asked about her health history with a focus on previous pregnancies and their outcomes. The woman will also be asked about her medical, surgical, psychological, social, and family/genetic history. A risk assessment is made based on questions related to family history, immunizations, nutrition, exercise, tobacco, alcohol, or illicit drug use, environmental or work hazards, and domestic violence. The woman should be asked about any prescription or over-the-counter drugs she may be currently taking, and it must be determined if the medication is absolutely necessary. If the risk of the drug outweighs the benefit is should be discontinued and an alternative treatment may be considered. The information that is collected from a client's history and physical exam help guide the plan of care and the interventions during pregnancy.

A complete physical exam is performed, including a pelvic and breast exam. Initial laboratory studies that are done include blood type Rh factor and antibody screen; complete blood count, including hemoglobin and hematocrit; varicella and rubella titers; hepatitis B screen; syphilis screening by RPR or VDRL; HIV screen; urinalysis; gonorrhea and chlamydia screening; and Pap smear. Genetic carrier screening may be done depending on the state laws, the ethnicity of the parents, or at the request of the parents, and include genetic tests for inherited disorders such as sickle cell anemia, cystic fibrosis, Down syndrome, or Tay-Sachs disease. Information regarding routine prenatal tests and genetic screening should be explained to the woman. (Prenatal screening is explained in detail in Chapter 10). A three-generation family pedigree can be done to identify inherited diseases in the mother or father (see Chapter 13). If a genetic disease or trait is identified on a pedigree or a genetic screen is positive for a genetic disease or trait, the woman may need a referral to a genetic counselor.

Prenatal care is an excellent example of preventive care and should focus on keeping the mother and fetus healthy throughout the pregnancy and birth, and on educating the client and her partner and/or family. Counseling a pregnant woman on normal discomforts of pregnancy, proper nutrition and expected weight gain, exercise, sleep, sexual activity, and working while pregnant may contribute to a healthy pregnancy and possibly prevent potential problems. The woman should be informed about the schedule for routine prenatal care throughout the pregnancy, including ultrasound scheduling, and information should be given on any childbirth preparation or newborn care classes that are available. The client may not know about potential teratogens and their affect on prenatal development; therefore, an early prenatal visit is an opportune time for teaching about the dangers of exposures to certain substances.

Nurses are in a position to establish a rapport with a pregnant woman and to collect heath history and pedigree information that can contribute to a complete prenatal assessment. The nurse can set priorities for the client depending on the gestational age of the fetus and focus on education and preventive care. Since education is a vitally important part of prenatal care, the nurse is tasked to perform ongoing assessments of well-being, identify and discuss concerns that the pregnant woman has, and provide education for her throughout the pregnancy and postpartum period to ensure continuity of care.

Fetal Loss

Pregnancy loss can be a catastrophic event for a couple who are anticipating a healthy baby. Spontaneous abortion (**SABO**) is the most common complication of pregnancy and up to 50% of pregnancies end in SABO (miscarriage), including pregnancies from the period of conception (Paidas & Hossain, 2009). Pregnancy loss has been defined as SABO if it occurs before 20 weeks gestation and it is defined as stillbirth when there is fetal death after 20 weeks. The causes of pregnancy loss vary depending on the gestational age. Most cases of pregnancy loss are sporadic; however, some women experience recurrent miscarriages. If the parental karyotypes are normal and fetal loss occurs due to fetal aneuploidy, it is assumed to be sporadic with minimal recurrence risk. Recurrent pregnancy loss (**RPL**) is defined as three or more pregnancy losses and no more than one live birth. Several etiologies are implicated in the causes of fetal loss for both sporadic and recurrent loss, which include morphologic abnormalities, genetic causes, endocrine disorders, environmental substances, uterine abnormalities, immunologic disorders, and infection (Warren & Silver, 2008).

Fifty to seventy percent of SABO are caused by cytogenic abnormalities, the most common being fetal aneuploidy. Autosomal trisomies occur in 60% of losses followed by monosomy X in 20% of cases and polyploidy in 20% of cases. The trisomies are caused by meiotic nondisjunction during gametogenesis. The most common trisomy is 16 and it accounts for 20% to 30% of trisomy losses seen in postmortem fetal specimens (Warren & Silver, 2008).

Anembryonic loss refers to loss before the development of an embryo, commonly known as a blighted ovum and usually occurring during the first three weeks. The rate of chromosomal abnormalities in an anembryonic loss is 90%. The rate of an abnormal karyotype in specimens of spontaneously aborted specimens is higher earlier in gestation and decreases as gestation increases (Warren & Silver, 2008).

Advanced maternal age is associated with an increased risk of aneuploidy. Low maternal folate levels may be a factor in meiotic nondisjunction as they have been found in women who experience loss due to aneuploidy (Paidas & Hossain, 2009). Other genetic causes of fetal loss that have been identified are single gene disorders such as hemoglobinopathies, thrombophilias, and metabolic disorders. **Consanguinity** may also be a factor since there is an increased risk single gene disorders if both parents carry the same autosomal recessive mutation. When multiple male fetal losses occur, a lethal X-linked dominant disorder may be suspected and is usually associated with third trimester fetal demise.

Heritable thrombophilias in women have been associated with RPL and occur because of damage to chorionic vessels, reduced trophoblast invasion, apoptosis and impaired uteroplacental circulation due to thrombosis. Other mutations associated with RPL are (a) hyperhomocysteinemia, an autosomal recessive trait; (b) skewed X inactivation, a hemizygous X-linked mutation; (c) human leukocyte antigen genotype (HLA-G) deficiency; and (d) confined placental mosaicism (**CPM**). However, outcomes depend on several factors. The worst outcomes connected with CMP are associated with chromosomal involvement—for example, trisomy 16, which results in a high rate of pregnancy loss (Warren & Silver, 2008).

Exposure to environmental substances can also be connected to fetal loss. Contaminants in drinking water such as selenium, nitrates, and arsenic are associated with pregnancy loss. Drinking water can contain by-products of chlorine-based treatments such as trihalomethanes (THMs): chloroform, bromoform, bromodichloromethane (BDCM), and dibromochloromethane). Other chemicals found in drinking water include the haloacetic acids: monochloroacetic acid, dichloroacetic acid, monobromoacetic acid, and dibromoacetic acid. A chlorinated pesticide used in the United States before 1972 was dichlorodiphenyltrichloroethane (DDT), which was shown to cause spontaneous abortion. More recently, bisphenol-A (BPA), a compound used in the production of polycarbonate plastics and dental sealants with a chemical structure similar to that of estrogen, has been implicated in recurrent first trimester pregnancy loss (Stillerman et al., 2008).

Genetic evaluation and counseling are recommended for all couples who experience fetal loss and especially RFL (recurrent fetal loss). It is essential for the nurse to obtain a complete, detailed medical, surgical, reproductive, social, and family history that will aid in determining the cause of fetal loss. Fetal autopsy; maternal, paternal, and fetal karyotyping; and placental evaluation are recommended following any pregnancy loss. Also, laboratory tests in addition to routine pregnancy blood tests such as screening for antiphospholipid antibodies should be performed to help determine the cause of recurrent loss. The nurse should be sensitive to the couple's grief and acknowledge the emotional impact on the woman and her family. The nurse may assist with understanding the reason or results of any tests that may be necessary and encourage resources such as support groups for the woman and her family. Finally, the nurse can assist the woman with any referrals she may need.

SECTION FOUR REVIEW

1. Components of preconception counseling include all of the following EXCEPT
   A. family history.
   B. history of preexisting conditions.
   C. partner's educational background.
   D. partner's medical history.
2. Prenatal care should ideally begin
   A. before the first missed menstrual period.
   B. after the first missed menstrual period,
   C. after the second missed menstrual period.
   D. after the third missed menstrual period.
3. Prenatal care is more than just health care.
   A. True
   B. False
4. Which of the following statements in NOT true about pregnancy loss?
   A. Fifty percent of pregnancies end in spontaneous abortion.
   B. Most cases of pregnancy loss are sporadic.
   C. Advance maternal age is associated with an increased risk of aneuploidy.
   D. Consanguinity is not considered a factor in fetal loss.
5. Recurrent fetal loss
   A. includes only losses when a genetic abnormality has occurred.
   B. does not require examining a parent's karyotype.
   C. is defined as having three pregnancy losses and no more than one live birth.
   D. has nothing to do with maternal or paternal age.

Answers: 1. C; 2. B; 3. A; 4. D; 5. C

POSTTEST

1. During which phase of the menstrual cycle does the endometrium thicken in preparation for ovulation and fertilization?
   A. Menstrual
   B. Proliferative
   C. Secretory
   D. Ischemic
2. A couple who wants to use natural family planning to try to conceive needs to know that the ovum is considered fertile for ___.
   A. 8 hours
   B. 24 hours
   C. 2–3 days
   D. 1 week
3. In order for fertilization to occur, what part of the sperm must penetrate the egg?
   A. Entire sperm
   B. Tail
   C. Head
   D. Both head and tail
4. The pre-embryonic stage occurs during
   A. week 3–8.
   B. the week of the last monthly period (LMP).
   C. the first 14 days following conception.
   D. the first 4 days after fertilization.
5. The hormone primarily responsible for maintaining the pregnancy is
   A. progesterone.
   B. human chorionic gonadotropins (hCG).
   C. human placental lactogen (hPL).
   D. gonadotropins releasing hormone (GnRH).
6. A baby is born with a congenital heart defect. At what point would this anomaly occur?
   A. Between the third and fifth week of development.
   B. In the first 2 weeks of development.
   C. During the eighth week of development.
   D. 14 days after fertilization.
7. Based on Nagele's rule, if the last monthly period (LMP) was 5/7/12, the expected date of birth would be
   A. December 30, 2012.
   B. February 14, 2013.
   C. June 1, 2013.
   D. August 23, 2013.
8. At what time in embryonic development do the male and female genital organs begin to differentiate?
   A. Week 4
   B. Week 8
   C. Week 12
   D. Week 18
9. A woman with a family history of twins has a high chance of having
   A. identical twins.
   B. monozygotic twins.
   C. triplets.
   D. dizygotic twins.
10. If studies in animals or pregnant women demonstrate evidence of fetal abnormality or risk, or if the potential for fetal risk clearly outweighs any possible benefit of the drug, the Food and Drug Administration (FDA) category for this drug is
    A. B.
    B. C.
    C. D.
    D. X.

Posttest answers are located in the Appendix.

CHAPTER SUMMARY

An ovum remains viable for 6 to 24 hours and sperm are healthy and viable for about 24 hours in the female genital tract. Fertilization normally takes place in the ampulla of the fallopian tube. It takes 72 to 96 hours for the fertilized ovum to travel to the uterus. After implantation, it releases human chorionic gonadotropin (hCG), which signals the corpus luteum to secrete progesterone to maintain the pregnancy until the placenta is large enough to secrete progesterone.

Gender is determined immediately at fertilization. Females have two X chromosomes and males have one X and one Y chromosome. X chromosomes are larger and contain more genes than the Y chromosome; therefore, there are more X-linked traits.

During organogenesis the three germ layers (the ectoderm, the endoderm, and the mesoderm) give rise to many specific tissues and organs. This occurs in the 3rd to the 8th week of development and is also known as the embryonic period.

The critical time of the embryonic period is when the embryo is most vulnerable to substances or agents known as teratogens. Toxins, radiation, infections, and genetic abnormalities are some of the things that can cause congenital anomalies or serious birth defects in the developing embryo and fetus.

Twins can be either dizygotic (fraternal) or monozygotic (identical). Twins that originate from two oocytes fertilized by two separate sperm are dizygotic. Twins who

CHAPTER SUMMARY (*Continued*)

develop from a single oocyte fertilized by a single sperm are monozygotic.

The fetal period begins in the 9th week (based on dates calculated using the last menstrual period) and continues for 40 weeks gestation. Development during the fetal stage is concerned with rapid growth and differentiation of organs, tissues, and systems.

Women should begin prenatal care as soon as possible after the first missed menstrual period. Ideally, women would seek care and counseling prior to becoming pregnant to identify risk factors for complications with pregnancy.

Recurrent fetal loss (RFL) is defined as three or more miscarriages and no more than one live birth. Several etiologies are implicated in the causes, including genetic causes.

CRITICAL THINKING CHECKPOINT

L.B. is a 28-year-old Caucasian woman who has polycystic ovarian syndrome and irregular periods. She recently discovered that she was pregnant. She went to her first prenatal visit and was diagnosed by ultrasound as being 11 weeks gestation. She tells the nurse that she has a family history of cleft lip—her younger brother and her uncle were born with cleft lip and palate. She also has a cousin who has Down syndrome. Two weeks ago she attended a wedding and drank three beers at the reception and later joined some friends in a hot tub. She stated that she sat in the hot tub for only 5 minutes because she started feeling nauseated. She is worried that she may have hurt her baby by drinking the beers.

1. What factors related to this pregnancy could put the fetus at risk?
2. Can testing be done to determine if the fetus has a cleft lip? If so, when?
3. What potential effect could the alcohol have on the fetus?
4. What topics should the nurse consider discussing with this woman?

Answers are provided in the Appendix

Pearson Nursing Student Resources

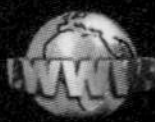

Find additional review materials at nursing.pearsonhighered.com

Prepare for success with additional NCLEX®-style practice questions, interactive assignments and activities, web links, animations, videos, and more!

ONLINE RESOURCES

Behavioral Genetics http://www.ornl.gov/sci/techresources/Human_Genome/elsi/behavior.shtml

Childhealth Explanation http://www.childhealth-explanation.com/genetics.html

Fetal Development http://childdevelopment.howtoinfo-247.com/fetal-developm

REFERENCES

American College of Obstetrics and Gynecology. (2002; Reaffirmed 2009). ACOG Committee Opinion No. 267: Exercise in pregnancy and the postpartum period.*Obstetrics and Gynecology, 99,* 171–173.

American College of Obstetrics and Gynecology. (2005). ACOG Committee Opinion No. 313: The importance of preconception care in the continuum of women's health care. *Obstetrics and Gynecology, 106,* 665–6.

Broussard, C. S., Rasmussen, S. A., Reefhuis, J., Friedman, J. M., Jann, M. W., Riehle-Colarusso, T., & Honein, M. A. (2011). Maternal treatment with opioid analgesics and risk for birth defects. *American Journal of Obstetrics and Gynecology, 204*(4), 314.e1–314.e11.

Center for Disease Control and Prevention. (CDC; 2010). *Cytomegalovirus (CMV) and congenital CMV infection.* Retrieved June 28, 2012, from http://www.cdc.gov/cmv/congenital-infection.html

Czeizel, A. E., & Banhidy, F. (2011). Vitamin supply in pregnancy in prevention of congenital birth defects. *Current Opinion in Clinical Nutrition and Metabolic Care, 14*(3), 291–296.

Gabbe, S. G., Biebyl, J. R., & Simpson, J. L. (2007). *Obstetrics: Normal and problem pregnancies.* (5th ed.). Philadelphia, PA: Elsevier.

Green, R. F., Devine, O., Crider, K. S., Olney, R. S., Archer, N., Olshan, A. F., & Shapira, S. K. (2010). Association of paternal age and risk for major congenital anomalies. *Annals of Epidemiology, 20*(3), 241–249.

Gunatilake, R. P., & Perlow, J. H. (2011). Obesity and pregnancy: Clinical management of the obese gravida. *American Journal of Obstetrics and Gynecology, 204*(2), 106–119.

Heron, M., Hoyert, D. L., Murphy, S. L., Hx, J., Kochanek, K. D., & Tejada-Vera, B. (2009). Deaths: Final data for 2006. *National Vital Statistics Report, 57*(14), 1–135. Retrieved June 28, 2012, from http://www.cdc.gov/ncbddd/birthdefects/data.html

Knupple, R. A. (2007). Maternal-placental-fetal unit: Fetal & early neonatal physiology. In A. H. DeCherney, L. Nathan, T. M. Goodwin, & N. Laufer (Eds.). *Current diagnosis & treatment: Obstetrics & gynecology* (10th ed.). New York, NY: McGraw-Hill, pp. 159–186.

Koch, R., Hanley, W., Levy, H., Matalon, K., Matalon, R., Rouse, B., et al. (2003). The maternal phenylketonuria study international study: 1984-2002. *Pediatrics, 112* (6), 1523–1529.

Lau, C., Rogers, J. M., Desai, M., & Ross, M. G. (2011). Fetal programming of adult disease: Implications for prenatal care. *Obstetrics & Gynecology, 117*(4), 978–984.

Lewis, R. (2008). *Human genetics: Concepts and applications*. New York, NY: McGraw-Hill.

Little, C. M. (2010). One consequence of infertility treatment: Multifetal pregnancy. *The American Journal of Maternal/Child Nursing (MCN), 35*(3), 150–155.

Moore, K. L., & Persaud, T. V. N. (2011). *The developing human: Clinically oriented embryology*. (9th ed.). Philadelphia, PA: W.B. Saunders.

Murin, S., Rafii, R., & Bilello, K. (2011). Smoking and smoking cessation in pregnancy. *Clinics in Chest Medicine, 32*(1), 75–91.

Paidas, M .J., & Hossain, N. (2009). Embryonic and fetal demise. In R. K. Creasy, R. Resnik, & J. D. Iams (Eds.). *Creasy and Resnik's maternal-fetal medicine: Principles and practice*. Philadelphia, PA: Saunders, pp. 619–633.

Rand, L., & Lee, H. (2009). Complicated monochorionic twin pregnancies: Updates in fetal diagnosis and treatment. *Clinics in Perinatology, 36*(2), 417–430.

Sadler, T. W. (2010). *Langman's medical embryology.* (11th ed.). Baltimore, MD: Lippincott Williams & Wilkins.

Stillerman, K. P., Mattison, D. R., Giudice, L. C., & Woodruff, T. J. (2008). Environmental exposures and adverse pregnancy outcomes: A review of the science. *Reproductive Sciences, 15*(7), 631–650.

Thalidomide. (2010). National Toxicology Program, Department of Health and Human Services. http://cerhr.niehs.nih.gov/common/thalidomide.html

Toriello, H. V., & Meck, J. M. (2008). Statement on guidance for genetic counseling in advanced paternal age. *Genetics in Medicine, 10*(6), 457–460.

Warren, J. E., & Silver, R. M. (2008). Genetics of pregnancy loss. *Clinical Obstetrics and Gynecology, 51*(1), 84–95.

Wlodarczyk, B. J., Palacios, A. M., Chapa, C. J., Zhu, H., George, T. M., & Finnell, R. H. (2011). Genetic basis of susceptibility to teratogen induced birth defects. *American Journal of Medical Genetics Part C (Seminars in Medical Genetics), 157*(3), 215–226.

PART 3

Ethical, Legal, and Social Implications

CHAPTER 9 Ethical, Legal, and Social Implications of the Human Genome Project

Judith A. Lewis

LEARNING OUTCOMES

Following the completion of this chapter, the learner will be able to

1. Identify the relevance of ethical, legal, and social issues related to genetics and genomics.
2. Discuss selected social policy implications of the Human Genome Project.
3. Describe the importance of ethical, legal, and social issues related to genetics and genomics in the provision of appropriate care to clients.

The sequencing of the human genome has had, and will continue to have, profound ethical, legal, and social implications for society. Unlike assisted reproductive technology, where the scientific discoveries occurred before the public policy implications were addressed, the leaders of the Human Genome Project were proactive in addressing the policy issues that would arise from the genomic era of health care. From the outset, a minimum of 5% of each year's annual budget was set aside to fund studies that could help us address the ethical, legal, and social implications of the genetic discoveries. Dr. Elizabeth Thomson, a registered nurse, led the **ELSI** division of the Human Genome Project for many years (http://www.genome.gov).

Just as anesthesia and surgery were the watershed developments of the 19th century, and immunizations and antibiotics helped redefine health and illness in the 20th century, the 21st century will be defined by genetics and genomics. The public policy issues arising from this new paradigm are, fortunately, being discussed concurrently with the development of the science. This chapter will discuss several public policy issues: privacy and confidentiality, informed consent, newborn screening, reproductive decision making, presymptomatic genetic testing, and reimbursement issues. The landmark legislation known as the Genetic Nondiscrimination Act, or GINA, is discussed in Chapter 12.

PRETEST

1. Professional nursing has a code of
   A. social policy.
   B. legal regulations.
   C. financial rules.
   D. ethics.
2. Nurses have a social contract with
   A. doctors.
   B. hospitals.
   C. each other.
   D. society.
3. An example of a specialty that developed technical advances without concurrent ethical guidelines is
   A. assisted reproductive technology.
   B. pharmacology.
   C. surgery.
   D. orthopedics.
4. The regulations that mandate the privacy of personal health care information are known as
   A. GINA.
   B. HIPAA.
   C. Dodd-Frank.
   D. the Affordable Health Care Act.
5. Public policy implications of the Human Genome Project are
   A. mandated by law.
   B. promulgated by regulation.
   C. unique to genetics.
   D. important sequelae of the scientific genetic discoveries.
6. Genetic testing on newborns
   A. is standardized across the country.
   B. is universal across the globe.
   C. varies from state to state.
   D. is covered by all forms of health insurance.
7. Nurses' actions related to patient confidentiality
   A. are directed by individual institutional policy.
   B. are discussed in the Code of Ethics.
   C. are regulated by the State Boards of Nursing.
   D. is based on the individual nurse's understanding of the specific situation.

8. Testing of children for definitive diagnosis of a genetic condition
   A. requires informed parental consent.
   B. is a routine practice that does not require informed parental consent.
   C. can be performed if the child agrees to the procedure.
   D. is not allowed under any condition.
9. Women consenting to prenatal genetic testing
   A. use the information from testing to make informed decisions related to the future course of the pregnancy.
   B. always terminate the pregnancy if they learn that the fetus is affected with a genetic condition.
   C. always need to have the consent of the father of the baby before making the decision to terminate a pregnancy.
   D. always need to have the consent of the father of the baby before undergoing genetic testing.
10. People who have a family history of an adult-onset genetic condition
   A. are required to have genetic testing before they can purchase health or life insurance.
   B. face significant discrimination in the workplace unless they can document they are not at risk for the condition.
   C. should be required to have genetic testing before they attempt to become pregnant.
   D. should be encouraged to make an informed decision about whether or not to be tested for the condition.

Pretest answers are located in the Appendix.

SECTION ONE: Privacy, Confidentiality, and Informed Consent

We all have the expectation that our personal health information will remain private and confidential. This expectation is codified in the HIPAA regulations, and every health care employee is expected to abide by these regulations. When an individual first seeks care from a provider or health care institution, they are required to acknowledge that the organization has shared its privacy policies with them, and that they are aware of any situations that might require the sharing of such personal information, such as when insurance claims are filed or referrals are made. Patients have the right to refuse to have specific information shared. Also, we all have the right to determine whether to share our personal information with others, including family members.

This is not always possible with genetic information. If a person discovers that he or she is a carrier of a particular gene, then that person knows that at least one parent also is a carrier of the gene. Thus, parents who may not choose to be tested still have had their personal health information become known.

Do health care professionals have a duty to share this confidential health care information with those who have no idea that they may carry a mutation for a serious illness so that these relatives can make personal health care decisions for themselves? It always is best if the involved individuals share their personal health information with each other, but there are some family constellations where this does not happen, either because of interpersonal dynamics or unusual family structures.

Ethical conflicts can clearly arise in this situation. Your patient expects you to keep all personal health information private and confidential. Yet, others may be harmed if they remain ignorant of information that could affect their health and the health of any future offspring.

The process of informed consent is an important concept. It is more than signing a document authorizing the conduct of a test or procedure. Informed consent should always be the end point of informed decision making. Health care providers are obligated to provide consumers with information that includes the type of test or procedure to be performed, the risks associated with the procedure, and the risks associated with not having the procedure performed. The information needs to be presented at an appropriate level to ensure comprehension. The person actually performing the procedure needs to be assured that the patient knows the risks and benefits of the procedure, including any adverse consequences. Only after the procedure has been fully explained should a signature be obtained.

All too often, consent forms are completed by admissions clerks, office managers, or technicians. In some cases, such as that of newborn screening, tests are done without the signed consent of the parent. These procedures are often included in global documents and are considered "routine" by both clinicians and patients. It is only when a positive test result is presented to the patient along with the need for further diagnostic procedures that the patient truly realizes the nature of the "routine" test to which they have consented.

Routine global consent forms are often long, wordy, and difficult to understand. The clerk obtaining the consent often is not knowledgeable about the scope of the consent, and may be ill-prepared to answer questions. The patient who asks questions, who wishes to modify the consent form, or who appears unwilling to sign the standard form is often seen as a troublemaker rather than as a patient who is exercising the right to self-advocacy.

Genetic testing may be very expensive. Accurate testing may require obtaining samples from family members who carry the gene of concern. If testing a family member with a specific condition, such as cancer, is necessary to determine whether another individual is at risk for that specific cancer, whose insurance should pay for the family member's test? The individual wishing for the information may find that his or her personal insurance may not cover the costs of testing others. Also, who owns the test results?

SECTION ONE REVIEW

1. A man who is the son of a woman with Huntington disease has what chance of having inherited the disease for this condition?
   A. 1 in 4
   B. 1 in 2
   C. 2 in 3
   D. 1 in 3
2. Personal health care information
   A. is not private.
   B. is not confidential.
   C. may never be revealed to another entity under any circumstances.
   D. may become known to others as the result of genetic testing.
3. Before signing a consent form, the patient should
   A. consult their attorney.
   B. read the document carefully and ensure that all parts of it are understood.
   C. insist on seeing the patient ombudsperson.
   D. be premedicated for the procedure.

Answers: 1. B; 2. D; 3. B

SECTION TWO: Newborn Screening and Genetic Testing of Children

Newborn screening is a public health initiative performed on the entire population to identify those at risk for certain congenital disorders. Many of these conditions, such as phenylketonuria (PKU), are treatable with dietary modifications in early infancy. Left untreated, PKU causes irreversible mental retardation. These tests are routinely performed on newborns before hospital discharge, and in most states they do not require signed parental informed consent.

Little and Lewis (2008) discuss several ethical concerns related to newborn screening, including the use of test results to deny access to health insurance, unequal access to diagnostic and treatment facilities based on health care disparities, and the anxiety created by positive screening results. Since there is variability among the states related to the panel of tests included in routine newborn screening, infants in some parts of the United States will be screened for more conditions than infants in states where the newborn screening panel is less robust. Given the mobility of people, infants may end up living in states where there are no diagnostic or treatment programs for positive test results that were obtained in the state where they were born.

There also is the question of parental rights to make health care decisions for themselves and for their children. When does the good of public health trump the autonomy of parents? Most of the conditions included in newborn screening panels are not contagious so infants who have these conditions do not pose a direct threat to the public health.

Another issue raised by newborn screening is the retention of test samples. This means that the testing agency has the newborn's DNA stored. Do parents know this? Do they have a right to refuse to have their infants tested or the residual sample stored? If these samples are used for research purposes, is informed consent obtained from the parents?

Emerging Evidence

As the political climate in the United States debates critical social issues, it is important to ensure that the rights of the individual are balanced with the rights of society. Legislation and judicial review play an important part in providing safeguards that ensure technology is applied in a manner that protects these safeguards and ensures the appropriate incorporation of this technology into society. We as health care providers and informed citizens need to ensure that our voices are heard and that we educate those elected to represent us in issues related to the incorporation of this new information in a way that is responsive, responsible, and ethical.

The issue of genetic testing of children is complicated by the fact that children cannot provide informed consent. They are not aware of the complexities of genetic testing or of the potential life-altering consequences of the test results. Parents may wish to know whether their children are at risk for conditions that run in the family. Do they have the right to know? Will this knowledge alter the parent–child relationship? This is especially true of conditions for which there are no known preventions or treatments. It is suggested that testing be deferred until the child is sufficiently mature to provide informed consent. This may be a problem if the child becomes sexually active and runs the risk of transmitting the condition of concern to offspring before they are sufficiently mature to determine when, or whether, they will be tested themselves.

In some cases, testing of children may be justified. If a child is at risk for congenital colon cancer, the standard screening for early detection is an annual colonoscopy, perhaps beginning as young as 10 years of age. If a child undergoes genetic testing and is found not to carry the candidate gene, then the child is spared this annual invasive procedure.

SECTION TWO REVIEW

1. Newborn screening
   A. is performed only after written parental informed consent.
   B. is a population-based screening program undertaken by state health departments.
   C. provides definitive diagnoses.
   D. may be performed any time during the first year of life with equally valid results.
2. Genetic testing of minor children
   A. requires written informed consent from the child.
   B. is never justified.
   C. is not recommended as a general rule.
   D. is not covered by parental health insurance.

Answers: 1. B; 2. C

SECTION THREE: Reproductive Decision Making; Presymptomatic Genetic Testing

There are many opportunities for genetic testing during pregnancy. Genetic tests can be used to screen for conditions such as Down syndrome and spina bifida, to diagnose conditions such as trisomy 21, and to inform parents of the gender of the fetus. Pregnant women, as autonomous persons, have the right to decide what, when, or whether they will undergo prenatal screening tests or diagnostic procedures. Some of these tests may occur before pregnancy begins, and others may occur during the first and second trimesters of pregnancy.

Women use the results of preconception and prenatal testing for a variety of purposes. Some women use the information to determine whether to continue or terminate a pregnancy. Others use the information to delay pregnancy, hoping for science to provide them with additional treatment options. Others use this information to avoid pregnancy entirely, or to become pregnant using donor eggs or sperm. Still others use the information to learn about the condition affecting their fetus, to plan to deliver the fetus at a high-risk perinatal unit where facilities to treat the infant immediately upon birth are available, or to make plans for parenting an infant with special needs.

Many in society incorrectly assume that women who receive "bad news" about the pregnancy will use this information to terminate their pregnancy. The issue of abortion is a highly charged social issue; however, current legislation notes that this is a private decision, not one in which society has a right to dictate actions. It is a complex ethical issue. Women deserve to have accurate information delivered in a nonjudgmental fashion so that they, in consultation with those of their choice, can make an informed decision that is right for them and their family.

The same basic principles hold true in the case of presymptomatic genetic testing, especially in the case of conditions where there is neither prevention nor effective treatment. Some people wish to know whether they will develop a condition such as Huntington disease or Alzheimer disease later in life; others prefer not to find out. Some wish to ensure that they do not have a child at risk for the condition, even as they choose not to know their personal health history. This is possible through the use of IVF with the implantation only of embryos that do not carry the gene of concern, without telling the prospective parents whether there are embryos that do carry the condition.

These are highly personalized decisions that are easy for others to criticize. It is important, again, to provide care that is personalized, sensitive, and nonjudgmental.

SECTION THREE REVIEW

1. If a woman discovers that she is carrying a child with a lethal genetic condition she may
   A. choose to keep this information private and confidential.
   B. be forced to have the child against her wishes.
   C. be referred to an adoption agency.
   D. be denied insurance for the pregnancy.
2. Presymptomatic genetic testing
   A. is required as a part of preventive health maintenance.
   B. is required for life insurance policies.
   C. is a voluntary decision.
   D. requires informed consent of a person's spouse.

Answers: 1. A; 2. C

POSTTEST

1. Genetic testing can be used for
   A. determining insurability.
   B. determining whether a person will definitely develop a genetic condition later in life.
   C. providing services to individuals with disabilities.
   D. denying employment.
2. The branch of the Human Genome Project that studies ethical and social concerns is
   A. ELSI.
   B. AHRQ.
   C. CDC.
   D. FDA.
3. The federal prohibition on genetic discrimination is a part of
   A. ELSI.
   B. the FDA.
   C. GINA.
   D. the CDC.

Posttest answers are located in the Appendix.

CHAPTER SUMMARY

In addition to those discussed in this chapter, there are many other issues that have profound ethical, social, and legal implications. Direct-to-consumer marketing, the availability of genetic testing over the Internet, biobanking, cloning, stem cell research, and other innovations are rapidly adding to the issues that will require us to have serious conversations about the interface between scientific possibilities and their appropriate use in society.

The availability of genetic testing brings up many complex ethical, legal, and social issues. This chapter has raised several questions; it has provided few answers. The purpose of this chapter is to encourage thought, discussion, and reflection among clinicians, consumers, and policy makers. The GINA legislation discussed elsewhere in this book has gone a long way to creating a policy climate that is nonjudgmental and nonpunitive, but it also is important to create a public climate that is informed and questioning. At the turn of the 20th century, the science of eugenics was in vogue, making it acceptable to make decisions to ensure that social engineering would create a healthier society. It was considered acceptable to perform involuntary sterilizations on women who were considered unfit to reproduce, and eugenics was at the core of Hitler's atrocities as he attempted to create an Aryan master race. Genetic determinism could have the same risks if we do not engage in appropriate critical thinking and policy making as the benefits of the Human Genome Project is applied in the 21st century.

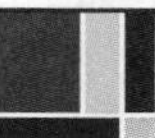

CRITICAL THINKING CHECKPOINT

After appropriate informed consent, Susan is screened for cystic fibrosis early in her pregnancy, and the test results indicate that she is a carrier for a common cystic fibrosis mutation. You share the results with her, and suggest that the next step would be to have her husband tested. She tells you that this pregnancy is a result of an extramarital affair. Her husband believes that he is the father, and the man with whom the affair occurred is not aware that he fathered Susan's baby.

1. What are your responsibilities to Susan?
2. Should you inform her husband that he is not the baby's father?
3. Do you have a responsibility to tell the baby's father of the situation so that he can be tested? If he agrees to be tested, whose insurance is responsible for paying for the test?
4. Do you have any obligation to the fetus?

Answers are provided in the Appendix

Pearson Nursing Student Resources

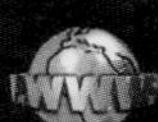

Find additional review materials at nursing.pearsonhighered.com

Prepare for success with additional NCLEX®-style practice questions, interactive assignments and activities, web links, animations, videos, and more!

ONLINE RESOURCES

Coalition for Genetic Fairness: http://www.geneticfairness.org/index.html Genetic Alliance: http://www.geneticalliance.org

Genetic Information Nondiscrimination Act of 2008: http://www.eeoc.gov/laws/statutes/gina.cfm

NIH ELSI Research Program: http://www.genome.gov/ELSI/

NIH Issues in Genetics: http://www.genome.gov/Issues/

NIH website with information about GINA: http://www.genome.gov/24519851

U.S. Department of Labor FAQs on the Genetic Information Nondiscrimination Act: http://www.dol.gov/ebsa/faqs/faq-GINA.html

REFERENCE

Little, C. M., & Lewis, J. A. (2008). Newborn screening. *Newborn and Infant Nursing Reviews, 8*(1), 3–9.

CHAPTER

10 Prenatal Testing and Screening

Judith A. Lewis, Carole Kenner

LEARNING OUTCOMES

Following the completion of this chapter, the learner will be able to

1. Describe genetic factors that contribute to inherited disorders.
2. Discuss prenatal screening and diagnostic procedures used to identify birth defects and genetic disorders.
3. Identify implications of prenatal testing and screening for pregnant women and families.
4. Describe the role of nurses and other health care professionals in providing information about prenatal screening and testing to pregnant women and their families.

This chapter presents the definitions of prenatal testing and screening and the application of these tools to childbearing women and their families, and it discusses how knowledge of genetics is intertwined in the nurse's role in health promotion and disease management. This chapter provides a brief overview of prenatal testing and screening and also focuses on routine prenatal screening and genetic testing and offers information on prenatal diagnostic tests. In addition, this chapter presents the risks and cautions of prenatal testing and screening and discusses the management of the woman and family undergoing prenatal testing and screening.

PRETEST

1. Autosomal refers to the
   A. chromosomes that are not related to sex/gender.
   B. chromosomes that are responsible for sex/gender.
   C. chromosomes that are broken.
   D. chromosomes that are X-linked.
2. Prenatal testing is
   A. required only for women who are at risk for producing an infant with a genetic problem.
   B. required for all women who are pregnant.
   C. recommended for all women planning a pregnancy.
   D. recommended for all women who are pregnant.
3. The ideal time to consider perinatal health is
   A. prenatally once pregnancy is confirmed.
   B. antepartally before the third trimester.
   C. intrapartally before the delivery.
   D. preconceptually before the pregnancy begins.
4. Chorionic villus sampling is usually done
   A. during the first trimester.
   B. during the second trimester.
   C. during the third trimester.
   D. at any time.
5. Mendelian inheritance patterns include
   A. autosomal dominant.
   B. autosomal recessive.
   C. mutations.
   D. Both A and B
6. A woman of advanced maternal age is one who is
   A. over the age of 30.
   B. over the age of 35.
   C. over the age of 40.
   D. over the age of 45.
7. A woman of advanced maternal age is at
   A. greater risk for producing an infant with a genetic problem than a younger woman.
   B. equal risk for producing an infant with a genetic problem than a younger woman.
   C. less risk for producing an infant with a genetic problem than a younger woman.
   D. unknown risk for producing an infant with a genetic problem.

8. X-linked conditions can be passed from fathers to their
   A. daughters.
   B. sons.
   C. Both A and B
   D. Neither
9. A screening test can be used to make a definitive diagnosis of a genetic condition.
   A. True
   B. False
10. Cultural beliefs and values affect the attitude towards prenatal testing and screening.
   A. True
   B. False

Pretest answers are located in the Appendix.

SECTION ONE: Introduction to Prenatal Screening and Testing

Prenatal **testing** and **screening** is not a new concept but one that has increased in importance as more is known about genetics and the importance of the prenatal period. Ironically, while this type of testing and screening refers to the prenatal period, the ideal time for beginning this care is before pregnancy begins, preconceptionally. Since no contraceptive is 100% effective, women of reproductive age who are sexually active with men are at risk for pregnancy. Data confirm that more than half of all pregnancies are unintended (Moos, 2004), meaning that the couple engaging in sexual activity did not intend for that particular act of coitus to result in a conception. Most women do not recognize that they are pregnant until several weeks after conception occurs. The first prenatal visit does not usually occur until at least 8 weeks gestation (Moos, 2003), at which time the embryonic development of most organs and body systems is nearly complete (Jones, 2008).

Sexually active women often visit health care providers only to undergo routine gynecologic examinations and to receive contraceptive devices or prescriptions. **Preconception health counseling** is an important part of these health promotion visits so that women may become aware of any genetic risk factors that exist in their personal or partner's family background. For example, a couple where both members are of Ashkenazi Jewish background should be educated about the importance of screening for **Tay-Sachs** disease (a Mendelian recessive condition) before attempting pregnancy so that they are aware of their risk as a couple for transmitting this condition to any future offspring. Individuals who have family histories of genetic or congenital abnormalities may benefit from preconception genetic counseling so they are aware of the heritability of the condition of concern and the availability of any genetic testing or screening that may be available. Preconception genetic counseling allows individuals and couples the opportunity to make informed decisions about family planning. **Interconceptual education** occurs in the time between pregnancies, when women are seen by their health providers and are open to learning about potential risks. Women and their partners have choices such as attempting, deferring, avoiding, and terminating the pregnancy and having appropriate prenatal genetic screening and testing.

Genetic Factors Contributing to Inherited Disorders

Genetic disorders can be inherited in Mendelian fashion. See Chapter 7 for a full description of the principles of Mendelian inheritance. Examples of conditions inherited in an autosomal recessive fashion include cystic fibrosis **(CF)**, Tay-Sachs disease, and **Factor V Leiden**. In most cases there is no previous family history of the condition. There is increased risk of autosomal recessive genetic disorders when both members of a couple have a common ancestor, which is known as consanguinity. Some cultures are more likely to have consanguineous relationships than others (Lewis, 2010).

Other genetic conditions, such as **neurofibromatosis** and **Huntington disease (HD)**, are transmitted in an autosomal dominant fashion. In many cases a family history of the condition is present; in other cases, the mutation is newly developed. According to Francomano (2006), more than 80% of cases of **achondroplasia** are caused by these de novo mutations.

Some genetic conditions such as **Duchenne muscular dystrophy (DMD)** and red-green color blindness are X-linked recessive conditions. These conditions are inherited by male offspring from a female carrier of the condition. While this female carrier most often is asymptomatic, there are conditions where the female carrier of **hemophilia A** may experience prolonged bleeding, or the carrier of Duchene muscular dystrophy may demonstrate some muscle weakness (Nussbaum, McInnes, & Willard, 2007). There are some conditions that are inherited from maternal mitochondrial DNA. These conditions usually involve the heart, skeletal muscles, and the brain, and can be quite complex. The risk of inheritance by offspring is variable and depends on the amount of abnormal mitochondrial DNA in the cytoplasm of the ovum (Lashley, 2005).

There are other issues that are important in assessing the genetic factors contributing to inherited disorders. Conditions such as Huntington disease, which is transmitted in an autosomal dominant fashion, may become more severe and may present earlier in offspring than in their parents. This phenomenon is called anticipation. Imprinting, where there is unequal expression of each allele, may result in conditions such as Angelman syndrome (**AS**) and Prader-Willi syndrome (**PWS**). Uniparental disomy, where an offspring receives both alleles from the same parent, may result in a child exhibiting symptoms of a Mendelian recessive disorder when only a single parent carries the gene for the condition.

SECTION ONE REVIEW

1. Which of the following is an example of imprinting?
   A. Duchenne muscular dystrophy
   B. Factor V Leiden
   C. Prader-Willi syndrome
   D. Tay-Sachs
2. Autosomal dominant is an example of which inheritance pattern?
   A. Anticipation
   B. De novo
   C. Imprinting
   D. Mendelian
3. Which of the following is true about recessive characteristics?
   A. One gene copy is necessary for the characteristic to occur.
   B. Two gene copies are necessary for the characteristic to occur.
   C. The characteristic will never cause a problem.
   D. The characteristic exists only in a carrier state.
4. Screening refers to
   A. genetic testing for a disease already known to be present.
   B. testing done to determine if there is a potential increased chance for a disease.
   C. a diagnostic tool that confirms a disease is present.
   D. a nursing assessment.
5. Preconception health counseling is
   A. health education done before, during, and after a pregnancy.
   B. health education done before and/or after a pregnancy.
   C. health education done during the pregnancy.
   D. health education done only for women.

Answers: 1. C; 2. D; 3. A; 4. B; 5. B

SECTION TWO: Genetic Tests: Routine Prenatal Screening

Perhaps the most informative screening tool is the three-generation **family history** (see Figure 10–1 ■). All nurses are expected to be proficient in eliciting a comprehensive family history (Consensus Panel, 2006) and depicting it graphically in a **pedigree**, using standard pedigree symbols (Bennett et al., 1995). Evaluation of the family history provides the nurse with information related to the specific risk factors for the individual. Ethnic background, along with conditions present among family members, provides the nurse with information that can be used to tailor prenatal screening and diagnostic tests for individual women and their partners (see Figure 10–2 ■).

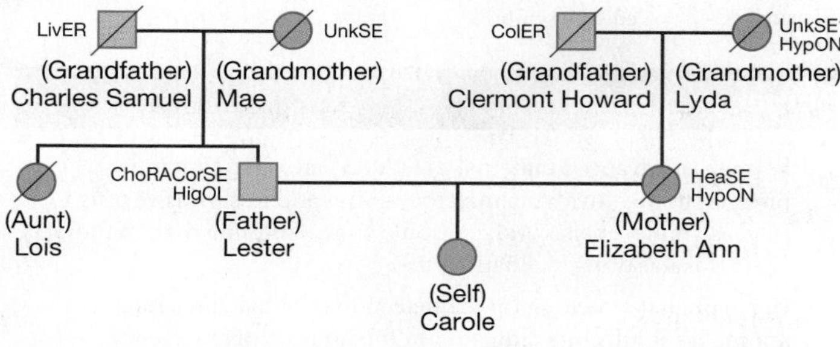

Figure 10–1 ■ Family history: three generations

Routine screening refers to **population-based screening** tests that are performed on healthy individuals with no history of the disease. The screening test is designed to detect those who may have or develop a disease. In other words, there are three basic elements to population-based screening: 1) the identification of persons likely to be at high risk for a specific disorder so that further testing can be done and preventive actions taken; 2) outreach to populations that have not sought medical attention for the condition, and 3) follow-up and intervention to benefit the screened persons (for example, newborn screening and prenatal maternal serum alpha-fetoprotein (**MSAFP**) multimarker screening). In the future, genetic information will increasingly be used in population screening to determine individuals who are susceptible to common disorders such as heart disease, diabetes, and cancer. Such screening will identify groups at risk so primary prevention efforts (e.g., diet and exercise) or secondary prevention efforts (early detection or pharmacologic intervention) can be initiated. Such information could lead to the modification of screening recommendations, which are currently based on population averages (e.g., screening of people over 50 years of age for the early detection of colorectal cancer). Not all women are aware that the "routine" prenatal tests may include tests that act as a screening tool for biological markers that suggest a genetic disorder. Screening tests are a first-level test, and, to be effective, must have acceptable sensitivity and specificity. **Sensitivity** refers to the test's ability to identify those who are at risk for the condition, and therefore need more in-depth **diagnostic testing**. **Specificity** refers to a test's ability to accurately predict those who are not at risk for a specific condition and who therefore do not necessarily require further diagnostic testing. Any test has **false positives** and **false negatives**; therefore, these test results must be explained to the woman and her partner in a way that presents the information accurately and identifies the limitations of the screening test. Laboratory calculations must be adjusted when a woman has diabetes or other metabolic or endocrine problems, as well as for weight and ethnicity, because these factors can affect the overall amount of metabolites present and change what is considered to be the "normal range" for that

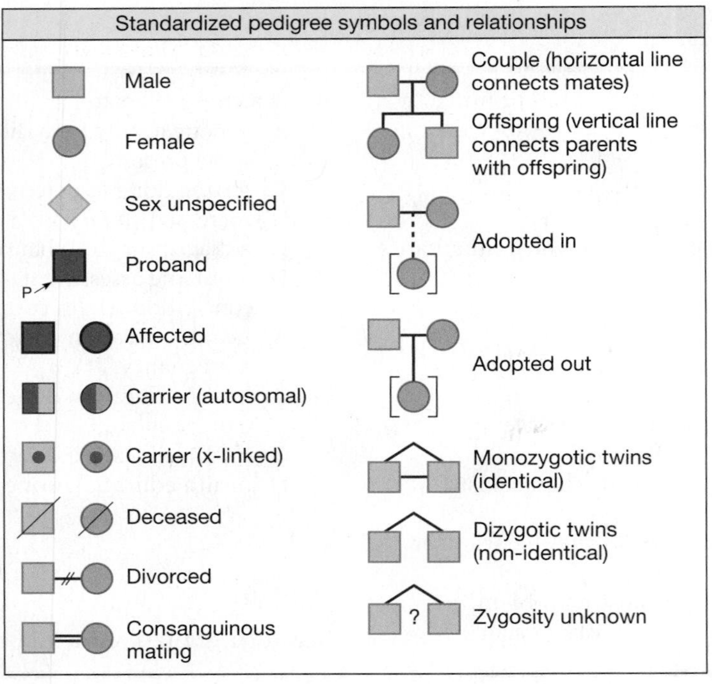

Figure 10–2 ■ Pedigree symbols

Emerging Evidence

- Women of advanced maternal age (AMA) are obtaining more prenatal testing involving maternal serum and less invasive tests such as amniocentesis and chorionic villus sampling than in the past (Nakata, Wang, & Bhatt, 2010).
- Using prental screening for the detection of lethal congenital anomalies results in a reduction in the number of emergency cesarian delivery rate (Dempsey, Breathnach, Geary, Fitzpatrick, Robson, & Malone, 2010). This is one study and it needs to be replicated.
- Prenatal carrier screening in Ashkenazi Jewish population who is at risk for the gene (trait) or disease such as Tay-Sachs appears to have promise for health promotion. Several mutations for recessive conditions has been identified. Since these are in the carrier state, health and genetic counseling can be used to prevent diseases and promote health (Scott, Edelmann, Liu, Luo, Desnick, & Kornreich, 2010).

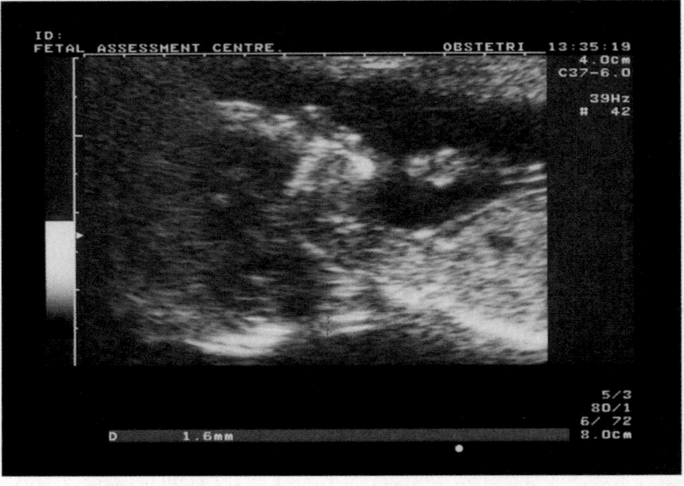

Figure 10–3 ■ Ultrasound demonstrating fetal nuchal translucency
SPL / Photo Researchers, Inc.

population. Women who have an out-of-normal range screening result but seem to be carrying a normally developing fetus may still have an increased risk of perinatal complications. These complications may include premature rupture of membranes, abrupt placenta, and pregnancy loss.

An **ultrasound** is often performed early in pregnancy to confirm a viable pregnancy and to provide accurate dating of the pregnancy. Screening ultrasounds may identify areas of concern as incidental findings. For example, a screening ultrasound may identify an abnormally large area of **fetal nuchal translucency** (see Figure 10–3 ■). An area of increased nuchal translucency is suggestive of **Down syndrome** or trisomy 21 and would indicate the need to perform **karyotype** testing via amniocentesis to determine chromosomal numbers. This ultrasound is only a screening test; therefore, additional tests are required before a definitive diagnosis can be made.

Full integrated screening is often used when conditions such as Down syndrome and trisomy 18 are suspected. This screening involves testing during the first and second trimesters, examining biological markers and ultrasounds. Use of this two-step process increases the likelihood that the condition will be detected accurately.

Other considerations are women who have had a child with a genetic problem that may or may not have been detected during the prenatal period. They may be at risk during subsequent pregnancies but they must be provided screening and testing options. For example, a woman who had a baby with Down syndrome in a previous pregnancy may opt to have screening in her next pregnancy before going directly to diagnostic testing.

Routine prenatal blood work often includes prenatal maternal serum screening, which identifies women whose fetuses are at increased risk for Down syndrome, **trisomy 18**, or **neural tube defects** such as **hydrocephalus** and **spina bifida**. The serum markers in a **triple screen** include maternal serum alpha fetoprotein (MSAFP), human chorionic gonadotropin (hCG), and maternal serum unconjugated estriol (uE3); **quad screening** also includes inhibin-A (**INH-A**). Results are compared to a scale that is calibrated by gestational age. Women who have abnormally high or low readings, which are measured in units called multiples of the median (**MoM**), are offered repeat screening. If the results remain in the abnormal range, more definitive diagnostic testing is offered. Nurses can be of assistance to pregnant women by explaining the nature of the screening test before the blood is drawn, reminding them that there are many reasons for false positives, including multiple gestation and inaccurate calculation of gestational age. Women should be offered the option of declining the test after receiving information that is sufficient to ensure informed decision making. The possibility of producing a child with a genetic condition such as trisomy 21 is increased in women of **advanced maternal age** (**AMA**), which is women who are 35 years of age or older when they become pregnant. These women should be tested with routine serum screening at the time of delivery, not at the time when they become pregnant, and may also receive further testing such as chorionic villus sampling or amniocentesis.

In 1997 the National Institutes of Health (NIH) issued a consensus statement recommending that prenatal care providers offer cystic fibrosis screening to adults with a family history of CF, to partners of those who have CF, to couples who are planning a pregnancy, and to pregnant women who present for prenatal testing (NIH, 1997). As of 2009, more than 1,400 mutations of the CF gene have been identified (Cystic Fibrosis Foundation, 2009) and the frequency of CF carriers in the U.S. population varies widely by race and ethnicity, from 1 in 29 in the Caucasian population to 1 in 90 in the Asian-American population. The sensitivity of the test also varies widely among population groups. For example, screening tests can more accurately identify potential carriers in the Ashkenazi Jewish population than in the African-American population. Another concern regarding CF screening is the variation in the presentation of the condition itself. Some children born with CF have profound illness and a remarkably shortened life expectancy, where in other individuals the condition presents itself in a much milder form and does not have significant impact on functional ability or life expectancy. The nurse can explain the spectrum of information about CF and help women and their partners make informed decisions about whether to avail themselves of the screening test. It must be remembered that CF screening has variable sensitivity in different populations because it only screens for a select number of mutations that are more common in some populations such as the Ashkenazi Jewish population. It is less common in African-Americans. It also must be remembered that some carriers do have mild symptoms, such as was described with a carrier for hemophilia A, who has prolonged bleeding but no other problems.

SECTION TWO REVIEW

1. Population-based screening is done on individuals who
   A. have a history of the disease for which the screening is aimed.
   B. have no history of the disease for which the screening is aimed.
   C. have symptoms of the disease for which the screening is aimed.
   D. have both a history and symptoms of the disease for which the screening is aimed.
2. ____________ refers to a test's ability to accurately predict those who are not at risk for a specific condition and who therefore do not need further diagnostic testing.
   A. Accuracy
   B. Reliability
   C. Sensitivity
   D. Specificity
3. ____________ refers to the test's ability to identify those who are at risk for the condition, and therefore need more in-depth diagnostic testing.
   A. Accuracy
   B. Reliability
   C. Sensitivity
   D. Specificity
4. Triple screen includes all of the following EXCEPT
   A. hCG.
   B. INH-A.
   C. MSAFP.
   D. uE3.
5. A carrier is a person who has one copy of the gene and
   A. exhibits no symptoms for the gene of interest.
   B. exhibits symptoms for the gene of interest but no disease.
   C. exhibits symptoms of the disease associated with the gene of interest.
   D. knows at some point the gene will cause illness in them.

Answers: 1. B; 2. D; 3. C; 4. B; 5. B

SECTION THREE: Prenatal Diagnostic Tests

While screening tests are population-based tests performed on healthy individuals with no known risk factors for disease, diagnostic tests are used to identify individuals who have specific conditions. **Diagnostic testing** is most often performed when there are indications that a condition may exist. Those indicators may come from personal or family history, results of screening tests, environmental exposures, or other factors that lead the patient or clinician to have concerns in a specific area.

Ultrasound testing can provide confirmation of suspected congenital abnormalities that are associated with specific genetic conditions, such as skeletal abnormalities, cardiac conditions and **congenital renal agenesis**. Ultrasound can also be used to locate the placenta, and it may be used in conjunction with other diagnostic procedures to guide instruments and locate pockets of amniotic fluid.

Amniocentesis involves the withdrawal and analysis of amniotic fluid. Fetal cells present in the amniotic fluid are cultured and examined. Amniocentesis is usually performed early in the second trimester of pregnancy, after enough fluid has developed for the procedure to be technically possible. Fetal karyotyping is performed to examine the structure and number of chromosomes and rule out the presence of trisomies as well as many other genetic conditions. This is not the only testing that can be done. Biochemical and DNA testing is also possible. Fetal gender also can be determined by karyotyping. A family history may determine specific conditions for which a test can be done; however, it is not technically possible to test for all known genetic conditions. Thus, a mother may be reassured if the fetus does not demonstrate a specific gene alteration, but she cannot be given a guarantee that her fetus is completely normal.

Chorionic villus sampling involves the removal of tissue from the chorionic sac and is performed during the first trimester. Fetal karyotyping is performed. The test provides information to pregnant women earlier in the gestation but does not yield the depth of information gleaned from amniocentesis. The test also carries a higher risk of unintended spontaneous abortion.

Prenatal diagnostic tests also can be done to determine if the parents are carriers of specific genetic conditions, and most often are done on members of specific ethnic groups. Couples where both members are of Ashkenazi Jewish descent may be tested for the gene for Tay-Sachs disease, a condition that is far more prevalent in this ethnic community. If both parents test positive, any pregnancy will have a 25% risk of producing a fetus with this condition. Conditions that are transmitted in an X-linked recessive fashion would carried by the mother, and it would be appropriate to determine her carrier status if there was a family history suggestive of this. Conditions that are inherited in a Mendelian dominant mode, such as Huntington disease, have a 50% transmission risk for each pregnancy if either parent is a carrier. In the example of the Ashkenazi Jewish population, there is a national group called Dor Yeshorium that facilitates genetic screening for a large number of Jewish young adults worldwide. This organization goes out into the community and collects blood samples. These samples are then coded and genotyped for several autosomal recessive diseases that are common to this group. Participants do not receive results. When two members with samples in the repository are contemplating marriage they contact the organization to see if they are a genetic "match." If they both carry a recessive allele for the same disease, the organization recommends the couple does not go through with the marriage. While the couple is still able to choose to marry, the community has responded positively and apparently applies significant pressure so that a marriage of two "matches" rarely happens. It has led to a substantial decrease in the frequency of Tay-Sachs within the community. This action however, has potentially serious ethical ramifications and is only given as an example of how genetic testing is being used. This type of repository and pressure on marriage plans will potentially grow; with this growth comes more ethical issues and considerations.

Another consideration is the woman who has a genetic condition such as Marfan syndrome or cystic fibrosis and who can now get pregnant and bear a child. A woman with one of these conditions should know firsthand the importance of getting diagnosed and treated early in life. They represent a growing population of childbearing women who need thorough, respectful, and nondirective genetic counseling. These women also may want to undergo other options for pregnancy.

Family history is an important consideration for any preconception prenatal plan. Taking a family history is discussed fully in Chapter 13. If there is significant family history of a condition that parents wish to avoid, it is possible to test an embryo prior to implantation.

Preimplantation genetic diagnosis involves the creation of an embryo using the technology of in-vitro fertilization (**IVF**) and then testing each embryo for the condition of concern. Since IVF involves ovarian hyperstimulation, there usually are multiple embryos created from each cycle. It is possible to identify those embryos that do not carry the gene of concern, and to implant one of those embryos back into the woman's uterus. Theoretically, it is possible to do this without informing the parents whether there were any embryos that carried the specific condition. This may be the choice of parents who know they are at risk of developing a condition with later adult onset. They can ensure that the condition will not be passed on to future offspring without finding out their own individual genotype. The procedure is extremely expensive, as it involves the costs of both genetic testing and IVF.

SECTION THREE REVIEW

1. Diagnostic tests are used to
   A. detect problems in individuals believed to have a condition.
   B. detect problems only in individuals who show no symptoms.
   C. detect only problems prenatally.
   D. detect problems only if screening has been done.
2. Pre-implantation genetic diagnosis involves
   A. an embryo already in the womb.
   B. an embryo before it has been placed in the womb.
   C. informed consent always.
   D. cost considerations.
3. Choronic villus sampling can be done
   A. earlier than amniocentesis.
   B. later than amniocentesis.
   C. any time during the pregnancy.
   D. after birth.
4. Ultrasound testing is used to detect
   A. chromosomal analysis.
   B. karyotype changes.
   C. structural anomalies.
   D. changes in DNA.
5. Fetal gender can be determined by
   A. amniocentesis.
   B. choronic villus sampling.
   C. karyotyping.
   D. changes in DNA.

Answers: 1. A; 2. B; 3. A; 4. C; 5. C

SECTION FOUR: Risks and Cautions

Genetic testing can provide women and their partners with valuable information that can lead to informed decision making regarding pregnancy outcome. There are, however, limitations to the technology as well as legal and ethical concerns.

One of the concerns is the inadvertent identification of wrongful paternity. It is possible that the presumptive father of the child is not the biological parent. This situation can raise serious issues for the couple. The nurse or physician will face challenges in communicating this information to the woman. There are also issues related to the male partner's right to know his genetic complement in the case that he has been or will be involved in fathering children with other partners. This is a complex ethical issue and relates to the identification of who the patient is and what her rights are, and what the rights are of any other involved individuals.

Providing information in a nonjudgmental, neutral fashion is more difficult than it seems. Conditions may be described in many ways, and the description may color how an individual perceives the severity of the condition. Past knowledge of individuals with a particular condition, television and Internet material, and other information may provide people with information that is less than scientifically accurate. It is important to help women and their partners sort through the vast amount of information available and separate science from sensationalism. It is also important to help couples discuss their individual tolerance for risk and which options are acceptable to them and to help patients and families understand how to select reliable Internet resources. For example, information from the International Society of Nurses in Genetics is a reliable, professional resource, and the Genetic Alliance is an excellent resource that includes links to disease-specific research and advocacy groups.

There is a difference between genotype and phenotype. While genetic testing can identify the genetic composition of an individual (the genotype), it may not be able to accurately determine what a person actually will look like (the phenotype). For example, Down syndrome has a wide variation in expression. Determining that an individual has three copies of chromosome 21 cannot predict whether the individual will be mildly or profoundly affected. While an ultrasound may be able to determine whether the fetus with trisomy 21 has congenital cardiac defects, it cannot determine the severity of mental developmental disability.

Another caution is in the use of genetic testing to determine fetal gender. While women and their partners may find this information nice to know, it can pose ethical dilemmas in cultures where there is a strong preference for a child of a particular gender (usually male). In China, with its one child per family policy, a significant unbalance between males and females is occurring. In cultures such as rural India, where female infanticide is still practiced, prenatal gender identification raises other dilemmas. In families where multiple pregnancies are attempted in the hopes of finally producing a child of a different gender than those already present, still other issues are present.

Finally, there have been published reports of families attempting pregnancy coupled with prenatal or pre-implantation genetic testing to produce a child who has the appropriate genetic composition to serve as a tissue donor for a current child who has a severe medical condition, such as **Fanconi's anemia (FA)**. In some states this can pose a potential legal liability for parents as this action can be considered a crime so they can be brought into a lawsuit.

Nurses who are aware of the complexities of prenatal testing can serve as informed patient educators and advocates. They can identify appropriate referral resources for their clients, provide culturally competent care, and use genetic literacy to help their clients navigate the health care system.

SECTION FOUR REVIEW

1. Genetic testing can determine paternity, which in turn can lead to
   A. unintended consequences of revealing a father other than the mother's partner.
   B. ethical dilemmas about how this information should be released.
   C. misinterpretation of the results.
   D. All of the above
2. Issues of getting pregnant to produce a child for tissue transplants is
   A. a personal decision.
   B. a potential legal liability.
   C. always an ethical dilemma.
   D. should never be done.
3. Understanding the mother and/or father's culture is important for genetic testing.
   A. True
   B. False
4. Prenatal testing can determine the severity of the fetal condition without question.
   A. True
   B. False
5. The nurse's role in prenatal testing unless certified as a Genetic Nurse or Counselor is to
   A. interpret the results.
   B. analyze the genetic risk.
   C. emotionally support the mother and/or father.
   D. ensure that no ethical dilemmas occur.

Answers: 1. D; 2. B; 3. A; 4. B; 5. C

SECTION FIVE: A Woman/Family Undergoing Prenatal Testing and Screening

Preconception health education should be considered a role of the nurse any time that she is working with a woman who has expressed an interest in becoming pregnant or who is sexually active. When making decisions about preconception or prenatal testing and screening, women and their families are often confused by what the physician may have told them. They rely on the nurse to help make the decision about such testing and screening (Park & Mathews, 2009). These women often also depend on Internet resources or advice from friends. A nurse can assist with finding credible resources and interpreting information about such testing and screening (Park & Mathews, 2009). Prenatal testing and screening is not always covered by health insurance, at least not all types of testing. Therefore the nurse can help a woman and family sort out which tests can be covered and what is available if there is no insurance (Tapon, 2010).

Another role that a nurse plays in the management of the woman undergoing testing is to prepare the woman physically for the test, to teach about the signs and symptoms of problems after the test such as cramping or bleeding following a chorionic villus sample, and to know when results can be expected. After the results are given to the woman and her family, the nurse can, at the very least, assist with understanding the results after the physician or genetic counselor reports the findings. In many instances today, the nurse is credentialed in genetic nursing and can provide genetic counseling services. If there is a decision to be made about the termination of pregnancy, the nurse can assist with active listening. If a problem is identified that indicates a baby is to be born who is at high risk for an early death or lifelong problems, the nurse can advocate for resources for the woman and family.

SECTION FIVE REVIEW

1. Preconceptual education is important because
   A. many pregnancies are unplanned; therefore, risks are undetermined.
   B. a woman needs to know about genetic risks prior to pregnancy.
   C. it promotes a healthy lifestyle in light of genetic risks.
   D. All of the above
2. Prenatal testing is always covered by health insurance.
   A. True
   B. False
3. The role of the nurse in prenatal testing and screening unless certified or educated as a genetic nurse specialist/counselor is as a(n)
   A. advocate.
   B. diagnostician.
   C. genetic counselor.
   D. practitioner.
4. Internet resources with health information are generally reliable.
   A. True
   B. False
5. Ethical decision making is part of the management of a woman undergoing prenatal testing and screening.
   A. True
   B. False

Answers: 1. D; 2. B; 3. A; 4. B; 5. A

POSTTEST

1. A recessive condition occurs when
   A. one parent has a copy of abnormal gene.
   B. both parents have a copy of the same abnormal gene.
   C. neither parent has a copy of an abnormal gene.
   D. a mutation in the genes occurs.
2. Prenatal screening is used for
   A. only women who are at risk for a genetic condition.
   B. only women who are advanced maternal age.
   C. only women who request the screening.
   D. all women who are pregnant.
3. Preconceptual screening is
   A. useful to promote health and disease prevention.
   B. a waste of time and money.
   C. reserved for high risk childbearing women.
   D. not recommended by any professional organizations.
4. Screening tests are used to
   A. determine risk.
   B. diagnosis a disease.
   C. make a treatment plan.
   D. teach women about genetics.
5. A woman who is at risk for producing a baby with a neural tube defect
   A. should undergo prenatal screening and testing for alpha fetoprotein and have an amniocentesis.
   B. must undergo prenatal screening and testing for alpha fetoprotein and have an amniocentesis.
   C. should wait until the baby is born to determine what diagnostic tests should be done.
   D. must wait until the baby is born to determine what diagnostic tests should be done.
6. Diagnostic tests are used to
   A. determine risk.
   B. diagnose a disease.
   C. make a treatment plan.
   D. teach women about genetics.
7. While genetic testing can identify the genetic composition of an individual, also known as the ___________, it may not be able to accurately determine what a person actually will look like, which is known as the ___________.
   A. genotype; phenotype
   B. phenotype; genotype
   C. phenotype; allele
   D. genotype; allele
8. Interconceptual education is important because
   A. many pregnancies are unplanned; therefore, risks are undetermined.
   B. a woman needs to know about genetic risks prior to pregnancy.
   C. the time between pregnancies is when women tend to see their provider.
   D. All of the above
9. Genetic testing is a new concept.
   A. True
   B. False
10. The family history tool is used
   A. only when a woman is pregnant.
   B. only when a woman is at risk for a genetic condition.
   C. throughout the lifespan for any person.
   D. throughout the lifespan for any person at risk for a genetic condition.

Posttest answers are located in the Appendix.

CHAPTER SUMMARY

Prenatal testing and screening is not a new concept but one that has increased in importance as more is known about genetics. Ironically, while this type of testing/screening refers to the prenatal period, the ideal time for starting prenatal care is before pregnancy begins.

Preconception health counseling is an important part of these health promotion visits so that women may become aware of any genetic risk factors that exist in their personal background or in their partner's.

The most informative screening tool is the three-generation family history.

Screening tests are a first-level test; to be effective, these tests must have acceptable sensitivity and specificity. Genetic testing can provide women and their partners with valuable information that can lead to informed decision making regarding pregnancy outcome. The nurse's role in prenatal testing and screening is one of educator and advocate.

CRITICAL THINKING CHECKPOINT

Zoe is a 38-year-old, Caucasian woman who is pregnant for the first time. She and her husband are excited about the pregnancy. Her husband appears to be scared and states that both sides of the family have experienced pregnancy losses. The pregnancy is approximately 12 weeks along.

1. What prenatal testing and screening would be appropriate for this woman?
2. Is a family history important in this case?
3. Are there any factors that put this woman at risk for a genetic problem?
4. What is the role of the nurse before and after the prenatal tests are done?
5. What follow-up care would be necessary?

Answers are provided in the Appendix

Pearson Nursing Student Resources

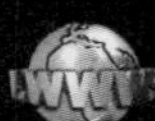

Find additional review materials at nursing.pearsonhighered.com

Prepare for success with additional NCLEX®-style practice questions, interactive assignments and activities, web links, animations, videos, and more!

ONLINE RESOURCES

Dor Yeshorium: http://www.modernlab.org/doryeshirum.html

Preconception Health: http://www.marchofdimes.com/pregnancy/getready_indepth.html

Prenatal Screening: http://www.marchofdimes.com/pregnancy/prenatalcare_routinetests.html

Prenatal Testing: http://www.nlm.nih.gov/medlineplus/prenataltesting.html

REFERENCES

Bennett, R. L., Steinhaus, K. Al, Uhrich, S. B., O'Sullivan, C. K., Resta, R. G., Lochner-Doyle, D., et al. (1995). Recommendations for standardized human pedigree nomenclature. *Pedigree Standardization Task Force of the National Society of Genetic Counselors, American Journal of Human Genetics, 56*(3), 745–52.

Consensus Panel on Genetic/Genomic Nursing Competencies. (2006). *Essential nursing competencies and curricula guidelines for genetics and genomics.* Silver Spring, MD: American Nurses Association.

Cystic Fibrosis Foundation. (2009). *About cystic fibrosis*. Retrieved from http://www.cff.org/aboutCF

Dempsey, M. A., Breathnach, F. M., Beary, M., Fitzpatrick, C., Robson, M., & Malone, F. D. (2010). Congenital anomalies: Impact of prenatal diagnosis on mode of delivery. *Irish Medical Journal, 103*(3), 88–89.

Dommering, C. J., van den Heuvel, M. R., Moll, A. C., Imhof, S. M., Meijers-Heijboer, H., & Henneman, L. (2010). Reproductive decision-making: A qualitative study among couples at increased risk of having a child with retinoblastoma. *Clinical Genetics,* Epub. Retrieved July 31, 2010, from http://www.ncbi.nlm.nih.gov/pubmed/20618349

Francomano, C. A. (2006). Achondroplasia. *GeneReviews*. Retrieved June 28, 2012, from http://www.ncbi.nlm.nih.gov/bookshelf/br.fcgi?book=gene&part=achondroplasia

Jones. S. L. (2008). Genetics, embryology, and preconceptual/prenatal assessment and screening. In S. A. Orshan (Ed.), *Maternity, newborn, & women's health nursing: Comprehensive care across the life span*. Philadelphia: Lippincott, Williams & Wilkins, pp. 355–428.

Lashley, F. R. (2005). *Clinical genetics in nursing practice*, (3rd ed.). New York: Springer.

Lewis, J. A. (2010). Genetic issues for perinatal nurses. (3rd ed.). White Plains, NY: March of Dimes.

Moos, M. K. (2003). *Preconception health promotion: A focus for women's wellness* (2nd ed.). White Plains, NY: March of Dimes.

Moos, M. K. (2004). Preconceptional health promotion: Progress in changing a prevention paradigm. *Journal of Perinatal & Neonatal Nursing, 18*(1), 2–13.

Nakata, N., Wang, Y., & Bhatt, S. (2010). Trends in prenatal screening and diagnostic testing among women referred for advanced maternal age. *Prenatal Diagnosis, 30*(3), 198–206.

National Institutes of Health (NIH) Consensus Development Conference. (1997). *Genetic testing for cystic fibrosis: Consensus development conference statement.* April 14–16; 15(4); 1–37.

Nussbaum, R. L., McInnes, R. R., & Willard, H. F. (2007). *Thompson & Thompson's genetics in medicine* (7th ed.). Philadelphia: Saunders.

Parker, A., & Mathews, M. (2009). Women's decisions about maternal serum screening testing: A qualitative study exploring what they learn and the role prenatal care providers play. *Women Birth, 22*(2), 73–78.

Scott, S. A., Edelmann, L., Liu, L., Luo, M., Desnick, R. J., & Kornreich, R. (2010). Experience with carrier screening and prenatal diagnosis for sixteen Ashkenazi Jewish genetic diseases. *Human Mutation,* Epub. Retrieved July 31, 2010, from http://www.ncbi.nlm.nih.gov/pubmed/20672374

Tapon, D. (2010). Prenatal testing for Down syndrome: Comparison of screening practices in the UK and USA. *Journal of Genetic Counseling, 19*(2), 112–130.

CHAPTER

11 Newborn Screening and Genetic Testing: Ethical Considerations

Michelle Beauchesne, Michele DeGrazia

LEARNING OUTCOMES

Following the completion of this chapter, the learner will be able to

1. Discuss the history and controversies of screening large-scale populations.
2. Describe the core conditions that are included in the newborn screen.
3. Discuss how newborn screening may differ between states.
4. Describe the role of the nurse and other health care professionals in the collection and interpretation of newborns screens.
5. Discuss ethical principles as they pertain to the newborn screen and other population-based screening programs.
6. Identify the proposed benefits and risks associated with the retention, storage, and use of newborn screening blood samples.
7. Discuss the proposed expansion of the newborn screening program.

Amid controversies, significant advancements in newborn screening have been observed during the last five decades in the United States. However, diverging viewpoints persist over the identification of serious genetic conditions (even if rare), genetic implications for family members, limitations of analytical and clinical screening tests, screening for maternal drug and alcohol use, and retaining samples for DNA analysis. This chapter provides an overview of the ethical principles and theories underlying population-based, public health screening, past and present recommendations for newborn screening, and the controversies associated with mass screening of newborns.

PRETEST

1. Civilians organized Boards of Health to address rampant spread of diseases to maintain healthy populations.
   A. True
   B. False
2. Which statement is true about a false positive screen?
   A. The individual has the disease or illness but the screen is negative.
   B. Further testing is not needed.
   C. The screen is positive and the individual has the disease or illness.
   D. The screen is positive but the individual does not have the disease or illness.
3. Which of the following statements is true about validity?
   A. It refers to whether or not an instrument, test, or screen accurately measures what it is supposed to measure.
   B. It refers to whether or not an instrument, test, or screen consistently measures what it is supposed to measure.
4. Mass spectrometry (MS/MS) has become the primary instrument for analyzing blood samples obtained from infants following birth.
   A. True
   B. False
5. Ethics is
   A. the examination of moral reasoning.
   B. guided by a set of longstanding principles that have served as the foundation for ethical decision making.
   C. categorized by profession (medicine, nursing, teaching) and by specialty (bioethics, biotechnology).
   D. All of the above

6. Cystic fibrosis
   A. usually presents in infancy.
   B. is a hereditary disease that primarily affects the lungs, pancreas, intestine, liver, sweat glands, and male reproductive tract.
   C. can be treated with a pancreatic enzyme, fat soluble vitamin, and salt supplementation, if detected by newborn screen.
   D. All of the above
7. Congenital hypothyroidism is
   A. not detected by newborn screen.
   B. a disabling and untreatable condition.
   C. associated with significant neurologic impairment.
   D. treated with human insulin.
8. The method used to ensure the voluntary participation of subjects is
   A. justice.
   B. beneficence.
   C. informed consent.
   D. fidelity.
9. If the parent declines the newborn screen after they have been thoroughly educated
   A. a refusal form may need to be completed depending upon the state or hospital of birth.
   B. the nurse will need to contact social services to report neglect.
   C. the nurse will obtain the newborn screen regardless of parental wishes because it is state law.
   D. None of the above
10. Some advocate for newborn screening of prenatal exposure to which of the following substances?
   A. Drugs
   B. Alcohol
   C. Nicotine
   D. All of the above

Pretest answers are located in the Appendix.

SECTION ONE: Public Health and Newborn Screening Programs

Concerted efforts to maintain healthy populations in the United States surfaced during the late 1800s and early 1900s. The U.S. military employed preventative medicine to halt the spread of infectious disease among troops, while civilians organized Boards of Health to address rampant spread of diseases such as small pox and yellow fever. Military and civilian teams employed basic concepts of preventative medicine resulting in the control of disease and environmental threats, reducing **morbidity** and **mortality**. These successful interventions served as the catalysts for the evolution of preventative medicine and population-based, public health screening (English Articles, 2011; Whayne, 1959). This evolution has led to a number of public health screening programs in place today.

Ethics is the branch philosophy that deals with values that pertain to human conduct. It is the examination of moral reasoning about what is right or what is wrong with regards to personnel and societal actions (Gillon, 1985). The study and practice of ethics is guided by a set of longstanding principles that have served as the foundation for ethical decision making. It is thought that by following the principles of ethics, one is led toward making the right or correct decision. Sometimes ethical theories, based upon ethical principles, are used to help guide individuals to make correct decisions when faced with an ethical dilemma (Rainbow, 2002). Many ethical theories and principles exist. Tables 11–1 and 11–2 include examples and brief descriptions of commonly encountered principles and theories (Ascension Healthcare, 2011; Davenport, 1997; Rainbow, 2002).

TABLE 11–1: Ethical Principles

Ethical Principle	Description
Autonomy	The capacity for self-determination or the right to determine what will happen to a person's own body.
Beneficence	To do good or to make sure people benefit from the most good.
Capacity	The ability to decide for oneself and to communicate this decision.
Competency	The possession of required skill, knowledge, qualification, or capacity.
Distributive Justice	In the context of health care, this means all have equal access to basic health care and resources.
Fidelity	The proposition that the health care provider prioritizes the patients' interest first above all others.
Informed Consent	A patient is entitled to receive adequate information to make a decision (includes risk, benefit, and alternatives).
Justice	The prescribed actions are fair to those involved.
Non-maleficence	This means to do no harm.
Self-determination	The ability to make a decision for oneself without outside influence or coercion.
Surrogate	One who stands in place of one who lacks capacity to decide for him- or herself.

TABLE 11–2: Ethical Theories

Ethical Theory	Description
Deontology	This states that people should adhere to their obligations and duties when analyzing an ethical dilemma. This provides a basis for special duties and obligations to specific people such as within one's own family or patients.
Utilitarianism	This is founded on the ability of one to predict the consequence of an action. For instance, when given several options, the one that yields the greater benefit for the most number of people is the correct choice.
Rights	Rights that are set forth by society are protected and given the highest priority. Rights are considered to be ethically correct and valid since a large or ruling population endorses them.
Casuist	This compares a current ethical dilemma against similar ethical dilemmas in order to come up with the best possible or correct solution.
Virtue	The idea that a person is judged by his or her usual character (including morals, reputation and motivation) rather than upon an irregular behavior or deviation from the norm.

The study of ethics is also further categorized by profession (medicine, nursing, teaching) and by specialty (bioethics, biotechnology). For instance medical ethics is the branch of ethics that deals with health care matters, examining the interaction between individuals, society, and the doctor and/or medical profession (Gillon, 1985). Similarly, nursing ethics deals with health care matters, examining the interaction between individuals, society, and the nurse and/or nursing profession (Wright & Brajtman, 2011). Moreover, each of these professions has its own code of ethics that has been established to help guide the discipline (American Medical Association, 1995–2011; American Nurses Association, 2001).

As members of a collaborative health care team, physicians and nurses recognize that ethics play a major role in the collective care they provide. Hence, a more modern interdisciplinary approach is taken towards examining ethical issues (Gaudine, LeFort, Lamb, & Thorne, 2011). Often all members of the health care team (medicine, nursing, respiratory therapy, social work, and others) take part in discussions when ethical dilemmas present (Wright & Brajtman, 2011). Ethical issues frequently faced by the collaborative health care team include end-of-life care, palliative care, and population-based public health issues (Gaudine et al., 2011; Sade, 2011).

Population-Based, Public Health Screening Controversies

Population-based, public health screening has experienced steady advancements in medical technology and screening for **genetic disorders**. Despite these advancements, not all identifiable illnesses have effective treatments or cures. Thus, controversies over the appropriateness of testing large-scale populations have been at the forefront of discussion. Dating back to the 1960s, debate over population-based, public health screening has had two central themes: the screening of asymptomatic individuals for illness and inequities in screening (Wilson & Jungner, 1968).

In the debate over screening asymptomatic individuals for illness, some believe that screening is unnecessary due to the lack of treatment or cure and therefore offers no direct benefit to the individual. In contrast, others believe that expanding screening programs will enable health care providers to learn more about disease so that one day a treatment or cure might be found (Wilson & Jungner, 1968). The former argument is based upon the principle of **autonomy**, which states individuals should have control over their own bodies (Ascension Healthcare, 2011; Rainbow, 2002), while the latter argument is based on the ethical principles of **beneficence** (Ascension Healthcare, 2011; Rainbow, 2002), which supports doing the most good for the most people.

The debate over inequality of screening for illness stems from observed differences in the availability of screening programs at the national (between states) and international levels (between nations). In the past and still today, some states and developed nations have well-established population-based screening programs, while other states and less developed nations have very little to offer with regards to screening programs (Wilson & Jungner, 1968). It is argued that these inequalities of screening practices directly conflict with the ethical principle of **justice**, which supports equality and fairness for all involved. Moreover, it is hypothesized that those with fewer financial resources remain more concerned with managing active disease rather than implementing methods for disease prevention (Baily & Murray, 2008).

Wilson and Jungner Classic Screening Criteria

In 1968, commissioned by the World Health Organization (**WHO**), Wilson and Jungner published a report titled *Principles and Practice of Screening for Disease.* The purpose of their work, based largely upon ethical principles, was to provide principles and practices to screen for disease in a clear and simple way (Box 11–1). The Wilson and Jungner report provides detail with regard to (1) types of screening population-based screening programs should consider (Table 11–3), and (2) criteria to consider before selecting a screening method (Table 11–4). The **Wilson and Jungner Classic Screening Criteria** was to serve as a guide for population-based, public health screening resource utilization (Wilson & Jungner, 1968). Furthermore, Wilson and Jungner intended to address

BOX 11–1 Wilson and Jungner Classic Screening Criteria

1. The condition sought should be an important health problem.
2. There should be an accepted treatment for patients with recognized disease.
3. Facilities for diagnosis and treatment should be available.
4. There should be a recognizable latent or early symptomatic stage.
5. There should be a suitable test or examination.
6. The test should be acceptable to the population.
7. The natural history of the condition, including development from latent to declared disease, should be adequately understood.
8. There should be an agreed policy on whom to treat as patients.
9. The cost of case finding (including diagnosis and treatment of patients diagnosed) should be economically balanced in relation to possible expenditure on medical care as a whole.
10. Case finding should be a continuing process and not a "once and for all" project.

Source: Wilson, Jungner, in *Principles and Practice of Screening for Disease*, Geneva: World Health Organization (1968). Reprinted with permission.

TABLE 11–3: Types of Screening

Screening Method	Description
Selective	High risk; may be large scale
Mass Public Health	Large scale; entire population; general public
Surveillance	Long term; methodical, group, or disease specific
Hospital Patients	High risk group; common disease or illness
Industrial Workers	Special industrial risks; early detection of disease that would impair ability of worker

ethical issues for population-based public health screening in adult medicine, though in retrospect it has been used in a broad spectrum of patient care settings, including pediatrics, and has served as a gold standard in ethical decision making (Crowe 2008). However, due to the dramatic growth of genetics, limitations in Wilson and Jungner's Classic Screening Criteria have been identified, and new criteria for population-based public health screening have emerged. These new criteria will be discussed in Section Three of this chapter.

TABLE 11–4: Criteria to Consider Prior to Screening

Criteria	Definition
Validity	Refers to whether or not an instrument, test, or screen accurately measures what it is supposed to measure
Reliability	Refers to whether or not an instrument, test, or screen consistently measures what it is supposed to measure
Yield	Relates to the prevalence of the disease in the population, and to the availability of use of medical facilities for treatment
Cost	Financial feasibility of conducting the screening program
Acceptance	Refers to whether or not the practitioners and population are willing to utilize the screening test

Newborn Screening: In the Beginning

In 1934, Dr. Asbjorn Folling identified the presence of phenylpyruvic acid in the urine of some patients with intellectual disabilities, and in the early 1960s Dr. Robert Guthrie developed a test to detect phenylpyruvic acid in the urine (known as pheylketonuria) of infants. These discoveries led the way for detection of illness, before infants demonstrated symptoms of the genetically transmitted disease (Crowe, 2008; Schuett, 2009). The discovery of these detection methods along with the development of special diets and food products have served as a template for the early detection and prevention of numerous genetically based disorders. In 1963, mass screening of newborns for pheylketonuria was initiated, and by 1967 more than half of the United States had laws in place for mandatory pheylketonuria screening (Schuett, 2009).

In the beginning, due to issues with **validity** and **reliability** of the testing instruments, several diagnostic tests were needed to identify a variety of problems through **newborn screening**. However since that time newborn screening has expanded and benefited from major technological advances. In fact, it has become possible to screen for many conditions using only one test (Pollitt, 2010). Today, tandem **mass spectrometry** (**MS/MS**) has become the primary instrument for analyzing the blood samples obtained from infants following birth. MS/MS works by weighing molecules. The molecules are then sorted and used for identification of specific disorders (The President's Council on Bioethics Washington, 2008). MS/MS has significantly reduced false positives and is the most reliable method available used to identify newborn disorders (Crowe, 2008).

SECTION ONE REVIEW

1. Classic population-based screening criteria include
   A. the test should be acceptable to the population.
   B. there should be a recognizable latent or early symptomatic stage of illness.
   C. facilities for diagnosis and treatment must be made available.
   D. All of the above
2. In 1934, Dr. Asbjorn Folling developed a test to detect phenylpyruvic acid in the urine (known as pheylketonuria) of infants.
   A. True
   B. False
3. The philosophical examination of moral reasoning about what is right or what is what wrong with regards to personnel and societal actions is called
   A. ethics.
   B. pride.
   C. justice.
   D. collective conscious.
4. A report titled *Principles and Practice of Screening for Disease,* written by Wilson and Jungner, was commissioned by the
   A. United States government.
   B. Department of Health and Human Services.
   C. WHO.
   D. Maternal Child Health Bureau (MCHB).
5. During the late 1800s and early 1900s U.S. military employed preventative medicine to halt the spread of infectious disease among troops, while civilians organized Boards of Health to address rampant spread of diseases to maintain healthy populations.
   A. True
   B. False

Answers: 1. D; 2. B; 3. A; 4. C; 5. A

SECTION TWO: Diagnostic and Genetic Testing

State-Based Newborn Screening Programs

The newborn screening program is one of the most established population-based, public health screening programs in the United States and serves as a model for genetic screening. Furthermore, the newborn screening program is heralded as one of the most successful public health prevention initiatives because of its ability to detect congenital disorders before developmental disability or death. While both federal and state governments have played a role in newborn screening policymaking, the role of the federal government remains limited. The federal government cannot mandate newborn screening; it can only make recommendations to the states (The President's Council on Bioethics Washington, 2008). Public health initiatives like the newborn screening programs remain under the jurisdiction of state governments; therefore, states maintain control over the panel of conditions for which newborns are to be screened and for ensuring that all parents of newborns within the states' jurisdictions are given the opportunity to have their newborns screened ("Overview newborn screening," n.d.).

Newborn Screen Procedure and Management

In the first days of life, a blood sample is obtained by impregnating a special filter with the blood, often from the newborn's heel, and it is then sent to the state laboratory for analysis. When the newborn screening laboratory identifies an infant with a positive newborn screen, the infant's primary care provider is contacted. The primary care provider (pediatrician, family physician, or nurse practitioner) is responsible for contacting the infant's family, providing initial counseling, arranging a subspecialty referral, and obtaining a repeat blood sample (if indicated).

Arranging for follow-up and providing initial counseling can be a daunting task. Many conditions identified through the newborn screen are rare; therefore, the pediatrician or primary care provider may not be adequately prepared to educate the family (DeLuca, Kearney, Norton, & Arnold, 2011; Kemper, Uren, Moseley, & Clark, 2006; Stark, Lang, & Ross, 2011). Most often the patient and his or her family are sent to a specialist for education and for additional confirmatory and severity testing. Confirmatory and severity testing is done because some disorders require additional testing to confirm the diagnosis and because identification of a disorder will not necessarily provide information about the severity of the illness (DeLuca et al., 2011).

Core Conditions

Newborn screening for congenital conditions began in the 1960s with Guthrie's original **filter paper** screening technique and has now been available for more than 50 years in the United States. However, not all states have kept pace with advancements and expansion with screening newborns for genetically based illness. Specifically, there have been notable differences in the number and quality of screens provided. Additionally, states differed on screening protocols, follow-up services, and who assumes costs (families versus state) (Bailey, Skinner, Davis, Whitmarsh, & Powell, 2008; Baily & Murray, 2008). When deciding upon on which screens to perform, states considered multiple factors, such as prevalence of the disorder, accuracy of detection, availability and outcomes of treatment, overall cost effectiveness of both short-term diagnostic procedures, long-term management, and follow-up services. Even with the advent of tandem mass spectroscopy, which decreased the cost of screening, only four disorders (classic phenylketonuria, congenital hypothyroidism, classic galactosemia, and sickle cell disease) had been commonly screened ("Overview newborn screening," n.d.).

In 1999, the American Academy of Pediatrics (**AAP**) called upon the federal government to support a national endeavor involving the government, professionals, and consumers to address disparities and to make recommendations for consistency and uniformity of state-based newborn screening programs. In response, the Maternal Child Health Bureau (MCHB) commissioned the American College of Medical Genetics (**ACMG**) to develop an expert panel to assess the strengths and weaknesses of individual state newborn screening programs and to develop recommendations for uniform screening policies, procedures, and processes for quality assurance and oversight. The resulting document, titled "Newborn Screening: Toward a Uniform Screening Panel and System," (2006) identified principles that guided (1) the decision-making process, (2) development criteria and categories for conditions considered for screening, and (3) development of a system for comparative analysis of conditions.

The expert panel was charged with conducting a review of the newborn screening program in an efficient manner to ensure that the findings were current and relevant. Transparency of the decision-making processes and providing evidence to support each decision was crucial to the expert panel. The expert panel utilized a decision-making algorithm to determine eligibility for inclusion on the newborn screening panel of **core conditions** and **secondary target conditions**. All conditions, including the original core conditions, classic phenylketonuria, congenital hypothyroidism, classic galactosemia, and sickle cell disease were evaluated using the same methods.

The expert panel reviewed a total of 84 genetic conditions to determine if scientific evidence was available to support screening of the various conditions according to the following criteria:

- Availability of a sensitive and specific screen for the condition within a 24–48 hour interval after birth
- Availability of effective/successful treatment
- An understanding of the history of the condition
- The potential for identification of a genetically transmitted disease or carrier state (Green et al., 2007)

Of the 84 genetically based conditions, 29 core conditions (see Tables 11–5 through 11–10) were recommended for uniform screening in every state, and a list of 26 secondary target conditions was also identified.

According to the "Newborn Screening" report, secondary targets may be clinically important and therefore should be obtained when the infant has his or her first newborn screen blood test or in follow-up testing if indicated. When combined, a total of 55 conditions were recommended for screening and 27 additional conditions were excluded because they either met too few evaluation criteria or lacked a screening test (Watson et al., 2006).

Review and Oversight

Periodic review of the core conditions and the secondary target conditions on the Uniform Panel of Screening Disorders was also recommended by the expert panel to ensure that newborn screening programs remain current. This periodic review was considered essential and would guarantee that the uniform panel is updated as new evidence emerges. They recommended that in addition to disease specific evidence, input from patients, family groups, and other stakeholders should be submitted as part of the evidence for the periodic reviews (Watson et al., 2006). The expert panel also called for national oversight and authority over newborn screening programs and for the implementation of ongoing performance improvement initiatives (Advisory Committee on Heritable Disorders and Genetic Diseases in Newborn and Children, 2006).

The Secretary's Advisory Committee on Heritable Disorders in Newborns and Children (**SACHDNC**) endorsed this report and its recommendations for a core panel.

The SACHDNC then became responsible for determining the process for nomination and evidence-based review of additional conditions to this initial core set (Calonge et al., 2010; Green et al., 2007). It established a rigorous process of systematic external review of nominations, separating them into three broad areas, similar to those used by the original ACMG expert panel. In addition, six key questions were developed to evaluate whether the current evidence is adequate enough to warrant inclusion in the core panel. (See Box 11–2.) Finally, a decision matrix was used based upon the level of certainty of the evidence to make recommendations to the Health and Human Services Secretary.

In 2008, upon recommendation of the ACMG, the Maternal Child Health Bureau (**MCHB**) of the Health Resources and Services Administration (**HRSA**), and the March of Dimes, a law was adopted recommending that all 50 states and the District of Columbia conduct mandatory screening of newborn infants for the 29 core conditions organized in the following general categories: metabolic disorders, endocrine disorders, hemoglobin disorders, and others (Kaye, 2006). The 29 serious genetic or functional disorders make up what is known as the uniform panel of core conditions. This landmark federal legislation, The Newborn Screening Saves Lives Act, was signed into law with the intent to strengthen the federal role in newborn screening policy, to improve the newborn screening infrastructure, and to decrease disparities between states ("Newborn screening law," 2011; "Overview newborn screening," n.d.).

In 2010, severe combined immunodeficiency was added to the uniform panel of core conditions by the SACHDNC, making a new total of 30 core conditions (Lipstein et al., 2010). As of 2010, all core conditions in the ACMG's uniform panel would now be obtained through a single blood sample obtained by heel stick, except for the newborn hearing screen. In 2010, Secretary of Health and Human Services Kathleen Sebelius adopted the SACHDNC recommendations for newborn screening, stating adoption would facilitate federal guidance to assist states to voluntarily bring their newborn screening programs into alignment with national standards and best practices. By 2011, all states were required to screen for these disorders with only a few minor exceptions ("Newborn screening overview," 2011). Furthermore, in September

2011, pulse oximetry for critical congenital heart disease (CCHD) was recommended for inclusion in state programs.

Core Conditions

The 30 Core Conditions recommended in routine newborn screening by the SACHDNC Recommended Uniform Screening Panel (RUSP) are grouped in four major categories based upon the cause of the disorder. These categories are metabolic disorders, endocrine disorders, hemoglobin disorders, and other. The metabolic category includes three subcategories: organic acid conditions, fatty acid oxidation disorders, and amino acid disorders. These conditions will be discussed in this order identified by name and assigned individual American College of Medical Genetics (AMCG) code (2011).

I. Metabolic Disorders

These conditions involve complex biochemical processes, in which enzymes convert essential amino acids, carbohydrates, and lipids to substances or energy that can be used at the cellular level. External nutrients, such as breast milk, formula, and food are transformed into energy through these metabolic pathways. Inherited metabolic disorders are called inborn errors of metabolism because they are caused by genetic alterations in the genes responsible for certain enzymes, which result in disruption of major metabolic pathways. Clinical consequences for the child can range from mild to severe. Most often these infants appear normal at birth with signs and symptoms presenting within a few days or months. In many cases, early identification and treatment with special diets or supplements can alleviate symptoms and prevent further problems.

Organic Acid Conditions Infants and children who have one of these types of metabolic disorders have a problem with processing branched-chain amino acids (leucine, isoleucine, and valine). Plasma concentrations of the branched-chain amino acids are significantly affected by dietary changes in amounts of calories, proteins, fats, and carbohydrates. Even one day of fasting or starvation can have untoward effects in these infants and children (See Table 11–5).

TABLE 11–5: Organic Acid Conditions

Condition and Code	Description	Clinical Manifestation
1. Propionic Acidemia (ACMG code=PROP)	An inherited disorder in which there is a defect in the processing of essential amino acids. As a result, abnormal toxic levels of propionic acid build up in the blood and tissues leading to health issues during the newborn period, usually due to intolerance to dietary protein.	Clinical manifestations: Episodic emesis, dehydration, and metabolic acidosis. Hematologic abnormalities such as neutropenia, thrombocytopenia, and hypogammaglobulinemia are common. Without treatment, brain damage, coma, and death can result. Treatment includes a low-protein diet and nutritional supplements. However, even with treatment, some affected children go on to exhibit intellectual disabilities, developmental delays, seizures, abnormal muscle tone, frequent infections, and cardiac problems.
2. Methylmalonic Acidemia (Methylmalonyl-CoA Mutase) (ACMG code=MUT)	An increase in methylmalonic acid that causes a variety of health problems.	Clinical manifestations: Failure to thrive, episodic dehydration, and hypotonia as well as central nervous system changes (dystonia, dysphagia, and dysarthria). Infants with methylmalonic academia have distinct facial dysmorphism.
3. Methylmalonic Acidemia (cobalamin disorders) (ACMG Code=Cbl A,B)	An inherited disorder in which there is a defect in the enzyme that processes four essential amino acids—isoleucine, methionine, threonine, and valine. As a result, abnormal accumulations of amino acids in the blood, urine, and tissues can lead to serious morbidity, and often mortality, in the first year of life. Two forms of this defect, Methylmalonic Acidemia CblA caused by a mutation in the MMAA gene and CblB caused by a mutation in the MMAB gene, are recommended for screening.	Clinical manifestations: Brain damage, seizures, paralysis, hepatic toxicity, and coma; often can begin as early as the first week of life. A minority of affected children exhibit no symptoms until later in life, often following an illness. Treatment includes a low-protein diet, vitamin B12, and nutritional supplements. However, even with treatment some infants die during the first year of life or develop serious lasting consequences.
4. Isovaleric Acidemia (ACMG Code=IVA)	A disorder caused by an inability to process the amino acid leucine resulting in abnormal levels of amino acids in the blood, urine, and tissues. The newborn form of the disorder often results in serious health concerns including coma, permanent neurologic damage, and death. Sometimes symptoms develop later in infancy and childhood, frequently following an illness or high dietary protein intake. Early diagnosis and treatment, including a low-protein diet and nutritional supplements, promote normal development in most infants and children.	Clinical manifestations: Recurrent episodes of emesis, dehydration, and severe metabolic acidosis, anorexia, listlessness, lethargy, neuromuscular irritability, and hypothermia.

TABLE 11–5: Organic Acid Conditions *(Continued)*

5. 3-Methylcrotonyl CoA Carboxylase 1 Deficiency (ACMG Code=3-MCC)	An inherited disorder in which a deficiency in the body has inadequate levels of an enzyme that helps to process the amino acid leucine. As a result, increased by-products of leucine processing lead to toxic levels.	Clinical manifestations: Brain damage, seizures, liver failure, and death in infancy. Some children exhibit no symptoms at all until later in life, often following an illness. Treatment includes a low-protein diet and nutritional supplements.
6. 3-Hydroxy-3-methylglutaric Aciduria (ACMG Code= HMG)	An inherited disorder in which the body is unable to process leucine properly due to a deficiency in lysase, an enzyme that is essential to leucine catabolism and ketone formation.	Clinical manifestations: Metabolic acidosis, hypoglycemia, and sometimes unexplained fevers. Encephalopathy such as somnolence, coma, malaise, hepatopathy, and sudden infant death may occur.
7. Holocarboxylase Synthase Deficiency (ACMG code=MCD)	An inherited disorder that interferes with effective utilization of the vitamin biotin. Biotin is essential to the normal production and processing of proteins, fats, and carbohydrates in the body. As a result, the body is unable to process nutrients properly, which can result in a variety of health problems.	Clinical manifestations: May be asymptomatic. Some newborns and infants will show signs of transient hypoglycemia, some will show degrees of hypotonia and may be lethargic.
8. ß-Ketothiolase Deficiency (ACMG code=BKT)	An inherited disorder that affects utilization of the amino acid isoleucine and interferes with the processing of ketones. This results in the body's inability to process proteins and fats properly, contributing to acidosis.	Clinical manifestations: Serious symptoms such as coma, brain damage, and death are most often seen in infants. Early diagnosis, recognition of signs of illness (which may trigger recurrent acidosis), and prompt subsequent treatment with glucose promotes normal growth and development. Additional treatments may vary but can include avoidance of protein-rich diets and long-term treatment with bicarbonate.
9. Glutaric Acidemia Type I (ACMG Code= GA1)	An inherited disorder with inadequate levels of an enzyme that processes the amino acids lysine, hydroxylysine, and tryptophan, resulting in excessive levels of these amino acids.	Clinical manifestations: Asymptomatic; normal development may occur into later infancy (up to 18 months) until symptoms are triggered by a mild viral illness or other health condition. Macrocephaly may present in the neonatal period or later in infancy before the onset of any neurologic symptoms. Other manifestations include neurologic symptoms (such as hypotonia and choreoathetosis), respiratory distress, unusual odor that is often described as "sweaty feet," and liver dysfunction. Without prompt treatment of the triggering illness, this disorder can lead to further neurologic symptoms and death within the first decade of life. Early diagnosis and treatment, which usually includes dietary protein restriction and supplementation with a nutrient called L-carnitine, may prevent severe consequences.

Source: Modified from Kaye, C. I. (2006). Newborn Screening Fact Sheets. *Pediatrics, 118*, e934.
Newborn Screening Clearinghouse Definitions Overview and National Newborn Screening and Genetics Resource Center: http://www.marchofdimes.com/peristats. New England Center for Newborn Screening: http://www.umassmed.edu/nbs/
ACMG. (2006). Nomenclature for Conditions is based on the report Naming and counting disorders (conditions) included in newborn screening panels. *Pediatrics, 117*(5), **Suppl:** S308–314.
ACMG and HRSA. (2006). Newborn screening: Towards a uniform screening panel and system. *Genet. Med 8*(5), Suppl S12–S252.

Fatty Acid Oxidation Disorders These conditions interfere with the utilization of fatty acids, which process stored body fat, the body's source of energy. As a result, these fatty acids accumulate in the blood. These infants and children are dependent upon external energy sources, particularly glucose from food. When nutritional sources are used up and no longer available, even for short periods of time, or when energy requirements increase during times of even minor illness, serious health problems occur. Early identification and treatment with special diets and supplements are essential to prevent morbidity and mortality.

Clinical manifestations: Symptoms and prognosis vary depending on the type of fatty acid oxidation disorder. Without treatment, these infants and children may experience periods of poor feeding, lack of energy, difficulty breathing, low blood glucose (sugar), and vomiting, leading to developmental delay, seizures, coma, and even sudden death. In many cases, therapy with a special diet and/or prescription medication is used (see Table 11–6).

TABLE 11–6: Fatty Acid Oxidation Disorders

1. Carnitine Uptake Defect /Carnitine Transport Defect (ACMG Code=CUD)	A condition in which transporter cells needed to carry carnitine are absent. Carnitine transfers fatty acids across the membranes of the mitochondria, the cells source of energy production. This results in reduced energy production and the cellular accumulation of unused fatty acids.	Clinical manifestations: Fasting hypoglycemia with seizures and coma, cardiomyopathy, arrhythmias, muscle weakness, and hepatomegaly/abnormal liver function.
2. Medium-chain acyl-CoA Dehydrogenase Deficiency (ACMG Code=MCAD)	An inherited condition that results from inadequate levels of an enzyme required to convert medium chain fatty acids to energy, particularly during periods without food. The resultant decreased energy production and increased cellular accumulation of unused fatty acids result in increased morbidity and mortality in infancy and childhood. Although may present in the neonatal period, the most common presentation is between 3 and 15 months of age with some children not exhibiting signs and symptoms until later childhood when triggered by periods of fasting or illness.	Clinical manifestations: No apparent symptoms at birth, but serious illness can occur very quickly in infants who are not feeding well. Early identification of children with this condition before they become ill is essential to avoid a crisis and subsequent serious consequences, which include hypoglycemia, failure to thrive, persistent vomiting, seizures, cardiomyopathy, arrhythmias, muscle weakness/rhabdomyolysis, and hepatomegaly/abnormal liver function coma and cardiac arrest. Intellectual and developmental disabilities, speech and language delay, behavioral problems, attention deficit hyperactivity disorder (ADHD), proximal muscle weakness, chronic seizure disorder, cerebral palsy, and failure to thrive are all identified potential chronic sequelae. Treatment includes close detection and monitoring, avoidance of fasting, strict dietary measures, and nutritional supplements before onset of symptoms. Safe time between meals lengthens as infants and children mature.
3. Very Long-Chain acyl-CoA Dehydrogenase Deficiency (AMCG Code=VLCAD)	An inherited condition that results from inadequate levels of an enzyme required to convert very long chain fatty acids to energy, particularly during periods without food. The resultant decreased energy production and increased cellular accumulation of unused fatty acids result in increased morbidity and mortality in infancy and childhood.	Clinical manifestations: Symptoms can first appear at any age from the newborn period through adulthood, but tend to be most severe in infants. Without treatment, affected infants often develop cardiac and liver failure. There is a high mortality rate during the first year of life. Treatment includes a high-carbohydrate/low-fat diet, nutritional supplements, avoidance of fasting, and prolonged exercise.
4. Long-Chain L-3 Hydroxyacyl-CoA dDehydrogenase Deficiency AMCG Code=LCHAD)	An inherited condition that results from inadequate levels of an enzyme required to convert long chain fatty acids to energy, particularly during periods without food. The resultant decreased energy production and increased cellular accumulation of unused fatty acids result in increased morbidity and mortality in infancy and childhood.	Clinical manifestations: Symptoms such as hypoglycemia, lethargy, hypotonia, and cardiomyopathy may present in the neonatal period, resulting in heart, lung, or liver failure and sudden death. In other cases, symptoms such as low muscle tone; developmental delay; heart, lung, or liver failure may develop later in infancy or childhood, usually triggered by an illness or periods of fasting. Early diagnosis and treatment effectively prevent life-threatening events, though some children may still develop symptoms. Treatment includes a high-carbohydrate/low-fat diet, nutritional supplements, and avoidance of fasting. Women who are pregnant with fetuses with LCHAD are at increased risk of developing acute fatty liver of pregnancy and other pregnancy complications.
5. Trifunctional Protein Deficiency (AMCG Code=TFP)	A condition in which inadequate levels of this enzyme interferes with the conversion of long-chain fatty acids into energy, especially during episodes of fasting. The resultant decreased energy production and increased cellular accumulation of unused fatty acids result in increased morbidity and mortality in infancy and childhood.	Clinical manifestations: May present as sudden sudden death in an otherwise well infant. Other infants may develop low muscle tone, cardiomyopathy, seizures, heart failure, and coma, following an illness or periods of fasting. Treatment is based on strict avoidance of fasting, a low-fat diet, and nutritional supplements.

Source: Modified from Kaye, C. I. (2006). Newborn Screening Fact Sheets. *Pediatrics, 118,* e934.
Newborn Screening Clearinghouse Definitions Overview and National Newborn Screening and Genetics Resource Center: http://www.marchofdimes.com/peristats. New England Center for Newborn Screening: http://www.umassmed.edu/nbs/

ACMG. (2006). Nomenclature for Conditions is based on the report Naming and counting disorders (conditions) included in newborn screening panels. *Pediatrics, 117*(5), **Suppl:** S308–314.
ACMG and HRSA. (2006). Newborn screening: Towards a uniform screening panel and system. *Genet. Med 8*(5), Suppl S12–S252.

Amino Acid Disorders These are a group of inborn errors of metabolism that interfere in the breakdown and utilization of amino acids. As a result, one or more amino acids accumulate in the blood and/or urine. Although majorities of these disorders present in the neonatal period, symptoms may not develop until later in infancy and childhood. Symptoms, which vary and range in severity, include metabolic disturbances such as acidosis and hematological and neurologic manifestations (see Table 11–7).

TABLE 11–7: Amino Acid Disorders

Disorder	Description	Clinical manifestations
1. Argininosuccinic Aciduria (ACMG Code=ASA)	A rare inherited disorder of the urea cycle due to inadequate levels of an enzyme that processes nitrogen removal from the body. As a result, nitrogen, in the forms of argininosuccinic acid and ammonia, accumulates in the blood.	Clinical manifestations: Symptoms, which generally present in the neonatal period, include failure to thrive, hepatic failure, unusual hair (trichorrhexis nodosa), and seizures. Brain swelling, coma, and eventually death may occur. Early diagnosis and treatment can prevent further morbidity and mortality. However, those children who recover often suffer permanent neurologic damage and may have recurrence in later infancy or childhood. Treatment consists of a low-protein diet, avoidance of fasting, medications to prevent ammonia buildup, nutritional supplements, and in some cases, liver transplant.
2. Citrullinemia, Type I (ACMG Code=CIT)	A rare inherited disorder of the urea cycle due to inadequate levels of citrulline, an enzyme that processes removal of nitrogen from the body. As a result, excessive levels of nitrogen, in the form of ammonia, and other toxic substances accumulate in the blood.	Clinical manifestations: Symptoms including seizures, coma, brain damage, and resultant death may present in the neonatal period or later infancy. Early diagnosis and treatment with a low-protein diet, medications to rid the body of amino groups to prevent ammonia buildup, and nutritional supplements may foster normal development.
3. Maple Syrup Urine Disease (ACMG Code=MSUD)	An inborn error of metabolism in which there is a deficiency in the branch chain decarboxylase enzyme needed in the metabolism of the amino acids leucine, isoleucine, and valine, which are present in many kinds of food. As a result, these amino acids and their by-products build up in the body leading to progressive neurologic problems, which if unrecognized and untreated can lead to death.	Clinical manifestations: Range from mild to severe. Infants who appear normal at birth usually develop symptoms within the first week of life. However, lower intake of protein, as in breastfeeding, can delay the onset of symptoms until the second week of life. Initial symptoms are lethargy, feeding difficulties, and failure to thrive. Progressive neurologic deterioration, alternating hypertonia and hypotonia, and dystonic posturing of the arms and eventually seizures and coma lead to death. Ketosis, acidosis, and a persistent lactic acidosis develop. The resulting characteristic of urine smelling like maple syrup, burnt sugar, or curry give the disorder its name. Without dietary treatment, severely affected babies do not survive the first month; even those who do receive treatment may have irreversible intellectual disability. Rapid diagnosis and treatment are major factors in survival and outcome. Treatment consists of strict low-protein diet, which will vary depending on severity of symptoms, and supplementation with the vitamin thiamin. Continued developmental monitoring and assessment are essential to leading normal lives.
4. Homocystinuria (ACMG Code=HCY)	An inherited biochemical condition in which the body is deficient in an enzyme responsible for converting the amino acid homocysteine into cystathionine, a requisite for normal brain development. The resultant high levels of amino acids in the blood, urine, and tissues lead to serious health problems.	Clinical manifestations: If undetected and untreated, homocystinuria leads to optical dislocation, intellectual disability, osteoporosis, and thromboembolism. With early detection, strict dietary management, vitamin supplements (B6 or B12), and other supplements such as betaine, growth and development can be normal.

TABLE 11–7: Amino Acid Disorders *(Continued)*

5. Classic Phenylketonuria (ACMG Code=PKU)	An inherited disorder in which the body cannot effectively process the essential amino acid phenylalanine, found in the protein of foods. The resultant accumulation of phenylalanine leads to serious health problems.	Clinical manifestations: Infants may appear normal in the first few months of life, but left untreated, PKU can cause intellectual and motor disability, microcephaly, poor growth rate, and seizures. With early detection and proper dietary treatment consisting of a low-phenylalanine diet at least throughout childhood and adolescence—and for females during pregnancy—growth and development should be normal.
6. Tyrosinemia, Type I (ACMG Code=TYR 1)	An inherited disorder in which the body has inadequate levels of an enzyme that metabolizes the amino acid tyrosine. The resultant accumulation of tyrosine and its by-products (particularly succinylacetone) in the blood, urine, and liver cause serious health conditions. There are acute and chronic forms of this condition.	Clinical manifestations: Type I tyrosinemia in the acute form is characterized by failure to thrive, vomiting, diarrhea, a cabbage-like odor, hepatomegaly, fever, jaundice, edema, melena, and progressive liver disease. If untreated, death from liver failure may occur in the first year of life. The chronic form is similar but with milder features characterized by hypophosphatemic rickets, hypertrophic obstructive cardiomyopathy, abdominal crises, polyneuropathy, hypertension, and hepatoma. Death occurs during the first decade of life.

Source: Modified from Kaye, C. I. (2006). Newborn Screening Fact Sheets. *Pediatrics, 118,* e934.
Newborn Screening Clearinghouse Definitions Overview and National Newborn Screening and Genetics Resource Center: http://www.marchofdimes.com/peristats. New England Center for Newborn Screening: http://www.umassmed.edu/nbs/
ACMG. (2006). Nomenclature for Conditions is based on the report Naming and counting disorders (conditions) included in newborn screening panels. *Pediatrics, 117*(5), **Suppl:** S308–314.
ACMG and HRSA. (2006). Newborn screening: Towards a uniform screening panel and system. *Genet. Med* 8(5), Suppl S12–S252.

Endocrine Disorders The endocrine system regulates growth, development, energy production, storage, and utilization. These conditions are caused by an alteration in the regulation of the normal feedback system that results in either hyposecretion or hypersecretion of one or more hormones. The interrelationship of the hypothalamic-pituitary-thyroid axis is disrupted in some way (see Table 11–8).

TABLE 11–8: Endocrine Disorders

1. Primary Congenital Hypothyroidism (ACMG Code=CH)	A condition in which there is an inability to produce adequate amounts of thyroid hormone from birth. The thyroid gland produces iodine-containing hormones necessary in regulating growth, brain development, and the rate of chemical reactions in the body. If untreated, congenital hypothyroidism can lead to intellectual disability and abnormal growth. If detected soon after birth, the condition can be treated simply with oral doses of thyroid hormone to permit normal development. Thyroid hormone deficiency at birth is one of the most common treatable causes of intellectual disability. There are multiple etiologies of this disorder, both heritable and sporadic, varying in severity. There is an inverse relationship between age at diagnosis and neurodevelopmental outcome; the later treatment is started, the more severe the intellectual disability.	Clinical manifestations: Approximately 5% of infants, generally those who are more severely affected, are shown in recognizable features at birth, including large fontanels and wide suturae, macroglossia, distended abdomen with umbilical hernia, and skin mottling. Most affected infants appear normal at birth, without obvious manifestations of CH up until 3 months of age, at which time maternal thyroid hormone is excreted and disappears, and clinical features gradually become apparent. These infants are slow to feed, constipated, lethargic; and sleep more, often needing to be awakened to feed; have a hoarse cry; may feel cool to touch; may be hypotonic with slow reflexes; and may have prolonged jaundice. Other long-term neurologic sequelae include ataxia, gross and fine motor incoordination, hypotonia and spasticity, speech disorders, problems with attention span, and strabismus. Approximately 10% of these infants will have an associated sensorineural deafness, and approximately 10% will have other congenital anomalies, most commonly cardiac defects. If detected early (before 3 weeks) and maintained on appropriate levels of thyroid hormone medication, infants diagnosed with CH should have normal growth and development. Levothyroxine is the treatment of choice.

TABLE 11–8: Endocrine Disorders *(Continued)*

2. Congenital Adrenal Hyperplasia (ACMG Code=CAH)	A group of inherited disorders resulting from inadequate levels of an enzyme needed in the synthesis of adrenal gland hormones, resulting in decreased cortisol and aldosterone production. This results in excess production of androgens, which can lead to abnormalities of sexual development. In female infants, CAH sometimes results in masculinization of the genitals. There are three forms of CAH ranging from the most severe salt-wasting, life-threatening type to a mild form.	Clinical manifestations: Newborns may initially appear normal, but neonates with the SW form can quickly develop symptoms of adrenal crisis during the 1st through 4th weeks of life, peaking at approximately 3 weeks of age. This manifests as poor feeding, vomiting, loose stools or diarrhea, weak cry, failure to thrive, dehydration, and lethargy. If untreated, then circulatory collapse, shock, and death are inevitable. Affected females have ambiguous genitalia (AG) (but normal internal reproductive anatomy), prompting a clinical diagnosis in many. Affected males have no obvious physical signs of CAH. Therefore, without newborn screening and in the absence of a positive family history, all male and a minority of female neonates are undiagnosed until adrenal crisis. If inadequately treated, postnatal virilization (girls), pseudo- or true-precocious puberty (boys), and premature growth acceleration (boys and girls) occur, leading to early growth cessation. Infants with milder forms of the disorder are at risk for reproductive and growth difficulties. Treatment includes salt replacement and hormone replacement. If detected early and maintained on appropriate doses of medication, infants diagnosed with CAH should have normal growth and development.

Source: Modified from Kaye, C. I. (2006). Newborn Screening Fact Sheets. *Pediatrics, 118,* e934.
Newborn Screening Clearinghouse Definitions Overview and National Newborn Screening and Genetics Resource Center: http://www.marchofdimes.com/peristats. New England Center for Newborn Screening: http://www.umassmed.edu/nbs/
ACMG. (2006). Nomenclature for Conditions is based on the report Naming and counting disorders (conditions) included in newborn screening panels. *Pediatrics, 117*(5), **Suppl:** S308–314.
ACMG and HRSA. (2006). Newborn screening: Towards a uniform screening panel and system. *Genet. Med* 8(5), Suppl S12–S252.

Hemoglobin Disorders Sickle cell diseases are inherited abnormalities that reduce the production of hemoglobin, the molecule in red blood cells that delivers oxygen to cells throughout the body. Atypical hemoglobin molecules called hemoglobin S distort red blood cells into a sickle, or crescent, shape. *Sickling* is the term referring to changes in the red blood cells causing them to become hard, sticky, and crescent shaped. This prevents the cells from moving smoothly through the body. These sickle cells do not last as long as normal, round, red blood cells, which leads to anemia (a low number of red blood cells) and repeated infections. The sickle cells also get stuck in blood vessels, blocking blood flow. Anemia can cause pale skin, weakness, fatigue, and more serious complications.

There are three types of sickle cell anemia included in routine screening: sickle cell anemia, sickle beta thalassemia, and sickle cell disease. Newborns appear normal, but anemia develops in the first few months of life, followed by increased susceptibility to infection, slow growth rates, and the possibility of life-threatening splenic sequestration. With appropriate care that includes penicillin prophylaxis, appropriate vaccinations, and long-term management, the complications of all sickle cell disorders can be minimized. The primary rationale for newborn screening and presymptomatic diagnosis is prevention of mortality from pneumococcal sepsis and splenic sequestration during infancy and childhood. Infants identified with the sickle cell trait typically will have few or no clinical symptoms (see Table 11–9).

TABLE 11–9: Hemoglobin Disorders

1. S.S Disease (Sickle Cell anemia) (ACMG Code= Hb SS)	The actual disease that affects hemoglobin, the molecule in red blood cells that delivers oxygen to cells throughout the body. People with this disorder have atypical hemoglobin molecules called hemoglobin S, which distort red blood cells into a sickle, or crescent, shape.	Clinical manifestations: Classic symptoms of anemia, periodic episodes of severe pain, damage to the vital organs, stroke, and sometimes death in childhood. Young children with sickle cell anemia are especially prone to dangerous bacterial infections such as pneumonia and meningitis. Treatment with penicillin, beginning in infancy, can dramatically reduce the risk of these adverse effects and the deaths that can result from them.
2. S, βeta-thalassemia (ACMG Code=Hb S/β Th)	In this form of sickle cell anemia, the child inherits one sickle cell gene and one gene for beta thalassemia, another inherited anemia.	Clinical manifestations: Symptoms that are often milder than for Hb SS, though severity varies among affected children. Routine treatment with penicillin may not be recommended for all affected children.

TABLE 11–9: Hemoglobin Disorders *(Continued)*

3. SC Disease (ACMG Code= Hb S/C)	A common single gene disorder that affects hemoglobin, the molecule in red blood cells that delivers oxygen to cells throughout the body. A form of sickle cell disease, in which the child inherits one sickle cell gene (hemoglobin S) and one gene for another abnormal type of hemoglobin called hemoglobin C (HbC), which can distort red blood cells into a sickle, or crescent, shape.	Clinical manifestations: anemia and repeated infections. As with Hemoglobin Hb S/Beta-Thalassemia (Hb S/Th), this form is often milder than the Hb SS, and routine penicillin treatment may not be recommended. These children are at increased risk for severe morbidity (hemolytic anemia, splenic dysfunction, pain crisis, and bacterial infections) especially during the first 3 years of life.

Source: Modified from Kaye, C. I. (2006). Newborn Screening Fact Sheets. *Pediatrics, 118,* e934.
Newborn Screening Clearinghouse Definitions Overview and National Newborn Screening and Genetics Resource Center: http://www.marchofdimes.com/peristats. New England Center for Newborn Screening: http://www.umassmed.edu/nbs/
ACMG. (2006). Nomenclature for Conditions is based on the report Naming and counting disorders (conditions) included in newborn screening panels. *Pediatrics, 117*(5), **Suppl:** S308–314.
ACMG and HRSA. (2006). Newborn screening: Towards a uniform screening panel and system. *Genet. Med 8*(5), Suppl S12–S252.

Other Core Conditions

This last group of conditions have varying causes including congenital infectious disease, genetic conditions, and enzyme deficiency. Refer to Table 11–10 for additional core condition and their manifestations.

TABLE 11–10: Additional Core Conditions

1. Biotinidase Deficiency (ACMG Code=BIOT)	An inherited autosomal recessive disorder caused by inadequate levels of biotinidase, an enzyme that recycles the water-soluble vitamin biotin needed to process fats, proteins, and carbohydrates effectively. This can result in serious complications including frequent infections, uncoordinated movement, hearing loss, seizures, and intellectual disability.	Clinical manifestations: Newborns appear normal at birth but present with clinical symptoms as early as the 1st week of life up to 10 years of age. The most commonly affected systems are the central nervous system and skin. Other symptoms include seizures, hypotonia, seborrheic or atopic dermatitis, partial or complete alopecia, and conjunctivitis. Developmental delay, optic nerve atrophy, sensorineural hearing loss, lethargy, ataxia, breathing problems, hepatosplenomegaly, coma, metabolic acidosis, and death may also occur. Early diagnosis and immediate treatment with daily biotin supplementation can completely prevent problems.
2. Cystic Fibrosis (ACMG Code=CF)	An inherited autosomal recessive disorder of the mucus glands due to an altered synthesis of a protein involved in the transport of chloride ions. The major clinical consequences are the production of abnormally thickened mucous secretions in the lungs and digestive systems of affected newborns.	Clinical manifestations: CF may present in the neonatal period with meconium ileus. Older infants present with failure to thrive secondary to exocrine pancreatic insufficiency, chronic respiratory symptoms, or both. Nutritional deficits can be severe at presentation and may lead to edema and hypoproteinemia from protein-calorie malnutrition. Infants may present with hypoelectrolytemia from sweat salt loss. The most common chronic respiratory symptoms are cough and wheeze. If infants are not diagnosed in the newborn period, they often undergo months of illness with concomitant stress on the parents. Patients are prone to chronic endobronchial infections with Pseudomonas aeruginosa, Staphylococcus aureus, and other characteristic bacteria throughout childhood. Recurrent intestinal blockages, severe liver disease, and diabetes may present in later childhood or adolescence. Treatment varies depending on severity of symptoms, but may include a high-calorie diet supplemented with vitamins and medications to improve digestion, respiratory therapy to help clear mucus from the lungs, and medications to improve breathing and prevent lung infections. With early detection and lifelong comprehensive treatment plans, infants diagnosed with CF can be expected to live longer and in a better state of health than in the past.

TABLE 11–10: Additional Core Conditions *(Continued)*

3. Classic Galactosemia (ACMG Code=GALT)	An autosomal recessive disorder due to inadequate levels of the liver enzyme needed to metabolize the simple sugar galactose, derived from the breakdown of the major sugar lactose in milk, into glucose, another simple sugar. This results in difficulty in processing various foods, including all dairy products and most formulas. Galactose accumulation in vital organs leads to severe consequences.	Clinical manifestations: Generally present within the first weeks after birth with a life-threatening illness. Feeding intolerance, vomiting and diarrhea, jaundice, hepatomegaly, lethargy, hypotonia, and excessive bleeding after venipuncture are characteristic findings. Laboratory studies indicate liver and renal tubular disease. Septicemia, particularly with Escherichia coli, is not uncommon. Bilateral cataracts are generally seen at presentation, but they may be mild in the first few weeks of life and only detectable with slit-lamp examination. Untreated, the disorder may result in blindness, severe intellectual disability, hepatomegaly, growth failure, infection, and death. Milk and other dairy products must be eliminated from the diet for life. Supportive care may include vitamin K supplementation and fresh-frozen plasma transfusions, antibiotics for presumed Gram-negative sepsis, and phototherapy for hyperbilirubinemia. After dietary galactose has been eliminated, most infants improve rapidly. Milk and milk products are excluded from the diet indefinitely, because significant ingestion of galactose at any age can be toxic. Because medications may contain galactose, medications need to be carefully screened before administering it to the child. Regular nutritional evaluation is necessary to ensure adequate calcium intake. Regular developmental evaluation and early speech assessment are also required. Girls should be monitored frequently in late childhood and adolescence for pubertal development.
4. Hearing Loss (ACMG Code=HEAR)	It is estimated that approximately 50% of congenital hearing loss is caused by genetic factors. Of these, approximately 77% of congenital nonsyndromic hearing impairment is autosomal recessive, 22% is autosomal dominant, and 1% is X-linked. Causes of congenital hearing loss that are not hereditary in nature include prenatal infections, illnesses, toxins consumed by the mother during pregnancy, or other acquired conditions.	Clinical manifestations: In children without risk factors, without early testing, hearing loss frequently escapes detection until the age when the child presents with delayed speech and language development. The goals of newborn screening are to identify those infants with hearing loss early for prompt intervention with hearing aids and/or auditory stimulation during the first 6 months of life as these are critical to development of speech and language skills.
5. Severe Combined Immunodeficiencies (ACMG Code=SCID)	A group of rare inherited disorders characterized by defects in two critical immune system cells that are normally mobilized by the body to combat infections.	Clinical manifestations: Also referred as the "bubble boy disease" because without treatment, infants with SCID are more susceptible to and can develop recurrent infections, leading to failure to thrive and often death. These infections are often caused by opportunistic organisms that ordinarily do not cause illness in people with a normal immune system. If not treated in a way that restores immune function, children with SCID usually live only a year or two. With treatment, including a bone-marrow transplant, infants live because they can make T cells that untreated SCID babies cannot.

Source: Modified from Kaye, C. I. (2006). Newborn Screening Fact Sheets. *Pediatrics, 118,* e934.

Newborn Screening Clearinghouse Definitions Overview and National Newborn Screening and Genetics Resource Center: http://www.marchofdimes.com/peristats. New England Center for Newborn Screening: http://www.umassmed.edu/nbs/

ACMG. (2006). Nomenclature for Conditions is based on the report Naming and counting disorders (conditions) included in newborn screening panels. *Pediatrics, 117*(5), **Suppl:** S308–314.

ACMG and HRSA. (2006). Newborn screening: Towards a uniform screening panel and system. *Genet. Med* 8(5), Suppl S12–S252.

BOX 11–2 Questions to Evaluate Evidence of New Nominations to the Panel

Key Question 1
Is there direct evidence that screening for the condition at birth leads to improved outcomes for the infant or child to be screened? Are there potential benefits for the child's family?

Key Question 2
Is there a case definition that can be uniformly and reliably applied? What is the incidence and prevalence of the condition? What are the natural history and the spectrum of disease of the condition, including the impact of early recognition and treatment verses later recognition and delayed or no treatment?

Key Question 3
Is there a screening test or screening test algorithm for the condition with sufficient analytic validity?

Key Question 4
Has the clinical validity of the screening test or screening algorithm, in combination with the diagnostic test or test algorithm, been determined and is that validity adequate?

Key Question 5
What is the clinical utility of the screening test or screening algorithm? What are the benefits associated with use of the screening and diagnostic test and the treatment? What are the harms associated with screening, diagnosis, and treatment?

Key Question 6
How cost effective is the screening, diagnosis, and treatment for this disorder compared with usual clinical case detection and treatment?

Screening for Hearing Loss

In the past decade, many states have implemented universal newborn hearing screening programs. These programs are made possible because of the combination of technological advances in **Auditory Brainstem Response** (**ABR**) and **Otoacoustic Emissions** (**OAE**) testing, which enable accurate and cost-effective evaluation of hearing in newborns. ABR audiometry is a neurologic test of auditory brainstem function in response to auditory (click) stimuli, and OAE measures the sounds produced by the cochlea (Bhattacharyya et al.).

According to the AAP, hearing loss is one of the most frequently occurring birth defects, affecting approximately 3 infants for every 1,000 live births. Infants requiring admission to intensive care units at birth present an even higher risk while others may acquire hearing loss during early childhood (American Academy of Pediatrics Task Force for Improving Newborn Hearing Screening, 2010).

If hearing loss is not detected and treated early, it can impede speech, language, and cognitive development. Over time, such a delay can lead to significant educational costs and learning difficulties (Nelson, Bougatsos, & Nygren, 2008).

The National Center for Hearing Assessment and Management (**NCHAM**) reports that detecting and treating hearing loss at birth is a cost-effective screening measure, costing approximately \$10–\$50 per infant and saving \$400,000 in special education costs alone from birth to high school graduation for one child (Prosser, Kong, Rusinak, & Waisbren, 2010; Russ, Hanna, DesGeorges, & Forsman, 2010).

The goal of Early Hearing Detection and Intervention (**EHDI**) is to maximize "linguistic competence and literacy development for children who have deafness or hearing loss." Evidence supports early identification of and intervention for hearing loss to maximize positive outcomes for children by providing opportunities for language acquisition, communication, cognition, reading, and social–emotional development (Nelson et al., 2008; Prosser et al., 2010; Shulman, Besculides, Saltzman, Ireys, & White, 2010).

The Joint Committee on Infant Hearing (**JCIH**) endorses early detection of and intervention for infants with hearing loss ("Year 2007 Position Statement," 2007).

According to the JCIH recommendations, screening should occur at no later than one month of age. Those who do not pass the initial screen should have a comprehensive **audiologic evaluation** at no later than 3 months of age. When hearing loss is detected it is graded as moderate, profound, or severe.

Infants with confirmed hearing loss should receive appropriate intervention at no later than 6 months of age from health care and education professionals with expertise in hearing loss and deafness in infants and young children. Regardless of previous hearing-screening outcomes, all infants with or without risk factors should receive ongoing surveillance of communicative development beginning at 2 months of age during well-child visits in the **pediatric health care home**. At least one ABR test is recommended as part of a complete audiology diagnostic evaluation for children younger than 3 years for confirmation of permanent hearing loss. Separate protocols are recommended for neonatal intensive care and well-infant nurseries. Neonatal intensive care infants admitted for more than 5 days are to have ABR included as part of their screening so that neural hearing loss will not be missed (American Academy of Pediatrics Task Force for Improving Newborn Hearing Screening, 2010).

As noted previously, of the 30 core conditions, hearing loss is the only newborn screen that is not identified by a blood test. Screening for this core condition adds additional costs for specially trained personnel and requires special equipment, and access to facilities to gain a diagnosis may be limited. Although not perfect, primary care providers prefer universal screening for hearing loss over individual screening because when neonatal hearing screening was limited only to high-risk groups (such as those requiring neonatal intensive care), approximately 50% of the infants with identified hearing loss had not been tested during the newborn period (Prosser et al., 2010).

States have taken a variety of approaches to screening for hearing loss: Some mandate that all hospitals or birthing centers screen infants for hearing loss before they are discharged, some mandate that insurance policies cover the cost of the screening, and others use state dollars to fund screening programs. Still other states require that information on hearing screening be available to parents before they leave the hospital. Fourteen states allow newborns to be exempt from universal hearing screening programs if a parent objects to the testing. As of May, 2011, 36 states require hearing screening for newborns.

A number of states have created task forces or advisory committees on newborn hearing screening ("Newborn hearing screening laws," 2011). According to the Centers for Disease Control (CDC), of the nearly 4 million infants born in the United States in 2005, 91.5% were screened for hearing loss ("Newborn screening," n.d.).

Newborn Screening Resources

In 2009, the first national Newborn Screening Clearinghouse (**NBSC**) was established with funding from HRSA genetic branch ("First national newborn screening clearinghouse," 2009). HRSA awarded a 5-year grant to Genetic Alliance and multiple partners that provide resources on newborn screening. The purpose of this free collaborative effort is to link parents, the public, industry representatives, and health care providers with coordinated key information about newborn screening with a goal to improve understanding and facilitate informed decision making. This site provides diverse information ranging from condition-specific facts to details of state-by-state services. For example, if interested in learning what is available in a specific state, there is a March of Dimes Quick Link (Peristats) that provides a map for finding out which states screen for a particular condition ("Newborn screening overview," 2011).

In 2011, Genetic Alliance announced the launch of BabysFirstTest.org, an interactive online newborn screening clearinghouse that includes a blog and Really Simple Syndication (**RSS**) of newborn screening news and tweets for discussion of key topics and activities on newborn screening. RSS allows republication of an article from its original source to other public sources such as a website or blog (Alliance, 2011).

SECTION TWO REVIEW

1. Early treatment of PKU is associated with improved intellectual outcome, and it is rarely diagnosed before 6 months of age without newborn screening.
   A. True
   B. False
2. The goals of screening for Congenital Adrenal Hyperplasia include
   A. preventing a life-threatening adrenal crisis.
   B. preventing male sex assignment to a virilized female.
   C. preventing short stature and psychosexual disturbances in both sexes.
   D. All of the above
3. Biotinidase deficiency is included on the newborn screen because it is a
   A. potentially tragic illness if not diagnosed.
   B. condition that has a low-cost treatment.
   C. rare and untreatable condition.
   D. Both A and B
4. Hearing loss is more common in infants
   A. delivered by cesarean section.
   B. admitted to intensive care units.
   C. Both A and B
   D. None of the above
5. Secondary targets should be obtained
   A. when the infant has his or her first newborn screen blood test.
   B. in follow-up testing if indicated.
   C. Both A and B
   D. None of the above

Answers: 1. A; 2. D; 3. D; 4. B; 5. C

SECTION THREE: Ethics and Ethical Concerns of Newborn Screening

Continued success and growth of the newborn screening program is threatened by a number of undesirable consequences inherent within population-based screening. Therefore, it is necessary for newborn care providers to understand the role of ethics as it pertains to the newborn screening program.

Ethics and the Newborn Screen

Initially, development of the newborn screening program was guided by Wilson and Jungner's classic screening criteria, and the fundamental rationale for screening was based on the principles that testing procedures are readily available, technically feasible, economically sound, and clearly beneficial to the affected newborns, their families, and to society. However, the newborn screening program has continued to experience logistical, social, and ethical problems (Kaye et al., 2001). Recently, the moral compass has shifted and Wilson and Jungner's classic screening criteria have become obsolete. The problems stem (in part) from advances in genetics screening. The rate of disease related to new gene identification is now surpassing the rate of newly available treatments or cures. Thus, there exists diverging viewpoints over the following issues:

1. Importance of identifying serious genetic conditions, even if rare
2. Implications of genetic information for family members
3. Need for analytical and clinical validity of screening tests
4. Possibility of interventions that offer reproductive options

In response to these problems, several new criteria for population-based public health screening have emerged (Andermann, Blancquaert, Beauchamp, & Dery, 2008). These criteria reflect a trend towards a less paternalistic belief system that offers informed choice and focuses on evidence-based health care, cost effectiveness, quality assurance, and accountability of decision makers (Table 11–11). Recent proposed changes to the newborn screening program at the local and national levels seem to fit nicely with these new criteria though it is too soon to evaluate their utility. The remainder of this section is devoted to discussing issues associated with these proposed changes.

TABLE 11–11: Newly Proposed Screening Criteria and Related Ethical Principles

Synthesis of Emerging Screening Criteria Proposed Over the Past 40 Years	Related Ethical Principle
1. The screening program should respond to a recognized need.	**Beneficence**
2. The objectives of the screening should be defined at the outset.	**Beneficence**
3. There should be a defined target population.	**Justice**
4. The program should integrate education, testing, clinical services, and program management.	**Informed Consent**
5. There should be quality assurance, with mechanisms to minimize potential risks of screening.	**Non-maleficence**
6. The program should ensure informed choice, confidentiality, and respect for autonomy.	**Informed Consent**
7. The program should promote equity and access to screening for the entire target population.	**Distributive Justice**
8. Program evaluation should be planned from the outset.	**Fidelity**
9. The overall benefits of screening should outweigh the harm.	**Non-maleficence**

Source: Adapted from Andermann, A., Blancquaert, I., Beauchamp, S., & Dery, V. (2008). Revisiting Wilson and Jungner in the genomic age: a review of screening criteria over the past 40 years. *Bulletin of the World Health Organization, 86*(4), 317–319.

Informed Consent

All newborns, regardless of which state or town they are born in, now have the opportunity to be screened for a minimum of 30 potentially treatable conditions or diseases. However, despite this great achievement, newborn screening is not perfect or without risk, even in situations where known treatments are available. Due to lack of sensitivity and specificity of testing, false negative and false positive screens can lead to increased parental anxiety and increased cost due to the need for additional testing and potentially unnecessary implementation of treatments in infants with only a mild disease state or inaccurate testing (DeLuca et al., 2011). These inaccuracies in newborn screens have given rise to debate over the right of parental consent in the U.S. and in other developed nations.

Originally, most newborn screening programs involved voluntary participation. However, as screening programs evolved many states made participation mandatory. Mandatory screening is controversial because many ethicists believe it interferes with **self-determination**, the ability to make a decision without outside influence (Ascension Healthcare, 2011). This is a concept that is closely linked with the principle of autonomy. In addition, these early screening programs were limited to screening for a few disorders requiring limited parental education. Now with advanced screening technologies for multiple disorders, the educational needs of parents to facilitate informed decision making have increased proportionately.

For some, the assumption that "no reasonable person would refuse" comes from a paternalistic viewpoint and demonstrates a lack of understanding associated with screens that may lack accuracy, despite the proven benefits. Because newborns do not possess the **capacity** to decide for themselves and communicate their decision to others, parents—if **competent**—serve as their babies' **surrogates** (Davenport, 1997). Thus, some parents, health care providers, and lawmakers contend that parental consent should be a component of newborn screening since this will enable the parent to make decisions about which screens make sense for their infant and to help educate parents as to the benefits and the limitations of the screening tests (Quinlivan & Suriadi, 2006).

Emerging Evidence

- At present, pilot studies are underway to explore the potential benefits and risks associated with screening for disorders with no known treatment. One such program is titled Prospective Assessment in Newborns for Diabetes Autoimmunity (**PANDA**), and another is titled The Environmental Determinants of Diabetes in the Young (**TEDDY**). Both programs screen for genetic markers for Type I diabetes and may be included in future newborn screening (Crowe, 2008).
- New DNA microchip technology promises to allow newborns to be screened directly, at even lower costs, and more accurately.
- Genotyping is not only used for secondary confirmation of many newborn screening conditions, but it also may be included in future recommendations with advances in DNA research technology.

Munson (2008), a medical ethicist, summarizes the moral dilemma and poses these questions: "Are screening programs so worthwhile that they justify the denial of individual choice entailed by required participation? What if parents don't want to know whether their child has the genes responsible for a particular disease? Is it legitimate for a state, in the interest of protecting the child, to require parents to find this out whether or not they want to know" (p. 280)?

With the acceptance of the revised screening criteria, where informed choice and respect for autonomy play a central role, it is likely that many states will make **informed consent** a requirement for newborn screening. Until this happens, health care providers need to know that parents of newborns retain the right to decline screening for religious reasons in some states. In these situations, health care providers are encouraged to identify the rationale for declining. Once the health care provider understands the rationale, it is the health care provider's responsibility to initiate a discussion about the benefits of screening and to ensure that the parents have a full understanding of the advantages and limitations of newborn screening (Bailey et al., 2008; Kemper et al., 2010). Recent studies have found that when provided with evidence of accurate screening and effective treatment, most parents are in support of population-wide screening for newborn disorders. However, parents are more likely to support optional screening when either screening or treatment is less effective (Lipstein et al., 2010; Plass, van El, Pieters, & Cornel, 2010).

If the parents still decline the newborn screen after they have been thoroughly educated, a refusal form may need to be completed depending upon the state or hospital of birth. In these situations, the refusal form can serve as documentation that the parents were informed about the possible adverse outcomes of declining the newborn screening and that they accept legal responsibility for the consequences of their decision. In states or hospitals that do not have a refusal form to sign, the health care provider should document the refusal and efforts made to educate the parents in the newborn's medical record. The AAP provides a sample refusal form for health care providers to use ("Newborn screening expands: Recommendations for pediatricians and medical homes - Implications for the system," 2008).

Screening When No Medical Intervention Is Possible

The incidence for most inborn errors of amino acid, fatty acid, and organic acid metabolism is < 1:100,000 infants in the United States (Crowe, 2008). Prior to the onset of newborn screening, most inborn errors of metabolism were detected after the nonspecific symptoms (including lethargy, vomiting, characteristic odors, tachypnea, seizures, profound acidosis, global developmental delay, and encephopathy) were present. Although the presenting symptoms for most disorders are often similar, the illness trajectories for these disorders are not. Some disorders have a slow onset, while others present acutely with life-threatening acidosis, necessitating swift intervention.

The challenge of newborn screening is to diagnose and intervene whenever possible, before the signs and symptoms of the disorder are present. Currently there are 30 core conditions, referred to as the uniform panel. An additional set of 25 conditions may be found as a result of screening for the uniform panel, with 42 of the 55 conditions detected by MS/MS. New markers and analytic methods for the detection of enzyme activity, steroids, organic acids, and bile acids are already being considered as future additions to the newborn screening panel. As a result many affected infants will never experience the symptoms of the disease for which they are genetically predetermined to develop.

Currently, some states give parents the opportunity for supplementary screening of their newborn for diseases to which there is no available treatment. Selecting to screen for conditions that have no known cure comes in response to new directives by decision makers who believe that the benefits of identifying a disorder without a known treatment outweighs the potential risks or undesired consequences (Box 11–3). However, decisions about which disorders will be added to the newborn screen panel should be approached with great caution. Decision makers must take into consideration the added responsibilities of the primary care provider, the possible negative impact to the family, and the societal burdens associated with the inclusion of additional screens, which can potentially be infinite in numbers (Hayeems et al., 2009; Kemper et al., 2010; Lloyd-Puryear et al., 2006; "Newborn screening expands: Recommendations for pediatricians and medical homes - Implications for the system," 2008; Perrin et al., 2010; Ross, 2009).

With the detection of untreatable conditions, health care providers and families will be faced with making ethical decisions sooner than ever before. Families will be confronted with decisions about withholding medical interventions for their infant with a known untreatable disorder earlier in the illness trajectory. However, decisions about withholding medical interventions should only be made once confirmatory testing is complete. Health care providers will need to develop strategies that include the utilization of all available resources to help families with life and death decisions. Hospital-based ethics teams can play an integral role in helping health care providers and families make sound decisions for the infant entrusted in their care (Acharya, Ackerman, & Ross, 2005; Therrell et al., 2006).

BOX 11–3 Benefits of Identifying Disorders With No Known Treatment

1. Once a child is diagnosed with a late onset disease, they can be monitored, helping the researchers learn more about the latent stages of the disease.
2. Society benefits from the advancement of science around a particular disorder by learning more about the latent stages of disease.

Costs as an Ethical Concern

Costs are a concern to most families and becomes an ethical consideration. How should genetic testing and newborn screening be made available to families, especially those without financial means or insurance to coverage such costs? The next section will discuss the context of this issue.

Equal Access to Basic Health Care and Resources

Traditionally, ethical ethicists have argued cost should not be considered when human life is at stake (Baily & Murray, 2008). However, others propose that costs are an ethical concern when determining fair and equitable allocation and distribution of resources to individuals, families, and the broader community (Arn, 2007; Hayeems et al., 2009; Moyer, Calonge, Teutsch, Botkin, & Force, 2008; Ross, 2009; Therrell et al., 2006).

Those holding this position propose that decisions regarding newborn screening need to involve systematic ways of reviewing the broader consequences based upon comparative effectiveness research and cost-benefit analysis. Realistically speaking, if monies are designated for newborn screening, then other resources may receive less money. Hence, newborn screening programs must take into account the costs of parental education, follow-up services, home visits, and prenatal care. Examples of areas that might be affected by cost cutting include prenatal preventive services and/or parental education and follow-up services for affected infants (Baily & Murray, 2008).

One study conducted on costs associated with expanded newborn screening concluded that it is a cost-effective health intervention. However, these authors found that the stress associated with negative quality of life issues may offset gains in quality from newborn screening. They caution decision makers to carefully review new disorders for expanded newborn screening panels and state that the potential for reduction in quality of life associated with treatment as well as the burden of treatment on children and parents should be included in the evaluation process (Prosser et al., 2010).

Screening for Drugs, Alcohol, and Nicotine

In addition to screening newborns for genetically transmittable disorders, it has been proposed that the newborn screening should expand to identify infants exposed to drugs, alcohol, and nicotine (found in tobacco smoke). Exposure to drugs, alcohol, and nicotine during pregnancy is preventable; when it occurs, it can have a negative impact and sometimes result in devastating consequences for the newborn infant (National Institute on Drug Abuse, 2011). However screening for drugs, alcohol, and nicotine may have major implications for the family, particularly if a false positive result were to occur.

Neonatal abstinence syndrome is the direct result of maternal substance use or abuse during pregnancy. It is a constellation of symptoms or problems that occur in the newborn that was exposed to addictive illegal or prescription drugs while in utero. Amphetamines, barbiturates, cocaine, diazepam, marijuana, and opiates (heroin, methadone, codeine) are some of the drugs to which a newborn can be addicted to at birth. Infants exposed to addictive substances in utero can develop birth defects, have low birth weight, deliver prematurely, have small head circumferences, and be at increased risk for sudden infant death syndrome (SIDS) (Best, Committee on Environmental Health, Committee on Native American Child Health, & Committee on Adolescence, 2009; Braun et al., 2010; Bruin, Gerstein, & Holloway, 2010; Washington State Department of Health & Maternal and Child Health Programs, 2010). Infants exhibit signs of withdrawal because following birth, they are no longer exposed to the substance. Signs and symptoms of withdrawal can begin between 1–10 days after birth. Factors such as the type of substance(s), length and frequency of exposure, and dose have an impact the severity of withdrawal. The symptoms of exposure are numerous and include loose stool, excessive or high-pitched crying, excessive sucking, fever, hyperactive reflexes and tremors, increased muscle tone, poor feeding, seizures, and sweating. Management of the substance-exposed infant is a challenge. Parents and health care providers can become distressed as they watch the infant withdraw. The treatment for withdrawal includes prescribing methadone, neonatal morphine solution, phenobarbital, and comfort measures. At present, screening for drug exposure can be accomplished through testing meconium stool, hair, and umbilical cord tissue (Braun et al., 2010; Goh et al., 2008; Gray et al., 2009; Liaquet et al., 2010; Montgomery et al., 2008).

Fetal alcohol spectrum disorder (**FASD**) is the direct result of maternal alcohol ingestion during pregnancy. FASD is further differentiated as Fetal Alcohol Syndrome (FAS), Alcohol-Related Neurodevelopmental Disorder (**ARND**), and Alcohol-Related Birth Defects (**ARBD**) according to the type of observed signs and symptoms. FAS is the most severe form of FASD and can result in fetal death. Typically, infants with FAS exhibit abnormal facial features and can have problems with growth, motor skills, learning, memory, attention span, communication, vision, and hearing. Infants that develop ARND have intellectual disabilities, perform poorly at school, and have difficulties with memory, attention, judgment, and impulse control. In contrast, infants that develop ARBD have problems with the heart, kidneys, or bones, and sometimes hearing. FASD is not diagnosed prenatally, and until recently diagnostic tests to detect for prenatal alcohol exposure were not available. Diagnosis was based upon maternal report, maternal prenatal testing for alcohol consumption, and infant physical and developmental characteristics (Centers for Disease Control and Prevention, National Center on Birth Defects and Developmental Disabilities, & Division of Birth Defects and Developmental Disabilities, 2006). Through technological advancements, screening for prenatal exposure to alcohol is now available by testing meconium stool for fatty ethyl esters, offering health care providers a new tool for diagnosis.

Likewise, extensive studies report that nicotine, a primary ingredient in tobacco, leads to undesirable effects upon the central nervous and vascular system of the developing fetus. Maternal tobacco use leads to intrauterine growth restriction. Infants with intrauterine growth restriction are born small and are at higher risk for emotional and behavioral disorders (Chiswick, 1985). Prenatal tobacco exposure is also thought to sensitize the fetal brain to nicotine, increasing the risk of addiction when the brain is exposed to nicotine later in life. Furthermore, infants exposed to maternal tobacco are reported to be at risk for the development of adult-onset diseases such as obesity, hypertension, and Type 2 diabetes (among other problems) during their adult years (Braun et al., 2010; Bruin et al., 2010). Similar to other drugs, nicotine can be detected in the newborn's hair, amniotic fluid, meconium stool, fetal cord blood, and neonatal urine (Liaquet et al., 2010).

Mounting evidence suggests that maternal use of drugs, alcohol, and nicotine have detrimental effects on the developing fetus. However, exposure to these substances is difficult to control and equally difficult to diagnose. This is because the presence of signs and symptoms often mimic other disorders. As previously discussed, new tests have been developed to screen for prenatal exposure to these substances. Moreover, some health care providers and parents advocate for the identification of newborns exposed to drugs, alcohol, and nicotine through newborn screening.

Those in favor of screening newborns for exposure to drugs, alcohol, and nicotine report that identification of exposed infants through newborn screening would allow for implementation of services early in the child's life to optimize outcomes. Others believe that early identification of exposed infants will invade the privacy of the mother, potentially lead to false accusations from false positive results, lead to destruction of a family unit, and increase health care costs. Moreover, disruptions to the family unit, from an inaccurate diagnosis, might result in irreparable harm. An inaccurate diagnosis from a false positive screen is in direct conflict with the ethical principle of **non-maleficence**, which means to do no harm.

For integration of screening newborns for drug, alcohol, and nicotine exposure to be successful, it requires programs to have sustainable mechanisms in place to ensure **fidelity**, confidentiality, respect for autonomy, and quality assurance, and to minimize the potential risks of screening. Furthermore, adequate public health programs will need to be available to service the mother, infant, and family (Hicks et al., 2009).

Retention and Use of Samples

While a great deal of attention has been paid to ethical issues surrounding equality of newborn screening and securing universal screening for infants, less attention has been placed on the appropriate use of newborn screening specimens after screening tests are finished. Yet a growing interest in using newborn screen specimens for **deoxyribonucleic acid (DNA)** analysis has intensified. This is because these samples have the potential to serve as a useful resource for scientists, administrators, and judicial officials. Thus, some researchers and public officials have considered putting mechanisms in place that require the retention of newborn screens for use in the future as DNA banks (Lewis, Goldenberg, Anderson, Rothwell, & Botkin, 2011; Ross, 2009; Therrell et al., 2006).

As one can imagine many issues have surfaced in response, such as cost, personal privacy and consent issues, lack of appropriate sample release procedures, validity issues around stored samples (degradation and reanalysis), and appropriateness of applications (legal proceedings are a few of the ethical, social, and legal concerns). In response to the growing interest of securing newborn screening samples for later use, the newborn screening program and governmental authorities need to develop guidelines that will ensure safe practices around the use of these samples beyond their original intent (Lewis et al., 2011).

Future Challenges

Another controversial ethical concern often discussed within the context of newborn screening is the storage and utilization of placenta or umbilical cord blood. Placenta or umbilical cord blood contains a high concentration of stem cells from which all blood cells develop. Recent technological advances allow placenta/umbilical cord blood to be stored for future use in **blood banks** similar to the way whole blood products are stored and utilized for blood transfusions. It has enabled placental/umbilical cord blood products to be used for hematopoietic reconstitution in patients with hematological malignancies, certain lysosomal storage and peroxisomal enzyme deficiency disorders, Hurler syndrome (MPS I), Krabbe disease (globoid leukodystrophy), X-linked adrenoleukodystropy, primary immunodeficiency diseases, bone marrow failure, and beta thalassemia, and can also be used for reproductive health. When stored, if placental/umbilical cord blood is used in recipients unrelated to the donor, it is called an **allogeneic** use. However, when the stored placental/umbilical cord blood is used in a first- or second-degree blood relative, it is called **autologous** use (ACOG Committee Opinion Number 399, 2008).

Most health care professionals agree that the public storage of cord blood (more formally known as cord hematopoietic stem/progenitor cells, cord HPC-C) may serve a public need similar to the way that the public benefits from the newborn screening. However, much like newborn screening, legal and ethical issues have arisen over usage and future research endeavors involving cord blood, including the following:

1. Determination of ownership
2. Informed consent processes
3. Commercialization of these blood banks

The United States Department of Health and Human Services Food and Drug Administration Center for Biologics Evaluation and Research recognizes these concerns and has begun to establish standards and guidelines for the use, storage, marketing, and commercialization of such banks for profit ("Guidance for Industry," 2009).

Summary

Comprehensive newborn screening programs involve much more than standardizing the initial screening process. Legislation must address the issue of informed consent, equitable payment, fair distribution and allocation of resources, privacy and confidentiality issues, parental education, accessibility of follow-up care, support, and treatment. Challenges regarding quality and safety of laboratory standards, including the storage, use, and disposal or retention of blood spots, must be considered.

SECTION THREE REVIEW

1. Justice as it relates to the newborn screen means
   A. screening of infants is based on socioeconomic groups.
   B. screening of infants must be undertaken with fairness and equity.
   C. screening of infants is the result of undue influence or coercion.
   D. disproportionate screening based on maternal age.
2. As a result of improved screening technologies, scientists can now screen for prenatal alcohol exposure.
   A. True
   B. False
3. A teenage mother delivers a sick newborn and the infant is admitted to your unit. Your state requires parental consent before a newborn screen can be obtained. The nurse caring for the sick newborn does not believe that the mother has the capacity to make a decision about the newborn screen for her newborn because she is a teen. The nurse obtains the newborn screen without asking for parental consent. Which ethical principle or concept did the nurse fail to acknowledge in this situation?
   A. Fidelity
   B. Surrogacy
   C. Informed consent
   D. All of the above
4. Proponents to the retaining of DNA blood samples for the entire population suggest that the scientific and medical benefits of retaining blood samples far outweigh the privacy risk. This viewpoint is an example of which ethics' principle?
   A. Autonomy
   B. Non-maleficence
   C. Self-determination
   D. Beneficence
5. When the health care provider fails to follow up on an abnormal newborn screen, which ethical principle did he or she fail to follow?
   A. Negligence
   B. Abuse
   C. Misconduct
   D. Non-maleficence

Answers: 1. B; 2. A; 3. D; 4. D; 5. D

POSTTEST

1. Results of a screen are considered to be false positive when
   A. results are interpreted as negative when actually positive.
   B. results are interpreted as positive when actually negative.
   C. results are interpreted as positive when actually positive.
   D. results are interpreted as negative when actually negative.
2. The degree to which a test measures what it claims to measure is called
   A. validity.
   B. reliability.
   C. accuracy.
   D. specificity.
3. In most newborn screens blood is taken from the infant by a(n)
   A. antecubital stick.
   B. heel stick.
   C. finger stick.
   D. arterial stick.
4. Ethics is the branch of philosophy that all includes of the following EXCEPT
   A. values that pertain to human conduct.
   B. moral reasoning about what is right actions.
   C. determination of punishment for immoral actions.
   D. correctness of personal and social actions.
5. Cystic fibrosis is an autosomal recessive disorder.
   A. True
   B. False

6. Congenital hypothyroidism falls into which of the following category of disorders?
   A. Endocrine
   B. Hematology
   C. Metabolic
   D. Other
7. Newborn screening programs fall under which level of governmental oversight?
   A. Federal
   B. State
8. The primary type of test used to analyze newborn screening results is
   A. Acumeter.
   B. MS/MS.
   C. Polymerase chain reaction (PCR).
   D. Radioallergosorbent test (RAST).
9. The only newborn screen not accomplished through a blood test is hearing.
   A. True
   B. False
10. A newborn disorder that is categorized in the core conditions as genetic is
   A. congenital adrenal hypoplasia.
   B. cystic fibrosis.
   C. homocystinuria.
   D. citrullinemia.

Posttest answers are located in the Appendix.

CHAPTER SUMMARY

The newborn screening program is one of the most established population-based, public health screening programs in the United States, and it serves as a model for genetic population-based screening programs. The challenge of newborn screening is to diagnose and treat the infant before the signs and symptoms of the disorder are present.

- In 2008, landmark legislation was passed that requires all 50 states and the District of Columbia to screen every newborn for 29 serious genetic or functional disorders on the uniform panel. This law made a significant impact on the inequities of newborn screening programs that had previously existed from state to state.
- Subsequent to the 2008 law, an additional screen was added to the uniform panel; now all states are recommended to perform a minimum of 30 screens.
- Despite significant advances in newborn screening, controversies over the appropriateness of testing remain at the forefront of discussions. Diverging viewpoints persist over identification of serious genetic conditions (even if rare), genetic implications for family members, limitations on analytical and clinical screening tests, screening for maternal drug and alcohol use, and retaining samples for DNA analysis.
- In response, clinical experts in the field of genetics and ethics, in collaboration with the newborn screening program and governmental authorities, are working to develop guidelines that will ensure safe practices around the use of the newborn screening blood samples.

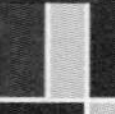

CRITICAL THINKING CHECKPOINT

Baby Girl M. is the 34-week gestation infant admitted to the NICU for low blood sugar and breathing difficulties. Upon admission of the infant, you are told that the mother refuses newborn screening along with vitamin K and ophthalmologic prophylaxis.

1. What is your responsibility as this patient's nurse as it pertains to the newborn screen?
2. Under what circumstances is it appropriate for the mother to decline the newborn screen?
3. How do you communicate your nursing interventions to others when a mother declines the newborn screen?
4. If the mother in this scenario changes her mind, when should the newborn screen be obtained and what is the method for obtaining the newborn screen?

Answers are provided in the Appendix

ONLINE RESOURCES

A Compendium of Resources on Newborn Screening Policy and System Development: http://www.medicalhomeinfo.org/downloads/docs/NBScategorizedcompend.doc

Centers for Disease Control: http://www.cdc.gov/ncbddd/pediatricgenetics/newborn_screening.html

Committee on Heritable Disorders in Newborns and Children: http://www.hrsa.gov/advisorycommittees/mchbadvisory/heritabledisorders/

Early Hearing Detection and Intervention Program (EHDI): http://www.cdc.gov/ncbddd/hearingloss

Genetic Alliance Collection of Newborn Screening Videos: http://www.youtube.com/geneticalliance#g/c/A6C56724C998F799

Hearing Screening: http://www.medicalhomeinfo.org/how/clinical_care/hearing_screening/

March of Dimes: http://www.marchofdimes.com/baby/bringinghome_recommendedtests.html

National Conference of State Legislatures (**NCSL**): http://www.ncsl.org/default.aspx?tabid=14382

National Newborn Screening and Genetics Resource Center: http://genes-r-us.uthscsa.edu/

Newborn Screening in Massachusetts: Answers for You and Your Baby: http://www.umassmed.edu/nbs/

Newborn Screening Translational Research Network (NBSTRN): http://www.nbstrn.org

Presidential Commission for the Study of Bioethical Issues: http://bioethics.gov/meetings/

The Parent's Guide to Newborn Screening: These Tests Can Save Your Baby's Life: http://mchb.hrsa.gov/pregnancyandbeyond/newbornscreening

Pearson Nursing Student Resources

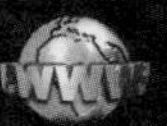

Find additional review materials at nursing.pearsonhighered.com

Prepare for success with additional NCLEX®-style practice questions, interactive assignments and activities, web links, animations, videos, and more!

REFERENCES

Acharya, K., Ackerman, P. D., & Ross, L. F. (2005). Pediatricians' attitudes toward expanding newborn screening. *Pediatrics, 116*, e476–484.

ACOG Committee Opinion Number 399: February 2008: Umbilical cord blood banking. (2008). *Obstetrics Gynecology, 111*(2), 475–477.

Advisory Committee on Heritable Disorders and Genetic Diseases in Newborn and Children. (2006, October 23). *Evidence-based evaluation and decision process for the advisory committee on hertiable disorders and genetics diseases in newborn and children: A workgroup meeting summary*. Washington, DC.

Alliance, G. (Producer). (2011, 4/1/11) Award-winning vendor selected to develop BabysFirst.org, the nation's first online clearinghouse of newborn screening information. Notice retrieved from http://www.geneticalliance.org

American Academy of Pediatrics (AAP) Task Force for Improving Newborn Hearing Screening, D. A. I. (2010). *Early Hearing Detection and Intervention (EHDI)*. Elk Grove Village, IL: AAP.

American Nurses Association. (2001). *Code of ethics for nurses*. Retrieved from http://www.nursingworld.org/about/01action.htm

Andermann, A., Blancquaert, I., Beauchamp, S., & Dery, V. (2008). Revisiting Wilson and Jungner in the genomic age: A review of screening criteria over the past 40 years. *Bulletin of the World Health Organization, 86*(4), 317–319.

Arn, P. (2007). Newborn screening current status. *Health Affairs, 26*(2), 559–566.

Ascension Healthcare. (2011). Key ethical principles. *Ascension Health's Ethics Resources*. Retrieved from http://www.ascensionhealth.org/index.php?option=com_content&view=article7id=47<emid=171

Bailey, D. B., Skinner, D., Davis, A. M., Whitmarsh, I., & Powell, C. (2008). Ethical, legal, and social concerns about expanded newborn screening: Fragile X syndrome as a prototype for emerging issues. *Pediatrics, 121*, e693–704.

Baily, M. A., & Murray, T. H. (2008). Ethics, evidence, and cost in newborn screening. *The Hastings Center Report, 38*(3), 23–31.

Best, D., Committee on Environmental Health, Committee on Native American Child Health, & Committee on Adolescence. (2009). Secondhand and prenatal tobacco smoke exposure. *Pediatrics, 124*, e1017–e1044.

Bhattacharyya, N., Megerian, C. A., Talavera, F., Gianoli, G. J., Slack, C. L., & Meyers, A. D. *Auditory brainstem response audiometry*. Retrieved June 30, 2012, from http://emedicine.medscape.com/article/836277-overview#showall

Braun, J. M., Daniels, J. L., Poole, C., Olshan, A. F., Hornung, R., Bernert, Y. X., et al. (2010). A prospective cohort study of biomarkers of prenatal tobacco smoke exposure: The correlation between serum and meconium and their association with infant birth weight. *Environmental Health, 9*(53), 1–13.

Bruin, J. E., Gerstein, H. C., & Holloway, A. C. (2010). Long term consequences of fetal and neonatal nictotine exposure: A critical review. *Toxicology Sciences, 116*(2), 364–374.

Calonge, N., Green, N. S., Rinaldo, P., Lloyd-Puryear, M. A., Dougherty, D., Boyle, C., et al. (2010). Committee report: Method for evaluating conditions nominated for population-based screening of newborns and children. [Commentary]. *Genetics in Medicine, 12*(3), 153–159.

Centers for Disease Control and Prevention, National Center on Birth Defects and Developmental Disabilities, & Division of Birth Defects and Developmental Disabilities. (2006). *FASD, Diagnosis*. Retrieved from http://www.cdc.gov/ncbddd/fasd/diagnosis.html

Chiswick, M. L. (1985). Intrauterine growth retardation. *British Medical Journal, 291*, 845–848.

Crowe, S. (2008). *A brief history of newborn screening in the United States*. The President's Council on Bioethics, 1–8. Retrieved May 6, 2011, from http://bioethics.georgetown.edu/pcbe/background/newborn_screening_crowe.html

Davenport, J. (1997). Ethical principles in clinical practice. *The Permanente Journal, 1*(1), 1–8. Retrieved from http://xnet.kp.org/permanentejournal/sum97pj/principles.html

DeLuca, J. M., Kearney, M. H., Norton, S. A., & Arnold, G. L. (2011). Parents experiences of expanded newborn screening evaluations. *Pediatrics, 128*, 53–61.

English Articles. (2011). History of public health in America. pp. 1–3. Available from http://www.englisharticles.info/2011/04/06/history-of-public-health-in-amercia/

First national newborn screening clearinghouse. (2009). Retrieved June 4, 2011, from http://www.geneticalliance.org/pr.nbs.clearinghouse

Gaudine, A., LeFort, S. M., Lamb, M., & Thorne, L. (2011). Clinical ethical conflicts of nurses and physicians. *Nursing Ethics, 18*(1), 9–19.

Gillon, R. (1985). Philosophical medical ethics. *British Medical Journal, 290*, 1890–1891.

Goh, Y. I., Chudley, A. E., Clarren, S. K., Koren, G., Orrbine, E., Rosales, T., et al. (2008). Development of canadian screening tools for fetal alcohol spectrum disorder. *Can J Clin Pharmacol, 15*(2), e344–366.

Gray, T. R., Kelly, T., LaGasse, L. L., Smith L. M., Derauf, C., Haning, W., et al. (2009). Novel biomarkers of prenatal methamphetamine exposure in human meconium. *Ther Drug Monit, 31*(1), 70–75. Retrieved from http://www.ncbi.nlm.nih.gov/pmc/articles/PMC2629503

Green, N. S., Rinaldo, P., Brower, A., Boyle, C., Dougherty, D., Lloyd-Puryear, M. A., et al. (2007). Committee report: Advancing the current recommended panel of conditions for newborn screening. [Brief report]. *Genetics in Medicine, 9*(11), 792–796.

Guidance for Industry. Minimally Manipulated, Unrelated Allogeneic Placental/Umbilical Cord Blood Intended for Hematopoietic Reconstitution for Specified Indications. (2009). *Federal Register, 74*(201), 53751–53752.

Guidelines for Pediatric Medical Home Providers. American Academy of Pediatrics American Medical Association. (1995–2011). *AMA's code of medical ethics*. Retrieved from http://www.ama-assn.org/ama/pub/physician-resources/medical-ethics/code-medical-ethics.page

Hayeems, R. Z., Miller, F. A., Little, J., Carroll, J. C., Allanson, J., Chakraborty, P., et al. (2009). Informing parents about expanded newborn screening: Influences on provider involvement. [Article]. *Pediatrics, 124*(3), 950–958.

Hicks, M., Tough, S. C., Premji, S., Benzies, S., Lyon, A. W., Mitchell, I., et al. (2009). Alcohol and drug screening of newborns: Would women consent? *J Obstet Gynaecol Can., 31*(4), 331–339.

Kaye, C. I. (2006). Introduction to the Newborn Screening Fact Sheets. *Pediatrics, 118*(3), 1304–1312.

Kaye, C. I., Laxova, R., Livingston, J. E., Lloyd-Puryear, M. A., Mann, M., McCabe, E. R. B., et al. (2001). Integrating genetic services into public health guidance for state and territorial programs from the national newborn screening and genetics resource center (NNSGRC). *Community Genetics, 4*, 175–196.

Kemper, A. R., Trotter, T. L., Lloyd-Puryear, M. A., Kyler, P., Feero, W. G., & Howell, R. R. (2010). A blueprint for maternal and child health primary care physician education in medical genetics and genomic medicine: Recommendations of the United States Secretary for Health and Human Services Advisory Committee on Heritable Disorders in Newborns and Children. [Editorial Material]. *Genetics in Medicine, 12*(2), 77–80.

Kemper, A. R., Uren, R. L., Moseley, K. L., & Clark, S. J. (2006). Primary care physician's attitudes regarding follow-up care for children with positive newborn screening results. *Pediatrics, 118*(5), 1836–1841.

Lewis, M. H., Goldenberg, A., Anderson, R., Rothwell, E., & Botkin, J. R. (2011). State laws regarding the retention and use of residual newborn screening blood samples. *Pediatrics, 127*(4), 703–712. doi:10.1542/peds.2010-1468

Liaquet, H., Pichini, S., Joya, X., Papseit, E., Vall, O., Klien, J., et al. (2010). Biological matrices for the evaluation to environmental tobacco smoke dring prenatal life and childhood. *Anal Bioanal Chem*(1), 379–399.

Lipstein, E. A., Nabi, E., Perrin, J. M., Luff, D., Browning, M. F., & Kuhlthau, K. A. (2010). Parents' decision-making in newborn screening: Opinions, choices, and information needs. *Pediatrics, 126*(4), 696–704. doi:10.1542/peds.2010-0217

Lloyd-Puryear, M. A., Tonniges, T., vanDyck, P. C., Mann, M. Y., Brin, A., Johnson, K., et al. (2006). American Academy of Pediatrics Newborn Screening Task Force Recommendations: How far have we come? *Pediatrics, 117*, S194.

Montgomery, D. P., Plate, C. A., Jones, M., Rios, R., Lambert, D. K., Schumtz, N., et al. (2008). Using umbilical cord tissue to detect fetal exposure to illicit drugs: A multicenter study in Utah and New Jersey. *J Perinatol, 28*(11), 750–753.

Moyer, V. A., Calonge, N., Teutsch, S. M., Botkin, J. R., & Force, U. S. P. S. T. (2008). Expanding newborn screening: Process, polity, and priorities. [Article]. *Hastings Center Report, 38*(3), 32–39.

Munson, R. (2008). *Intervention and reflection: Basic issues in medical ethics.* (8th ed.). Belmont, CA: Thomson.

National Institute on Drug Abuse. (2011). *Prenatal exposure to drugs of abuse*. Retrieved from http://www.nida.nih.gov/tib/prenatal.html

Nelson, H. D., Bougatsos, C., & Nygren, P. (2008). Universal newborn hearing screening: Systematic review to update the 2001US Preventive Services Task Force Recommendation. *Pediatrics, 122*, e266–e277.

Newborn hearing screening laws. (2011, May). Retrieved June 30, 2011, from http://www.ncsl.org/default.aspx?tabid=14382

Newborn screening. (May 19, 2011). Retrieved June 30, 2012, from http://www.cdc.gov/newbornscreening/

Newborn screening expands: Recommendations for pediatricians and medical homes—Implications for the system. (2008). [Article]. *Pediatrics, 121*(1), 192–217. Retrieved June 30, 2012, from http://pediatrics.aappublications.org/content/121/1/192.full

Newborn screening law. (2011). Retrieved June 30, 2012, from http://www.fsma.org/FSMACommunity/Legislative?FSMALegislation

Newborn screening overview. Retrieved July 1, 2011, from www.marchofdimes.com/Peristats/

Overview newborn screening. (n.d.). Retrieved May 2, 2011, from http://genes-r-us.uthscsa.edu/resources/newborn/overview.htm

Perrin, J. M., Knapp, A. A., Browning, M. F., Comeau, A. M., Green, N. S., Lipstein, E. A., et al. (2010). An evidence development process for newborn screening. [Review]. *Genetics in Medicine, 12*(3), 131–134.

Plass, A. M. C., van El, C. G., Pieters, T., & Cornel, M. C. (2010). Neonatal screening for treatable and untreatable disorders: Prospective parents' opinions. *Pediatrics, 125*, e99–e107. Retrieved from http://pediatrics.aappublications.org/content/125/1/e99.full.html. doi:10.1542/peds.2009-0269

Pollitt, R. J. (2010). New technologies extend the scope of newborn blood-spot screening, but old problems remain unresolved. *ACTA Paediatrica, 99*, 1766–1772.

Prosser, L. A., Kong, C. Y., Rusinak, D., & Waisbren, S. L. (2010). Projected costs, risks, and benefits of expanded newborn screening for MCADD. *Pediatrics, 125*, e286–294.

Quinlivan, J. A., & Suriadi, C. (2006). Attitudes of new mothers towards genetics and newborn screening. *Journal of Psychosomatic Obstetrics & Gynecology, 27*(1), 67–72.

Rainbow, C. (2002). Descriptions of ethical theories and principles. *Principles and Theories*, 1–6. Retrieved from http://www.biodavidson.edu/people/kabernd/indep/carainbow/Theories.htm

Ross, L. R. (2009). Ethical and policy issues in newborn screening: Historical, current, and future developments. [Ethics]. *NeoReviews, 10*(2), e71–e81.

Russ, S. A., Hanna, D., DesGeorges, J., & Forsman, I. (2010). Improving follow-up to newborn hearing screening: A learning-collaborative. *Pediatrics, 126*, S59–69.

Sade, R. M. (2011). The locus of decision making for severly impaired newborns. *The American Journal of Bioethics, 11*(2), 40–41.

Schuett, V. (2009). Celebrating 75 years since the discovery of PKU. *PKU News, 21*(2).

Shulman, S., Besculides, M., Saltzman, A., Ireys, H., & White, K. R. (2010). Evaluation of the Universal Newborn Hearing Screening and Intervention Program. *Pediatrics, 126*, S19–27.

Stark, A. P., Lang, C. W., & Ross, L. F. (2011). A pilot study to evaluate knowledge and attitudes of Illinois pediatricians toward newborn screening for sickle cell disease and cystic fibrosis. *American Journal of Perinatology, 28*(3), 169–176.

The President's Council on Bioethics. (2008). The changing moral focus of newborn screening: An ethical analysis by the president's council on bioethics. Washington, DC. Retrieved June 30, 2012, from http://bioethics.georgetown.edu/pcbe/reports/newborn_screening/

Therrell, B. L., Johnson, A., & Williams, D. (2006). Status of newborn screening programs in the United States. [Article]. *Pediatrics, 117*(5), S212–S252.

Washington State Department of Health, & Maternal and Child Health Programs. (2010). *Drug and alcohol screening*. Retrieved from http://www.doh.wa.gov/cfh/mch/DrugAlcohScreen.htm

Watson, M. S., Mann, M. Y., Lloyd-Puryear, M. A., Rinaldo, P., & Howell, R. R. (2006). Newborn screening: Toward a uniform screening panel and system. Executive summary. [Article]. *Genetics in Medicine, 8*, 1S–252S.

Whayne, T. F. (1959). The history of preventative medicine in World War II. *Public Health Reports, 74*(2), 170–174.

Wilson, J. M. G., & Jungner, G. (1968). *Principles and practice of screening for disease.* Geneva: World Health Organization.

Wright, D., & Brajtman, S. (2011). Relational and embodied knowing: Nursing ethics within the interprofessional team. *Nursing Ethics, 18*(1), 20–30.

Joint Committee on Infant Hearing. (2007). Year 2007 position statement: Principles and guidelines for early hearing detection and intervention programs *Pediatrics, 120*(4), 898–921.

CHAPTER 12 Genetic Information Nondiscrimination Act Legislations

Sharon Terry

LEARNING OUTCOMES Following the completion of this chapter, the learner will be able to

1. Identify the people who are covered by GINA.
2. Recognize the situations in which GINA protects an individual's genetic information.
3. Gain an understanding of why GINA is necessary and how the law came to pass.

This chapter begins by defining **genetic discrimination** as a central ethical, legal, and social issue impacting an individual's decision-making process in accessing genetic services. The chapter presents the key activities in the public and private sector that built momentum for federal protections against genetic discrimination. It provides an overview of the Genetic Information Nondiscrimination Act (GINA) of 2008, which offers a baseline of federal protections against genetic discrimination in health insurance and employment settings. The final section of the chapter presents practical applications of GINA in nursing practice, focusing on how the law interacts with family health history and reimbursement of genetic services as examples.

PRETEST

1. What is genetic discrimination? In what context does it happen?
2. In what two areas does GINA apply?
3. Who enforces the regulations outlined by GINA?
4. In what way are GINA and HIPAA related?
5. A patient's genetic test results indicate the she has a genetic disorder. Can health insurers use that information to raise her premiums?
6. A patient's genetic test results indicate the she has a high risk of developing a disease. Can health insurers use that information to raise her premiums?
7. An individual's boss accidentally found out that he has a gene common to those with a certain type of cancer. Can the individual be discriminated against?
8. Who is not covered by GINA's protections?
9. What specific insurance areas are not covered by GINA's protections?
10. In what situations does GINA apply to nursing practice?

Pretest answers are located in the Appendix.

SECTION ONE: Introduction to Genetic Discrimination

Genetic discrimination is the act of treating an individual differently based on their **genetic information**. Discrimination based on genetic information is similar in many respects to discrimination based on race or ethnicity. While race, ethnicity, and genetics have no effect on an individual's character, capabilities, or ability to work, an individual may be treated unfairly because of society's stigma.

An individual's genetic information includes a number of things beyond his or her genetic testing information. For example, much of the information about someone's personal and family health history is genetic information. The act of asking for genetic testing, receiving genetic testing, and participation in a clinical trial that includes genetic services are all also considered genetic information.

Genetic information, as defined by the GINA, does not include information about the age or sex of an individual, nor does it include information about common medical tests, such as common blood tests or cholesterol measurements (Regulations Under the Genetic Information Nondiscrimination Act, 2008). Gaining a thorough understanding of genetic information is critical to be able to recognize genetic discrimination when it happens.

How, Where, and When Can Discrimination Occur?

GINA covers genetic discrimination with regard to employees, job applicants, and health insurance applicants and enrollees. Genetic discrimination is possible in the workplace in many forms. Some examples include employers altering pay, promotions, job assignments, training, benefits, or any other term of employment because of assumptions about an employee's genetic information. In another example, a potential employer could discriminate against a job applicant if genetic tests indicate that he or she is at risk for a disease that normally requires high health care costs.

Genetic discrimination of health insurance applicants or enrollees is an equally important issue. This form of genetic discrimination may include denying coverage or charging higher premiums based on predictive genetic information, because of fear that the individual may be at higher risk for developing a condition in the future.

While GINA protections are limited to health insurance and employment, genetic discrimination is not limited to those areas. Section Five describes more about the people and situations not covered by GINA, and the other measures in place to prevent genetic discrimination.

Overview of GINA

GINA was passed in May of 2008 and is commonly referred to as the first major civil rights legislation of the 21st century. After scientists developed genome sequencing technology and sequenced most of the human genome in 2003, concerns began to mount about the use of such information. People feared that their genetic information could be misused, opening the potential for discrimination based on genetic information. In addition, the scientific community was concerned that a fear of genetic discrimination would deter individuals from undergoing beneficial clinical genetic testing or participating in genetic research. Various umbrella associations for employers and insurers mounted opposition and said GINA was "a solution in search of a problem." However, through strong support from the scientific community, the National Institutes of Health, the Coalition for Genetic Fairness, and staunch congressional support, GINA was proposed and passed in order to address many of these concerns.

GINA provides federal-level, broad, baseline protections to individuals' genetic information. However, these protections are limited to two areas: **Title I**, which prohibits discrimination by health insurers, and **Title II**, which prohibits discrimination in employment. Section Three details the specific protections and limitations of these two titles in GINA.

SECTION ONE REVIEW

1. Describe three ways in which genetic discrimination can occur at the workplace.
2. Explain why genetic discrimination has a negative effect on genetic research.
3. What are the two main areas addressed by the Genetic Information Nondiscriminatory Act?

Answers:

1. Employees may be discriminated against on the basis of pay, promotions, and job assignments.
2. Genetic discrimination would have a negative effect on genetic research because individuals would be afraid to participate in testing that would further this research.
3. GINA addresses employment and health insurance discrimination.

SECTION TWO: Evidence Supporting Federal Protections Against Genetic Discrimination

The passage of GINA is truly a cornerstone in today's world of technical advances in scientific research and health care, but reaching that achievement involved more than a decade of raising awareness and legislative development. Understanding the evidence and support that called for GINA underscores the importance of this law in today's society.

Concerns Rise

Although GINA was officially signed into law in 2008, public support for federal protections against genetic discrimination was introduced in 1995. The first document supporting a genetic nondiscrimination law was published in October 1995. Scientists, including Dr. Francis Collins, currently the Director of the National Institutes of Health (at that time the Director of the National Human Genome Research Institute [**NHGRI**]) and the prominent leader of the Human Genome Project, published an article reporting that the use of genetic information to exclude individuals from health care would severely limit the anticipated benefits of genetic research (Hudson, Rothenberg, Andres, et al., 1995). The article cited multiple cases of genetic discrimination and articulated the position that fear of genetic discrimination would drive people away from participating in research or sharing information. A few months later a member of the U.S. House of Representatives, Louise Slaughter (D-NY), introduced the first of many bills addressing genetic discrimination (see Table 12–1). She remained its most staunch advocate until its passage in 2008, an almost 13-year heroic effort.

To address some of these issues, the National Institutes of Health (NIH), Department of Energy (DOE), the Working Group on Ethical, Legal, and Social Implications (ELSI), and

TABLE 12–1: Legislative Timeline

December 1995	Rep. Louise Slaughter introduces H.R.2748.
April 1996	Sen. Olympia Snowe introduces S.1694.
January 1997	Rep. Slaughter introduces H.R.306 and Sen. Snowe introduces S.89.
July 1999	Rep. Slaughter introduces H.R.2457 and Sen. Tom Daschle introduces S.1322.
February 2001	Rep. Slaughter introduces H.R.602, Sen. Daschle introduces S.318, and Sen. Snowe introduces S.382.
March 2002	Sen. Snowe introduces S.1995.
May 2003	Rep. Slaughter introduces H.R.1910 and Sen. Snowe introduces S.1053.
October 2003	Senate passes S.1053.
February 2005	Sen. Snowe introduces S.306.
February 2005	Sen. passes S.306.
March 2005	Rep. Biggert introduces H.R. 1227.
January 2007	Rep. Slaughter introduces H.R.493 and Sen. Slaughter introduces S.358.
April 25, 2007	GINA passes in House.
April 24, 2008	GINA reintroduced in Senate and passes.
May 1, 2008	GINA reintroduced in House and passes.
May 21, 2008	President George W. Bush signs GINA.
May 21, 2009	Title I (insurance) takes effect.
November 21, 2009	Title II (employment) takes effect.

the National Action Plan on Breast Cancer (NAPBC) organized a workshop to evaluate the implications of the Human Genome Project and to examine the current state of genetic discrimination. Held in October of 1996, the workshop developed a series of recommendations for state and federal policy makers to protect against genetic discrimination in employment decisions. The recommendations stated that employers should be (1) prohibited from using genetic information to affect the hiring, terms, benefits, or termination of employment; (2) prohibited from requesting or requiring the disclosure of genetic information; (3) restricted from access to genetic information in medical records; and (4) prohibited from releasing genetic information without prior written authorization of the employee (National Institutes of Health, National Human Genome Research Institute, 1996). The workshop concluded by suggesting that violators of the recommendations be subject to strong enforcement measures.

That same month, another article was published that discussed the perceptions of members of genetic disease support groups. The study revealed multiple statistics about the individuals and families who believed they were denied health insurance or let go from a job as a result of a genetic disorder (Lapham, Kozma, & Weiss, 1996). The study results reinforced previous concerns that fear of discrimination would turn people away from genetic testing, and refuted the claim that there was no problem.

Months later, in January of 1997, the Department of Labor (**DOL**) released the report, *Genetic Information and the Workplace*. The goal of the report was to demonstrate why American workers deserved federal legislation to protect them from genetic discrimination in the workplace (Dept. of Labor, DHHS, EEOC, & Dept. of Justice, 1998). The report also reiterated that many Americans were reluctant to use breakthroughs in genetic testing because they felt that the potential for genetic discrimination outweighed the promises to improve health. The report concluded that most professional groups, including the American Medical Association (AMA), found it inappropriate to exclude workers due to predictive genetic characteristics and thought that the use of genetic testing and access to genetic information in the workplace should be either prohibited or severely restricted. Current laws at the time did not fully address the issue of genetic discrimination, and any existing protections were limited.

Support Gains Momentum

In the fall of 1996, at the American Society of Human Genetics annual meeting, a number of organizations, including the Alpha-1 Association, Genetic Alliance, Hadassah, National Partnership for Women & Families, National Society of Genetic Counselors, and the National Workrights Institute, met and discussed the need for a coalition to support a movement toward legislation. In the spring of 1997, the Coalition for Genetic Fairness (**CGF**) was founded, bringing together civil rights, disease-specific, and health care organizations as well as industry groups and employers. The Coalition, led first by the National Partnership for Women & Families, and later by Genetic Alliance, united more than 500 organizations and thousands of individuals as one voice against genetic discrimination. The groups aimed to address public concern about discrimination by employers and health insurers and to help inform Congress so that legislation could be seriously considered.

In the 11 years of advocacy, the bill faced strong opposition from the National Association of Manufacturers, the National Retail Federation, the Society for Human Resource Management, the United States Chamber of Commerce, and other members of the Genetic Information Nondiscrimination in Employment Coalition (GINE). GINE said that the proposed legislation was overly broad, and thought that it would create frivolous litigation. In addition, some of the early advocates of the legislation stepped away from support since they felt the bill lacked "teeth" (i.e., strong penalties) as it was revised in various compromises. Furthermore, the bill contained two titles (a title is a major part or heading of the U.S. Code of Law), amended several laws, and fell under the jurisdiction of three federal departments, all of which created enormous legal and political hurdles.

A few years later, in February of 2000, President Bill Clinton issued Executive Order 13145: To Prohibit Discrimination in Federal Employment. The executive order ensured that Executive branch employees were not subject to genetic discrimination and hoped to encourage employers in the private industry to adopt similar policies.

In 2001, the Equal Employment Opportunity Commission (**EEOC**) filed a lawsuit against Burlington Northern Santa Fe (BNSF) Railway Company regarding discriminatory use of employees' genetic information. As one of the few legal cases of genetic discrimination, the suit created even more momentum for legislation against genetic discrimination. Dave Escher, a former BNSF employee, was forced to undergo genetic testing without his knowledge or consent after he was diagnosed with work-related carpal tunnel syndrome. BNSF's intent was to reduce the medical and workers' compensation due to Mr. Escher, and had tried to use genetic tests to prove that the condition was genetic, rather than work related (Escher, 2007). The company reached a \$2.2 million settlement that was distributed to 36 BNSF employees who had been tested or asked to submit to genetic tests.

Publications continued to support the prohibition of genetic discrimination, particularly one such article in *Science* that specifically urged Congress to approve GINA and called genetic discrimination a civil rights issue (Collins & Watson, 2003). The authors emphasized that the success of U.S. scientific discovery and medicine would be at risk the longer the problem of genetic discrimination remained unsolved.

In the coming years, President George W. Bush would support the legislation by issuing two Statements of Administration Policies (SAP) (Bush, 2003; Bush, G., 2005), while the Secretary's Advisory Committee on Genetics, Health, and Society (**SACGHS**) would release multiple publications and letters of support for the legislation (Tuckson, 2005; NIH, n.d.; NIH, n.d.).

In January of 2007, President Bush again urged Congress to pass genetic nondiscrimination legislation, this time while visiting the NIH. Multiple news sources, including *NPR*, the *Washington Times*, and the *New York Times*, began to follow news surrounding GINA; as public awareness grew, there was growing pressure on Congress to pass the bill. Senators Ted Kennedy (D-MA) and Olympia Snowe (R-ME) remained active supporters of the bill through many years. Rep. Judy Biggert (R-IL) became a key supporter, building Republican support and creating a turning point for momentum in the House. On April 25, 2007, GINA finally passed in the House 420-9, but a hold put on it in the Senate by Tom Coburn (R-OK), due to concerns about the details of the proposed bill, prevented a vote in the Senate (see Figure 12–1 ■). Finally, the Senate voted almost a year later, on April 24, 2008, and passed the bill 95-0. (Five senators, including then candidates Obama, Clinton, and McCain, did not vote.) President Bush officially signed GINA into law on May 21, 2008.

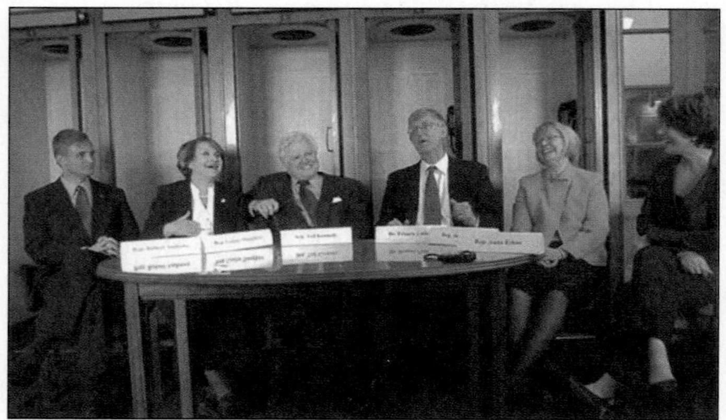

Figure 12–1 ■ The champions share a moment of levity after the passage of GINA in the House of Representatives: Robert Andrews (D-NJ), Rep. Louise Slaughter (D-NY), Senator Ted Kennedy (D-MA), Dr. Francis Collins (NIH Director), Rep. Judy Biggert (R-IL), and Rep. Anna Eshoo (D- CA).
Source: Photo courtesy of Diane Baker.

SECTION TWO REVIEW

1. How long had support for genetic nondiscrimination legislation existed before GINA was officially signed into law?
2. What role did the Coalition for Genetic Fairness (CGF) play in the passage of GINA?
3. Name four organizations that supported GINA and contributed to evidence supporting federal protections against genetic discrimination.

Answers:

1. Since 1995.
2. The CGF united organizations that aimed to address the public concern surrounding genetic information misuse by employers and health insurers. The CGF wanted to inform Congress about genetic discrimination so that legislation could be seriously considered.
3. National Institutes of Health (NIH), Department of Energy (DOE), Department of Labor (DOL), American Medical Association (AMA), Coalition for Genetic Fairness (CGF), Equal Employment Opportunity Commission (EEOC), Secretary's Advisory Committee on Genetics, Health, and Society (SACGHS)

SECTION THREE: The Law

"An Act to prohibit discrimination on the basis of genetic information with respect to health insurance and employment," Genetic Information Nondiscrimination Act of 2008 (GINA), Public Law 110-343 (2008).

The late Senator Edward Kennedy (D-MA), in a historic speech on the floor of the Senate the day GINA passed that chamber, said that GINA was the "first major new civil rights bill of the new century." The law's passage has empowered individuals and has profound effects in genetic research, health care, and society. Still, patients, providers, employees, and employers must first learn about the law and its titles on discrimination in health insurance (Title I) and in employment (Title II) in order to know how individuals are protected. A complete and technical understanding of GINA is critical in order to know the full scope and limits of the protections given in this law. This section discusses all this, and the next section builds on this knowledge to place GINA regulations in the context of nursing practice.

Definitions in GINA

Laws often define important terms quite technically, and even different provisions within one law may use different definitions. Knowing the distinctions is essential because terms often determine the boundaries of the law and specify who will be affected.

Genetic Information

The genetic information regulated by GINA includes four items:

1. Information about an individual's genetic tests
2. Information about the genetic tests of an individual's family members
3. Information about the manifestation of a disease or disorder in an individual's family members
4. Information about an individual's request for or receipt of genetic services or participation in clinical research that includes genetic services

Genetic information does not include information about an individual's gender or age. Additionally, genetic information does not include information about the manifestation of a disease or disorder in the individual.

Genetic Test

GINA defines a genetic test as the following:

1. An analysis of human DNA, RNA, chromosomes, proteins, or metabolites that detect genotypes, mutations, or chromosomal changes.
2. A test that excludes any analysis of proteins or metabolites that does not detect genotypes, mutations, or chromosomal changes.

Proteins and metabolites qualify as testable compounds for genetic tests because there are genetic disorders such as phenylketonuria (PKU) that can be effectively diagnosed by non-DNA-based analysis. However, GINA's definition of a genetic test also includes the subsequent exclusion noted in the preceding list in order to ensure that only very specific protein or metabolite analyses are regarded as genetic tests.

GINA also specifies *an additional exclusion* to the previous two-part definition when genetic tests are discussed with regard to Title I, the health insurance provisions:

3. (Applies only to Title I) Excluding any analysis of proteins or metabolites that is directly related to a manifested disease, disorder, or pathological condition that could reasonably be detected by a health care professional with appropriate training and expertise in the field of medicine involved.

The "manifested disease, disorder, or pathological condition" referenced in the preceding definition includes any medical diagnosis of any genetic disease or disorder, symptomatic or asymptomatic. In other words, Title I of GINA, regarding health insurance decisions, only covers predictive genetic information. Currently, GINA does not prevent health insurance providers from using genetic information about the current state of health to make **underwriting** decisions.

Since this second exclusion does not apply to Title II, employers are not allowed to use genetic information on an individual's current health status to make employment-related decisions. This protection follows the American Disabilities Act regulations, which prohibit discrimination based on disability in employment.

Manifest Disease

GINA defines **manifestation** specifically to be a state that has been or could reasonably be diagnosed as a disease, disorder, or pathological condition by a health care professional not based mainly on genetic information. In other words, test results alone are not evidence of a manifestation unless such results, used by a doctor, confirm a diagnosis for disease.

Genetic Services

Genetic services, as referenced in GINA, include genetic tests, genetic counseling, genetic education, and participation in a genetic research study.

Family Member

GINA defines a family member as any individual who is a first-degree, second-degree, third-degree, or fourth-degree relative. For example, an individual's aunt and grandfather are both second-degree relatives.

Underwriting

Title I of GINA describes underwriting in the context of health insurance offered in connection with a group health plan, and defines the term as having four purposes:

1. Making rules for or determining eligibility (including enrollment and continued eligibility) for health benefits
2. The computation of premium or contribution amounts
3. The application of any preexisting condition exclusion
4. Making rules for other activities related to the creation, renewal, or replacement of a contract of health insurance or health benefits

Genetic Monitoring

Genetic monitoring, as defined in GINA, is the periodic examination of employees to evaluate acquired modifications to their genetic material such as chromosomal damage or evidence of increased occurrence of mutations that may have developed in the course of employment due to exposure to toxic substances in the workplace, in order to identify, evaluate, and respond to the effects of or control adverse environmental exposures in the workplace. This term is only used in Title II of GINA.

Protections in Health Insurance

Title I of GINA outlines genetic nondiscrimination in health insurance and determines the unlawful use of genetic information. In the actual legislation, Title I of GINA is a collection of amendments to four already existing laws: the Employment Retirement Income Security Act (**ERISA**), the Public Health Service Act, the Internal Revenue Code, and the Social Security Act. Together, the amendments endow greater protections to individuals in obtaining and maintaining health insurance.

The "health insurance providers" referenced in GINA refer to those that offer plans through an individual's employer (i.e., a group plan) and those health insurance plans bought by individuals (i.e., an individual plan). GINA also applies to Medicare supplemental policies for individuals who have insurance through Medicare, but does *not* apply to those who receive health care from the military Tricare health system, Indian Health Service (**IHS**), or Federal Employees Health Benefits Plan (**FEHB**) (Regulation Under the Genetic Information Nondiscrimination Act, 2008).

GINA provides two main protections regarding the use and collection of genetic information by health insurance providers:

1. Health insurance providers may not make enrollment or coverage decisions or adjust premium or contribution amounts on the basis of predictive genetic information.
   - Recall the extra exclusion in the definition for genetic tests in Title I. Thus, insurance providers may still use genetic information about current health status to make decisions on enrollment, coverage, and premium or contribution amounts.
2. Health insurance providers may not request or require an individual or an individual's family member to undergo a genetic test except in two circumstances:
   - EXCEPTION: Health insurers may ask for the *minimum* amount of genetic information only to determine a medical need for a test, treatment, or procedure requested by the individual. Identification of a medical need is often a key decision factor in whether an insurer will cover the requested service.
   - EXCEPTION: Health insurers may request for, but not require, an individual to undergo a genetic test for research that (1) complies with protections on human subjects; (2) clearly indicates that compliance is voluntary and that noncompliance will have no effect on enrollment status, premium, or contribution amounts; (3) will not use any genetic information collected from research for underwriting; (4) has notified the federal government in writing with a description of activities conducted; and (5) complies with any future regulations that may be added to this provision.

Protections in Employment

Title II of GINA prohibits employment discrimination on the basis of genetic information. The law applies to employers, employment agencies, labor organizations, and training programs.

An employer, as regulated in GINA, includes not-for-profit organizations and for-profit corporations with at least 15 employees. Additionally, GINA protections do *not* apply to the U.S. military or employees of the federal government (Regulations Under the Genetic Information Nondiscrimination Act, 2008). The use of the term *employers* in the rest of this section refers collectively to employers, employment agencies, labor organizations, and training programs.

GINA outlines the unlawful use of genetic information in two components. Employers may not do the following:

1. Discriminate against any employee with respect to the hiring, termination, compensation, terms or conditions, or privileges of employment.
2. Limit, segregate, or classify employees in a way that would deprive or tend to deprive any employee of employment opportunities or otherwise adversely affect the individual's status as an employee because of genetic information.

Similar to Title I, Title II of GINA prohibits employers from requesting, requiring, or purchasing genetic information of an employee or the employee's family member. There are, however, certain circumstances where employers may legally gain or request access to an individual's genetic information:

1. *Inadvertent knowledge*. In some cases an employer may accidentally learn about an employee's genetic information whether through casual conversations at the workplace or if it is inadvertently included with the general medical information submitted to employers.
2. *Publicly available information*. An employer may learn the genetic information of an employee or the employee's family members if it is available in publicly available information sources, such as newspapers and periodicals but *not* medical databases or court records.
3. *Voluntary health services*. Some employers offer voluntary health or genetic services, such as employee wellness programs. If specific requirements are met and participation in the service is voluntary, then forms, questionnaires, or health care professionals treating employees as part of the service may request family health history or other genetic information.
4. *Family and Medical Leave Act (FMLA)*. Forms that employees must fill out as part of asking for time off from work to care for a sick family member may include questions about genetic information. Employees may need to provide this information for extended leave to be approved.
5. *Genetic monitoring*. Employers may request genetic information if the information is to be used for genetic monitoring of the biologic effects of toxic substances in the workplace, only when the employee provides voluntary and written authorization or when monitoring is required by federal or state law (in which case the employee must still be informed).

In all cases, employers are still prohibited from using the genetic information collected to discriminate against employees. Employers must also treat any collected genetic information as confidential medical records as prescribed by the Health Insurance Portability and Accountability Act (**HIPAA**). HIPAA and GINA regulations also add that genetic information may not be disclosed by an employer except at the employee's request or in response to a court order.

Implementation and Enforcement

Title I took effect on May 21, 2009, and Title II took effect on November 21, 2009. GINA provides baseline protections for individuals against genetic discrimination in health insurance and employment, so the law does not necessarily preempt state law. This is called a floor, and state laws trump it if the laws offer strong protections or penalties. Where a state's genetic discrimination law or regulations are more comprehensive, those state laws would still be in effect as long as they do not conflict with GINA.

GINA divides the responsibilities of enforcing Title I among three departments in the federal government: the Department of Labor, the Department of Health and Human Services, and the Department of the Treasury. The EEOC has been tasked with enforcing Title II, and the regulation guidance was released in 2010.

Emerging Evidence

GINA is a law based on the science of genetics as of 2008. It protects individuals from discrimination in employment and health insurance, using definitions of genetics and family history that rely on the available scientific evidence at the time of the bill's passage. It is likely that some of these definitions might evolve over the course of time as more genotype/phenotype correlations are made. It is possible that genetic information that indicates probable disease could become refined over time and be used in a diagnostic sense.

Further, at the time that GINA was written and passed, health insurance in the United States was connected to employment in many cases and provided by private insurance companies, except in the case of those covered by Medicare and Medicaid. It is possible in the future that new methods and forms of health insurance will arise, and these protections would be redundant for health insurance. This is true for countries in which healthcare is a right and is offered to all citizens by the government. Discrimination based on genetic information cannot impact health care coverage in those countries.

SECTION THREE REVIEW

1. How do Title I and Title II of GINA define genetic test differently? Why does this matter?
2. At what point does a disease become manifest, according to the use of the term in GINA?
3. What services are included in GINA's definition of genetic services?
4. a) Name one exception when an employer may request the genetic information of an employee.
   b) Name one exception when a health insurance provider may request the genetic information of an individual.
5. What entity or entities has regulatory responsibilities over the enforcement of GINA Title I and Title II?

Answers:

1. In Title I, a genetic test excludes analysis of proteins or metabolites that are related to manifest disease, and therefore covers only predictive genetic information. In Title II, this exclusion does not exist. The essential difference is that health insurers are allowed to use genetic information related to current health status to underwrite, while employers are not allowed to use that current health status information to discriminate among employees or job applicants.
2. The term manifest disease is used to describe any disease, disorder, or pathology that can be reasonably diagnosed by a health care professional.
3. The services included in GINA's definition of genetic services include genetic tests, genetic counseling, genetic education, and participation in a genetic research study.
4. a) Employers can ask for their employees to undergo periodic examination if they have been exposed to toxic substances in the workplace, including changes in genes.
   b) Insurers can ask for genetic information to determine if a medical test is needed.
5. The Department of Labor, the Department of Health and Human Services, and the Department of the Treasury oversee Title I, and Title II is enforced by the EEOC.

SECTION FOUR: Applications of GINA

Advances in genomics and medicine are rapidly changing the landscape of health care, driving it toward more effective and personalized therapies. GINA was created to ensure that legal protections keep pace with clinical advances. Given the novel and sometimes intimidating applications of genomics in health, it can be complicated to inform individuals and families about the protections included in GINA and to clarify the misconceptions that some may have about genetic tests and genetic counseling. Seeing GINA as an element in a patient-centric environment will enable these individuals to make informed decisions about the collection and sharing of their genetic information without fear of discrimination by employers or insurers.

GINA in Nursing Practice

Nurses constitute the front line of health care delivery, often consulting with patients about genetic services and communicating genetic test results or other genetic information. Thus, the nurse should be ready to inform the patient of the protections and limits provided by GINA. It is also important to remember that GINA is not the only form of protection against genetic discrimination. There are states that provide even more comprehensive protections against discrimination, and patients must also be aware of those additional protections. While it is impossible to anticipate every situation when GINA may be relevant, there are several common scenarios that may occur in nursing practice.

Family Health History Consultation

Reviewing a family health history is always an important part of an initial intake for a patient. It entails several steps before and after consultations. Ensuring that patients are aware of their protections at each step of the process will allow them to make decisions with greater confidence and gain the most benefit out of the results. These are some key areas where patients should be informed about GINA:

- *Before consultation.* Patients are commonly concerned with the potential misuse of family health information and how their employers and health insurers may interpret family members' genetic information to reflect the health status of the patient. GINA prohibits those employers and health insurers from discriminating based on family members' genetic information. Additionally, even the knowledge of the patient's request or receipt of any counseling about genetics is protected from discrimination.
- *After consultation.* Results from family health history consultations may reveal a risk for a certain disease or disorder. Patients must be assured that this information collected from a family health history consultation is protected as genetic information. GINA protects information all the way into the fourth generation; it places strict limits on the ability of employers and health insurers in accessing that information.

Genetic Testing

The protections afforded by GINA for genetic testing vary depending on the context of the use of that information. Thus, patients must be given a clear and comprehensive understanding of how their genetic test information can be used. Like genetic counseling or consultations, any knowledge of the patient's request or receipt of genetic tests is protected from discrimination. However, the patient must also understand the specific ways in which genetic test information may be used.

- *By employers*. Regardless of the context or nature of the results, employers are not allowed to discriminate based on information from genetic tests. Only in very rare circumstances may they gain access to this information (see Section Three), and they may not require employees to undergo any genetic test.
- *By health insurers*. If the genetic test results are predictive and reveal risk for developing a certain condition, health insurers are prohibited from using that information to underwrite. However, GINA does not prohibit health insurers from using a disorder or other condition to adjust premiums, deny or limit coverage, or use for other underwriting purposes—although other laws may prohibit this use. If the patient plans to make a reimbursement claim to cover the cost of the test, GINA does not prevent health insurers from requiring the individual to pay for the test. The individual may also be asked to prove the medical necessity of the test in order to have the test costs reimbursed.

Prenatal Testing

Another key application of GINA relates to prenatal testing. When a mother receives prenatal testing results, it is important to communicate information about GINA. If a fetus tests positive for a condition in utero and that condition has a phenotype (physical manifestations), GINA ensures a fair employment future for the child, but GINA cannot prohibit health insurers from using that information to determine coverage for the child. Further, infants in the United States are exempt from any preexisting condition limitations in insurance conditions. If the expectant mother or father is discovered to be a carrier of the condition, her or his health care coverage is not affected. Knowledge of this protection can help expectant parents make very important decisions during their pregnancy and prepare them to make the best possible health decisions for their babies after birth.

SECTION FOUR REVIEW

1. Identify the common situation where a health insurance provider may request genetic test information.
2. A patient arrives saying that her recent employment at a private company requires her to take a genetic test. Which title of GINA should you discuss with her?
3. Do patient–provider discussions about GINA mainly occur before or after the receipt of genetic services?
4. Identify another situation, not discussed in this list, where GINA would apply in nursing practice.

Answers:

1. Health insurance providers may request genetic test information when it is part of the diagnosis of a manifest disease.
2. If a patient arrives saying that her recent employment at a private company requires her to take a genetic test, you should counsel her about Title II of GINA, which is the employment title.
3. Patient–provider discussions about GINA should occur before and after the receipt of genetic services.
4. GINA would also apply in other nursing practice scenarios. For example, when a child is suspected to have a genetic problem, the family needs to understand the protections that GINA gives them; or when civilian nurses give care in a military hospital or health care related setting, they need to know the limitations of GINA for this population and be ready to advocate for the patient and family.

SECTION FIVE: Genetic Discrimination and Future Considerations

While GINA does protect the general population against genetic discrimination in health insurance and employment, there are certain areas in which it does not apply. GINA does not apply to life insurance, disability insurance, or long-term care insurance. During the long years of struggle to pass the bill, there were some who wanted to bring these other insurance products into protection under the law. There were others who felt that these products, usually based more closely on risk pools, would reduce the possibility of the bill passing to nil.

GINA is not applicable to the military, federal employees enrolled in the Federal Employees Health Benefits program (FEHB), veterans obtaining health care through the Veteran's Administration, employers with fewer than 15 employees, and individuals covered under the Indian Health Service. In most cases, GINA does not apply in these scenarios because there are similar discrimination policies already in place in protect the aforementioned groups (see Table 12–2).

TABLE 12–2: GINA Exclusions

People	Areas
Military	Life insurance
Federal employees enrolled in FEHB	Disability insurance
Veterans obtaining health care through the VA	Long-term care insurance
Employers with fewer than 15 employees	
Individuals covered by Indian Health Service	

Life Insurance, Disability Insurance, and Long-Term Care Insurance

GINA does not currently apply to life insurance, disability insurance, or long-term care insurance. Protection against discrimination in these areas varies according to state laws. As of 2011, only seven states prohibit genetic discrimination in life insurance without actuarial justification. Even fewer include protection against genetic discrimination in disability and long-term care insurance. A list of the states and their individual protections can be found online at the National Conference of State Legislatures website.

Military

GINA ensures that individuals' genetic information is kept private from employers and health insurance providers, but the military's policy requires personnel to disclose their genetic information in order to protect their well-being while serving and prevent any health concerns from disrupting military operations. For example, the Department of Defense (**DOD**) collects military personnel's genetic samples and tests them for sickle cell anemia and glucose 6-phosphate dehydrogenase (G6PD) deficiency (Baruch & Hudson, 2008). Military personnel who test positive for these two medical conditions have their test results recorded in their files, stated on their identification tags (dog tags), and represented by red armbands worn to distinguish themselves during military operations. In doing so, these service members may be identified prior to entering an environment that could trigger the symptoms of their condition. Genetic samples are also used by the military to identify service members, should positive identification be needed.

Genetic samples that have been taken from military personnel and stored in the repository are used for other purposes such as research. This practice has drawn criticism from some service members who demanded privacy of their genetic information, citing a violation of their Fourth Amendment rights. Despite these criticisms, federal courts have found that the use of this genetic information for research does not violate protections against unlawful search and seizure (Mayfield v. Dalton, 1995). Thus, genetic information from the repository continues to be used for purposes beyond standard military operations, although service members may choose to destroy their samples once they leave the military.

SECTION FIVE REVIEW

1. What types of insurance does GINA not apply to?
2. What groups are excluded from the protections offered by GINA?
3. For those groups that are excluded, are they left without protection from genetic discrimination?
4. For what reasons does the military collect genetic information from military personnel?

Answers:

1. GINA does not apply to disability, long-term, or life insurance.
2. Groups that are excluded from the protections offered by GINA are military, federal employees enrolled in FEHB, veterans obtaining health care through the VA, employers with fewer than 15 employees, and individuals covered by Indian Health Service.
3. For the groups that are excluded, most are covered by other laws, except individuals who work for companies with fewer than 15 employees.
4. The military collects information on active duty individuals to assess their well-being while serving and prevent any health concerns from disrupting military operations.

POSTTEST

1. Why did genetic discrimination become a major issue for U.S. citizens?
2. Define genetic information and how it differs between Titles I and II.
3. What are the two circumstances in which a health insurance provider may request genetic information or for an individual to undergo a genetic test?
4. Regarding this chapter's discussion of Title II, the term *employers* is used to collectively address what groups of people?
5. Name two of the five circumstances where employers are legally allowed to gain or request access to an individual's genetic information.
6. A health insurance provider discovers that a young beneficiary has several older relatives with cardiovascular disease. Can the insurer use this information to raise the beneficiary's premium?
7. A woman arrives at a wellness checkup as part of a voluntary service her company provides, but she complains that her employer should not be allowed to request that she give them her genetic information. Is her statement correct? Why or why not?
8. The woman from Question 7 arrives again a month later, after giving her genetic information to her employer, complaining that she was refused a pay raise because of her genetic condition. If she was refused the pay raise because of genetic information, is the employer out of compliance with GINA's regulations?
9. For what purpose are the stored genetic samples of military men and women most commonly used? When can servicemen decide to destroy those samples?
10. A federal employee arrives at the clinic. He is concerned that GINA does not apply to the genetic test results he just received. Can he be discriminated against based on his genetic information?

Posttest answers are located in the Appendix.

CHAPTER SUMMARY

Genetic discrimination is the act of treating an individual differently based on their genetic information. Due to the stigma that society has placed on certain genetic conditions, discrimination could have been a major issue in employment and health insurance. Fear of genetic discrimination may deter individuals from taking advantage of beneficial genetic tests and services and participating in important genetic research studies.

Concern about genetic discrimination rose throughout the years due to the sequencing of the human genome and as potential clinical uses of genetics increased. Numerous studies and reports revealed that both public perception and the reality of genetic discrimination were real issues that affected the use of breakthrough genetic tests and the support of further genetic research. Public support for federal protections against genetic discrimination began in the mid-1990s and culminated in 2008, when GINA was passed by the U.S. Congress and signed by President Bush.

GINA's definition of terms is a key concept that determines the boundaries of the law. The law outlines baseline protections for nearly all who are employed and for those with the most common forms of health insurance plans; however, there are important exceptions. Title I, which addresses health insurance, is enforced by DOL, HHS, and the DOT. Title II, addressing employment, is enforced by EEOC.

Nurses have a responsibility to inform patients of the protections and limits provided by GINA when discussing genetic tests or services. Patients are most often concerned with the misuse of their genetic information, and nurses can offer an accurate and comprehensive explanation of a patient's protections depending on the context of the situation. Employers and health insurance providers are only allowed to request or access a patient's genetic information in specific, rare circumstances. GINA, while comprehensive, does not apply to the U.S. military, federal employees enrolled in FEHB, veterans obtaining health care through the VA, employers with fewer than 15 employees, and individuals covered by the Indian Health Service. It does not apply to life, long-term care, or disability insurance. It offers a floor, or baseline, law regarding genetic discrimination. States may have more stringent laws that would trump this federal law.

CRITICAL THINKING CHECKPOINT

SMA and Health Insurance

Anne is a young woman who is 6 months pregnant with her first son. In her checkups at the hospital, she discloses that she had a cousin with cystic fibrosis (CF). She is concerned that she and her husband, who has a brother with CF, may be carriers, which would increase the probability of her own child inheriting CF. Anne worries that if her health insurance provider finds out that she took a genetic test it might impact her coverage. In response, you explain that GINA would prohibit her health insurance provider from adjusting her plan just because she decided to take a genetic test. However, you also remind her that the genetic test for CF could confirm diagnosis, meaning GINA would not prevent health insurers from using positive CF test results to make coverage decisions. After much consideration, Anne decides to go through with the genetic test for both her baby and herself.

After you receive the results, you inform Anne that she is in fact a carrier of CF and that her son tested positive for the disease. Anne's immediate concerns about the health consequences of the diagnosis are followed by anxiety over how to pay for her son's future health care needs. You assure her that she cannot be denied health care coverage and that her employment status should not be affected by this new genetic information. Unfortunately, you tell to her that since her baby has manifested CF, GINA does not stop insurance companies from underwriting the coverage of her child based on his newly discovered health status. Further, certain states have additional protections against health insurance discrimination based on health conditions. You check policy resources and encourage Anna to follow up with her state insurance department.

The Difference Between Disease Information and Manifestation

Kathleen is a 36-year-old woman who receives health insurance benefits from her employer, a large private company. Kathleen has a family history of breast cancer, and her sister, Debbie, has recently been diagnosed with the disease. While Kathleen has not been diagnosed with breast cancer, she is still concerned. Having heard about the recent development of the genes associated with increased risk for breast cancer from the news, she visits her health provider for more information.

At the clinic, her health provider clarifies that the genes associated with breast cancer are called *BRCA1* and *BRCA2.* The genetic test is in fact tests for mutations of each of these genes. Recent studies have found that mutations in the *BRCA1* and 2 genes are associated with increased risk for breast and ovarian cancer. After discussing her options, Kathleen and Debbie both decide to take the genetic test. When results come back, Kathleen discovers that she and her sister both have mutations in the *BRCA1* gene. Debbie's health insurance coverage increased costs when she was diagnosed with breast cancer. Kathleen did not face those higher costs as a result of her *BRCA* test. Neither sister's employment status changed.

1. Why didn't Kathleen's health insurance costs increase even though the *BRCA* test results placed her at a higher risk to develop breast cancer?
2. Why is it that Debbie's employment status did not change while her health insurance did change?
3. Kathleen later developed breast cancer like her sister. Would GINA still protect Kathleen from health insurers raising her premiums at that point?

The author acknowledges extensive research and writing assistance from Catherine Dokurno, Aileen Palmer, Dana Mariani, and Natalie Kwok, interns at Genetic Alliance, summer 2011.

ONLINE RESOURCES

Coalition for Genetic Fairness: http://www.geneticfairness.org

GINA Information Help: http://www.GINAhelp.org

NCHPEG: http://www.nchpeg.org

NHGRI: http://www.genome.gov

NCSL list of U.S. states and their respective genetic discrimination protections: http://www.ncsl.org/default.aspx?tabid=14283

Text of the Law: http://www.eeoc.gov/laws/statutes/gina.cfm

REFERENCES

Baruch, S., & Hudson, K. (2008). Civilian and military genetics: Nondiscrimination policy in a post-GINA world. *The American Journal of Human Genetics, 83*, 435–444. doi:10.1016/j.ajhg.2008.09.003

Bush, George W. (2003). *Statement of administration policy: S.1053 - Genetic Non-discrimination Act of 2003*. Executive Office of the President, Washington, DC: Retrieved June 30, 2012, from http://georgewbush-whitehouse.archives.gov/omb/legislative/sap/108-1/s1053sap-s.pdf

Bush, George W. (2005). *Statement of administration policy: S.306 - Genetic Non-discrimination Act of 2005*. Executive Office of the President, Washington, DC: Retrieved June 30, 2012, from http://georgewbush-whitehouse.archives.gov/omb/legislative/sap/109-1/s306sap-s.pdf

Collins, F. S., & Watson, J. D. (2003). Genetic discrimination: time to act. *Science, 302*(5646), 745. doi: 10.1126/science.302.5646.745

Escher, D., & United States House of Representatives Committee on Ways and Means, Subcommittee on Health. (2007). *Testimony of David Escher*. Retrieved June 30, 2012, from http://www.geneticalliance.org/ksc_assets/publicpolicy/hr493wmhearingeschertestimony.pdf

Hudson, K. L., Rothenberg, K. H., Andrews, L. B., Kahn, M. J., & Collins, F. S. (1995). Genetic discrimination and health insurance: An urgent need for reform. *Science, 270*(5235), 391–393. doi:10.1126/science.270.5235.391

Lapham, V. E., Kozma, C., & Weiss, J. O. (1996). Genetic discrimination: perspectives of consumers. *Science, 274*(5287), 621–624. doi:10.1126/science.274.5287.621

Mayfield v. Dalton, 901 F. Sup. 300 (D. Haw 1995), Vacated as moot, 109 F. 3d 1423 (9th Cir. 1997).

National Institutes of Health, National Human Genome Research Institute. (2010, November 3). *Cases of genetic discrimination*. Retrieved June 30, 2012, from http://www.genome.gov/12513976

National Institutes of Health, National Human Genome Research Institute. (1996). *National Institutes of Health - Department of Energy, ELSI Working Group and National Action Plan on Breast Cancer Workshop on Genetic Discrimination and the Workplace: Implications for Employment, Insurance and Privacy.* Bethesda, MD: Retrieved June 30, 2012, from http://www.genome.gov/10001746

National Institutes of Health, Office of Biotechnology Activities. (n.d.). *Genetic discrimination.* Retrieved from http://oba.od.nih.gov/SACGHS/sacghs_focus_discrimination.html

Regulations Under the Genetic Information Nondiscrimination Act of 2008; Final Rule, 75 Fed. Reg. 68912 (2010) (to be codified at 29 CFR Part 1635).

Secretary's Advisory Committee on Genetics, Health and Society, Public Perspectives on Genetic Discrimination September 2004-November 2004 (2005), Retrieved June 30, 2012, from http://www4.od.nih.gov/oba/sacghs/reports/Public_Perspectives_GenDiscrim.pdf

Tuckson, R. V., Department of Health and Human Services, Secretary. (2005). *SACGHS letter to Secretary Leavitt supporting H.R.1227.* Bethesda, MD: Retrieved June 30, 2012, from http://oba.od.nih.gov/oba/sacghs/reports/letter_to_Sec_05_03_2005.pdf

United States Department of Labor. (1998). *Department of Labor, Department of Health and Human Services, Equal Employment Opportunity Commission, & Department of Justice: Genetic information and the workplace.* Retrieved June 30, 2012, from http://www.dol.gov/oasam/programs/history/herman/reports/genetics.htm

PART 4

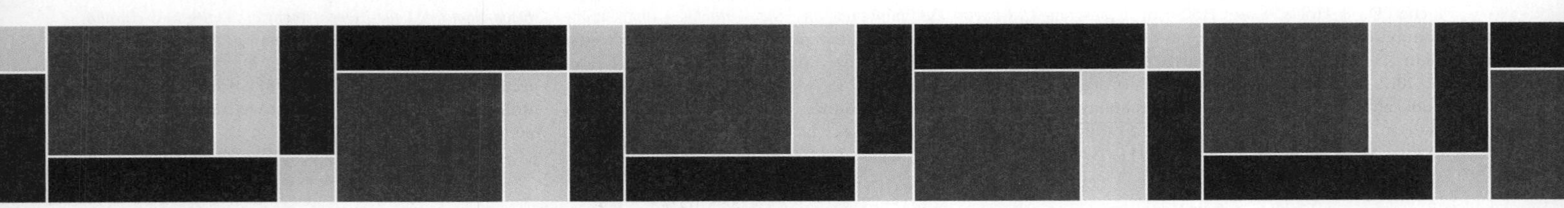

Assessment

CHAPTER

13 Family History Tool

Cindy M. Little

LEARNING OUTCOMES

Following the completion of this chapter, the learner will be able to

1. Describe the essential components of a family health history.
2. Identify current barriers to obtaining a comprehensive family history.
3. Discuss the components of a genetic pedigree and their meanings.
4. Demonstrate skill in constructing a third- and fourth-generation pedigree (genogram) using standardized pedigree symbols.
5. Discuss essential competencies expected of nurses related to obtaining a family health history, creating a pedigree, and referring individuals and families for genetic counseling.

This chapter provides knowledge to obtain a complete family health history and create a family pedigree. The chapter consists of three sections. The first section covers general information about and components that should be included in a family health history. Section Two provides the standardized symbols that are used in creating a family pedigree and instructions on how to use the symbols based on the family history. Finally, Section Three describes Punnett squares and demonstrates how to determine basic risk of transmission of a genetic disease or trait.

PRETEST

1. A family history can do all of the following, EXCEPT
   A. help to establish a pattern of inherited disorders.
   B. assist in identification of individuals who are at risk for genetic diseases.
   C. determine who is a carrier of a genetic disease.
   D. determine when someone will develop symptoms for a genetic disease.
2. The primary purpose of an individual's health history is to
   1. gather sound information to help develop diagnoses and assessments.
   2. establish a pattern of disease.
   3. assist in identifying individuals at risk for developing inherited disorders.
   4. determine how an individual responds to treatment.

   A. 1 and 2
   B. 1, 2, and 3
   C. All of the above
   D. None of the above
3. What is not considered a cultural factor?
   A. Language
   B. Health beliefs
   C. Skin color
   D. Religion
4. A health history on a 2-year-old child should include
   A. mother's menstrual history.
   B. father's surgical history.
   C. prenatal and birth history.
   D. mother's infertility history.
5. An example of consanguinity is when a child is born to a woman who is married to her uncle.
   A. True
   B. False
6. A pedigree is a graphic presentation of a family history using the following EXCEPT
   A. pictures.
   B. words and numbers.
   C. abbreviations.
   D. symbols.
7. The occurrence of affected individuals in every generation in a family suggests a __________ trait.
   A. autosomal dominant
   B. autosomal recessive
   C. random assortment
   D. sex-linked
8. A family pedigree is considered a confidential and private document that must be protected.
   A. True
   B. False

9. A Punnett square is
   A. a symbol used in a pedigree that indicates a female.
   B. a mathematical tool used to predict the due date in a pregnancy.
   C. a diagram that shows all possible genetic combinations of two parents.
   D. a tool used to predict height of children based on their parents' stature.

10. A professional nurse with specialized education and training in genetics may be credential as a genetic clinical nurse (GCN).
    A. True
    B. False

Pretest answers are located in the Appendix.

SECTION ONE: When Conducting an Interview For a Family History

A family health history is one of the most important tools used in diagnosing and assessing for common diseases. The family history contains pertinent information about the health of the entire extended family including family members who have died. A positive family history for a heritable disease has been recognized as a risk factor for that disease in related individuals. Many individuals are unaware of their relatives' medical histories since many people feel their own medical histories are a private matter not to be shared with anyone but their closest relatives or their spouse. A family history helps to establish a pattern of inherited disorders and traits, and assists in identifying individuals who are at risk for developing specific genetic diseases that may have modifiable or preventable risk factors. Genetically susceptible individuals may be revealed by the family history and may benefit from preventive interventions. A family history is considered the first step before genetic testing can be done. Clinicians can target personalized services and genetic counseling for patients once an inheritable disorder has been identified.

The family health history is one part of an individual's medical history. The origins of the family history can be traced to ancient storytelling, which was used as a means of preserving family information (Hinton, 2008). Biologic relationships and milestones such as marriages, births, and deaths were recorded in the family Bible. The family history also has its origins in genealogy, the study of families and their **kinship** in determining relationships to nobility. Hippocrates has been credited with using the family history as well as the clinical evaluation in diagnosing diseases that appeared to run in families (Hinton, 2008). Murray Bowen, a family systems theorist, developed the **genogram**, which he used in analyzing family structure. Later, McGoldrick and Gerson (1985) attempted to standardize the genogram to be used by other professionals who were working with families. Today, the family health history has become the most important tool in diagnosing and assessing risk of genetic diseases.

Information and Tips for Obtaining a Health History

The primary purpose of an individual's health history is to gather sound information to help develop diagnoses and assessments, screen for other existing or potential health problems, establish a relationship between the provider and the client, and develop a health care plan. The family health history allows the provider to collect data to determine familial transmission of diseases, which aids in diagnosis and can identify other family members who might be at risk. During the interview, the health care provider has the opportunity to observe family interactions and communication among family members. More commonly, the family history is obtained from the individual client who may have a lack of knowledge about the health history of his or her relatives. Obtaining a comprehensive health history is a standard competency required of all nurses (Consensus Panel, 2009).

Before the interview, the nurse should choose a location where the client is comfortable and is assured that the information will be kept in strict confidence. If there is another family member or spouse with the client, the nurse should acknowledge that person and indicate if it is appropriate for that person to be in the room. The nurse can allow some time to "get to know" the client, building trust and developing rapport before gathering personal information. It is important to be courteous and respectful at all times. The nurse should use good eye contact and provide good lighting. It is best to begin the interview by explaining why the questions are asked and how the data will be used and continue with the least threatening questions and explain to the client the purpose of the questions. The nurse must start the interview with open-ended questions to obtain the best information possible. Questions should be directed from general to specific. It is important that the nurse avoid leading questions and not be judgmental in any way. Asking one question at a time is preferred since compound questions may confuse the client and elicit incorrect information. The interviewer should avoid using euphemisms or medical terms that the client may not understand, and should define technical terms, such as *hypertension*, that are included in the questions. If the client is shy and tends to not offer much information, the nurse should offer gentle prompts. If the client becomes tired, it may be necessary to schedule another appointment to complete the interview.

During an interview the nurse must be acutely aware of cultural factors. The relationship between **culture** and communication is complex and includes language, nonverbal communication, customs, and perceived values. First, the nurse must know if English is spoken in the home and how well the language is understood by the client and the family. The nurse should request the use of a translator if necessary to ensure that accurate information is understood and collected. The way a client defines health and illness and methods used to maintain health or treat illness may be different than the nurse's, and communication may be restricted if the nurse is not aware of the client's cultural beliefs. Health beliefs and illnesses are shaped by cultural and/or religious beliefs. Symptoms and diseases may not be recognized as such within a specific culture. During the interview, the nurse must ask more specific questions to clarify meaning and facilitate understanding of the client's beliefs. If the nurse does not understand the cultural meaning of the symptoms, he or she can create undue stress as well as cause invasive and unnecessary tests. For example, there is no literal translation in Chinese for the word *depression* and the client may describe it as "heaviness of the heart," which could be interpreted as cardiovascular disease (Andrews & Boyle, 2003). Specific questions should be asked about how the client defines health and illness, what methods the client uses to maintain health, what methods are used to treat illness, what health topics are considered taboo, what attitudes the client has about mental illness, and whether there are any special religious or belief practices specific to a client's culture that may affect health care.

Health History for Each Member of the Family

A health history for an infant or a child is modified according to the age of the infant or child. The parent is usually the historian for the child, but if a nanny, grandparent, or other caretaker provides the history it must be reviewed and validated by the parent(s) whenever possible. The health history of an infant or child frequently needs to be updated as the child grows. The history should begin with the mother's pregnancy of that child including the mother's health during pregnancy and the extent of prenatal care. It is important to note the mother's and father's ages. A woman who is age 35 at the time of delivery is considered advanced maternal age (AMA) and there is an increased risk of Down syndrome. Information on weight gain, course of pregnancy, gestation, and any complications during pregnancy should be documented. Complications would include conditions such as hypertension, preeclampsia, diabetes, bleeding, infections, or loss of pregnancy. Medications, including **over-the-counter** (**OTC**) drugs, hormones, and vitamins should be recorded. Diet, general nutritional status, and any gastrointestinal problems such as hyperemesis gravidarium should be documented. Other information related to the pregnancy should include exposure to teratogens (such as X-rays or viruses), medications, cigarette smoking, alcohol use, and any illicit substance use (Seidel et al., 2010).

The next part of the child's health history includes the birth experience, length of labor, anesthesia, the characteristics of the delivery (e.g., Cesarean or vaginal), the condition of the infant, the Apgar score, and the birth weight. Questions should be asked about any complications during the neonatal period that include congenital anomalies, feeding characteristics, illnesses, medical care, and medications. A child who has been diagnosed with a congenital anomaly may have an unspecified syndrome or other hidden major anomaly (Spahis, 2002). The provider should ask about current eating habits, whether the infant was breast- or bottle-fed, if the child has allergies or reactions to certain foods, and if there are cultural variations of diet. Prenatal history is not as important in older children unless there is a significant factor that contributed to the child's well-being.

At all ages from infant to adolescence, developmental milestones are important to document to assess a child's behavior and physical and emotional health, and to determine if she or he is appropriate for her or his age. Physical growth characteristics such as height and weight and physical features should be documented as well as dentition and sexual development. Other important items to include are any communicable diseases, childhood immunizations, illnesses, injuries, and any history of mental illness including depression, or hospitalizations. For deceased infants or children, the cause of death, the age of death, date, and specifics surrounding death including prenatal history if applicable are also necessary. It is especially important to identify children who were adopted as their medical history is unrelated to the client's medical history (Seidel et al., 2010).

Older children and adolescents need to be asked about school performance and grades, learning disabilities, or other problems with school. The provider should ask about substance abuse including cigarette smoking and use of any performance-enhancing drugs or steroids. The patient should be asked about their friends and social life, involvement in school sports or other activities, and sexual attitudes and behavior. It is especially important to be respectful and sensitive when interviewing children and adolescents and to continuously remind them that this information will be kept private and confidential.

During pregnancy the health history should include details about the current pregnancy as well as any previous pregnancies. Once the pregnancy has been confirmed, the following information should be documented: age, ethnicity, gravidity, parity, last menstrual period (LMP), **estimated date of delivery** (**EDD**), current employment, race, marital status or relationship, partner's occupation, religion, and education. Attitudes about pregnancy and physical symptoms should be included. Information about illnesses, infections, injuries, or accidents since conception should be discussed. Exposure to any teratogens such as radiation, viruses, chemicals, fever, hot tubs, or medications should be discussed in detail as they can cause varying complications. A complete gynecologic and obstetric history should also be obtained. Obstetric history includes detailed information on any pregnancy regardless of length, date of pregnancy, complications during pregnancy, gestational age, weight and gender of infant, length of labor, type of delivery, spontaneous (miscarriage) or elective abortion, any complications in labor or during postpartum, and current status of infant. Pregnancy loss is a common occurrence in 25% of pregnancies; while most are sporadic cases, recurrent losses need to be investigated for genetic abnormalities (Warren & Silver, 2008). Gynecologic history includes age of **menarche**, characteristics of the menstrual cycle, associated symptoms, sexual history, contraception, history of **sexually transmitted infection (STI)**, infertility, in-vitro fertilization (IVF), gynecologic surgery, and results of the most recent Pap smear as well as the history and previous results of Pap smears (Seidel et al., 2010).

An adult health history usually includes a history of the present illness, past medical history, surgical history, obstetric and gynecologic history, sexual or reproductive history, psychiatric history, personal and social history, and family history. The history of the present illness requires a detailed explanation of the events that surround the reason for the client's visit. This includes the onset of the problem and the chronological list of events since the onset. The nurse may need to know the location, the duration, the character, and the severity of the problem as well as aggravating or relieving factors. The nurse must ask specifically about hidden and obvious concerns and seek to understand the client's perspective about his or her current problem and past medical history.

The past medical history may be helpful in assessing the client's current problem. This should include a description of the client's past general health, up until the time of the present illness. Childhood diseases such as measles, mumps, chicken pox, and immunizations are included. Any major adult illnesses the client has previously been diagnosed with such as diabetes; hypertension; heart disease; liver disease; kidney disease; gallbladder disease; stomach or intestinal diseases; genitourinary disease; pulmonary disease; cancer; asthma; anemia or other blood disorders; infectious diseases including hepatitis, HIV, or tuberculosis; autoimmune disorders, neurologic disorders; psychiatric disorders; and allergies should be documented in detail. Any previous surgeries should include the date, surgical procedure, hospital, and any complications. Blood transfusions including the date, amount, and any reactions should be acknowledged. Complete documentation should be done on any serious injuries, limitations, or disabilities and if these have physically or psychologically affected the client's health. Other information to be collected includes medications (past, current and most recent), home remedies, nonprescription drugs, and allergies to medications, foods, or environmental substances. Recent screening tests such as Papanicolaou test or Pap smear, mammogram, prostate-specific antigen (PSA), glucose, or cholesterol should be documented (Seidel et al., 2010).

A reproductive or sexual history for a woman should be part of the obstetric and gynecologic history. Other information that should be asked of both men and women includes sexual orientation, frequency of sexual activity, number of partners (currently and lifetime), libido, type of sexual activity, sexual practices, sexual satisfaction, use of contraception, history of STIs and treatments, and any history of sexual abuse. Other information to be asked of male clients includes puberty onset, erections, libido, emissions, testicular lumps or pain, and history of infertility (Seidel et al., 2010).

The psychological history should include past and current psychiatric problems and illnesses including history of anxiety, depression, mood swings, suicidal thoughts, hallucinations, nervousness or irritability, and/or sleep disturbances. The client should be asked about taking any psychotropic medications and whether she or he has been hospitalized for a psychiatric illness or has received any therapy or counseling for mental illness. A history of learning problems or developmental disabilities is especially significant. Revealing personal habits such as frequent abuse of alcohol or drugs (illegal or prescription) or a history of sexual or physical abuse may lead to a more accurate mental health diagnosis (Seidel et al., 2010).

Questions related to the personal and social history are important in that they may reveal lifestyle habits that influence the client's health. The personal information includes birthplace, cultural and ethnic background, level of education, home conditions, marital status or partner status, socioeconomic status, and sources of support. It is important to know the client's ethnicity or ancestry of origin as many genetic diseases are more prominent in certain groups of people. It is also helpful to identify the client's interests, hobbies, sources of stress, and general satisfaction with life. Habits such as eating and sleeping patterns, cigarette smoking, exercise, leisure activities, use of caffeinated beverages, and dietary supplements should be included. Occupational information includes current job, job history, military service, and exposure to chemicals and industrial toxins. Finally, spiritual beliefs and/or religious affiliation and any religious concerns or restrictions about medical care are important to document (Seidel et al., 2010).

The Family History

The family history is considered the first risk assessment in primary care. It is universally accessible and is a comparatively inexpensive first genetic screen. A positive family history identifies affected family members and those who may be at risk for a heritable disease. Relatives to include in a family history are children, siblings, nieces, nephews, parents, aunts, uncles, cousins, and grandparents. The information obtained from a family history can be used to raise awareness of personal disease risk and promote a healthy lifestyle to reduce risk, prevent disease, or delay adverse outcomes. The family health history reflects the complex interactions between genetic, environmental, and behavioral factors and is an excellent determinant of disease risks.

In 2004, the *Surgeon General's Family History Initiative* was announced in an effort to inform Americans of the importance of the Family Health History. Every year since 2004, the Surgeon General has declared Thanksgiving Day to be National Family History Day. This is a day when many families gather together and so are encouraged to discuss and record health problems or diseases that tend to run in their families. This helps to organize the family health history that family members can share with their health care providers. The Surgeon General has created a computer program titled, "My Family Health Portrait" that allows an individual to generate a "sophisticated portrait" of their family's health history (USDHHS, 2004). The Utah Department of Health has developed a Family Health History Toolkit to assist individuals in collecting pertinent information from family members (Utah Department of Health, 2005). The American Medical Association (AMA) has identified red flags in a family health history that suggest a genetic disorder or a disease risk. These include several relatives who are affected with the same or related disease, a disorder with an early age of onset especially if there are multiple affected family members, sudden death of an individual, a woman with three or more pregnancy losses, and children whose parents are closely related (consanguinity). Individual red flags include someone with dysmorphic features or physical anomalies, a child with congenital deafness, blindness, or cataracts, someone with disproportionate short stature, an individual with learning disabilities or behavioral problems, and someone with a history of unexplained infertility (American Medical Association, 2004).

Information on first, second, and third-degree relatives is necessary to determine a pattern of risk. **First-degree relatives**, including siblings, children, and parents, have the most in common genetically with the client and indicate the greatest genetic risk. **Second-degree relatives** include nieces, nephews, aunts, uncles, and grandparents. First cousins and great-grandparents make up **third-degree relatives**. Medical conditions or diseases for each family member and the age of onset of the disease should be recorded. Individuals should be asked about common disorders such as cancer (especially breast, colon, and prostate), diabetes, vision or hearing loss, dementia or Alzheimer disease, hypertension, heart disease, or stroke. It may be necessary to interview multiple individuals within a family to obtain accurate detailed data such as age at onset of the disease. The family health history is a dynamic medical record that changes over time and must continuously be revised and updated (American Medical Association, 2004).

Barriers to Obtaining a Family Health History

There are significant barriers to obtaining and using the family health information. Many people do not know their family history and may not understand its relevance in health care diagnosis and management. Some relatives may not be forthcoming with their health information and may want to keep their health history private. Family members may not want to reveal sensitive information such as alcoholism, mental illness, or consanguinity. Clients frequently have poor recall of a diagnosis or understanding of their own health problems and limited knowledge of their family's health. Parents may not know or understand the congenital disorders or chronic diseases that were diagnosed in their children. In a small family, it may be difficult to identify disease patterns and risks since the trait may not be severe enough to impair fertility.

Genetics specialists allege that the family history is underused in primary care. Currently, there are time constraints in most health care practices that do not allow time for the completion of a comprehensive individual and family health history. Any history is usually selectively performed and not well maintained or updated. Many health care providers, including nurses and physicians, do not have formal training in genetics and are not comfortable with counseling patients about genetic risk (Hinton, 2008). Many health care providers perceive genetics as a low priority and may not feel confident in identifying clients who need to be referred (Beery & Shooner, 2004).

Sending a detailed questionnaire for a client to complete prior to his or her visit may eliminate the need for extra time during the visit. The nurse can review the document with the client to confirm that the information is correct and to clear up any uncertainties. The clinical validity of the family health history depends on the accuracy of the information that has been collected. The health history's accuracy "usually decreases as the degree of relatedness decreases" (Wattendorf & Hadley, 2005, p. 444). The provider should indicate the source of the information as the client, a family member, or a medical report. It may be necessary to interview family members to obtain the information for creating an accurate family health history. If family members are deceased or unavailable, information may be gathered from government records for birth, marriages, or deaths, or from family records such as baby books or a family Bible.

SECTION ONE REVIEW

1. The family health history has become the most important primary tool in diagnosing and assessing risk of genetic diseases.
   A. True
   B. False
2. A woman is considered "advanced maternal age" and her risk of having a child with Down syndrome increases at what age?
   A. 25
   B. 35
   C. 45
   D. None of the above
3. The Surgeon General chose Thanksgiving Day as National Family History Day for all of the following reasons EXCEPT
   A. it is a day when families gather together.
   B. family members can discuss their wills.
   C. family members can discuss and record health problems.
   D. families can organize their family history.
4. One of the problems with the family history tool is that
   A. it can be used and maintained on the Internet.
   B. genetic specialists feel that it is underused in primary care.
   C. some family members may be deceased.
   D. the nurse will have to review the document with the individual or family.
5. A barrier to obtaining a family health history is
   A. a husband can report his wife's medical history.
   B. a mother can recall her labor and delivery experience.
   C. a family member may not be forthcoming with his health history.
   D. a family member may not be able to recall his immunizations.

Answers: 1. A; 2. B; 3. B; 4. B; 5. C

SECTION TWO: The Pedigree Analysis

A pedigree is a graphic presentation using symbols, words, abbreviations, and numbers that illustrate an individual's extended family health history, and genetic relationships. It is a resourceful way to assess genetic inheritance patterns and predict genetic risk. A pedigree is organized to illustrate basic relationships among family members and extends over at least three generations. Other generations should be included if the patient has relevant health information about those more distant relatives. Similarities in health information between the **proband**, who is usually the client, and other family members can be visualized. The pedigree includes family and individual health information, dates, diagnoses of disease, and any genetic information.

Components of a Pedigree

A pedigree is made up of lines that connect shapes, primarily squares designating males and circles designating females. A lesbian or gay couple is displayed as two circles or two squares with a triangle inside the circle or square. Diamond shapes indicate individuals of unspecified sex and can be used for transgendered individuals or persons with congenital disorders of sex development. If an individual is affected with a condition or trait, the square or circle should be shaded. Occasionally, when someone has more than one condition, the symbol can be divided into two to four sections and a different color or design should be used within the divided symbol (see Figure 13–1 ■).

The letter "P" (meaning pregnancy) is written in a circle or square if the sex of the baby is known; if not, a diamond with a "P" is used. The designation for a stillbirth is a circle or square if the gender is known, or a diamond symbol if it is not, with a diagonal line through the symbol and the gestational age of the infant written below the symbol. Triangles signify a pregnancy event such as a spontaneous or elective abortion or an ectopic pregnancy. A diagonal line should be drawn through the triangle for a termination of pregnancy or ectopic pregnancy. The triangle should be shaded if the fetus has been diagnosed with a genetic condition and the gestational age and diagnosis as well as the gender, if known, should be written below the triangle. In the case of an ectopic pregnancy, the letters "ECT" should be listed below the symbol (Bennett, French, Resta, & Doyle, 2008).

Emerging Evidence

- Oncology nurses need to be familiar with the components of a cancer risk assessment, a comprehensive process that includes all factors in cancer risk and diagnosis. An individual and family health history, environmental factors, lifestyle factors, and physical features influence cancer risk. Nurses can contribute to the assessment of cancer risk and can personalize a health care plan that includes counseling and testing (Aiello-Laws, 2011).
- In a study using a four-generation pedigree, researchers determined that sleepwalking is an inherited sleep disorder that may be transmitted as an autosomal dominant disorder with reduced penetrance (Licis, Desruisseau, Yamada, Duntley, & Gurnett, 2011).
- The perception of health care providers in using patient-generated family health histories is that they appreciate the potential benefits; however, they are underused because of concerns about accuracy of the information and time limits in a routine office visit. Nurses and genetic counselors are in a position to promote the use of patient-generated health histories in primary care (Fuller, Myers, Webb, Tabangin, & Prows, 2010).

	Male	Female	Gender not specified	Comments
1. Individual	b. 1925	30y	4 mo	Assign gender by phenotype (see text for disorders of sex development, etc.). Do not write age in symbols
2. Affected individual				Key/legend used to define shading or other fill (e.g., hatches, dots, etc.). Use only when individual is clinically affected.
			With ≥2 conditions, the individual's symbol can be divided, showing each segment shaded with a different color or shade fill and defined in legend.	
3. Nonpenetrant carrier, may manifest disease				
4. Obligate carrier, will not manifest disease				
5. Multiple individuals, number known	5	5	5	Number of siblings written inside symbol. (Affected individuals should not be grouped).
6. Multiple individuals numbers unknown or unstated	n	n	n	"n" is used in place of "?".
7. Deceased individual	d. 35	d. 4 mo	d. 60's	Indicate cause of death if known. To avoid confusion, when notating death, do not use the cross (†) symbol which can be mistaken for the symbol for evaluation positive (+).
8. Consultand				Individual(s) seeking genetic counseling/testing
9. Deceased				
10. Proband	P	P		Affected family member consulting independently of other family members.
11. Stillbirth (SB)	SB 28 wk	SB 30 wk	SB 34wk	Include gestational age and karyotype, if known.
12. Pregnancy (P)	P LMP- 7/1/2007 47,XY,+21	P 20 wk 46,XX	P	Gestational age and karyotype below symbol. Light shading can be used for affected; define in key/legend.
13. Dizygotic twins				
14. Monozygotic twins (identical)				
15. Sex unspecified				

Pregnancies not carried to term	Affected	Unaffected	
16. Spontaneous abortion	17 wks female cystic hygroma	< 10 wks	Below the symbol write the gestational age/gender, if known. Key/legend used to define shading.
17. Termination of pregnancy	18 wks 47,XY,+18		Other abbreviations (e.g., TAB, VTOP) not used for sake of consistency.
18. Ectopic pregnancy			Write ECT below symbol.

Instructions:
Key should contain all information relevant to interpretation of pedigree (e.g., define fill/shading)

For clinical (non published) pedigrees include:
(a) Name of consultand (client) and/or proband
(b) Family name/initials of relatives for identification, where appropriate. Limit identifying information to maintain privacy and confidentiality.
(c) Name and title of recorder
(d) Historian (person relaying history information)
(e) Date of intake of update
(f) Reason for recording pedigree (list abnormal test result, familial disease or disorder
(g) Ancestry of both sides of the family

Recommended order of information placed below symbols
(h) Age
(i) Evaluation (see figure 13-4)
(j) Pedigree number

Figure 13–1 ■ Common pedigree symbols, definitions, and abbreviations

The paternal section of the pedigree should go on the left and the maternal on the right of the page. Roman numerals on the left of the diagram indicate generations, and Arabic numbers are used across the generation from left to right for each individual. Vertical lines connect generations and a horizontal line between two shapes represents mating of that couple. That horizontal line connects vertically to a second horizontal line that displays the **sibship**. (Occasionally a diagonal line is used for convenience). Siblings should be drawn in order of birth starting with the oldest on the left. Twins are drawn from a single vertical line that splits into two shapes depending on the sex of the twins. If the twins are monozygotic, a horizontal line is placed between the two (diagonal) lines that split. A horizontal line with two forward slashes indicates the relationship has ended, as in a divorce. If one of the partners begins another relationship the horizontal line is extended to add that partner. An individual must always be closer to his or her first partner and then to the second and third partner (if any) and so on. According to Bennett et al. (2008), if there are multiple previous partners, there is no need to include them in the pedigree if they do not affect the genetic assessment. In a consanguineous mating or marriage, there

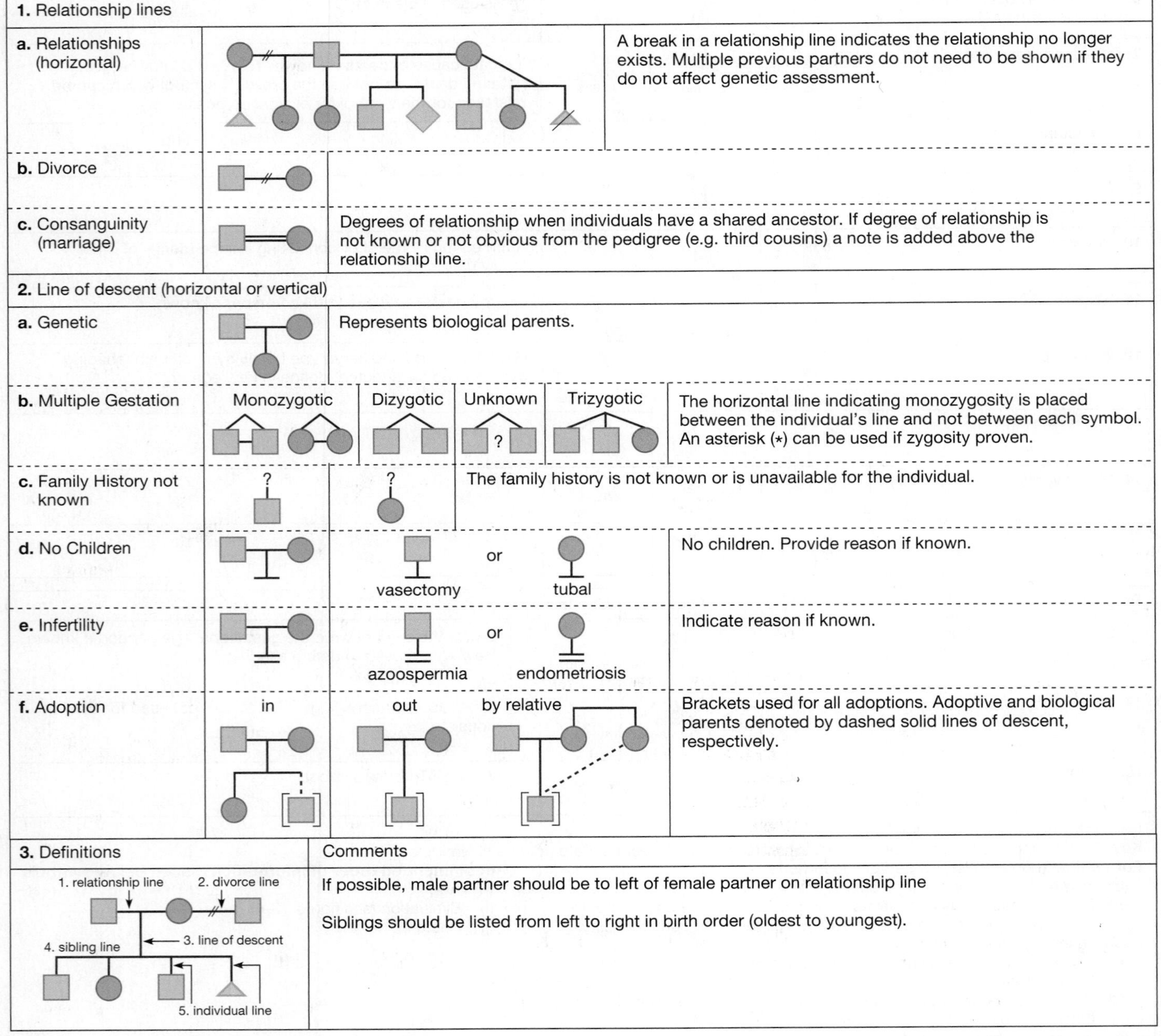

Figure 13–2 ■ Pedigree line definitions

should be a double horizontal line connecting the individuals. If there are multiple siblings in a sibship the number of siblings is written in a circle, square, or diamond; however, affected individuals should be listed individually. If the number of siblings is unknown, the letter "n" is written in the symbol. A diagonal line drawn through the circle or square indicates that person is deceased. The cause and date (year) of death should be written below the symbol (see Figure 13–2 ■).

There are special circumstances where certain designations need to be used such as in a case of infertility or when a couple has no children by choice. If a couple has no children by choice or if the reason is unknown, a short vertical line connected to a short horizontal line is used. If the cause is known, it should be written under the appropriate symbol. A short vertical line with two short horizontal lines should be used when it is necessary to indicate that the couple or an individual has been diagnosed with infertility. The cause, if known, should be written under the symbol. A set of brackets are used around a circle or square to indicate that the individual has been adopted. Other special information that may need to be displayed is when an individual is a sperm or ovum donor, or when a surrogate mother is part of the reproductive history (Bennett et al., 2008) (see Figure 13–3 ■).

Other important information for the pedigree include the name of the proband or **consultand**, the person who is relaying the information (historian), the person who is recording the information, the date when the information is being collected, and the indication for the referral. Initials or first names of family members should be recorded on the drawing for identification. An asterisk (*) or the letter "E" is used to indicate that an individual has been evaluated or has had any diagnostic testing for a disease. Clinical findings or results of genetic testing should be written in parentheses under the individual's symbol. The year of birth rather than the age should be used because the birth date never changes and it is considered private and protected information. The cause and year of death should be listed under the appropriate individual's symbol and would be more compliant with the Health Insurance Portability and Accountability Act (HIPPA) than using the full date of death (Bennett et al., 2008).

Possible Reproductive Scenarios		Comments
1. Sperm donor	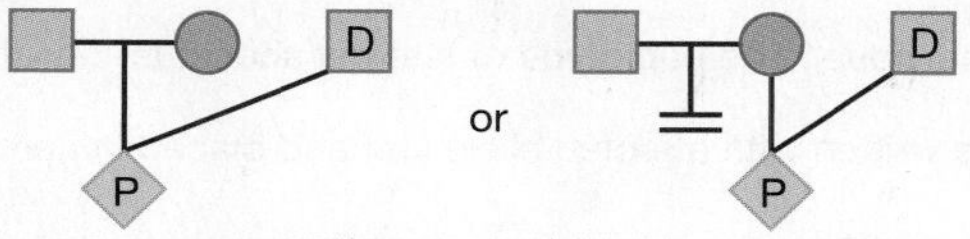 D, P, or, D, P	A couple in which the woman is carrying a pregnancy using donor sperm. No relationship line would be shown between the woman carrying the pregnancy and the sperm donor.
2. Ovum donor	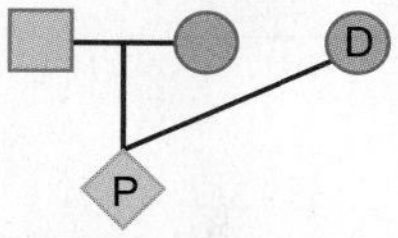 D, P	A couple in which the woman is carrying a pregnancy using a donor egg and partner's sperm. The line of descent from the birth mother is solid because there is a biological relationship (father's sperm) that may affect the fetus (e.g., teratogens).
3. Surrogate only	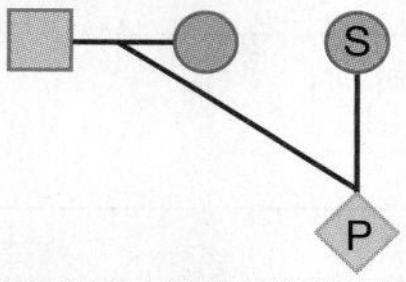 S, P	A couple whose gametes are used to impregnate a surrogate who carries the pregnancy. The line of descent from the surrogate is solid because there is a biological relationship (father's sperm and mother's egg) that may affect the fetus (e.g., teratogens).
4. Surrogate ovum donor	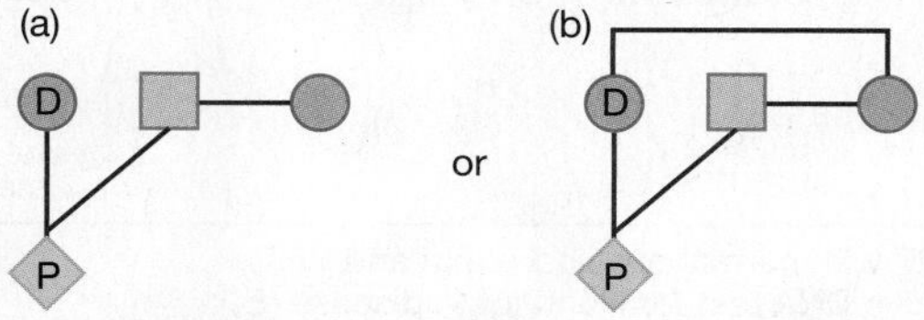 (a) D, P or (b) D, P	Couple in which male partner's sperm is used to inseminate (a) an unrelated woman or (b) a sister who is carrying the pregnancy for the couple.
5. Planned adoption	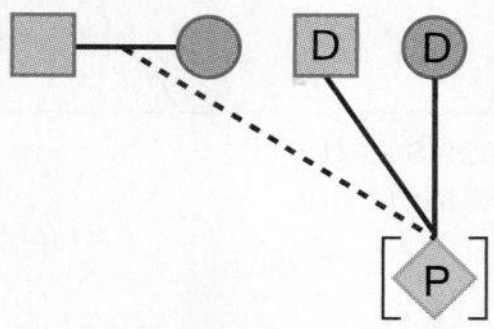 D, D, [P]	Couple contracts with a woman to carry a pregnancy using ovum of the woman carrying the pregnancy and donor sperm.

Instructions:

- D represents egg or sperm donor
- S represents surrogate (gestational carrier)
- If the woman is both the ovum donor and surrogate, for the purpose of genetic assessment, she will only be referred to as a donor (See examples 4 and 5); the pregnancy symbol and its line of descent are positioned below the woman who is carrying the pregnancy
- Available family history should be noted for the gamete donor and/or gestational carrier

Figure 13–3 ■ Assisted reproductive technology symbols and definitions

An arrow is used to designate the proband (the affected individual for whom the pedigree is being created) or the consultand (the person who is seeking genetic counseling). All affected individuals in the pedigree are illustrated by shading of the circle or square. When there is more than one condition, the individual's symbol can be divided into two to four sections and shaded differently. All symbols, lines, and shadings that are used in the drawing must be illustrated and defined in the **key** or **legend**. The key is used for "ease of reading by multiple users" (Bennett et al., 2008, p. 431). The pedigree must be updated periodically as individuals are born or adopted into the family, as family members become symptomatic, as new diseases are diagnosed, and as other family members pass away. One of the most important principles for using the pedigree with standardized symbols is communication between the client, the relatives of the client, and the health care team (see Figure 13–4 ■).

Internet Resources

The Internet has several resources that help individuals and families learn the skill of obtaining a family history. The Surgeon General created a computerized tool titled *My Family Health Portrait* that consumers and health providers can use to record family health information. The tool is available in English, Spanish, Portuguese, and Italian. All files are kept confidential and can be transferred to a CD or memory stick. The information from this program can also be transferred to an individual's electronic medical record (**EMR**) or it can be printed out and filed in a client's medical folder. Genetic Alliance, a health advocacy organization that includes a network of more than 1,000 genetic-disease specific organizations, offers a booklet entitled *Does It Run in the Family? A Guide to Family Health History* and a *Family Health History Questionnaire*.

Instructions:

- E is used for evaluation to represent clinical and/or test information on the pedigree
  - (a) E is to be defined in key/legend
  - (b) If more than one evaluation, used subscript (E_1, E_2, E_3) and define in key
  - (c) Test results should be put in parentheses or defined in key/legend
- A symbol is shaded only when an individual is clinically symptomatic
- For linkage studies, haplotype information is written below the individual. The haplotype of interest should be on left and appropriately highlighted
- Repetitive sequences, trinucleotides and expansion numbers are written with affected allele first and placed in parentheses
- If mutation is known, identify in parentheses

Definition	Symbol	Scenario	
1. Documented evaluation (*) Use only if examined/evaluated by you or your research/clinical team or if the outside evaluation has been reviewed and verified.	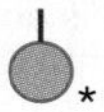 *	Woman with negative echocardiogram.	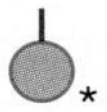 * E- (echo)
2. Carrier–not likely to manifest disease regardless of inheritance pattern.		Male carrier of cystic fibrosis by patient report (* not used because results are not varified).	
3. Asymptomatic/presymptomatic carrier–clinically unaffected at this time but could later exhibit symptoms.		Woman age 35 with negative transvaginal ultrasound and positive BRCA1 DNA test.	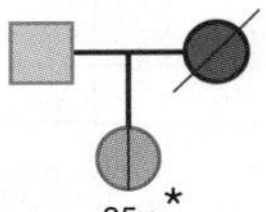 * 35y E_1– (transvaginal ultrasound) E_2+ (5385insC BRCA1)
4. Uninformative study (u)	Eu	Man age 27 with normal physical exam and uninformative DNA test for Huntington disease (E_2).	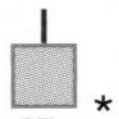 * 27y E_1– (physical exam) E_2u (36n/18n)
5. Affected individual with positive evaluation (E+)	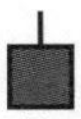 E+	Woman with symptomatic cystic fibrosis and positive mutation study; only one mutation has currently been identified.	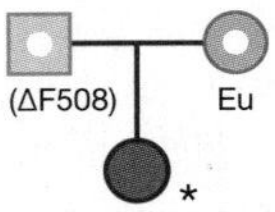 E+ (ΔF508) Eu * E+ (ΔF508/u)
		10 week male fetus with a trisomy 21 karyotype.	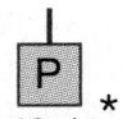 P * 10wk E+ (CVS) 47,XY,+21

Figure 13–4 ■ Pedigree symbols of genetic evaluation/testing information

Genetic Alliance's website also lists other programs that are focused on the family health history including *The Family Health History for Prenatal Providers* and the *Community Centered Family Health History*.

There are several other Internet resources and tutorials on how to collect family health information (refer to the online resources list at the end of this chapter). The Utah Department of Health has created a Family Reunion Packet to assist an individual in collecting family information when the family is able to gather together. The Center for Disease Control has a Family History page with tools, fact sheets, guidelines, and other information for collecting a family health history. The Utah Department of Health has developed a 20-page booklet called the Family Health History Toolkit that can assist individuals in compiling a family health history. Several other websites exist to assist families and health care providers collect significant family information that may aid in identifying individuals who may be at high risk for developing a heritable disease.

Privacy and Confidentiality

All personal information should be protected for privacy and confidentiality including the health history and family pedigree. It is important for the nurse to recognize the family health history and the pedigree as sensitive information since the well-being of some of the family members may be at risk. The health care provider may be faced with whether he or she should disclose or withhold genetic information, including findings in a pedigree. Genetic information poses some challenges because the information is shared between family members. Ideally, family members would sign an informed consent prior to genetic testing or pedigree analysis and receive genetic counseling in advance. The dilemma occurs when an individual decides not to inform his or her immediate biologic relatives that he or she is considering genetic testing. In 1998, the American Society of Human Genetics issued a position paper on the duty to warn. It stated physicians may disclose confidential genetic information when the following criteria is met: (a) The client fails to disclose the information to his or her family members, (b) harm is likely to occur, (c) the relative(s) at risk are identifiable, and (d) the disease is preventable or treatable. Disclosure is not permitted for a disease that is not treatable (Knoppers et al., 1998). Health care providers "must determine if their duty to warn the relative in question outweighs their obligation to keep specific patient information private" (Schneider et al., 2006, p. 499).

Another concern related to the privacy of pedigree or family history information is when the pedigree is published in a scientific journal. There have been cases of families recognizing their pedigrees, and the concern is that the condition or illness illustrated in the pedigree, such as Alzheimer disease, may carry a stigma. A published pedigree may also find its way onto the Internet where it may be recognized by a family member. Relatives who have not been notified of the information found in the pedigree, such as risk for a disease, may suffer psychological anguish in learning of their own risk of disease. Bennett et al. (2000) states that publishing or otherwise exposing the family's health history may be viewed as an intrusion on the family's privacy. To protect privacy, authors have altered or masked pedigrees to make them more obscure and unrecognizable. However, some scientists believe that by doing so, pertinent information may be omitted, which this may hinder the advancement of genetic science (Bennett et al., 2000).

Examples of Human Pedigrees

The following are examples of pedigrees that illustrate family relationships and transmission of genetic diseases or traits. Note the use of the pedigree nomenclature published by the National Society of Genetic Counselors that has become a national standard (Bennett et al., 2000).

1. Criteria for an autosomal dominant trait
   - A dominant trait is expressed when only one copy (heterozygosity) of an autosomal allele is present.
   - Males and females transmit the trait with equal frequency.
   - A dominant trait does not skip generations.
   - If no one in a generation is affected, the transmission of the trait stops.
   - Affected individuals have a 50% chance of passing the gene to each of their children.

An illustration of an autosomal dominant disorder can be found on page 60, in Figure 7–1.

2. Criteria for an autosomal recessive trait
   - A recessive trait is expressed when two copies (homozygosity) of an autosomal allele is present.
   - Individuals who are heterogyotes (having two different alleles of a gene) for the gene are carriers of that trait.
   - Children born to parents who are carriers of the gene (heterozygous) have a 25% chance of having the disease, a 25% chance of not having the disease and not being a carrier, and a 50% chance of being a carrier.
   - Males and females can be affected.
   - Affected males and females can transmit the disease if they live long enough to reproduce.
   - The trait can skip generations.

An illustration of an autosomal recessive trait can be found on page 63, in Figure 7–6.

3. Criteria for an X-linked dominant trait
   - X-linked dominant traits are rare.
   - These are characterized by disorders whose causative genes are carried on the X chromosome.
   - These are seen more often in males because they have only one copy of the gene.
   - These may be more severe or fatal in males.
   - These pass from father to all daughters but not to sons.

An illustration of an X-linked dominant trait can be found on page 66, in Figure 7–8.

4. Criteria for an X-linked recessive trait
   - X-linked recessive traits are almost always expressed in the male.
   - An affected father and a mother who is affected or is a carrier can pass the trait to a daughter.
   - Females would need two copies of the gene (homozygous) to express the X-linked trait.
   - The trait is passes from a heterozygous or homozygous mother to son.

An illustration of an X-linked recessive trait can be found on page 64, in Figure 7–7.

5. Consanguinity
   - Consanguinity is the mating of individuals who are "blood" relatives.
   - This increases the likelihood that harmful recessive traits will be combined and passed on to children.
   - Genetic diversity is decreased in a population that practices consanguinity.

(Figure 13–5 ■ depicts a pedigree of consanguinity.)

Punnett Squares

A Punnett square is an illustration used to predict Mendelian inheritance patterns and all possible combinations of alleles that can result when genes are combined. It can be used as a predictive tool in calculating risk of gene transmission to offspring. The combination of genotypes can be done only if the genotypes of the parents are known.

The Punnett square is drawn on a 2-by-2 grid. The genotypes of the parents are represented by using letters of the alphabet that signify each allele that could be passed from the parents. Uppercase letters signify dominant traits and lowercase letters represent recessive traits. The letters from the mother's genotype are inserted in the top two columns and the father's genotype is listed on the left side of the two rows as seen in Figure 13–6 ■. The letter from each column is combined with each letter from each row in the corresponding square. The two-letter combinations show the possible genotypes of the offspring, specifically the two allele possibilities for that trait. This means that with each pregnancy, the child that is conceived has the probability or not of inheriting that specific trait.

The genotypes of the mother and father are both heterozygous for the cystic fibrosis gene, meaning they each are Cc. Figure 13–6 illustrates that the risk of each child inheriting the trait for cystic fibrosis is 1 in 4 or 25%, the risk of being a carrier (having one recessive and one dominant allele for that trait) is 2 in 4 or 50%, and the chance of not having the disease and not being a carrier is 1 in 4 or 25%.

The father has been diagnosed with nonpolyposis colorectal cancer and is heterozygous for the trait, which is typical for an autosomal dominant trait (Figure 13–7 ■). The mother does not have the trait. The risk of each child inheriting the trait for the disease is 2 in 4 or 50% and the chance of each child not being affected is 2 in 4 or 50%.

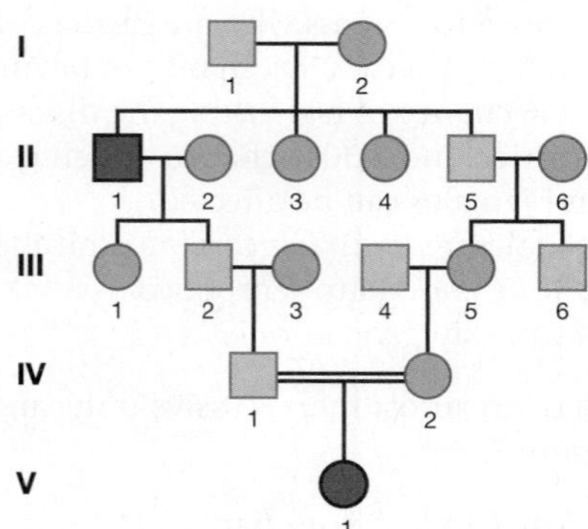

Figure 13–5 ■ Pedigree: consanguinity

Autosomal Recessive

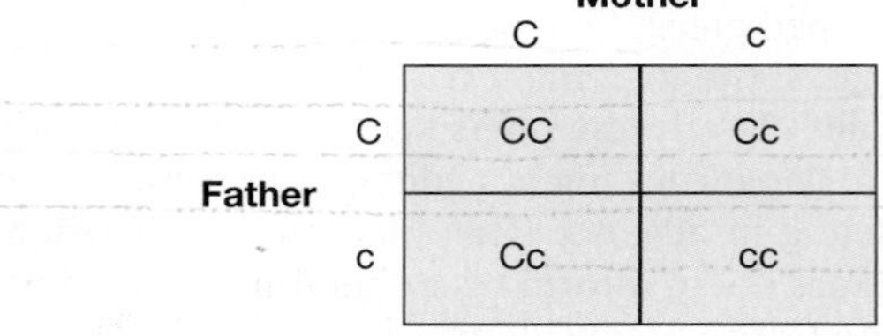

Figure 13–6 ■ Punnett square: cystic fibrosis (autosomal recessive)

Autosomal Dominant

Father \ Mother	C	c
c	Cc	cc
c	Cc	cc

Figure 13–7 ■ Punnett square: hereditary nonpolyposis colorectal cancer (autosomal dominant)

SECTION TWO REVIEW

1. In order to protect confidentiality, the birth year rather than the entire birth date of an individual is used in a pedigree.
   A. True
   B. False
2. A horizontal line in a pedigree indicates
   A. a relationship.
   B. a generation.
   C. consanguinity.
   D. adoption.
3. The paternal section of a pedigree should go on the right and the maternal section should go on the left.
   A. True
   B. False
4. An illustration used to predict the likelihood of inheriting a particular genetic trait or disease is called a
   A. pedigree.
   B. karyotype.
   C. Punnett square.
   D. dihybrid cross.
5. The horizontal line in a pedigree connects vertically to a second horizontal line that displays the __________.
   A. marriage.
   B. grandparents.
   C. sibship.
   D. adoption.

Answers: 1. A; 2. A; 3. B; 4. C; 5. C

SECTION THREE: Nursing Implications

Obtaining a detailed, accurate family health history and understanding its importance is one of the most important contributions a nurse can make with respect to genetics and health care. The nurse is usually the first health care provider that the patient meets; therefore, nurses need good communication skills to develop a rapport with the client, to educate the client, and to assist in client decision making. Competencies and curricula guidelines for nursing were established by a consensus panel and were published by the American Nurses Association. (Consensus Panel, 2009). Nurses are now expected to incorporate genetic knowledge and skills into their practices. Collecting a health history and constructing a pedigree are two of the essential competencies that apply to all professional nurses (Consensus Panel, 2009). Nurses need to understand the impact that genetics has on their patients and be knowledgeable enough to discuss choices and options with their patients.

The nurse may be expected to coordinate referrals and follow-up services for the client. The family health history and the pedigree can be tools for genetic diagnosis and risk assessment. When appropriate, the nurse may facilitate a referral to a genetic professional such as a genetic counselor, a geneticist, or a genetic nurse for counseling, determining disease risk, genetic testing, and intervention or treatment. A genetics nurse is a professional nurse with specialized education and training in genetics who may be credentialed as a **genetic clinical nurse** (GCN). The nurse should assess the client's knowledge and perceptions of genetic information and clarify any misconceptions or misinformation the client may have about his or her diagnoses or prognosis. Finally, the nurse must preserve individual and family confidentiality and privacy. The family health history and pedigree is private information as is the patient's medical record. The information should be protected and not shared with family members until informed consent is obtained and genetic specialists are available for counseling.

SECTION THREE REVIEW

1. Obtaining a comprehensive health history is a standard competency required of all nurses.
   A. True
   B. False
2. In working with clients who are seeking genetic information and/or counseling, nurses need the following skills EXCEPT
   A. communication.
   B. education.
   C. decision making.
   D. diagnosing.
3. The National Coalition for Health Professional Education in Genetics and the American Nurses Association lists the following expected competencies for nurses EXCEPT
   A. obtaining a family history.
   B. constructing a three-generation pedigree.
   C. ordering specific genetic tests.
   D. facilitating referrals for specialized genetic services.
4. It is the nurse's responsibility to inform family members of genetic risks.
   A. True
   B. False
5. A Genetics Clinical Nurse (GCN) is a registered nurse with a baccalaureate degree who has specialized education and training in genetics.
   A. True
   B. False

Answers: 1. A; 2. D; 3. C; 4. F; 5. A

POSTTEST

1. Tips for obtaining a comprehensive family health history include which of the following?
   A. Ask specific questions of the individual and family.
   B. Use leading questions to help the client remember the information.
   C. Explain the purpose of the questions to the client.
   D. Do not waste time socializing with the client before the interview.
2. A red flag in a family health history includes all of the following EXCEPT
   A. several relatives who are affected with the same disease.
   B. early sudden death of an individual.
   C. a disorder that occurs later in life.
   D. a child whose parents are closely related.
3. An example of a second-degree relative is a
   A. mother.
   B. grandfather.
   C. cousin.
   D. daughter.
4. The family history is considered the first risk assessment or genetic screen in primary care.
   A. True
   B. False
5. Barriers to obtaining a family health history include the following EXCEPT
   A. many people do not know their family history.
   B. multiple family members may want to contribute to the history.
   C. family members may not want to reveal sensitive information such as alcoholism.
   D. it may be difficult to identify disease patterns in small families.
6. In the pedigree of an individual with an autosomal dominant trait, one would observe
   A. it is always inherited from the mother.
   B. it does not skip generation.
   C. it only affects females.
   D. it only affects males.
7. Related individuals who have children together have a higher risk of having a child who is affected with a(n) __________ condition.
   A. mosaic
   B. autosomal dominant
   C. autosomal recessive
   D. None of the above
8. A couple who are both carriers for sickle cell disease, an autosomal recessive disorder, is pregnant. What is the probability that their unborn child will be affected?
   A. 0%
   B. 25%
   C. 50%
   D. 100%
9. Consanguinity is displayed in a pedigree by
   A. a double vertical line.
   B. a double forward slash.
   C. a double horizontal line.
   D. a single back slash.
10. A pedigree that has only male family members (squares) who are affected is probably displaying a(n) __________ disorder.
   A. autosomal dominant
   B. autosomal recessive
   C. Y-linked
   D. X-linked

Posttest answers are located in the Appendix.

CHAPTER SUMMARY

The family health history is one of the most important diagnostic tools for assessing risk of common diseases. The family history may identify individuals who are at risk for developing specific genetic diseases that may be treated or prevented. It is considered the first "genetic screen" and is underused in primary care. The purpose of an individual health history is to collect information to help develop diagnoses and assessment, screen for existing or potential health problems, establish a relationship with the client, and develop a health care plan.

The family pedigree is a graphic representation of an individual's extended family health history and genetic relationships and is a means to assess genetic inheritance patterns and predict risk for genetic disease.

Nurses are expected to incorporate genetic knowledge into their practice. Collecting an individual and family health history and constructing a family pedigree are two of the essential competencies expected of all nurses.

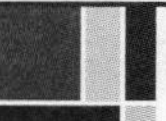

CRITICAL THINKING CHECKPOINT

Figure 13–8 ■ illustrates a family pedigree with a strong history of sickle cell disease. Emma is the proband; her parents are bringing her to the genetics clinic to determine if she has sickle cell disease. She is 3 weeks old but appears healthy and is thriving. The nurse begins by taking a family history and determining Emma's risk of having the disease.

1. What mode of inheritance is sickle cell disease?
2. What are the characteristics of this mode of transmission?
3. It is determined that Emma does not have sickle cell disease. What are the chances that she is a carrier of the sickle cell trait?
4. Who else in this pedigree are probable carriers of the trait? Why?
5. Are there any other patterns of inheritance in this pedigree? What would be needed to determine if anyone was at risk for other diseases?
6. What is the role of the nurse once the pedigree has been created?

Answers are provided in the Appendix

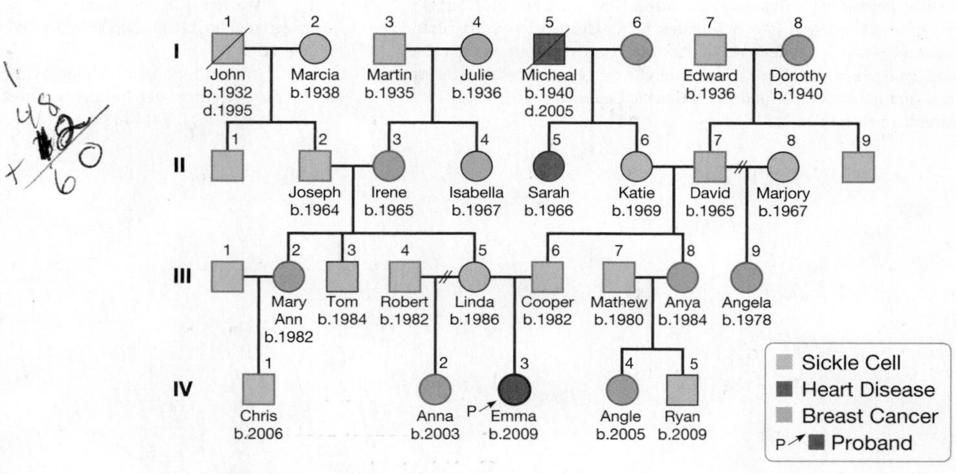

Figure 13–8 ■ Family pedigree of sickle cell disease

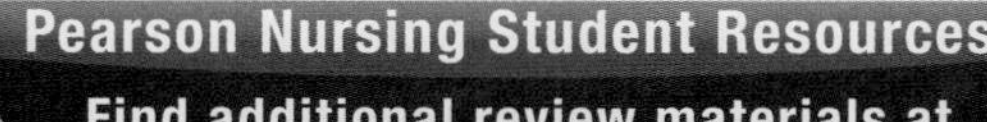
Pearson Nursing Student Resources

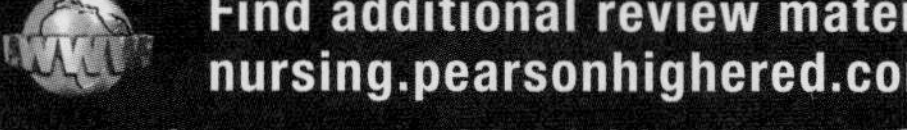
Find additional review materials at nursing.pearsonhighered.com

Prepare for success with additional NCLEX®-style practice questions, interactive assignments and activities, web links, animations, videos, and more!

ONLINE RESOURCES

Centers for Disease Control Family History: http://www.cdc.gov/genomics/famhistory/resources/fs_web.htm

Genetic Alliance Family Health History: http://www.geneticalliance.org/fhh

My Family Health Portrait: https://familyhistory.hhs.gov/fhh-web/home.action

Utah Department of Health Chronic Disease Genomics Program: http://www.health.utah.gov/genomics

Utah Department of Health Chronic Disease Genomics Program Family Reunion Packets: http://health.utah.gov/genomics/familyhistory/familyreunion.html

Utah Department of Health Family Health History Toolkit: http://health.utah.gov/asthma/pdf_files/Genomics/new%20entire%20toolkit.pdf

REFERENCES

Aiello-Laws, L. (2011). Genetic cancer risk assessment. *Seminars in Oncology Nursing, 27*(1), 13–20.

American Medical Association. (2004). *Family medical history in disease prevention.* Chicago, IL: American Medical Association. Retrieved January 6, 2011, from http://www.ama-assn.org/ama1/pub/upload/mm/464/family_history02.pdf

Andrews, M. A., & Boyle, J. S. (2008). *Transcultural concepts in nursing care* (5th ed.). Philadelphia, PA: Wolters Kluwer/Lippincott Williams and Wilkins.

Beery, T. A., & Shooner, K. A. (2004). Family history: The first genetic screen. *The Nurse Practitioner, 29*(11), 14–25.

Bennett, R. L. (2000). Pedigree parables. *Clinical Genetics, 58*(4), 241–249.

Bennett, R. L., French, K. S., Resta, R. G., & Doyle, D. L. (2008). Standardizing human pedigree nomenclature: Update and assessment of the recommendation of the national society of genetic counselors. *Journal of Genetic Counseling, 17*, 424–433.

Consensus Panel on Genetic/Genomic Nursing Competencies. (2009). *Essentials of genetic and genomic nursing: Competencies , curricula guidelines, and outcome indicators*. (2nd ed.). Silver Spring MD: American Nurses Association.

Fuller, M., Myers, M., Webb, T., Tabangin, M., & Prows, C. (2010). Primary care providers' responses to patient-generated family history. *Journal of Genetic Counseling, 19*(1), 84–96.

Hinton, R. B. (2008). The family history: Reemergence of an established tool. *Critical Care Nursing Clinics of North America, 20*, 149–158.

Knoppers, B. M, Strom, C., Clayton, E. W., Murray, T., Fibisons, W., & Luthers, L. (1998). ASHG statement. Professional disclosure of familial genetic information: The American society of human genetics social issues subcommittee on familial disclosure. *American Journal of Human Genetics, 62*(2), 474–483.

Licis, A. K., Desruisseau, D. M., Tamada, K. A., Duntley, S. P., & Gurnett, C. A. (2011). Novel genetic findings in an extended family pedigree with sleepwalking. *Neurology, 76*(1), 49–52.

McGoldrick, M., & Gerson, R. (1985). *Genograms in family assessment*. New York, NY: Norton.

Schneider, K. A., Chittenden, A. B., Branda, K. J., Keenan, M. A., Joffe, S., Patenaude, A. F., et al. (2006). Ethical issues in cancer genetics: Whose information is it? *Journal of Genetic Counseling, 15*(6), 491–503.

Seidel, H. M., Ball, J. W., Dains, J. E., Flynn, J. A., Solomon, B. S., & Stewart, R. W. (2010). *Mosby's guide to physical examination*. St. Louis, MO: Mosby Elsevier.

Spahis, J. (2002). Human genetics: Constructing a family pedigree. *American Journal of Nursing, 102*(7), 44–49.

U.S. Department of Health and Human Services [USDHHS]. (2004). *The surgeon general's family health history initiative: My family health portrait tool*. Retrieved July 9, 2012, from www.hhs.gov/familyhistory

U.S. Department of Health and Human Services [USDHHS]. (1996). *Health information privacy: Genetic information*. Retrieved January 29, 2011, from http://www.hhs.gov/ocr/privacy/hipaa/understanding/special/genetic/

Utah Department of Health. (2005). *Family health history toolkit*. Retrieved July 9, 2012, from http://www.health.utah.gov/genomics

Warren, J. E., & Silver, R. M. (2008). Genetics of pregnancy loss. *Clinical Obstetrics and Gynecology, 51*(1), 84–95.

Wattendorf, D. J., & Hadley, D. W. (2005). Family history: Three-generation pedigree. *American Family Physician, 72*(3), 441–448.

CHAPTER

14 Risk Assessment

Diane Seibert, Ann Maradiegue

The opinions expressed herein are those of the author(s), and are not necessarily representative of those of the Uniformed Services University of the Health Sciences (USUHS); the Department of Defense (DOD); or the United States Army, Navy, or Air Force.

LEARNING OUTCOMES

Following the completion of this chapter, the learner will be able to

1. Assess protective and predictive factors, including genetics, which influence the health of individuals, families, groups, communities, and populations.
2. Recognize the relationship of genetics and genomics to health, prevention, screening, and diagnostics using family history information and other risk assessment tools.
3. Describe the nursing role associated with the risk assessment process.

This chapter presents the definition of risk assessment, and the application of this construct to patient populations. It provides a brief historical perspective on risk assessment, as well as focuses on the attributes of risk assessment. This chapter also provides information on how a risk assessment is conducted and offers information on the future directions of genetics and genomics.

PRETEST

1. Nurses need to be able to
   A. identify red flags.
   B. collect a three-generation pedigree.
   C. diagnose genetic diseases based on pedigree patterns.
   D. lead multidisciplinary health care teams to manage the patient care.
2. The nurse's role in assessing risk for genetic disease is complex and includes which of the following?
   A. Ordering genetic tests
   B. Interpreting genetic test results
   C. Providing genetic counseling for specific diseases
   D. Being aware of new technologies and how they may impact health care
3. Which of the following is true of virtually all disease?
   A. Genes are almost always involved.
   B. Environmental exposures cause disease, regardless of genetics.
   C. Lifestyle plays a very minor role in disease.
   D. Being born with a risk gene or predisposition for a particular disease is responsible for almost all disease.
4. An individual's age is the least important factor when calculating risk for disease.
   A. True
   B. False
5. Genetic testing is now recommended before prescribing which of the following drugs?
   A. HCTZ (hydrochlorothiazide) for blood pressure
   B. Tylenol (acetaminophen) for mild pain
   C. Coumadin (warfarin) for clotting
   D. Amoxil (amoxicillin) for infection
6. Consanguinity is more commonly practiced in which of the following sociocultural groups?
   A. Germany
   B. United States
   C. Egypt
   D. Australia
7. Explaining risk to patients can be difficult, because words are easily misinterpreted or misunderstood. Which of the following words is suggested as a good substitute for the word *risk* when counseling a person about genetic disease?
   A. Chance
   B. Probability
   C. Hazard
   D. Consequence
8. Which of the following is a breast cancer red flag?
   A. Mother diagnosed with breast cancer at age 75.
   B. Family history reveals only one woman with breast cancer.

C. Father diagnosed with breast cancer at age 75.
D. Second cousin (female) once removed diagnosed with breast cancer at age 40.

9. What percentages of stillborn infants have anomalies that may inform future pregnancy risks?
   A. 1%
   B. 2.5%
   C. 10%
   D. 15%

10. Which ethnic group is at increased risk for inheriting a sickle cell mutation?
    A. Asian
    B. African
    C. Scandinavian
    D. Ashkenazi Jewish

Pretest answers are located in the Appendix.

SECTION ONE: Historical Background

Nursing programs began the process of seriously integrating genetics into curricula in the early 1980s. This effort began to accelerate in the 1990s, yet there is little progress in nurses' application of genetics at the bedside (Lashley, 2007; Calzone et al., 2010). In the past, risk assessment associated with genetic disorders was connected with the basic identification of dominant and recessive disorders. Today, as scientists begin to understand the complexity and heterogeneity of disease, concepts of penetrance, age of onset, and the interaction of genes and environment, it becomes clear a more in-depth understanding of the genetics/genomics of disease is required for the risk assessment process (Young, 2007). New genomic discoveries have gone from the treatment of rare, single gene disorders to using genetic testing for prescribing medications and the identification of common chronic diseases. There are three major changes that affect the way genetic information is handled. First, patients with diseases known to be genetic (Treacher-Collins, Tay-Sachs, cystic fibrosis, etc.) were once diagnosed and managed almost exclusively by medical geneticists and specialists. This is gradually changing because more genetic disorders are being recognized, and milder forms of some diseases (such as cystic fibrosis) that do not require intensive therapy but need to be monitored for emerging symptoms are now being managed in primary care settings. Second, genetic testing, once the end point in care, is now being used to prevent disease and promote healthy outcomes. Finally, the sheer volume of genetic information is overwhelming, and all health care professionals need to have a basic understanding of genetics to guide, inform, and assist patients optimize outcomes (Institute of Medicine, 2009). The role of the nurse at the bedside has never been more important.

The role of the nurse in risk assessment is complex. This includes being aware of new technology and its impact on health care, and the affect it has on individuals, families, and communities. All nurses and many other health care disciplines are familiar with collecting a family history. As part of the risk assessment process, nurses need to be able to identify red flags that pose a threat to health during the family history collection process, understand the collection of a three-generation pedigree, recognize disease patterns, and collaborate with a multidisciplinary health care team to manage the patient care (Lea, Skirton, Read, & Williams, 2011). It is speculated by experts that in the future patients will have a copy of their genetic map, and nurses will help them navigate it in order to identify health interventions based on their genomic tendencies for disease and drug sensitivities (Keuhn, 2011). Virtually all disease has a genetic/genomic component influenced by environment, lifestyle, and other factors. This makes a nurse's ability to conduct a genetic risk assessment crucial, no matter what the setting.

SECTION ONE REVIEW

1. Nurses will not have to know much about genetics when they practice because genetic health care is addressed primarily by genetic specialists such as genetic counselors.
   A. True
   B. False
2. The nurse's role in assessing risk for genetic disease includes which of the following?
   A. Ordering genetic tests
   B. Interpreting genetic test results
   C. Providing genetic counseling for specific diseases
   D. Being aware of new technologies and how they may impact health care
3. Managing patients with a genetic condition is exclusively done by genetic specialists.
   A. True
   B. False
4. Which of the following is incorrect?
   A. Patients with genetic diseases are often managed in primary care settings.
   B. Genetic testing can be used to prevent disease and promote healthy outcomes.
   C. Nurses still play a minor role in genetic health care.
   D. Family history is considered by many to be the first genetic test.

Answers: 1. B; 2. B; 3. B; 4. C

SECTION TWO: Defining Risk

Risk is the probability that something will go wrong, or the likelihood of developing a disease. This implies that risk can be measured. In genetic testing it is not acceptable to determine risk as high or low due to the uncertainty involved with testing and the evolving process of new discovery that can change the meaning of results (Young, 2007). There are three categories of risk: **population risk**, **high risk**, and **extremely high risk**. (See Table 14–1.)

Risk assessment involves recognition of personal and family medical history characteristics associated with increased disease risk for any given individual. Risk stratification is a process that assigns a level of risk for all individuals *within a population* based on personal and family medical history associated with increased disease risk. This process is conducted by considering the presence or absence of disease in family members in first, second, and (when necessary) third-degree relatives. Risk considerations are a family member with two or more related conditions, disease occurring in the less often affected sex (e.g., male breast cancer), a more severe phenotype including multifocal disease, individuals who refractory to usual treatment or prevention strategies, and recognition of a pattern of disease within a family consistent with a Mendelian disorder (Yoon, Scheuner, Jorgensen, and Khoury, 2009).

Genetics and genomics have made the possibility of early disease identification and prevention a reality for many diseases. With this new reality comes new responsibility, which includes knowing when to refer and collaborate with genetic experts. Risk assessment is traditionally defined in statistical terms, such as probability. Nurses need to have a clear understanding of risk in order to explain to individuals and family members the process of genetic testing, along with the uncertainty that surrounds testing, and must consider all of the ethical, cultural, and personal concerns (Young, 2007). Conducting a risk assessment is a step-wise process that should include genetics as part of the assessment process. The process of risk assessment includes identifying factors that predispose individuals to adverse health outcomes that can cause harm or injury. A personal risk evaluation incorporates all the personal and environmental risk factors and is part of the process of assimilating and incorporating this information into a personalized plan of care. An example of an evidence-based risk assessment tool currently in use is the Gail model. This risk assessment tool is designed to be used by health professionals to estimate a woman's lifetime risk for developing breast cancer by assessing several risk elements: age, family history (first-degree relative with breast cancer), personal history (history of ductal hyperplasia), **ethnicity**, and surgical history (breast biopsy) to estimate her 5-year and lifetime (to age 90) risk for developing invasive breast cancer (National Cancer Institute [NCI], 2008).

TABLE 14–1: Defining Risk

Population Risk	These individuals have no family history or known lifestyle or environmental risks. The recommendations for care would be based on the screening and management recommendations for the general population. For example, the American Cancer Society recommends all individuals have a colonoscopy at age 50.
High Risk	Individuals who have a red flag for family history and/or lifestyle or environment, but do not fit the criteria for genetic risk. For example, an individual whose father died at age 55 from cardiovascular disease may benefit from more frequent hypertension and cholesterol screening.
Extremely High Risk	Individuals with more than one red flag in their family history and lifestyle or environment. For example, a woman with multiple family members with breast and ovarian cancer should start her mammograms and other screenings 10 years earlier than the earliest diagnosis of cancer in her family and be referred to a genetic specialist for consultation and intervention strategies.

Source: National Coalition for Health Care Professionals in Genetics (n.d.)

Attributes of Risk

There are several **attributes** that expose an individual to genetic risk. These include inherited (e.g., heritability, ethnicity), environmental, moderating (e.g., socioeconomic status), lifestyle (e.g., cultural practices, diet), ethnicity, and epigenetic factors. All of these attributes are a part of genetic risk assessment. **Heritability** refers to the genetic makeup that is transmitted from one generation to the next. **Phenotypic** traits of individuals are influenced by both the inherited genes from the parents and the environment in which the individual was raised. When the individuals within a population differ in a phenotypic trait, the population is said to exhibit variation for that trait (Braveman, Egerter, & Williams, 2011).

Environment includes all factors that an individual will be exposed to from conception to death, such as climate, disease, and accidents. **Socioeconomic status (SES)** can also influence phenotypic presentation by affecting nutrition and exposure to more toxins in the environment. Neighborhood conditions for those of lower SES include exposure to lead paint and facilities that produce more hazardous substances. Environmental factors can change an individual's disease risk and are important because these factors are not genetically transmitted from parent to child. Factors such as environment and behavior can influence phenotypic disease presentation. The individual's phenotype is the interaction of his or her genes and the environment. For example, scientists know that there is a genetic predisposition to alcoholism, but if an individual never drinks, he or she will not become an alcoholic.

Many diseases are caused in whole or in part by environmental factors. Environmental and dietary factors have been shown to affect the **epigenetic** pathways, causing cellular damage identified in Table 14–2. Epigenetic pathways are the cellular mechanisms that initiate and maintain the inherited pathways of gene expression and gene function. Epigenetic pathways include methylation and histone modification. When too much or too little methylation occurs it can negate a genes function or cause unwanted alterations in the cell—for example, proliferation of cancer cells. Histones are the proteins that make up the nucleotides. Histones influence how loosely or tightly packed the chromatin is during the transcription process, thereby influencing if genes can be expressed. Inappropriate levels of gene expression can lead to diseases. DNA methylation is responsible for cancer and cell aging. Evidence that epigenetic change is responsible for the development of diseases (such as neurodevelopmental disorders, cardiovascular diseases, Type 2 diabetes, obesity, and infertility) is increasing (vanVliet, Oates, & Whitelaw, 2007). Dietary practices have also been linked to alterations in the epigenetic pathway. The fungus containing fumonisin, called *huitlacoche* in Mexico, grows on corn and is often eaten as a delicacy in Mexico with quesadillas, tamales, and other dishes. Fumonisin is a toxin that blocks one of the transporters that folic acid needs to enter cells, inhibiting the vitamin's role in ensuring that the neural tube closes properly and causing severe neural tube defects (Gelineau-van Waes et al., 2005). This illustrates the role that cultural practices play in dietary practices leading to a predisposition to genetic disorders. Cultural practices are often a more difficult genetic risk factor to overcome.

TABLE 14–2: Epigenetic Pathways and Risk Examples

Environmental/ Dietary Factor	Cellular Action	Outcomes
Folate and methionine	Supply methyl groups needed for DNA methylation; can change the expression of growth factor genes.	Birth defects
Cigarette smoking	Stimulate demethylation of metastatic genes.	Lung cancer, bladder cancer, prematurebirth, low birth weight, asthma
Pesticides	Alter DNA methylation.	Birth defects
Heavy metals	Disrupt DNA methylation.	Birth defects

Consanguinity is a cultural practice that can have a profound effect on genetic outcomes, increasing the risk for autosomal recessive disorders. Consanguinity is a common cultural practice in many populations, including the Amish community in the United States and many Middle Eastern cultures—particularly the countries of Turkey, Iran, Pakistan, India, and Muslim countries in North Africa (Tadmouri et al., 2009). First-cousin unions are the most common form of consanguineous marriage and occurrence rates vary by country. The prevalence of consanguineous unions is highest in Arab countries, with rates that vary from 20% to > 50% (Tadmouri et al., 2009). These marriages are felt by the families to foster social bonds from one generation to the next and are an integral part of cultural practice (Tadmouri et al., 2009). Careful histories that include family relationships are an important part of the risk assessment process. It is important to recognize the definition of family may vary by cultural groups and may differ from the health care provider (Berg et al., 2009). See Figures 14–1 ■ and 14–2 ■ for more details.

Ethnicity is another important part of risk assessment for a number of reasons. One such reason is inherited risk is more common within certain ethnic groups and cultural practices, which may place individuals at higher risk for genetic disorders. Examples of diseases that are more common within ethnic groups include sickle cell disease in those of African-American and Hispanic ancestry. Those of Ashkenazi Jewish heritage are at risk for early-onset breast and ovarian cancer due to the founder mutations BRCA1 and BRCA2 found in this population (Berliner & Fay, 2007). Families carrying these mutations

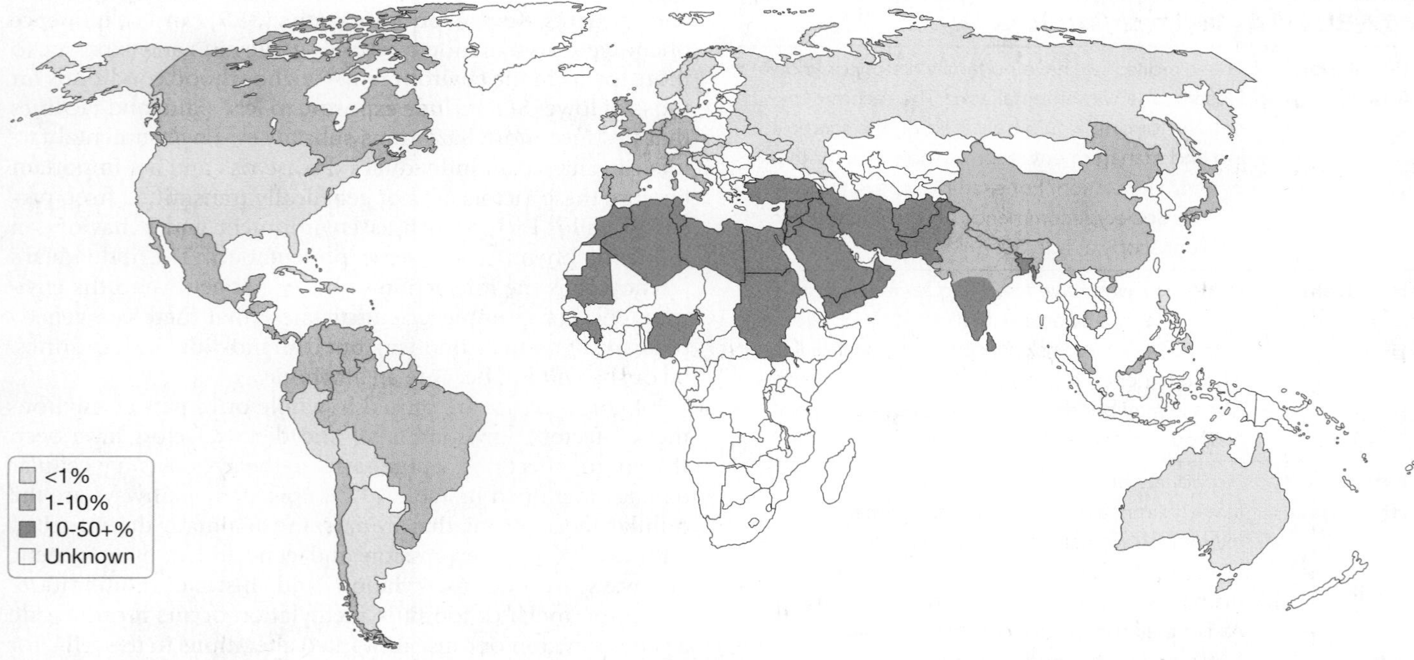

Figure 14–1 ■ Global consanguinity rates

Source: A. H. Bittles and M. L. Black, Consanguinity, human evolution, and complex diseases. PNAS January 26, 2010 vol. 107 no. suppl 1 1779-1786. Reprinted by permission of the National Academy of Sciences.

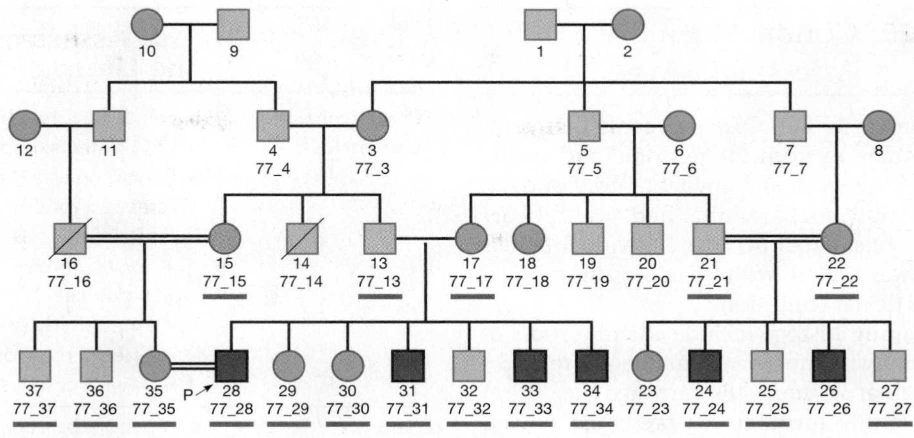

Figure 14–2 ■ Consanguinity pedigree example

can elect to undergo genetic testing; if found to have one of these gene mutations, the family members are able to become candidates for genetic testing so that prevention strategies can be implemented. Many risk models have been developed to facilitate the risk assessment and interpretation process.

Risk models that incorporate age, ethnicity, and sex provide a constellation of health care information, allowing for a stratified risk assessment. Age is an important part of the risk constellation (Chung et al., 2008). For example, approximately 180,000 to 250,000 individuals in the United States will suffer sudden cardiac death. Nurses knowledgeable in genetics/genomics can help people avert sudden cardiac death by conducting a thorough family history that includes the age of occurrence and death among family members with heart disease, thus establishing potential risk in other family members for an early onset of cardiac disease and possible sudden death. Nursing plays a key role in translating information about the family history in the clinical environment and can reduce the incidence of sudden cardiac death hemorrhage by collecting this important information and discussing it with the individual and family (Campbell & Berger, 2006).

Interpreting Risk

Individuals may calculate their risk very differently than a professional so these are important discussions to have with the patient and family members. Significant factors from the patient perspective are how this information is communicated. When discussing the possibility of acquiring a disorder, choosing a word such as *chance* is less threatening than the word *risk*. Trained genetic professionals need to carefully explain information to an individual who is at extremely high risk for a genetic disorder, as well as to his or her family members, with the information put into context so all can understand. For example, "women in the general population have a 1 in 11 chance of developing breast cancer, but in your family there is a 1 in 4 chance of developing breast cancer because you have inherited a gene mutation that increases your risk."

SECTION TWO REVIEW

1. Which of the following environmental attributes increase an individual's risk for an adverse health outcome?
   A. Exercising for 30 minutes a day, 6 days a week
   B. Maintaining a healthy body weight
   C. Being raised from birth to age 5 in a home built in 1928
   D. Wearing seatbelts
2. An individual's age is the least important factor when calculating risk for disease.
   A. True
   B. False
3. Genetic testing is now recommended before prescribing which of the following drugs?
   A. HCTZ (hydrochlorothiazide) for blood pressure
   B. Tylenol (acetaminophen) for mild pain
   C. Coumadin (warfarin) for clotting
   D. Amoxil (amoxicillin) for infection
4. Consanguinity is more commonly practiced in which of the following sociocultural groups?
   A. Germany
   B. United States
   C. Egypt
   D. Australia
5. Explaining risk to patients can be difficult, because words are easily misinterpreted or misunderstood. Which of the following words is suggested as a good substitute for the word *risk* when counseling a person about genetic disease?
   A. Chance
   B. Probability
   C. Hazard
   D. Consequence

Answers: 1. C; 2. B; 3. C; 4. C; 5. A

SECTION THREE: Conducting a Risk Assessment

The genetic risk assessment is a multistep process that gathers and interprets information from the personal and family history, the physical examination, and any laboratory or diagnostic test results. The individual's cultural and health belief system should also be considered, because individual beliefs and values do not always align with mainstream medical understanding for a particular condition.

Red flags in the family history include identification of more than one close family member (e.g., first-degree relative) with a disease that began at an unusually early age (i.e., colon cancer in 30-year-old family member) or presented unusually (e.g., breast cancer in a male relative or multiple relatives with several types of related cancers). These may indicate an increased risk for genetic disease. Risk assessment supports the development of a personalized plan of care that encompasses all of the patient characteristics including the family history; cultural, behavioral and environmental factors; diagnostic tests and laboratory values; and genetics/genomics.

Risk assessment is currently based on disorders for which specific populations are at increased risk (e.g., men over age 50 are screened for heart disease, and postmenopausal women are screened for breast cancer), not on what disorders an individual might be at increased risk for developing (Table 14–3). As genetic advances continue, it is highly likely that in the near future, risk assessment will evolve from identifying and screening particular populations to screening individuals based on their unique genetic, familial, and environmental risks. It is speculated that within the next 5 years it may become possible to sequence an entire human genome for less than $1,000 (Darr, 2010). When that price point is achieved, it will become financially feasible to screen a person's entire genome, and assess what disorders an individual is, or is not, at increased risk for. Although environmental exposures and lifestyle will continue to play a role in disease (high fat diets will still influence obesity, and radiation exposure will still predispose to cancer), screening, interventions, and medications could be specifically tailored to meet the unique needs of individuals. For example, based on her genome profile you know that Jane Smith has inherited a gene that decreases her risk for colorectal cancer (**CRC**), but she has also inherited a gene that slightly increases her risk for Type 2 diabetes mellitus (**DM**). Jane's sister, Sarah inherited genes that place her at population risk for CRC but she has not inherited the Type 2 DM risk gene. Despite their shared childhood environment, lifetime risk for CRC and Type 2 DM are different. Jane may never need a colonoscopy but should receive regular counseling about weight maintenance and exercise to help prevent the development of Type 2 DM. Sarah, on the other hand, should receive routine CRC screening (colonoscopy starting at age 50) but much less emphasis would need to be placed on education and screening for Type 2 diabetes. Risk assessment becomes personalized health care.

Family histories often contain surprises because families are complex and dynamic social organizations. Biological relationships may not be disclosed, health care problems may not be shared, and the person providing the information may be obscuring the information or may be misinformed. Because gathering a history can be complicated, nurses should familiarize themselves with institutional policies regarding how to handle complex family relationships before suggesting genetic testing. Nurses must also be prepared to respond to patient questions regarding stigmatization, insurance, and discrimination issues. One of the biggest concerns in genetic screening is misattributed parenthood, usually paternity. Nurses need to be prepared to deal with these challenges and respond in an ethical manner (Lashley, 2007).

A detailed family history should be collected early in life and updated periodically. In addition to these routine evaluations, there are specific time points when more detailed risk assessment should be performed, which may prompt referral to a genetic specialist (Jenkins & Lea, 2005). These time points include, but are not limited to, the preconception or prenatal period, the newborn and pediatric period, and adulthood to identify emerging disease.

During the preconception or prenatal counseling visit, risk assessment focuses on identifying actual or potential genetic conditions that may affect the pregnancy or the fetus. Collecting a detailed past family and personal obstetric history is important because many people may fail to mention a pregnancy that ended in miscarriage or stillbirth, either because they forgot, or don't appreciate the importance of that information. Fully 15% to 20% of stillborn infants have anomalies that may be important to screen for in future pregnancies.

TABLE 14–3: Risk Assessment Across the Lifespan

Preconception / Obstetrics	■ Family history (attention to miscarriage, birth defects, and childhood disorders) ■ Education about genetic disorders screened for during preconception or prenatal periods ◆ Cystic fibrosis ◆ Sickle cell ◆ Aneuploidy (trisomy 21, 18, and 13) ◆ Special risks for certain populations ◆ Jewish couples
Newborn/ Pediatric Screening	■ Newborn screening ■ Screening at every visit for milestones and developmental delays ■ Diabetes and cardiovascular testing based on family history
Adult	■ Family history (attention to common chronic diseases) ■ Identify individuals ◆ High risk for earlier interventions ◆ Extremely high risk for genetic referral
Geriatrics	■ Alzheimer testing ■ Hereditary and environmental influences for chronic disease (e.g., smoking)

During the newborn or pediatric visit, the focus is on identifying genetic factors that may have caused or contributed to a congenital anomaly. Approximately 2% to 3% of live-born infants have congenital anomalies that are present and identified at birth. As children continue to develop, more anomalies become evident, and by age 7, approximately 8% to 9% of children will be diagnosed with one or more major anomalies. As genetic science evolves from the identification of single gene disorders (e.g., cystic fibrosis, Fragile X syndrome, BRCA mutations) and moves toward identifying individuals with diseases now understood to have strong genetic component (e.g., Parkinson disease, Alzheimer disease, heart disease, and diabetes), adults may be diagnosed and referred more frequently for genetic counseling and testing.

Current Risk Assessment Tools

By far the most important tool in assessing an individual's risk for disease is to collect a detailed, accurate medical family history. If conducted methodically and updated regularly, the medical family history can provide important insights into shared familial and environmental risks. Several tools are available (see the online resources listed at the end of this chapter) in the collection of this important information. Perhaps the one that people are most familiar with is the Surgeon General's Family History Tool. This web-based tool was first introduced on National Family History Day (Thanksgiving Day) in 2004, with the goal of encouraging families to share information when gathered together to celebrate the holiday. The tool has undergone substantial revisions and refinements since 2004. It is now completely web based (no need to download anything) and free to use, and none of the data is stored on any website. The tool is available online in English and Spanish and the paper version (**PDF**) is available in English, Spanish, Chinese, French, Polish, and Portuguese. The tool helps users families organize and record health history information that, once recorded, can be emailed to other family members and printed out or uploaded into an electronic health record so it can be shared with a provider. For more detailed information on the family history tool, refer to Chapter 13.

Risk Models

In addition to family history tools, several risk assessment models have been developed to more accurately predict health outcomes for individuals. Some online risk assessment tools, such as Your Disease Risk (launched in 2000), offer the individual an opportunity to assess several different diseases from one interface. Originally developed as the Harvard Cancer Risk Index, the tool was renamed in 2007 when it migrated to the Washington University School of Medicine in St Louis. The site contains modules that assess risk for several types of cancers as well as for a number of common diseases (diabetes, heart disease, stroke, and osteoporosis). The target audience is the lay public and the goal is to improve knowledge through education and empower people to make healthy lifestyle choices.

Two additional risk assessment tools (cardiac risk and breast cancer risk) used by clinicians will be described in detail here, but other tools are either in development or available and nurses should use them when appropriate.

Heart disease is the leading cause of death in the United States for both men and women, and several cardiac risk scoring models (i.e., Reynolds, SCORE, QRISK, QRISK2, and Calcium and Framingham Risk Calculators) have been developed to estimate individual risk for developing heart disease (Vasan, Sullivan, & Wilson, 2005). There are a number of differences between the tools, but they all estimate risk for an early adverse cardiac event. The Framingham Risk Calculator was developed in a collaborative effort between the U.S. Preventive Services Task Force (**USPSTF**) and the American Heart Association. The Framingham Risk Assessment calculates a 10-year risk score for individuals considered to be at population risk for developing an adverse cardiac event (myocardial infarction and coronary death) within the next decade. The score can then be used to encourage individuals to modify their lifestyle and adhere to preventive treatment, and to identify people at increased risk for future cardiovascular events. Individuals considered to be at population risk have a Framingham Score of 10% or less. Those at high risk have a score between 10% and 20%, and people at extremely high risk have a 10-year risk of 20% or greater for an adverse cardiac event. The tool should not be used to calculate risk in people already known to be at extremely high risk for heart disease (e.g., individuals with diabetes, peripheral arterial disease, abdominal aortic aneurysm, carotid artery disease, or documented heart disease) because their 10-year risk is already greater than 20%. The calculator is available online and is free and easy to use.

Several cancer risk prediction models are available. The Gail and Claus models are both used to assess risk for breast cancer and are commonly used in clinical practice. Others such as the online Colorectal Cancer Risk Assessment Tool are currently being used primarily in oncology or genetics settings, but may become more commonplace in primary care settings.

The Gail model was developed by (and named after) Dr. Mitchell Gail from the National Cancer Institute (NCI). Dr. Gail and his colleagues used data from two major studies (the Breast Cancer Detection Demonstration Project [**BCDDP**] and the NCI's Surveillance, Epidemiology, and End Results [**SEER**] Program) to develop the model. The model gathers information on a woman's first-degree female relatives, her personal reproductive history, and her medical history to estimate her risk for developing invasive breast cancer over specific periods of time. Originally, the model was reliable only for Caucasian women, but it has recently been updated to assess risk for African-American women, although it may still underestimate risk for African-American women who have had a breast biopsy (Gail, Costantino, & Pee, et al., 2007). There are some significant limitations to the Gail model: It has not yet been validated in ethnic groups other than Caucasian and African American, it does not assess the age of onset of breast cancer, and it includes only first-degree female relatives. These limitations may result in a significant underestimation of risk, particularly in families of mixed ancestry, who have cancer in the paternal side, or whose family members have developed early onset breast cancer (Evans and Howell, 2007).

Claus and his colleagues developed a breast cancer risk assessment model based on data from a large case-control study conducted by the Centers for Disease Control during the 1980s. The Claus model is primarily used in genetic specialty clinic settings to assess cancer risk in individuals from families that do not have known hereditary breast cancer susceptibility genes but have numerous occurrences of breast and ovarian cancer. Unlike the Gail model, one advantage of the Claus model is that it includes the age at breast cancer diagnosis of first- or second-degree relatives and paternal family history. The Claus model has some major limitations. It does not include any nonhereditary risk factors (e.g., mantle radiation exposure) and its risk tables reflect breast cancer risk for American women in the 1980s, which are lower than the current incidence. As mentioned earlier, it is best used in genetic clinics because experience in primary care settings found that it substantially underestimated risks (Evans & Howell, 2007).

In the late 1990s Drs. Parmigiani, Berry, and Aguilar from Duke University published a breast cancer risk assessment tool called **BRCAPRO** that calculates the likelihood that an individual carries a BRCA1 or BRCA2 mutation. The model applies to both men and women, and incorporates family history, any known BRCA genetic information, personal history of cancer, and the known cancer penetrance in anyone with a BRCA mutation. The advantage of the BRCAPRO model is that it considers both affected and unaffected relatives, and estimates the likelihood of an individual having BRCA1 or BRCA2 mutations. Some major problems with the model are that none of the non-hereditary risk factors (no history of breastfeeding, early menarche, radiation, etc.) can be incorporated, and no other genetic mutations are accounted for (Cowden syndrome, etc.). As a result, the BRCAPRO tool underestimates risk in families who only have breast cancer (note breast and ovarian cancers are both commonly found in BRCA1 and 2 mutations).

The Tyrer-Cuzick model incorporates family history, estrogen exposure (breastfeeding, early menarche) as well as benign breast disease in its calculations. The model is unique in that it can capture the impact of multiple breast cancer causing genes, not just the BRCA1 and 2 genes. The Tyrer-Cuzick model therefore addresses many of the shortcomings of the other models and provides the most accurate breast cancer risk estimation for high risk patients. This model is complex and should be used by individuals with specialized training.

SECTION THREE REVIEW

1. Which of the following is a breast cancer red flag?
   A. Mother diagnosed with breast cancer at age 75.
   B. Family history reveals only one woman with breast cancer.
   C. Father diagnosed with breast cancer at age 75.
   D. Second cousin (female) once removed diagnosed with breast cancer at age 40.
2. What percentage of stillborn infants has anomalies that may inform future pregnancy risks?
   A. 1%
   B. 2.5%
   C. 10%
   D. 15%
3. The Surgeon General's Family History Tool is available in which of the following languages?
   A. Chinese
   B. Polish
   C. Portuguese
   D. All of the above
4. The Your Disease Risk assessment tool assesses a variety of individual health risks. Who was the tool developed for?
   A. Physicians
   B. Nurses working in outpatient clinics
   C. The lay public
   D. Social workers
5. Which of the four breast cancer risk assessment models should only be used by individuals with specialized training?
   A. Gail
   B. Claus
   C. BRCAPRO
   D. Tryer-Cuzick

Answers: 1. C; 2. D; 3. D; 4. C; 5. D

SECTION FOUR: Future Directions in Risk Assessment

Almost every disease, injury, or illness has a genetic component. While the relationship between cancer and genetics has been clear for many years, and rare single gene disorders such as sickle cell, Huntington disease, and cystic fibrosis are familiar to nurses, scientists have only recently begun to unravel the complex web of interconnections between genetics and the environment in the development of common diseases such as heart disease and diabetes. As more becomes known about the genetic contribution to common disease, nurses must be prepared assist patients understand their risks while helping them develop and implement strategies to reduce that risk. The 2011 "Future of Nursing; Leading Change, Advancing Health" report by the Institute of Medicine clearly identifies the need for nursing educators to include genetics and genomics content to prepare nurses for a genomic future.

An expansion in scientific understanding has increased the number and decreased the cost of genetic tests, but genetic testing is not a novel 21st century concept. Prenatal screening has been offered to expectant couples for nearly 25 years, and newborns have been routinely screened for genetic disorders for over five decades. Each year in the United States, over 4 million newborns are screened for a selected number of genetic disorders. In 2000, newborns were screened for an average of 8 disorders. One decade later, the number had tripled. In the 2011, the average newborn was screened for over 29 disorders, and in some states they are tested for as many as 50 disorders. Many experts predict that within the next 20 years, the cost for sequencing an entire genome will drop below that of newborn screening. When that moment occurs, it will finally become possible to offer truly personalized health care.

Genetic testing, particularly at the whole genome level, comes with an almost infinite number of ethical, legal, and clinical issues. One of the important issues that nurses must often help patients work through is the impact of new genetic information on the family. In a family being screened for inherited breast cancer, for example, one daughter may learn that she did not inherit the mutation, and is at normal (or average) lifetime risk for breast cancer, while her two sisters learn that they carry the mutation. That daughter may now feel somewhat isolated or guilty because she does not face the same decisions and challenges as her sisters. There are some other considerations as well. While most gene mutations only increase disease risk slightly and often involve an environmental trigger (smoking, a risk gene, and lung cancer, for example), in some disorders such as Huntington disease, progression is inevitable and there is no cure. In these cases, people may not seek genetic testing because they prefer not to know, or they may choose to pay for the testing without telling their health care provider because they don't want their health insurer or employer to find out. Nurses must be prepared for a variety of different reactions when genetic testing is discussed because an individual's response is dependent not only on the perceived likelihood of it occurring to them, but also on the perceived seriousness of the event. Chapter 9 discusses many of the ethical, legal, and social issues inherent when considering testing an individual for a genetic disease or predisposition to disease.

SECTION FOUR REVIEW

1. Which of the following diseases is likely to have been influenced by genetics?
   A. Cancer
   B. Heart disease
   C. Accidents
   D. All of the above

2. How many genetic disorders were most newborns being screened for in 2011?
   A. 19
   B. 29
   C. 39
   D. 49

Answers: 1. D; 2. B

POSTTEST

1. Which is NOT a health risk category?
   A. Low risk
   B. Population risk
   C. High risk
   D. Extremely high risk
2. Risk assessment for nurses involves
   A. identifying all the attributes of risk.
   B. gathering information about the risk.
   C. developing a personalized plan of care.
   D. All of the above
3. Which of the following environmental attributes increase an individual's risk for an adverse health outcome?
   A. Exercising for 30 minutes a day, 6 days a week
   B. Maintaining a healthy body weight
   C. Being raised in a home built in 1928
   D. Wearing seatbelts
4. Epigenetic pathways
   A. initiate and maintain gene expression and function.
   B. cause mutations to occur.
   C. are only active during embryogenesis.
   D. are not influenced by diet.
5. Which ethnic group is at increased risk for inheriting a BRCA mutation (increasing risk for breast cancer)?
   A. Asian
   B. African
   C. Hispanic
   D. Ashkenazi Jewish
6. In the near future, it is expected that risk assessment is likely to evolve from population-based screening to
   A. genome sequencing.
   B. mitochondrial patterning.
   C. karyotyping.
   D. pharmacogenomics.
7. Mary Rogers completed a detailed family history at age 12, and that baseline document is now part of her medical record. In addition to periodic updates, there are times when a more detailed genetic risk assessment should be considered. Which of the following times would it be appropriate to conduct a more detailed genetic risk assessment?
   A. When she is considering pregnancy.
   B. After her first baby is born.
   C. When her sister is diagnosed with breast cancer at age 36.
   D. All of the above

8. What is the percentage of children that are diagnosed with one or more major anomalies by age 7?
   A. 8%
   B. 16%
   C. 24%
   D. 32%
9. The Framingham Heart Disease Risk Calculator is a good tool to use in people who have already had a heart attack, because it accurately predicts their risk for having another cardiac event.
   A. True
   B. False

10. Which risk model is more appropriate to use if many members of the family on the paternal side have had breast or ovarian cancer?
   A. Gail
   B. Claus

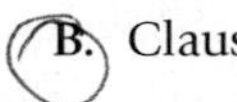

Posttest answers are located in the Appendix.

CHAPTER SUMMARY

The concept of risk assessment in health care emerged in the United States in the mid-1970s, and since then a number of reliable risk assessment models have become available. The intended use for all of them is to identify at-risk individuals or populations before illness or injury occurs. Risk assessment using genetic information is the most recent addition to the health care risk assessment toolkit. It is anticipated that as more is learned about the genetics of different diseases, more tools that are based on genetic markers will be developed to help identify individuals at increased risk for disease years or decades before the disease develops.

Nurses are expected to assume several different roles in genetic health care. Nurses are expected to be lifelong learners so that they can remain knowledgeable about advances in health care. They must consider how diseases and pre-symptomatic testing might impact the physical and mental health of individuals, families, and communities. Nurses should recognize red flags in the family history, be able to create a three-generation pedigree, and recognize disease patterns. Above all, nurses must be prepared to engage in the interdisciplinary health care system of the future to optimize health outcomes for all individuals.

CRITICAL THINKING CHECKPOINT

The following cases illustrate risk assessment for breast cancer in four different scenarios. Each case has familial red flags that the nurse should try to identify before progressing through the case.

In addition, the cases demonstrate how complex risk assessment can be, and the importance of understanding the strengths/weaknesses and intended uses of various risk assessment tools.

Case 1

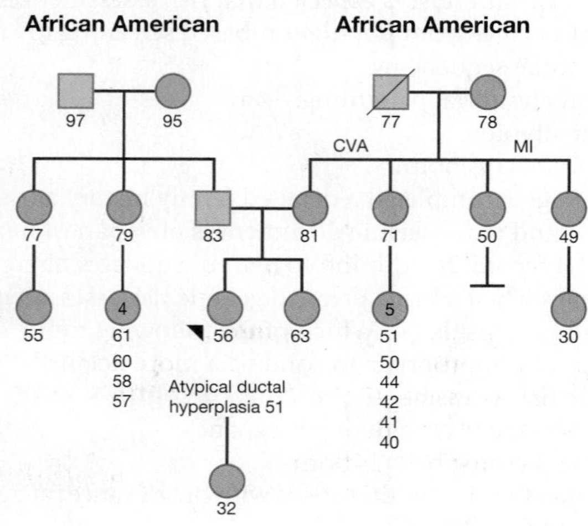

- 56-year-old female of African descent
- Menarche age 12; menopause at age 49; first pregnancy age 24
- No family history of breast cancer
- Two breast biopsies: one benign, one atypical ductal hyperplasia

Question 1: Which risk model is most appropriate to use in this case (Gail or Claus?)

- Cannot use the Claus model because there is no family history of breast cancer.
- The Gail model is appropriate because it takes reproductive history AND breast biopsy history into account.

Question 2: Calculate the 5-year and lifetime Gail scores (http://www.cancer.gov/bcrisktool)

- 5-year: 1.93%; lifetime: 11.18

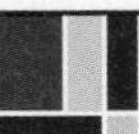

CRITICAL THINKING CHECKPOINT

Case 2

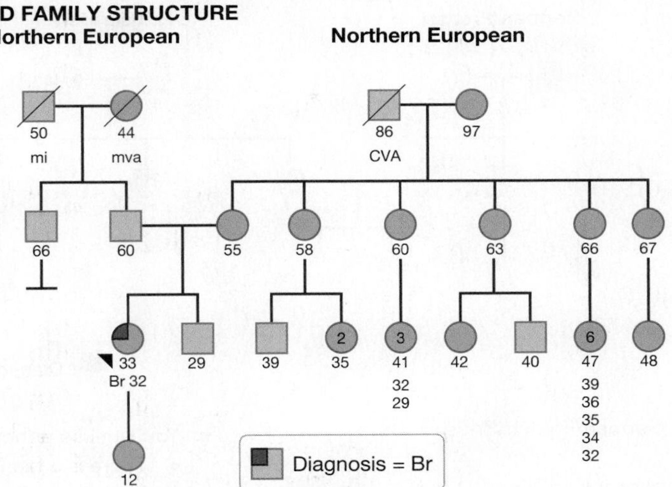

- 33-year-old woman of Northern European descent
- Menarche age 13; not menopausal
- First birth age 21
- Personal history of breast cancer; Dx: age 32
- No family history of breast cancer

Question 1: Which risk model is most appropriate to use in this case (Gail or Claus?)

- Cannot use either model:
  - There is a personal history of breast cancer—there's no point in calculating "risk" when the individual already has the disease.
  - The abbreviated family history is also a red flag and should generate a referral.

Case 3

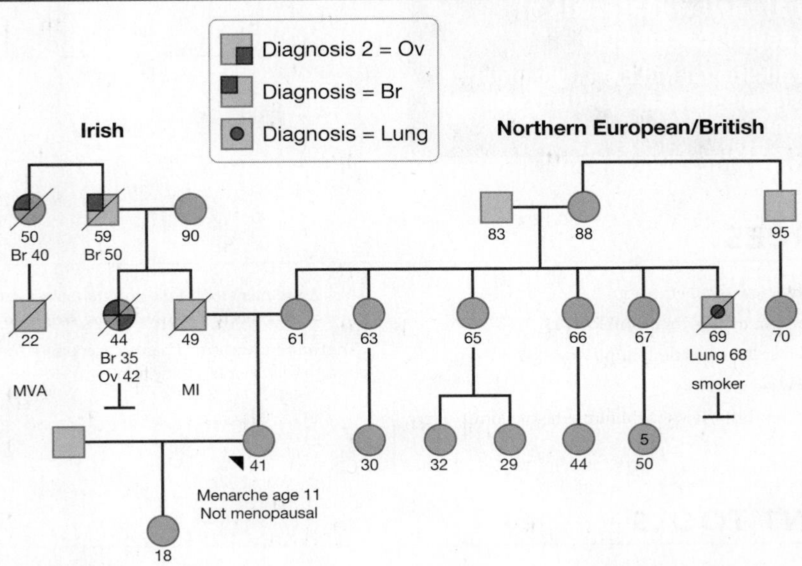

- 41-year-old female of Irish/British descent
- Menarche age 13; not menopausal; first pregnancy age 23

Paternal History:

- Aunt: breast cancer Dx 35; ovarian cancer Dx 42; died 44
- Grandfather: breast cancer Dx: 50; died age 59
- Great Aunt: breast cancer age 40; died age 50

Maternal history:

- Uncle: lung cancer age 68 (deceased age 69)

Question 1: Which risk model is most appropriate to use in this case (Gail or Claus?)

- You cannot use either model.
  - Male breast cancer is an automatic referral (so you can't use the Claus model)
  - The disease is on the paternal side (so you can't use the Gail model)

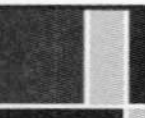

CRITICAL THINKING CHECKPOINT *(Continued)*

Case 4

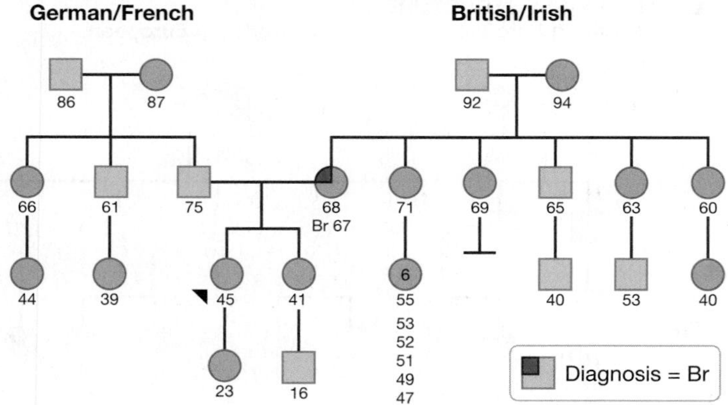

- 45-year-old woman of German/French/British/Irish descent
- Menarche 14; not menopausal; no biopsies
- First birth age 22
- Mother age 68 with BRCA; Dx: age 67

Question 1: Which risk model is most appropriate to use in this case (Gail or Claus?)

- You can use either one.
  - There is a family history so you can use Claus
  - The disease is on the maternal side and the patient has no personal history of breast cancer so you can use Gail

Question 2: What are the empiric risk estimates?

- You calculate them both and use the highest estimate.

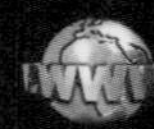

Pearson Nursing Student Resources

Find additional review materials at nursing.pearsonhighered.com

Prepare for success with additional NCLEX®-style practice questions, interactive assignments and activities, web links, animations, videos, and more!

ONLINE RESOURCES

Center for Jewish Genetics: http://www.jewishgenetics.org

Genes and Disease: http://www.ncbi.nlm.nih.gov/books/nbk22183

Genetics/Genomics Competency Center for Education: http://www.g-2-c-2.org

Gene Tests/Gene Reviews: http://www.genetests.org

Online Mendelian Inheritance in Man: http://www.ncbi.nlm.nih.gov/entrez/query.fcgi?db=OMIM

Risk Assessment tools for colorectal cancer: http://www.cancer.gov/colorectalcancerrisk/tool.aspx; http://digestive.ccf.org/scores/go

The Future of Medicine, Pharmacogenomics: An Online Course: http://www.lithiumstudios.com/fda/Sample_Home.htm

RISK ASSESSMENT TOOLS

Center for Disease Control and Prevention: Family Health History: http://www.cdc.gov/genomics/famhistory/index.htm

Genetic Alliance: Family Health History: http://www.geneticalliance.org/fhh

Surgeon General's Family Health History Initiative: My Family Health Portrait Tool: http://www.hhs.gov/familyhistory/portrait/index.html

REFERENCES

Arar, N., Seo, J., Abboud, H., Parchman, M., & Noell, P. (2010). Providers' behavioral beliefs regarding the delivery of genomic medicine at the Veterans' Health Administration. *Personalized Medicine, 7*(5), 385–494.

Berg, A., Baird, M., Botkin, J., Driscol, D., Fishman, P., Guarino, P, & Willaims, J. (2009). National Institutes of Health State-of-the-science Conference Statement: Family history and improving health. *Annals of Internal Medicine, 151*(12), 872–877.

Berliner, J., & Fay, M. (2007). Risk assessment and genetic counseling for hereditary breast and ovarian cancer: Recommendations of the National Society of Genetic Counselors. *Journal of Genetic Counselors, 16*(3), 241–260.

Braveman, P., Egerter, S., & Williams, D. (2011). The social determinants of health: Coming of Age. *Annual Public Health Reviews, 32*, 381–398.

Budnitz, D. S., Shehab, N., Kegler, S. R., & Richards, C. L. (2007). Medication use leading to emergency department visits for adverse drug events in older adults. *Annals of Internal Medicine, 147*(11), 755–765.

Calzone, K., Cashion, A., Feetham, S., Jenkins, J., Prows, C., & Wung, S. (2010). Nurses transforming health care using genetic and genomics. *Nursing Outlook, 58*(1), 26–35.

Campbell, R., & Berger, S. (2006). Preventing pediatric sudden cardiac death: Where do we start? *Pediatrics, 118*(2), 802–804.

Centers for Disease Control and Prevention. (2011). *Pediatric Genetics*. Retrieved on July 5, 2012, from http://www.cdc.gov/ncbddd/pediatricgenetics/genetics_workshop/detecting.html

Chugh, S. S., Reinier, K., Teodorescu, C., Evanado, A., Kehr, E., Al Samara, M., & Jui, J. (2008). Epidemiology of sudden cardiac death: Clinical and research implications. *Progress in Cardiovascular Disease, 51*(3), 213–228.

Connor, C. A., Wright, C. C., & Fegan, C. D. (2002). The safety and effectiveness of a nurse-led anticoagulant service. *Journal of Advanced Nursing, 38*(4), 407–415.

Darr, A. S. (2010). Vision of a personal genomics future. *Nature, 643*(21), 298–299.

Evans, D. G. R., & Howell, A. (2007). Breast cancer risk-assessment models, *Breast Cancer Research* 9. 213.

Gail, M. H., Costantino, J. P., Pee, D., Bondy, M., Newman, L., Selvan, M., et al. (2007). Projecting individualized absolute invasive breast cancer risk in African American women. *Journal of the National Cancer Institute, 99*(23), 1782–1792.

Gelineau-van Waes, J., Starr, L., Maadoc, J., Aleman, F., Voss, K., Wilberding, J., & Riley, R. (2005). Maternal fumonisin exposure and risk for neural tube defects: Mechanisms in an in vivo mouse model. *Birth Defects Research, 73*(Part A), 487–497.

Human Genome Project Information. (2011). *Potential benefits of the Human Genome Project research*. Retrieved on July 5, 2012, from http://www.ornl.gov/sci/techresources/Human_Genome/project/benefits.shtml

IOM (Institute of Medicine). (2009). *Innovations in service delivery in the age of genomics*. Washington, DC: The National Academies Press.

IOM (Institute of Medicine). (2011). *The future of nursing: Leading change, advancing health*. Washington, DC: The National Academies Press. Retrieved July 5, 2012, from http://www.nap.edu/catalog.php?record_id=12956

Jenkins, J., & Lea, D. H. (2005). *Nursing care in the genomic era: A case based approach*. Sudbury, MA: Jones and Bartlett.

Keuhn, B. (2011). Scientists see promise and challenges in translating genomics into the clinic. *JAMA, 305*(13), 1285–1286.

Lashley, F. (2007). *Essentials of clinical genetic practice*. New York: Springer.

Lea, D., Skirton, H., Read, C., & Williams, J. (2011). Implications for education the next generation of nurses on genetics and genomics in the 21st century. *Journal of Nursing Scholarship, 43*(1), 3–12.

National Coalition for Health Care Professionals in Genetics (n.d., a). *Communicating risk fact sheet*. Retrieved July 5, 2012, from http://www.nchpeg.org/index.php?option=com_content&view=article&id=58:communicating-risk-fact-sheet&catid=36:point-of-care&Itemid=76

National Coalition for Health Care Professionals in Genetics (n.d., b). *Assigning risk categories and modifying management*. Retrieved July 5, 2012, from http://www.nchpeg.org/index.php?option=com_content&view=article&id=169&Itemid=64

Seibert, D. (2010). Genetics and health promotion/disease prevention: Complimentary or contradictory? *The Journal for Nurse Practitioners, 6*(7), 507–515.

Shimabukuro, T. T., Kramer, J., & McGuire, M. (2004). Development and implementation of a nurse-managed anticoagulation program. *Journal of Healthcare Quality, 26*(1), 4–12.

Tadmouri, G., Nair, P., Obeid, T., Ali, M., Al Khaja, N., & Hamamy, H. (2009). Consanguinity and reproductive health among Arabs. *Reproductive Health, 6*(17). Retrieved July 5, 2012, from http://www.reproductive-health-journal.com/content/pdf/1742-4755-6-17.pdf

vanVliet, J., Oates, N., & Whitelaw, E. (2007). Epigenetic mechanisms in the context of complex diseases. *Cellular and Molecular Life Sciences, 64*(12), 1531–1538.

Vasan, R. S., Sullivan, L. M., Wilson, P. W., Sempos, C. T., Sundström, J., Kannel, W. B., et al. (2005). Relative importance of borderline and elevated levels of coronary heart disease risk factors. *Annals of Internal Medicine, 142*, 393–402.

Wadelius, M., & Pirmohamed M. (2007). Pharmacogenetics of warfarin: Current status and future challenges. *The Pharmacogenomics Journal, 7*(2), 99–111.

Yoon, P. W., Scheuner, M. T., Jorgensen, C., & Khoury, M. J. (2009). Developing family healthware: A family history screening tool to prevent common chronic diseases. *Preventing Chronic Disease, 6*(1), A33.

Young, I. (2007). *Introduction to risk calculation in genetic counseling* (3rd ed.). New York: Oxford University Press.

PART 5

Genetics of Cancer

CHAPTER 15 Immunogenetics

Linda K. Bennington

LEARNING OUTCOMES

Following the completion of this chapter, the learner will be able to

1. Deliberate aspects of nursing practice that can influence the immune system.
2. Explain the difference between natural and acquired immunity.
3. Describe the general characteristics of the immune system.
4. Discuss the structure of the immune system, types of immune cells, and their products.
5. Review the implications of understanding the genetics of the immune system.
6. Describe the influence of immunogenetics in understanding immune diseases.

This chapter presents the definitions of terms related to immunology and immunogenetics and reviews the general characteristics of the immune system. The chapter focuses on aspects of nursing practice that can influence the immune system. It covers basic immunologic mechanisms, including natural and acquired immunity, and elaborates on the characteristics of the immune system and its structure, type of immune cells, and their products. This chapter also offers a review of the genetics of the immune system and an introduction to immune diseases as potentially influenced by genetics.

PRETEST

1. The first line of defense in protecting the body from infection includes all the following components EXCEPT
   A. unbroken skin.
   B. normal microbial flora.
   C. phagocytic leukocytes.
   D. secretions such as mucus.
2. Natural immunity is characterized as being
   A. innate or inborn.
   B. able specifically to recognize exogenous or endogenous agents.
   C. able selectively to eliminate exogenous or endogenous agents.
   D. part of the first line of body defenses against microbial organisms.
3. Delayed hypersensitivity is also referred to as
   A. humoral immunity.
   B. cell-mediated immunity.
   C. B-cell hypersensitivity.
   D. cytotoxic hypersensitivity.
4. The most immediate and severe manifestation of immediate hypersensitivity reaction is
   A. anaphylaxis.
   B. anaphylactoid.
   C. itching.
   D. sneezing.
5. Immediate hypersensitivity consists of the reactions primarily mediated by the ______ class of immunoglobulins.
   A. IgM
   B. IgG
   C. IgE
   D. IgA
6. Components of the cellular natural immune system include
   A. mast cells, neutrophils, and lymphocytes.
   B. macrophages, mast cells, and neutrophils.
   C. neutrophils, mucus, and mast cells.
   D. mast cells, interferons, and neutrophils.
7. Components of the humoral natural immune system include
   A. complement, lysozyme, and interferons.
   B. lysozyme, mucus, and complement.
   C. macrophages, complement, and lysozyme.
   D. complement, lymphocytes, and lysozyme.
8. Another term for adaptive immunity is
   A. antigenic immunity.
   B. acquired immunity.
   C. lymphocyte reactive immunity.
   D. phagocytosis.

9. Humoral components of the adaptive immune system include
   A. T lymphocytes.
   B. B lymphocytes.
   C. antibodies.
   D. saliva.

10. Which type of antibody is capable of placental transfer?
   A. IgM
   B. IgG
   C. IgA
   D. IgD

Pretest answers are located in the Appendix.

SECTION ONE: Nursing Practice and the Immune System

In the preface of her *Notes on Hospitals,* Florence Nightingale stated, "It may seem a strange principle to enunciate as the very first requirement in a Hospital that it should do the sick no harm (1863, p. iii)." With the present day focus on improving safety in health care, Nightingale's words are as pertinent today as they were almost 150 years ago. Interestingly, Nightingale's influence on nursing practice as to the proper use of "fresh air, light, warmth, cleanliness, quiet, and the proper selection and administration of diet—all at the least expense of vital power to the patient (1859, p. 6)" is also relevant in today's practice of nursing because these actions can serve to boost the immune system. Extrapolating Nightingale's philosophy to present day nursing, evidence-based research offers strategies that can be used to facilitate healing through nurse/patient interactions.

Research has scientifically established that the link between mind and body is not only intuitive but also physiological. Biochemical substances termed **neuropeptides** function as neuroendocrine messengers that journey from the brain to each cell in the body, where they bind to receptor sites found on the surface. Neuropeptides assist in the functioning of the body's autonomic nervous system to regulate primarily involuntary processes that include the immune system and endocrine system as well as other bodily functions, such as pulse, respiration, perspiration, digestion, and blood circulation. This system of messenger molecules and receptors represents the physiological connection between mind, body, and emotions, and these chemicals are found in every cell in the body. Therefore, the body's structure can be viewed as a single neuroendocrine system, which regulates the internal state through nutrition, metabolism, excretion, water and salt balance, reaction to external stimuli, regulation of growth, development, reproduction, and reduction or storage of energy (Pert, 1997; Kiecolt-Glaser, McGuire, Robles, & Glaser, 2002; Cousins Center for Psychoneuroimmunology, 2011).

From this viewpoint, it is perceived that the neuroendocrine system serves to protect the body from threats, whether inside or outside; the hormones that are the most active in achieving this goal are stress hormones. **Psychoneuroimmunology (PNI)** has studied these stress interactions between psychological processes and the nervous and immune systems, but this new research goes a step further to include not only the physical environment, but the social as well. Thus, the positive and negative effects of stress hormones, prenatally and through the end of life, have forged research in a field termed *social genomics*.

While it is known that our genes can directly influence health and behavior, it has also become obvious that the environment affects genes, forcing some to turn on and others to turn off. When the human genome was completely mapped at the beginning of this century, it was believed that we now had deciphered the code for building all parts of the body. It was soon discovered, however, that the genome was only half the story. There are two modifications that affect DNA, and one includes the biochemical modification termed *methylation*. The other involves the fact that DNA is wrapped around proteins called histones, which are covered with chemical tags. This second structural layer is called the **epigenome**, which shapes the physical structure of the genome. It tightly wraps inactive genes, making them unreadable, and relaxes active genes, making them easily accessible. Different sets of genes are active in different cell types. The DNA code remains fixed for life but the epigenome is flexible. Epigenetic tags react to signals from the outside world such as diet and stress and thus control the inheritance phenomenon of being switched on or off. The epigenome adjusts specific genes in our genomic background in response to our rapidly changing environment, which, in turn, affects our phenotype (University of Utah, 2012).

In an examination of how chronic adversity (stress, poverty, and loneliness) affects immune function at the genetic level, Azar (2011) determined that it leads to health problems in the long term, including an increased risk of heart disease and some types of cancer. Further research revealed those genes, which were overexpressed in chronically lonely people and adults who experienced childhood adversity, originated in a myeloid line of immune cells that are quite old in evolutionary terms. These cells scan the body for damaged tissue and mount inflammatory responses as a first line of defense against infections. An additional finding was that genes in B-lymphocytes, which are cells that typically fight viruses and are evolutionarily young, were less active. Research such as this, to determine the effects of environmental triggers on gene expression, can be extrapolated to what some scientists believe is a paradigm shift in examining the epigenome. The chemical tags on the epigenetic structure have been found to play a significant role in disease formation and are passed on from our ancestors.

Research does exist that has examined the existence of transgenerational responses to environmental triggers and, specifically, from census data with linked periods of famine during a paternal grandfather's life to the mortality risk ratio of his grandson. Likewise, a paternal grandmother's food supply was associated with the granddaughter's mortality risk ratio. An additional transgenerational study found that early paternal smoking initiated before the age of 11 was associated not only with an earlier birth, but also with a higher body mass index in sons (but not in daughters). These transgenerational effects were observed with exposure during the slow growth period of both grandparents or fetal/infant life (grandmothers) but not during either grandparent's puberty. It was postulated that these responses add a new dimension to the study of gene–environment interactions in development and health (Pembrey et al., 2006).

Epidemiological investigators at Washington State University have provided evidence that environmental exposures early in life can cause a predisposition to disease in later life. Furthermore, these environmental effects seem to be passed on through subsequent generations, which could lead to disease phenotypes (Jirtle & Skinner, 2007). The implications of this research is that the exposure of a grandmother to a **toxin** is passed on to her grandchild. The lives of our ancestors are passed on to us and reach into every aspect of our own lives. Therefore, as Marcus Pembrey said, "Live your life as a guardian of your genome." (BBC, Horizon Interview, 2009).

To work within the domain of social genomics, it is beneficial to develop methods of dealing with stress as one environmental trigger. A review of the lines of evidence for mind–body communication can be simplified into an understanding of neuropeptides and the neuroendocrine system:

1. Nerve endings are embedded in the tissues of the immune system, so it follows that changes in the central nervous system (brain and spinal cord) would alter immune responses.
2. Likewise, when an immune response is triggered, central nervous system activity is also altered.
3. Changes in hormone and neurotransmitter levels will similarly alter immune activity, and immune activity will alter hormone and neurotransmitter levels.
4. Lymphocytes can produce both hormones and neurotransmitters.
5. Activated lymphocytes produce neuropeptides recognized by the central nervous system.
6. Psychosocial factors alter the susceptibility to or progression of autoimmune and infectious diseases.
7. Immunologic reactivity can be influenced by stress.
8. Immunologic reactivity can be influenced by relaxation techniques, hypnosis, and biologically targeted imagery.
9. Immunologic reactivity can be modulated by classical conditioning.
10. Psychoactive drugs and drug abuse influence immune function.
11. Stress can interfere with the effectiveness of immunizations.

The implications for nursing inherent within this research is to not only have a basic understanding of the immune system and how it works but also to be aware of stressors that could affect a patient's status. The nursing theorist Jean Watson emphasized being aware of caring and intentionality in any given moment at an individual and system level as a means to enhance the well-being of patient and caregiver. A nurse should not only be aware of the state of mind embedded within her or his thought processes but recognize the thought processes and circumstances of the individual being for whom they are caring. The research being done in social genomics is opening a new realm of possibilities for healing as it pertains to the environment in which we live, work, and are cared for when ill.

Several activities have been suggested as a means of strengthening the immune system, and they would work well for both the caregiver and the patient. These activities include the following and are discussed in detail in this section.

a. Nutrition
b. Laughter
c. Music
d. Group support
e. Counseling
f. Journaling

Nutrition

What we eat, how we eat, and when we eat are all factors that influence the state of our bodily functions. Throughout the past decades, there have been proponents of various diets claiming to possess the panacea of a healthy life, but they generally faded into oblivion. In an attempt to establish a scientific basis for dietary claims, José Ordovas, director of the Nutrition and Genomics Laboratory at Tufts University, began to research the connection between our genes and how we live: i.e., environmental triggers that include nutrition. Popularly known in the media as the DNA diet, this new field of nutrigenomics has demonstrated that broad dietary recommendations are not necessarily good for all people and could in some cases do harm. Dr. Ordovas asserts, based on cases studied thus far, that appropriate dietary or behavioral changes can cancel increased risks for disease and he envisions this becoming a practical application and routine approach to therapy (Bambrick, 2011). With this background knowledge, nurses can encourage patients to keep a daily food diary that includes not only what they eat, but when they eat and why they eat. With the understanding that environmental triggers can precipitate disease, the nurse and patient can collaborate on dietary changes that include not only food consumption but how and where it is consumed as indicated by the food diary.

Laughter

In 1964, Norman Cousins, former editor of the *Saturday Review,* was diagnosed with anklyosing spondylitis, a connective tissue disease considered to be incurable at that time. Refusing to accept this fact, Cousins went on to try various other means to overcome his condition, one of which was laughter. His case was published in the *Journal of the American Medical Association* in 1989, which lent some credibility to his strategies. With the advent of social genomics, it is now recognized that stress plays a large role in health and disease, and techniques that serve as stress reducers do promote healthy outcomes.

Vascular research involving laughter stimuli demonstrated a 22% increase in blood flow via vasodilatation while stress decreased blood flow by 35% (Vascular Medicine, 2006). Laughter has also been shown to affect the release of various immune mediators, such as interferon, through the hypothalamic-pituitary-adrenal (HPA) axis and neural supply of lymphoid tissues (Martin, 2002). More recent research encourages clinicians to incorporate laughter history into their general medical history taking as a means of documenting a correlation between laughter and emotional well-being (Hasan & Hasan, 2009). Whether or not it is possible to provide means of laughter via funny videos or books, the nurse can certainly intercede to reduce stressful stimuli for each individual with whom contact is made by maintaining a caring and sincere attitude.

Music

The power of music therapy has come to the forefront due to its role in helping Congresswoman Gabrielle Giffords recover from her serious brain injury. Scientific research has shown that music therapy helps stroke patients regain speech, may improve heart and respiratory rates and blood pressure, reduce anxiety and pain in cancer and leukemia patients, and actually impact the structure of the brain (Ifill & Johnson, 2012). Nursing researchers have noted the significance of the therapeutic use of music with and without a nurse's presence for cancer patients. Whereas it was beneficial in each scenario, it was found to be more beneficial when a nurse was present with the patient (Hui-Ling, Yin-Ming, & Li-Hua, 2012). This speaks to nursing presence as an essential component to holistic care, especially when implementing various forms of interventions.

Support Groups

The importance and benefits of support groups have long been noted not only in the nursing literature but also by social workers, psychologists, and other medical providers. Nurses should research areas for support groups and provide information about peer support through not only traditional face-to-face support groups but also in online communities.

Counseling

It is important for the nurse to understand that the spectrum of inheritable genetic illness challenges individuals and their families not only in the aspect of health management but also on a very personal level. It is an intensely complex emotional experience that can produce guilt and ambiguity in terms of family planning. Genetic counseling is covered in Chapter 11.

Journaling

Journal writing is an active means of providing focus and insight on issues and concerns within one's life. It provides a channel of self-exploration and introspection to deepen the process of self-reflection regarding actions, ideals, and principles that support life's choices. Additional alternatives that nurses could suggest are blog sites dedicated to various related topics, as well as support groups.

SECTION ONE REVIEW

1. Stress can alter the functioning of the immune system prenatally as well as after birth.
   A. True
   B. False
2. Neuropeptides are all of the following EXCEPT
   A. short chains of amino acids.
   B. neurotransmitters.
   C. modulators of synaptic activity.
   D. proteins with quaternary structures.
3. All of the following can strengthen the immune system EXCEPT
   A. music.
   B. laughter.
   C. pain.
   D. writing.
4. Genes and the environment are separate entities.
   A. True
   B. False
5. Social genomics will provide insight into how early life conditions relate to health and behavior.
   A. True
   B. False

Answers: 1. A; 2. D; 3. C; 4. B; 5. A

SECTION TWO: Basic Immunologic Mechanisms

Historically, the science of immunology arose from the knowledge that those who survived a common infectious disease of the past rarely contracted the disease again. The function of the immune system is to basically recognize self from nonself in order to defend the body against nonself. **Immunity** or the **immune response** is a reaction to foreign substances, which include microbes as well as macromolecules (such as proteins and polysaccharides) regardless of the physiologic or pathologic consequences of the reaction. Immunology is the study of the molecules, cells, **organs**, and systems responsible for the recognition and disposal of the nonself material and, in a broader sense, of the cellular and molecular events that occur after an **organism** encounters microbes and other macromolecules. Immunogenetics is the scientific discipline that studies the genetic control of those moieties that elicit the immune response—i.e., an individual's ability to respond to a foreign substance within the body.

First Line of Defense

Recognition of the human body as an ideal setting for the growth of microbes, such as bacteria, viruses, **parasites**, and fungi, leads to the understanding that the body has a variety of barrier-assisting defenses to protect against the invasion of these organisms. The first barrier to these infections is intact skin and mucosal membrane surfaces. Not only does the keratinization of the skin's upper layer prevent invasion, but the common flora microorganisms that normally inhabit the skin serve to deter penetration or facilitate elimination of foreign microbes. Fatty acids in sweat also serve to inhibit the growth of bacteria on skin. Thus, skin is generally penetrable only through cuts or tiny abrasions. The secretions of mucus-adhering membranes in the nose and nasopharynx likewise serve to trap microorganisms, which can then be expelled through coughing or sneezing. Additionally, tears and saliva have chemical properties that defend the body in the form of the enzymes lysozyme and **phospholipase**, which attack and destroy the cell wall of susceptible bacteria—in particular, gram positive bacteria.

Microbes that do breach the body's frontline defenses would next encounter the walls of the digestive, respiratory, or urogenital passageways, which are lined with tightly packed epithelial cells covered in a layer of mucus. This mucus layer effectively blocks the transport of many pathogens into deeper cell layers. Mucosal surfaces secrete a special class of an immunoglobulin antibody called IgA, which in many cases is the first type of antibody to encounter an invading microbe. IgA is also one of the protective substances found in tears and saliva. Additional factors in the frontline defense include defensins, which are low molecular weight proteins found in the lung and gastrointestinal tract that possess antimicrobial activity; and surfactants in the lung, which act as **opsonins** (substances that promote **phagocytosis** of particles by phagocytic cells).

In the event an organism is successful in penetrating the body's physical barriers, an evolved network system of cells, tissues, and organs initiate a defense against this invasion.

Innate Immunity

Innate (natural or inborn) **immunity** comprises the cellular and biochemical defense mechanisms that are in place even before infection occurs. It is primed for a rapid response to infections through receptor molecules located on the surfaces of innate immune system cells that identify distinctive structures of pathogens not found in the host. These mechanisms respond only to microbes and not to noninfectious substances. They respond in essentially the same manner to repeated infections because they are specific for features shared by groups of related microbes. Consequently, the innate system may not be capable of recognizing every possible antigen, but may focus on a few large groups of microorganisms that possess **pathogen-associated molecular patterns** (**PAMPS**). The receptors that discern these PAMPS are called **pattern recognition receptors** (**PRR**); an example is **toll-like receptors** (**TLR**). TLRs are a class of proteins with single membrane spanning receptors that identify structurally conserved molecules that have been derived from microbes. Elements of innate immunity include phagocytic cells, **complement**, and **natural killer cells** (**NKC**). Despite their limited specificity, these components are vital because they are primarily responsible for natural immunity to many environmental microorganisms.

Phagocytic cells, which serve to engulf invading foreign material, constitute the major cellular component of the innate system. Complement proteins, which are peptides in the blood that produce inflammatory effects and lysis of cells, are the major **humoral** component. Other humoral components include lysozymes and **interferons** (**IFNs**), which belong to a large class of glycoproteins called **cytokines** and are produced rapidly by many cells in response to viral infection.

Adaptive Immunity

In the event the innate immune system is overwhelmed by infection, a more specialized component of the immune response known as the adaptive (acquired) immune system is activated. In contrast to innate immunity, **adaptive immunity** is not only stimulated by exposure to infectious agents, but the response increases in magnitude and defensive abilities with each consecutive exposure. As its name implies, this part of the immune system is capable of changing, or adapting, to features of the invading microorganism in order to mount a more effective response. Significant characteristics of adaptive immunity include its exacting specificity for distinct molecules as well as the capacity to remember and respond more vigorously to repeated exposures of the same microbe. Additionally, it is capable of recognizing and reacting to a large number of microbial and nonmicrobial substances and has the amazing ability to distinguish among different, even closely related, microbes and molecules. Foreign substances that induce specific immune responses or are the targets of such responses are called **antigens**.

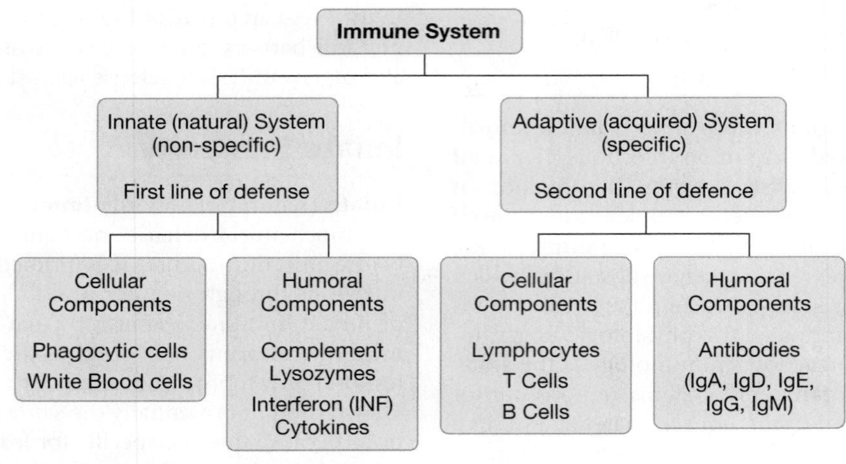

Figure 15–1 ■ Overview of the immune system

The major cellular component of acquired immunity is the **lymphocyte**, and the major humoral component is the **antibody**. Lymphocytes selectively respond to nonself materials—i.e., antigens—which leads to immune memory and a permanently altered pattern of response or adaptation to the environment. Thus, when an individual lymphocyte interfaces an antigen that binds to its unique antigen receptor site, activation and propagation of that lymphocyte occur. This is referred to as **clonal selection** and is responsible for the basic properties of the adaptive system.

The majority of actions within these two categories, **cell-mediated immunity (CMI)** and **humoral immunity**, are exerted by the interaction of the phagocytic cells (natural immunity) and of **T cell lymphocytes** with macrophages (CMI) and antibodies with complement (humoral). It is in this manner that the innate and adaptive responses are components of an integrated system of host defense in which numerous cells and molecules function cooperatively (Figure 15–1 ■).

Protective immunity against a microbe may be induced by the host's response to the microbe or by the transfer of antibodies or lymphocytes specific for the microbe. **Active immunity** refers to immunity that is induced by exposure to a foreign antigen because the host had an active role in responding to the antigen. The purpose of a vaccine is to stimulate active immunity and to create an immune memory so that exposure to the active disease microorganism will stimulate an already primed immune system to fight the disease. Most vaccines can be divided into two types: live, attenuated vaccines and nonreplicating vaccines. Traditionally prepared vaccines were preparations of inactivated (killed) or live, attenuated (weakened) microbes. Newer synthetic vaccines use subunit vaccines, conjugate vaccines, and DNA vaccines. The subunit vaccines are those consisting of components of the pathogens together with adjuvants, which serve to amplify the immune response. Immunity can also be conferred to an individual by transferring serum antibodies from a specifically immunized person. This is referred to as **passive immunity** and it occurs naturally when a mother's antibodies are transferred to the fetus.

Immune Tolerance

As previously noted, the ability of the immune response to distinguish between what is self and what is nonself is an essential process that serves to protect the host. Every cell in the host's body carries a pattern of self-markers, a set of distinctive surface proteins that serve to discern between self and nonself. This coexistence between the immune system and other body cells is known as a state of **self-tolerance**. This set of unique markers on human cells is called the **major histocompatibility complex (MHC)**. MHC marker proteins are as distinct as blood types and come in two categories: MHC Class I and MHC Class II. The MHC is referred to as the **human leukocyte antigen (HLA)** system in humans because its gene products were originally identified on white blood cells. The MHC has six genes that encode the class I molecules HLA-A, HLA –B, HLA-C, HLA-E, HLA-F, and HLA-G. Among these, HLA-A, HLA –B, and HLA-C are the most important. Five loci encode the class II molecules, and they are designated as HLA-DP, HLA –DQ, HLA-DR, HLA-DM, and HLA-DO. Among these, HLA-DP, HLA –DQ, and HLA-DR are the most important (Mayer & Nyland, 2011). These antigens are second only to the ABO antigens in influencing the survival or **graft rejection** of transplanted organs.

Those foreign substances, antigens, that trigger an immune response, can be a whole nonself cell, a bacterium, a **virus**, an MHC marker protein, or even a portion of a protein from a foreign organism. The distinctive markers on antigens that trigger an immune response are called **epitopes**. When tissues or cells from another individual enter a body carrying these antigenic nonself epitopes, an immune response is triggered. Thus, transplanted tissues are construed as being foreign, antibodies bind to them, and they are rejected.

Self-tolerance can be brought about in at least two ways—central **tolerance** and peripheral tolerance. Central tolerance occurs during lymphocyte development when an immune cell is exposed to many of the self-molecules in the body. Should an encounter occur prior to maturation, an internal self-destruct pathway is activated and the immune cell dies. This process, called **clonal deletion**, ensures that those T cells and B cells, which could develop the ability to destroy the body's own cells, do not mature and attack healthy tissues.

With peripheral tolerance, circulating lymphocytes may recognize a self-molecule but be incapable of responding to it due to an absence of chemical signals required to activate the T or B cell. This is termed **clonal anergy** and it keeps potentially harmful lymphocytes switched off. An additional means of peripheral tolerance involves a special class of regulatory T cells that inhibit helper or cytotoxic T-cell activation by self-antigens.

SECTION TWO REVIEW

1. A pathogen is an antigen.
   A. True
   B. False
2. Immediately following a break in the skin, phagocytes engulf bacteria within the wound. This is an example of an _________ immune response, which is _________ against a pathogen.
   A. adaptive; specific
   B. innate; specific
   C. innate; nonspecific
   D. adaptive; nonspecific
3. An synonym for an antigenic determinant is
   A. immunogen.
   B. epitope.
   C. binding site.
   D. polysaccharide.
4. Antigenic substances can be composed of
   A. large polysaccharides.
   B. proteins.
   C. glycoproteins.
   D. All of the above
5. The immunogenicity of an antigen depends greatly on
   A. its biochemical composition.
   B. being structurally unstable.
   C. its degree of foreignness.
   D. having low molecular weights.

Answers: 1. A; 2. C; 3. B; 4. D; 5. C.

SECTION THREE: Structure of the Immune System

The structure of the immune system involves organs that are positioned throughout the body (Figure 15–2 ■). They are termed **lymphoid organs** because they serve as home to lymphocytes, which are the small, white blood cells crucial for the functioning of the immune system. Within these organs, the lymphocytes grow, develop, and are deployed. The definitive source of all blood cells, including lymphocytes, is the bone marrow, which is the soft tissue in the hollow center of bones. These white blood cells, also referred to as **leukocytes**, are much less numerous than red cells with a ratio between the two of approximately 1:700. Unlike red blood cells, leukocytes have nuclei and participate in protecting the body from infection. Lymphocytes are one of the five kinds of leukocytes circulating in the blood. Although mature lymphocytes appear to be very similar under the microscope, they are extraordinarily diverse in their functions. The most abundant lymphocytes are the **B lymphocytes (B cells)** and the T lymphocytes (T cells), and both have their origin in the bone marrow. The precursors of T cells, however, leave the bone marrow and mature in the thymus, an organ that lays behind the breastbone—hence the term *T lymphocytes*, or just *T cells* (See "Cells of the Immune System," later in this chapter).

The spleen is a flattened organ located in the upper left of the abdomen. Like the **lymph nodes**, the spleen contains specialized compartments where immune cells gather and confront antigens. Unlike other lymphoid tissue, however, red blood cells flow through the spleen as it helps regulate the amount of blood and blood cells that circulate through the body to assist in the destruction of damaged cells. In addition to these organs, clumps of lymphoid tissue are found in many parts of the body, especially in the linings of the digestive tract and the airways and lungs—i.e., the tonsils, adenoids, and appendix.

The immune system organs are connected with one another and with other organs of the body by a network of **lymphatic vessels**, which carry **lymph**, a clear fluid that bathes the body's tissues (Figure 15–3 ■). Lymph is composed of water, protein molecules, salts, glucose, urea, lymphocytes, and other substances. Lymphocytes travel throughout the body using blood vessels as well as a system of lymphatic vessels that closely parallel the body's veins and arteries. Cells and fluids are exchanged between blood and lymphatic vessels, which enable this system to monitor the body for invading microbes.

Lymph nodes are round or kidney-shaped, range in size from very tiny to 1 inch in diameter, and are made of a mesh-like network of tissue. They are usually found in groups in different places throughout the body, including the neck, armpit, chest, abdomen, pelvis, and groin (Figure 15–4 ■). About two-thirds of all lymph nodes and lymphatic tissue are within or near the gastrointestinal tract. Lymph enters the lymph node via incoming lymphatic vessels or the lymph nodes' tiny blood vessels and works its way through passages called sinuses. Each lymph node contains specialized compartments where immune cells congregate and encounter antigens. After these substances have been filtered out,

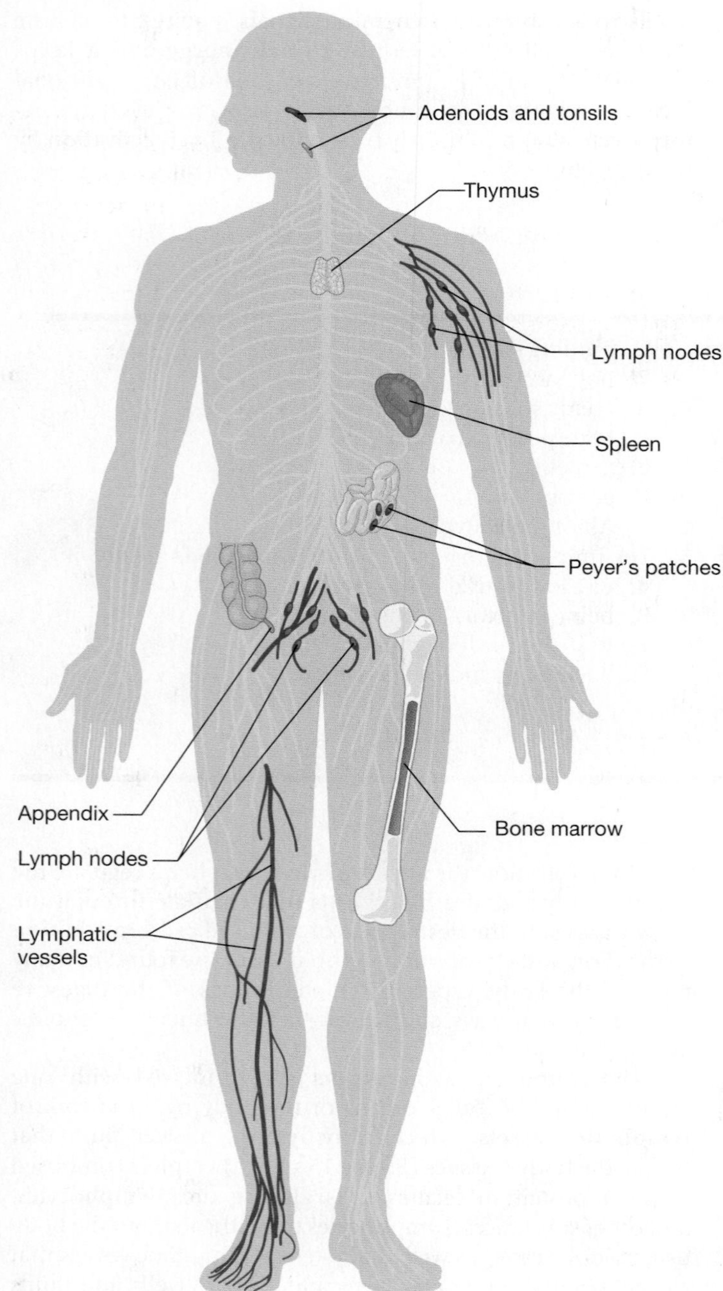

Figure 15–2 ■ Organs of the immune system

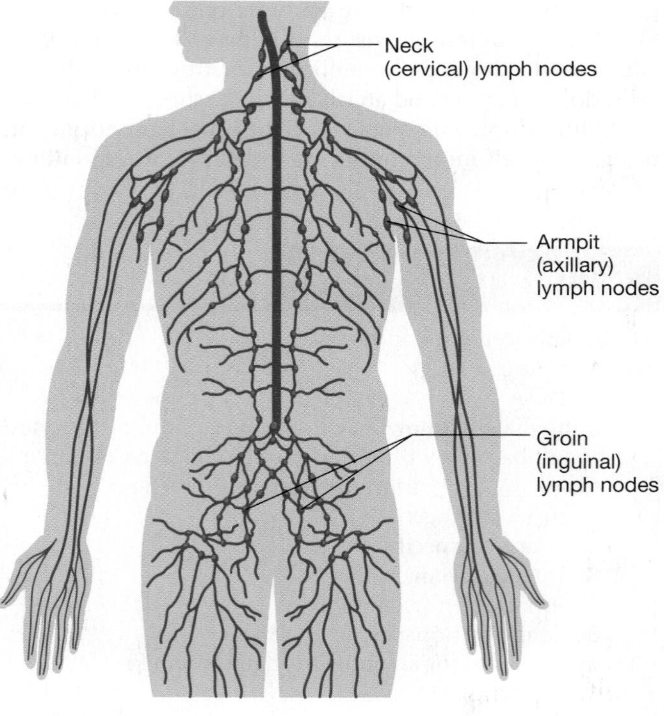

Figure 15–3 ■ Lymphatic system

the lymph then leaves the nodes and returns to the veins, where it reenters the bloodstream. All lymphocytes exit lymph nodes through outgoing lymphatic vessels. Once in the bloodstream, they are transported to tissues throughout the body, where they patrol for foreign antigens, then gradually drift back into the lymphatic system to begin the cycle all over again.

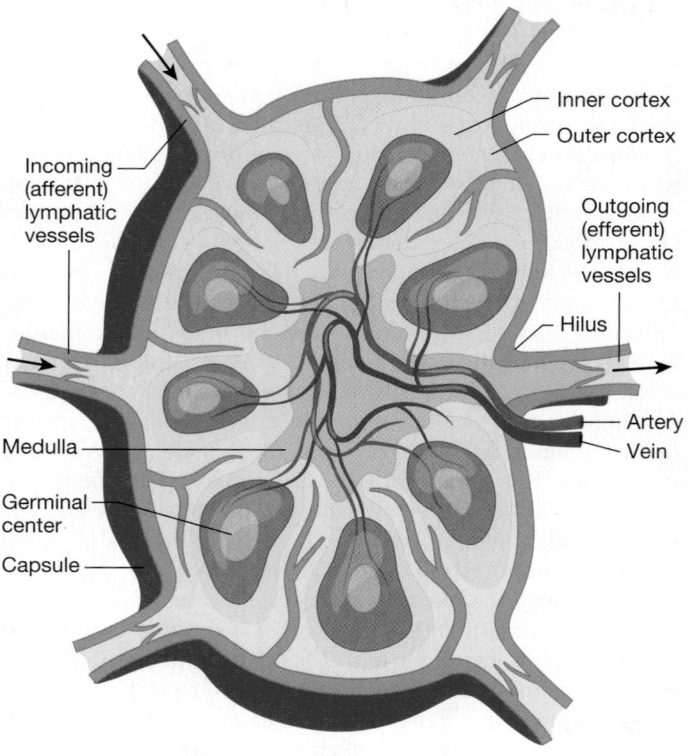

Figure 15–4 ■ Lymph node

Cells of the Immune System

All cellular blood components are derived from hematopoietic stem cells in the bone marrow, which gives rise to three major lineages, an erythroid progenitor (stem) cell, a myeloid progenitor (stem) cell, and a lymphoid progenitor (stem) cell. The erythroid progenitor gives rise to the oxygen carrying red blood cells. The myeloid progenitors develop into myeloid cells (**monocytes**, macrophages, **dendritic cells**, **meagakaryocytes**, and **granulocytes**), which respond early and nonspecifically to infection. The lymphoid progenitors develop into lymphoid cells (lymphocytes, T cells, B cells, and natural killer [NK] cells), which respond later in infections. These cells make up the cellular components of the innate (natural) and adaptive (acquired) immune systems (Figure 15–5 ■).

Cellular Components of the Innate Immune System

Cells of the innate immune system consist of phagocytic cells (monocyte/macrophages, neutrophils, and dendritic cells) and the leukocytes (NK cells, **basophils**, **mast cells**, **eosinophils**, and platelets). These cells possess receptors that are designated as pattern recognition receptors (PRRs), which are proteins expressed by cells of this system to recognize broad molecular patterns found on pathogens (PAMPS). The **inflammatory response** is the initial reaction of the body to harmful stimuli and is achieved by an influx of plasma containing polymorphonuclear leukocytes and macrophages. These cells are the main line of defense in the innate (nonspecific) immune system.

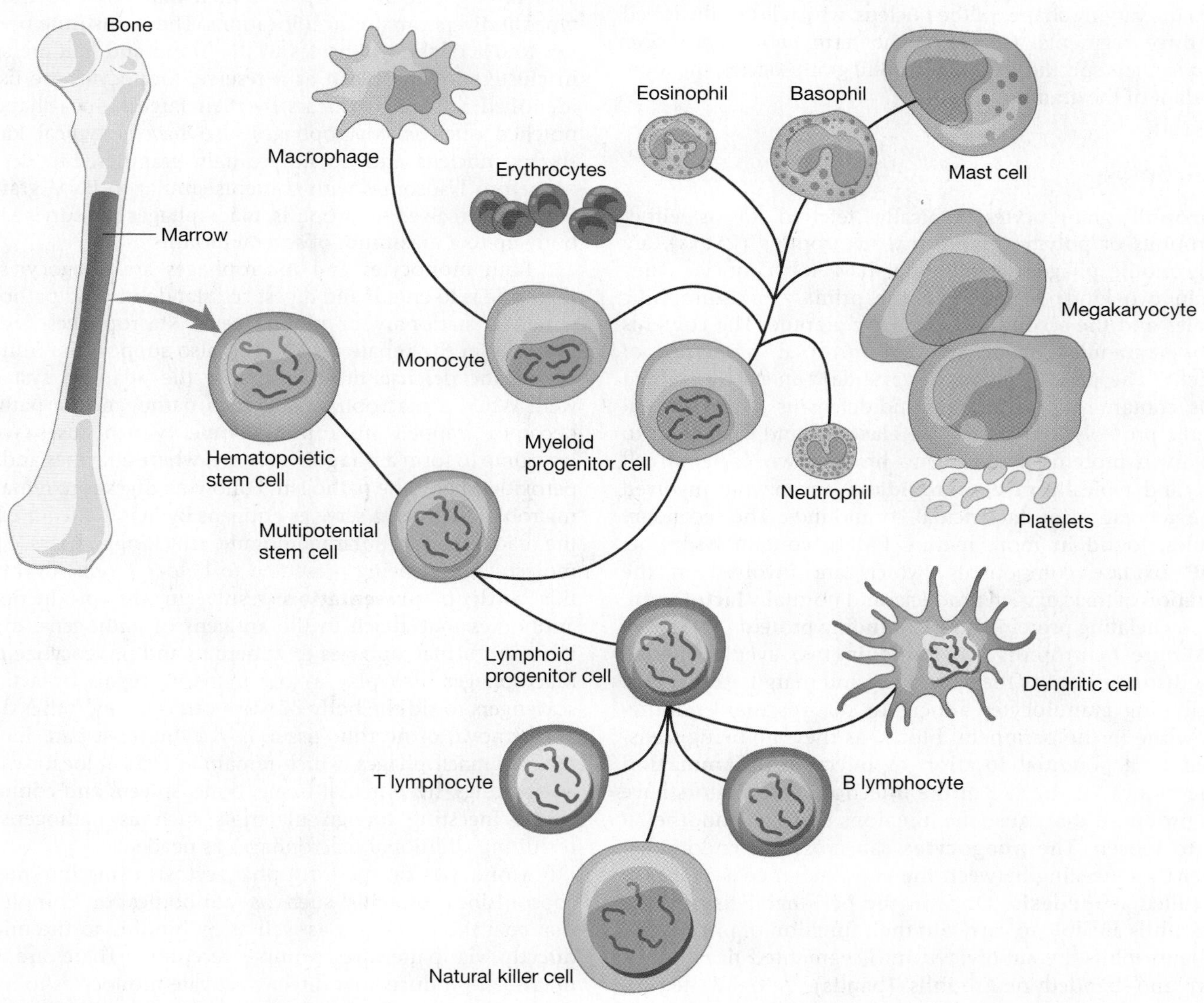

Figure 15–5 ■ Cells of the immune system

Emerging Evidence

A study determining that IL28B SNPs was associated with a sustained viral response of HCV treatment with ribavirin and pegylated interferon suggests that this knowledge could be used to provide novel guidelines in determining optimal treatment duration with interferon-based therapies. Noting that IL28B SNP had a significantly higher frequency in Asian populations than in populations with African and Caucasian ancestry origins, it was suggested that a longer period of treatment may be necessary in individuals without the advantageous IL28B SNP (Chen, 2011).

All **white blood cells** (**WBC**) are known as leukocytes, which are not closely associated with a particular organ or tissue and, therefore, function analogous to independent, single-celled organisms. Granulocytes are a category of WBC characterized by the presence of **granules** in their cytoplasm. They are also called **polymorphonuclear leukocytes** (**PMN**) due to the varying shapes of the nucleus, which is usually lobed into three segments. Generally, the term *polymorphonuclear leukocyte* refers specifically to neutrophil granulocytes, the most abundant of the granulocytes.

Neutrophils

Neutrophil granulocytes, typically referred to as either neutrophils or polymorphonuclear neutrophils (PMNs), are highly motile phagocytic cells that have lobed nuclei. They contain two kinds of granules: the primary or azurophilic granules and the secondary or specific granule. The contents of these granules define the antimicrobial properties of the cells. The primary granules, abundant in newly formed PMNs, contain cationic proteins and defensins, which can kill bacteria; proteolytic enzymes like **elastase**, and **cathepsin** to breakdown proteins; lysozyme to break down bacterial cell walls; and typically **myeloperoxidase**, an enzyme involved in the generation of bactericidal compounds. The secondary granules, found in more mature PMNs, contain lysozyme; **NADP** oxidase components, which are involved in the generation of toxic oxygen products; and normally **lactoferrin**, an iron chelating protein and B12-binding protein.

Mature neutrophils are found in two evenly divided pools distinguished as the circulating and marginating pools. Marginating granulocytes adhere to the vascular endothelium while in the peripheral blood, as they are being transported to a potential location of infection/**inflammation** in the tissues. At the site of the infection, vasodilators have been produced that cause the junctions between endothelial cells to loosen. The **phagocytes** can cross the endothelial barrier by squeezing between the endothelial cells in a process called **diapedesis**. Once in the peripheral tissues, the neutrophils are able to carry out their function of phagocytosis. Neutrophils are subdivided into segmented neutrophils (segs) and banded neutrophils (bands). A band neutrophil is one that is undergoing granulopoiesis to become a mature granulocyte and is characterized by having a curved nucleus instead of lobar. A count of band neutrophils is used to measure inflammation; an excess is termed **bandemia**. Neutrophils comprise approximately 50%–70% of the WBC and have an average lifespan, nonactivated, of about 5 days. When activated they undergo a process termed **chemotaxis**, which allows them to migrate toward sites of infection or inflammation. This takes place due to the presence of cell surface receptors that detect chemical gradients of molecules, i.e., **interleukin** or interferon. The formation of the inflammatory exudate (pus) develops rapidly in an inflammatory response and is composed primarily of neutrophils and monocytes. Interestingly, the cell nucleus of a neutrophil from a female subject shows a small additional X chromosome structure, known as a "neutrophil drumstick."

Monocytes/Macrophages

Macrophages are the progeny of monocytes after they have circulated in the bloodstream for 1 to 3 days, moved into tissues throughout the body, and then matured into different types at diverse anatomical locations. They constitute between 3% to 8% of the leukocytes in the blood and half are stored in clusters in the spleen as a reserve. Monocytes are usually identified in stained smears by their large kidney-shaped or notched nucleus. Macrophages also have a typical kidney-shaped nucleus and do not contain granules, but do have numerous lysosomes with contents similar to PNM granules. Unlike short-lived neutrophils, macrophages can survive in the body up to a maximum of several months.

Both monocytes and macrophages are phagocytes and their role is to engulf and digest cellular debris and pathogens, either as stationary or mobile cells. Macrophages function not only in the innate system, but also support the initiation of specific defense mechanisms in the adaptive system as well. When a macrophage ingests a pathogen, the pathogen becomes trapped in a **phagosome**, which fuses with a lysosome to form a **phagolysosome**, where enzymes and toxic peroxides digest the pathogen. Following digestion, remaining microbial fragments serve as antigens by being integrated into the macrophage cellular membrane, attaching to Class II MHC molecules, and being presented to helper T cells. Eventually, this **antigen presentation** results in the production of antibodies that attach to the antigens of pathogens, making it easier for macrophages to adhere to and phagocytize them. Macrophages also play a role in tissue repair by acting as scavengers to rid the body of worn-out cells and other debris. The removal of necrotic tissue is, for the most part, handled by fixed macrophages, which remain at tactical locations such as the lungs, liver, neural tissue, bone, spleen, and connective tissue, ingesting foreign materials such as pathogens and recruiting additional macrophages as needed.

Monocytes can perform phagocytosis using intermediary (opsonising) proteins such as antibodies or complement that coat the pathogen, as well as by binding to the microbe directly via pattern-recognition receptors. There are some microbial products that directly activate monocytes to lead to the production of pro-inflammatory and anti-inflammatory cytokines, which are small cell-signaling protein molecules secreted by numerous cells of the immune system and used extensively in intercellular communication. Typical cytokines produced by monocytes are **tumor necrosis factors** (**TNF**), IL-1 interleukin-1 and IL-12 interleukin-12.

Dendritic Cells

The primary function of dendritic cells is to process antigen material and present it on the surface to other cells of the immune system; i.e., they function as antigen-presenting cells. Thus, they act as messengers between the innate and adaptive immune systems. They are present on tissues that come into contact with the external environment, the skin, and inner linings of the nose, lungs, stomach, and intestines. Immature dendritic cells are called veiled cells because they display large cytoplasmic veils rather than the long dendritic projections of mature cells. Once activated, they migrate to the lymph nodes where they interact with T cells and B cells in order to manipulate the adaptive immune system. At certain developmental stages they grow branched projections—the dendrites that give them their name.

Natural Killer Cells (NK) and K-Type Lymphocytes

A total of 70% to 80% of NK cells have the appearance of large granular lymphocytes (**LGLs**) because they resemble lymphocytes in their morphology, except that they are slightly larger and have numerous granules. On the other hand, almost 75% of LGLs function as NK cells (Turgeon, 2009). Natural killer cells destroy target cells through an extracellular, nonphagocytic mechanism that is termed a *cytotoxic reaction, MHC unrestricted cytolysis*; i.e., the cell membrane is ruptured with the release of the cellular cytoplasm as a response to an MHC marker protein. NK cells have been found in various body tissues, in particular in the lung and liver, where they are thought to play a role in inflammatory reactions and host defense against certain viruses: e.g., cytomegalovirus (CMV) and hepatitis. Although NK cells are capable of killing virus-infected and malignant target cells, they are relatively inefficient in doing so. Upon exposure to interleukin-2 (IL-2) and interferon (IFN)-gamma, however, NK cells become **lymphokine-activated killer (LAK) cells**, which are capable of killing malignant cells. Continued exposure to IL-2 and IFN-gamma enables the LAK cells to kill transformed as well as malignant cells. The mechanism of LAK cells is distinctive from that of NK cells because they can lyse cells that NK cells cannot and they are also capable of acting against cells that do not display the MHC complex. NK and LAK cells can nonspecifically kill virus-infected and tumor cells. These cells are not part of the inflammatory response but they are important in nonspecific immunity to viral infections and tumor surveillance.

NK and LAK cells have two kinds of receptors on their surface that enable them to distinguish a normal cell from a virus-infected or malignant cell—a killer-activating receptor (**KAR**) and a killer-inhibiting receptor (**KIR**). When the KAR meets its **ligand**, a killer-activating ligand (**KAL**), on the target cell, the NK or LAK cells can kill the target. However, if the KIR binds to the ligand, then killing cannot occur even if KAR binds to KAL. KIR's ligands are MHC-class I molecules; therefore, any target cell that expresses Class I MHC molecules will not be killed by NK or LAK cells, even if the target also has a KAL that could bind to KAR. Although normal cells constantly express MHC Class I molecules on their surface, virus-infected and malignant cells downregulate their expression. Through this mechanism, NK and LAK cells selectively kill virus-infected and malignant cells and spare normal cells.

NK cells can be identified by the presence of CD56 and CD16 and absence of CD3 specific markers on their cell surface (Mayer, 2011). **Cluster of differentiation (cluster of designation)** (**CD**) molecules are markers on the cell surface, as recognized by specific sets of antibodies, used to identify the cell type, stage of differentiation, and activity of a cell. It has become a standard protocol to be used for the identification and investigation of cell surface molecules present on white blood cells, providing targets for immunophenotyping of cells.

K Cells

Killer (K) cells lack morphological distinction and are known as any cell that mediates **antibody-dependent cellular cytotoxicity** (**ADCC**). In ADCC, an antibody (typically IgG) acts as a link to bring the K cell and the target cell together to enable its destruction. The surface of K cells possesses a particular antibody receptor that can recognize, bind, and kill target cells coated with that antibody. These receptors are essentially proteins found on cell surfaces that have been named according to their binding specificity for a particular part of an antibody known as the **Fc** (Fragment, crystallizable) region. Those K cells, which contain **Fc receptors**, include NK, LAK, and macrophages. Macrophages have an Fc receptor for IgG antibodies and eosinophils, which have an Fc receptor for IgE antibodies.

Eosinophils

In normal individuals, eosinophils comprise approximately 1%–6% of white blood cells, persist in circulation for 8–12 hours, and can survive in tissue for an additional 8–12 days in the absence of stimulation. Eosinophils are considered to be a homeostatic regulator of inflammation in that they strive to suppress an inflammatory reaction to prevent its excessive spread. The presence of more than 500 eosinophils per microliter of blood is called eosinophilia and is typically seen in people with a parasitic infestation of the intestines, a collagen vascular disease (rheumatoid arthritis), malignant diseases (Hodgkin disease), extensive skin diseases (exfoliative dermatitis), Addison's disease, in the squamous epithelium of the esophagus in the case of reflux esophagitis, and with the use of certain drugs such as penicillin.

Following activation by an immune stimulus, eosinophils degranulate to release cytotoxic granule cationic proteins capable of inducing tissue damage and dysfunction. These include major basic protein (**MBP**), eosinophil cationic protein (**ECP**), eosinophil peroxidase (**EPO**), and eosinophil-derived neurotoxin (**EDN**). The eosinophil MBP is a potent enzyme against helminthes and causes the release of histamine from mast cells and basophils, activates neutrophils and alveolar macrophages, and is directly implicated in epithelial cell damage, exfoliation, and bronchospasm in asthma. ECP and EDN are ribonucleases with antiviral activity. EPO provides a potent mechanism by which eosinophils kill multicellular parasites (e.g., nematode worms) as well as certain bacteria (e.g., tuberculosis bacteria). However, the oxidizing compounds produced by EPO have been implicated in the inflammatory pathology of several disease states, including asthma.

Basophils

The least common of the granulocytes, basophils represent about 0.01% to 0.3% of circulating white blood cells. When stained, their large cytoplasmic granules can obscure the cell nucleus under the microscope; however, when unstained, the nucleus is visible and usually has two lobes. Like all circulating granulocytes, basophils can be diverted from the blood into tissue when needed. Basophilic degranulation occurs when an antigen such as pollen binds to two adjacent immunoglobulin E antibody molecules (IgE) located on the surface of mast cells. The result of this granulocytic release includes increased vascular permeability, smooth muscle spasm, and vasodilation, which, if severe, can result in **anaphylactic shock**. The substances released during degranulation include histamine, proteoglycans (e.g., heparin and chondroitin), and proteolytic enzymes (e.g., elastase and lysophospholipase), which all contribute to inflammation. Histamine and proteoglycans are prestored in the cell's granules while the other secreted substances are newly generated. Basophils are an important source of the cytokines, interleukin-4 (IL-4), which is considered one of the critical cytokines in the development of allergies and the production of IgE antibody by the immune system. Basophilia, an excess of basophilic cells, is quite uncommon but may be seen in some forms of leukemia or lymphoma.

Basophils also secrete lipid mediators like **leukotrienes**, and several cytokines. Leukotrienes act principally on a subfamily of G protein–coupled receptors (**GPCR**), which comprise a large protein family of transmembrane receptors that sense molecules outside the cell and activate inside signal transduction pathways and, ultimately, cellular responses. The ligands that bind and activate these receptors include light-sensitive compounds, odors, pheromones, hormones, and neurotransmitters, and vary in size from small molecules to peptides to large proteins. GPCRs are involved in many diseases and are the research target of approximately 30% of all modern medicinal drugs; e.g., Clarinex and Zantac (Overton, Al-Lazkani, & Hopkins, 2006).

Mast Cells

Mast cells are large tissue cells with basophilic granules containing amines and heparin. Direct injury (either physical or chemical), cross-linking of IgE receptors, or activated complement proteins can stimulate these cells to degranulate. IgE is the least common serum **Ig** because it binds very tightly to Fc (fragment, crystallized) receptors on basophils and mast cells even before interacting with antigen. As a result of this binding to basophils and mast cells, IgE is involved in allergic reactions. **Allergens**, typically proteins or polysaccharides, bind to the antigen-binding sites, situated on the variable regions of the IgE molecules that are bound to the mast cell and/or basophilic surface. In allergic reactions, mast cells remain inactive until an allergen binds to IgE, which is already in association with the cell. Other membrane activation events can either prime mast cells for subsequent degranulation or act in synergy with the IgE Fc signal. The clustering of the intracellular domains of the cell-bound Fc receptors, which are associated with the cross-linked IgE molecules, causes a complex sequence of reactions inside the mast cell that lead to its activation. This system of reactions is best understood today as it relates to allergens; but since IgE plays a role in parasitic helminth diseases, it is also evident that this had a more prominent part in earlier times. Since serum IgE levels rise in parasitic diseases, a measurement of their levels is helpful in diagnosing parasitic infections. Eosinophils, as noted previously, have Fc receptors for IgE, and a binding of eosinophils to IgE-coated helminths results in the destruction of the parasite. Increases in IgE levels are associated with atopic skin diseases such as eczema, hay fever, asthma, anaphylactic shock, and IgE-myeloma. Decreases in IgE levels are associated with congenital agammaglobulinemia and hypogammaglobulinemia due to faulty metabolism or synthesis of immunoglobulins (Mayer, 2011).

Platelets

Some products of the coagulation system can contribute to the innate immune system by their ability to increase vascular permeability and act as chemotactic agents for phagocytic cells. Moreover, some products of the coagulation system are directly antimicrobial; e.g., beta-lysine, a protein produced by platelets during coagulation, can cause lysis of many gram-positive bacteria by acting as a cationic detergent. Numerous acute-phase proteins of inflammation are involved in the coagulation system. Likewise, increased levels of lactoferrin and transferrin inhibit bacterial growth by binding iron, an essential nutrient for bacteria.

Humoral Components of the Innate Immune System

Complement proteins are the major humoral component of innate immunity. Traditionally, serum complement referred to a heat labile substance that was able to lyse (inactivate) bacteria through the process of heating, but this serum protein is now known to assist host defenses in other ways. Complement embraces over 20–30 different serum proteins produced by a variety of cells including hepatocytes, macrophages, and gut epithelial cells. Some complement proteins bind to immunoglobulins or to membrane components of cells. Others are **proenzymes** that, when activated, cleave additional complement proteins to yield fragments that activate cells, increase vascular permeability, or opsonize bacteria.

Complement system proteins are named with a capital "C" followed by a number. A small letter after the number indicates that the protein is a smaller protein resulting from the cleavage of a larger precursor by a protease. Several complement proteins are cleaved during activation of the complement system; these fragments are designated with lowercase suffixes, such as "C3a" and "C3b." Usually the larger fragment is designated "b" and the smaller fragment "a." The exception is the designation of the C2 fragments, where the larger fragment is designated "C2a" and the smaller fragment is "C2b."

Mayer (2011) presents complement activation as being divided into four pathways: the classical pathway, the lectin pathway, the alternative pathway, and the membrane attack (or lytic) pathway. Since, however, both the classical and alternative pathways lead to the activation of C5 **convertase** to produce C5b, which is the essential activation point for the membrane attack pathway, the initial activation still begins with the classical pathway, the lectin pathway, and the alternative pathway; i.e., three pathways as presented in prior publications (Turgeon, 2009; Abbas, Lichtman, & Pillai, 2010).

Recognition of microbes by complement occurs in three ways. The classical pathway uses a C1 plasma protein to detect **IgM**, **IgG**1, or IgG3 antibodies bound to a microbe surface or other structure. The alternative pathway is elicited by direct recognition of specific microbial surface structures, which is characteristic of innate immunity. The lectin pathway is prompted by a plasma protein called mannose-binding lectin (**MBL**), which identifies terminal mannose residues on microbial glycoproteins and glycolipids. MBL bound microbes activate a protein of the classical pathway, in the absence of antibody, by the action of an accompanying **serine protease**.

Discernment of microbes by any of these pathways results in ongoing conscription and assembly of additional complement proteins into protease complexes. The central protein of the complement system, C3, is cleaved, and its larger C3b fragment is placed on the microbial surface where complement is activated. C3b develops covalent attachment to microbes and functions as an opsonin to promote their phagocytosis. A smaller fragment, C3a, is released to stimulate inflammation by serving as a chemoattractant for neutrophils. C3b binds other complement proteins to create a protease, which cleaves a C5 protein, generating a secreted peptide (C5a) and a larger fragment (C5b) that remains attached to the microbial cell membranes. C5a stimulates the influx of neutrophils to an infection site as well as the vascular component of acute inflammation. C5b initiates the formation of a complex of complement proteins (C6, C7, C8, and C9), which are assembled into a membrane pore causing lysis of the cells where complement is activated.

Activation of complement causes the production of several biologically active molecules, which contribute to resistance, anaphylaxis, and inflammation. **Kinin** production occurs through the formation of C2b during the classical pathway of **C-activation** in the form of prokinin, which becomes biologically active following enzymatic alteration by **plasmin**. Excess C2b production is prevented by limiting C2 activation with a C1 inhibitor (C1-INH), also known as serpin, through a displacement process. A genetic deficiency of C1-INH results in an overproduction of C2b and is the cause of hereditary angioneurotic edema. C4a, C3a, and C5a (in increasing order of activity) are all **anaphylotoxins**, which cause basophil/mast cell degranulation and smooth muscle contraction followed by a release of vasoactive amines. C5a and **membrane attack complex** (**MAC**) (C5b67) are both chemotactic. C5a is also a potent activator of neutrophils, basophils, and macrophages, and causes induction of adhesion molecules on vascular endothelial cells. C3b and C4b serve as opsonins in the surface of microorganisms and attach to the C-receptor (CR1) on phagocytic cells to promote phagocytosis. C-reactive protein is a plasma protein identified and named because of its ability to bind to the capsules of pneumococcal bacteria. It belongs to the pentraxin family of plasma proteins, so termed for containing five identical globular subunits. Its physiological role is to bind to phosphocholine expressed on the surface of dead or dying cells (and some types of bacteria) in order to activate the complement system via the C1Q complex.

The complement system participates in both specific and nonspecific resistance and creates a number of products of biological and pathophysiological significance. There are known genetic deficiencies of most individual C complement components, but C3 deficiency is the most serious and fatal. Complement deficiencies also occur in immune complex diseases (e.g., SLE) and acute and chronic bacterial, viral, and parasitic infections.

Interferons

Interferons (IFNs) are one of the body's natural defense responses to foreign components; i.e., viruses, bacteria, parasites, tumor cells, and antigens. They belong to a large class of glycoproteins known as cytokines. Additional functions of IFNs include the activation of immune cells, such as NK cells and macrophages, and recognition of infection or tumor cells by means of antigen presentation to T lymphocytes. They are among the most expansive active physiologic regulators, enhancing the expression of specific genes, inhibiting cell proliferation, and augmenting immune effector cells. Specific body symptoms, such as aching muscles and fever, are related to the production of IFNs during infection.

Type 1 IFNs mediate the early innate immune response to viral infections and consist of two distinct groups of proteins, IFN-α and IFN-β, that are significantly different structurally. They both, however, bind to the same cell surface receptor and induce similar biologic responses. Interferon-gamma (IFN-γ) is the primary macrophage-activating cytokine and it serves a vital function in innate immunity and specific cell-mediated immunity as well. It stimulates the expression of MHC class I and class II molecules and co-stimulates antigen-presenting cells (APCs). Additionally, IFN-γ acts on B cells to promote switching to certain IgG subclasses, activates neutrophils, and stimulates the cytolytic activity of NK cells. It is often antagonistic to interleukin (IL-4).

Interleukins/Cytokines

Cytokines are polypeptide products of activated cells that control a variety of cellular responses in order to regulate the immune response. Because so many cytokines are made by leukocytes, they were initially referred to as interleukins (**IL**), a descriptive but imperfect term. Nonetheless, this original term is employed in the standard nomenclature as more cytokines are discovered; i.e., they are assigned a number to the abbreviation, IL-1. Other terms commonly used to describe particular kinds of cytokines include **monokines**, cytokines produced by mononuclear phagocytic cells; **lymphokines**, cytokines produced by activated lymphocytes; and **chemokines**, small cytokines primarily responsible for leucocyte migration.

Many cytokines are released in response to specific antigens; however, cytokines are nonspecific in that their chemical structure is not determined by the stimulating antigen and they do not bind antigens. Cytokines have a variety of roles in the line of defense. In innate immunity, cytokines mediate early inflammatory reactions to microbial organisms and stimulate adaptive immune responses. In contrast, in adaptive immunity, cytokines stimulate proliferation and differentiation of antigen-stimulated lymphocytes and activate specialized effector cells, such as macrophages. They are especially potent in minute concentrations and their action is usually limited to affecting cells in the local area of their production, although they can have systemic effects as well.

Role of Innate System in Stimulating Adaptive Immune System

As mentioned previously, innate and adaptive immune responses are constituents of an integrated system of host defense in which numerous cells and molecules function supportively. There are two significant connections between innate immunity and adaptive immunity. The first connection involves molecules produced during innate responses that serve to not only stimulate the adaptive system but also to influence the nature of its response. Secondly, adaptive immune system responses use many of the innate effector mechanisms to eliminate microbes and, in turn, they often function by enhancing the antimicrobial activities of the innate defense mechanisms.

This second response is often referred to as cell-mediated immunity (CMI), which is typically defined as an immune response that does not involve antibodies or complement but rather involves the activation of macrophages, natural killer cells (NK), antigen-specific cytotoxic T-lymphocytes, and the release of various cytokines in response to an antigen. Molecules produced during the initial innate response that serve as a signal for the adaptive system include **co-stimulators**, cytokines, and complement breakdown products.

Co-stimulators are membrane proteins expressed on a specialized subset of cells called **antigen-presenting cells (APCs)**. These cells are a heterogeneous population of leukocytes that play a crucial role in innate immunity and similarly serve as a tie to the adaptive immune system by participating in the activation of helper T cells. These cells include dendritic cells and macrophages. A distinctive feature of APCs is the manifestation of a cell surface molecule encoded by genes in the major histocompatibility complex, referred to as class II MHC molecules. Although not considered part of the innate system, B lymphocytes also express class II MHC molecules that function as APCs. There are additional cells (e.g., thymic epithelial cells) that can manifest class II MHC molecules and thereby function as APCs.

An example of CMI, using these connections, includes macrophages being activated by microbes and by INF to produce co-stimulators that enhance T cell activation and IL-12, which stimulates IFN production by T cells and the development of IFN-producing effector T cells. Similarly, as discussed earlier in the complement section "Humoral Components of the Innate Immune System," complement fragments generated by the alternative pathway provide second signals for B cell activation and antibody production. This latter example, however, does not involve CMI because of the presence of antibodies and complement.

Cellular Components of the Adaptive Immune System

Cells involved in the adaptive immune responses are antigen-specific lymphocytes, specialized antigen-presenting cells (APCs) that display antigens and activate lymphocytes, and **effector cells** that serve to eradicate antigens. Lymphocytes, one of the five WBCs circulating in the blood, are the only cells in the body capable of precisely identifying and differentiating wide-ranging antigenic determinants (epitopes). Additionally, they are responsible for the two essential characteristics of the adaptive immune response: specificity and memory. Lymphocytes consist of distinct subsets that are extraordinarily diverse in their functions and protein products, but are morphologically indistinguishable.

The most abundant lymphocytes are B lymphocytes (B cells), which attain full maturity in bone marrow, and T lymphocytes (T cells), which mature in the thymus. These lymphocytes go through complex maturational stages during which they express antigen receptors and acquire the functional and phenotypic characteristics of mature cells. When matured, they leave the marrow or thymus, enter the circulation, and inhabit the peripheral lymphoid organs. These mature cells are called naïve lymphocytes. A stable group of naïve lymphocytes is maintained in a state of equilibrium by the formation of new cells from bone marrow progenitors and the destruction of cells that do not encounter antigens.

B cells are primarily responsible for humoral immunity (i.e., they provide antibodies), and T cells are involved in cell-mediated immunity (CMI). Each B and T cell is specific for a particular molecular structure in an antigen and this specificity of binding is present in a receptor for that antigen—i.e., B cell receptor (**BCR**) and **T cell receptor** (**TCR**). The specificity of the adaptive immune system response resides within these receptors, which share certain properties: They are made before the cell ever encounters an antigen. They are present in thousands of identical copies at the cell surface. They have unique binding sites, which bind to a portion of the antigen called antigen determinant or epitope (i.e., each receptor is structurally unique). They are **integral membrane proteins (IMP)**, which means they are permanently attached to the biological membrane. They differ in their structure, the type of epitope to which they bind, and the genes that encode them.

They also differ in that BCRs are divalent and TCRs are monovalent, which means BCRs can have their antigen receptors cross-linked by antigen but TCRs cannot. This creates differences in how they are activated as well. During the process of antigen presentation, the function of these cells is to recognize specific non-self-antigens. After an intruder is identified, the cells develop precise responses that are designed to eliminate specific pathogens or pathogen infected cells.

As the immature T cells migrate to the interior of the thymus, they present varied cell surface receptors. After arrival in the gland, those T cells that do not attack the lining cells, which are covered with self antigens, begin to mature; whereas those that harmed the lining die by **apoptosis**. Thus, those T cells that recognize self are sustained while those that cause harm are eradicated.

Various sorts of T cells are differentiated by the types and patterns of receptors on their surfaces and by their functions. **Helper T cells (Th)** recognize foreign antigens on macrophages, stimulate B cells to produce antibodies, secrete cytokines, and activate another kind of T cell termed **cytotoxic T lymphocyte** (**Tc** or **CTLs**). There are numerous subsets of Th cells that secrete various cytokines to facilitate a different type of immune response. Th cells are also known as CD_4 (cluster of differentiation) cells because they express the CD_4 protein on their surface. Naïve Th cells become activated when they encounter peptide antigens by MHC class II molecules that are on antigen presenting cells (APCs) and subsequently produce cytokines. These cells have no cytotoxic or phagocytic activity and cannot destroy infected cells, but they do oversee the immune response by directing other cells to perform these tasks.

CTLs are a subgroup of T cells with CD_8 receptors, which induce the death of cells that are infected with viruses or other pathogens or are otherwise damaged or dysfunctional. Naïve cytotoxic CTLs are primed for activation when their TCR strongly reacts with a peptide-bound MHC class I molecule. A second signal is required for the CTL to become fully mature: the secretion of cytokines by Th cells, primarily IL and IFN. Following activation, CTL undergoes a process called **clonal expansion** in which it gains functionality and divides rapidly to produce a massive attack. Activated CTL will then travel throughout the body in search of cells bearing that unique MHC Class I peptide. It must come in contact with the infected cells in order to recognize the target antigen. It then releases perforin and granulysin, which are cytotoxins that produce pores in the target cell's plasma membrane. These pores allow the influx of ions and water that causes the cell to lyse. CTLs also release granzyme, a serine protease that enters the cell through the pores to induce apoptosis. To limit extensive tissue damage, CTLs are tightly regulated and do require a strong signal before responding. These cells are not injured when they lyse cells and are capable of destroying sequentially numerous target cells. Once the infection is cleared, these effector cells either die off or are phagocytized; however, a few do remain as **memory cells**.

An additional T cell about which little is known is the gamma delta T cell. This represents a small subset of T cells that possess a structurally distinct TCR on their surface. They are found primarily in the gut mucosa, within a population of lymphocytes known as intraepithelial lymphocytes (**IELs**).

T regulatory cells (**T_{reg}**) are a component of the immune system that suppress immune responses of other cells. They do not prevent initial T cell activation; but they seem to inhibit a sustained response and prevent chronic and potentially damaging responses. These cells are involved in regulating immune responses that may potentially attack one's own tissues—i.e., autoimmunity. They come in many forms, but the way they function has still not been elucidated, although there is the consideration that it may be related to cytokines as they are known to be either positive or negative regulators of the immune response.

Following antigen exposure, B and T lymphocytes undergo further differentiation to assist in establishing a reserve for the immune response. They form effector lymphocytes, which function to eliminate an antigen by releasing antibodies (B cells) or cytotoxic granules (CLTs) or by signaling other cells of the immune system (Th cells). Memory cells are created during these processes and remain in the peripheral tissues and circulation for an extended time ready to respond to the same antigen upon future exposure.

Humoral Components of Adaptive Immunity

B cells are derived from the progenitor cells through an antigen-independent maturation process occurring in the bone marrow and **GALT**. Participation of B cells in the humoral immune response is accomplished by reacting to antigenic stimuli through division and differentiation into **plasma cells**, whose primary function is the production of antibodies. Plasma cells are the end product of B cell differentiation.

When an antigen-presenting macrophage activates a T cell, an antibody response has begun. The next step involves this cell contacting a B cell with surface receptors that can bind the type of foreign antigen the macrophage presented. The B cell population in the immune system is so large, with innumerable combinations of surface antigens, that there should always be one that would correspond to a specific foreign antigen. There is a large daily turnover of these B cells because millions are destroyed in the lymph nodes and spleen while millions more are being created in the bone marrow, each with a unique arrangement of surface molecules.

Once the activated T cell has paired with the B cell match, it releases cytokines, which stimulate the B cell to divide into two kinds of cells. Plasma cells are the first to be formed and are the antibody producers. Each cell secretes anywhere from 1,000 to 2,000 identical antibodies per second into the bloodstream for the cell's short lifespan of a few days. This is the primary immune response. Plasma cells derived from different B cells secrete different antibodies with each type corresponding to a specific portion of the pathogen in what is called a **polyclonal antibody** response. Memory cells are the second type of B cell descendant, which are fewer in number and usually dormant. These cells would respond to this foreign antigen faster and stronger if it should appear again—this is a secondary immune response.

Immunoglobulins are glycoprotein molecules that are produced by plasma cells in response to an **immunogen** and that function as antibodies. Antigen binding by antibodies is immunoglobins' primary function, which can result in protection of the host. Binding occurs through the detection of specific antigenic determinants. The valency of an antibody refers to the number of antigenic determinants an individual antibody molecule can bind; for all antibodies this is at least two and sometimes more. The antibody–antigen binding may inactivate a pathogen or neutralize the toxin it produces. They can clump pathogens, making them more visible to macrophages, which then destroy them. Antibodies can also activate complement, thereby extending the innate immune response.

The basic antibody molecule is comprised of several polypeptides and is, therefore, encoded by several genes. It has four polypeptide chains connected by disulfide bonds forming a shape like the letter Y. Larger antibody molecules may have as many as five Ys joined together. Within the Y structure, the two longer polypeptides are called heavy chains and the other two are called light chains. The lower portion of each chain is an amino acid sequence, which is very similar in all antibody molecules. The region where the arms of the antibody form a Y is called the hinge region because there is some flexibility at this point. This area is also referred to as the constant region and provides the activity of the antibody. The amino acid sequences of the upper portions of each polypeptide chain are the variable regions and they can differ greatly among antibodies. These are the parts that provide the specificities of certain antibodies to individual antigens. The three-dimensional shapes of the tips of the variable regions are antigen-binding sites, and the areas that actually contact the antigen are called **idiotypes**. The parts of the antigens the idiotypes bind are the epitopes. The antibody contorts to form a pocket around the antigen.

The immunoglobulins can be divided into five different classes (Figure 15–6 ■), based on location, function, and differences in the amino acid sequences in the constant region of the heavy chains. Within each class there are subclasses based on small differences in the amino acid sequences in the constant region of the heavy chains. Immunoglobulin fragments produced by proteolytic digestion have proven very useful in elucidating structure/function relationships in immunoglobulins. In particular, the Fab fragment contains the antigen-binding site of the antibody, and Fc, which refers to the antibody's ability to crystalize, mediates the effector functions.

IgG

IgG is referred to as a gammaglobulin; all IgGs are monomers. The subclasses differ in the number of disulfide bonds and the length of the hinge region. IgG is the most versatile because it is capable of carrying out all of the functions of immunoglobulin molecules. It is the major antibody in serum with 75% of the composition and it is also the primary Ig in extra vascular spaces. This is the only class of Ig that crosses the placenta. Transfer is mediated by a receptor on placental cells for the Fc (fragment, crystalized) region of IgG and is capable of fixing complement; however, not all subclasses cross equally well. Not all subclasses bind well to cells but a consequence of binding to the Fc receptors on PMNs, monocytes, and macrophages is that the cell can now internalize the antigen better and thus

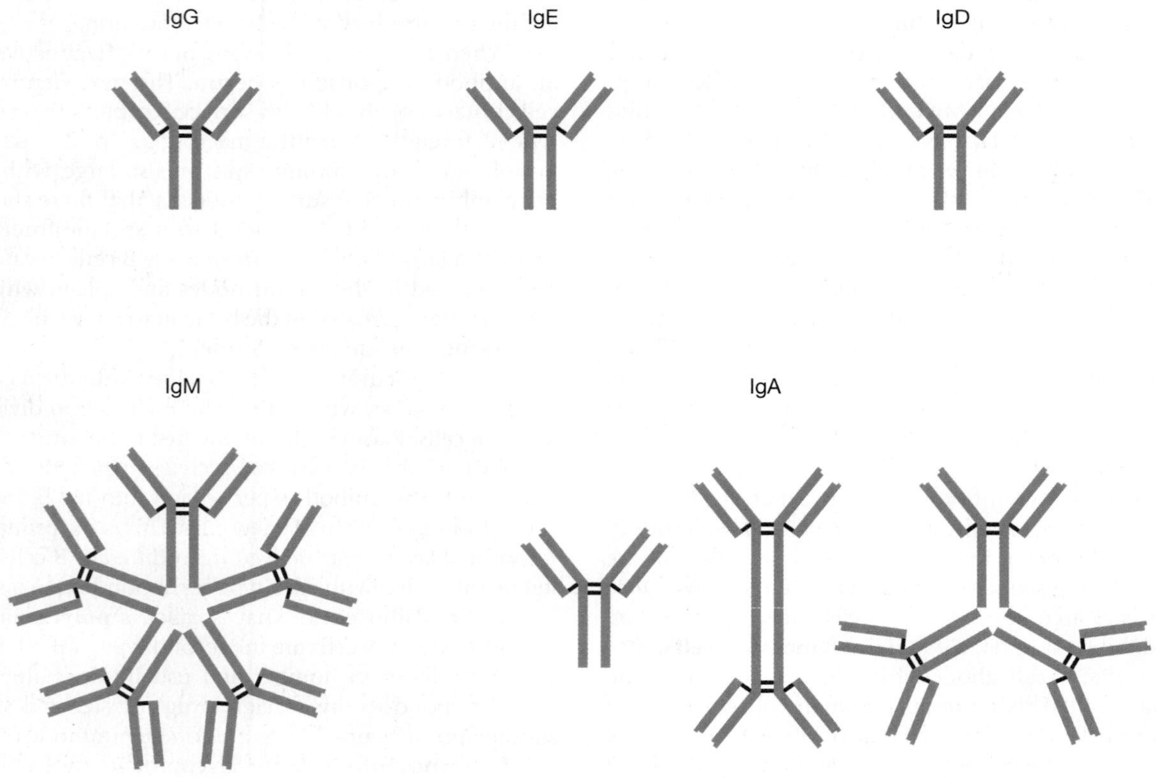

Figure 15–6 ■ Basic structure of five classes of immunoglobulins

prepare it for eating by the phagocytic cells, which makes it a good opsonin. The binding of I21 > IgM.

The Mu gammaglobulin normally exists as a pentamer but it can be a monomer as well. It is the third most prevalent Ig. It is the first to be made by the fetus and the first to be made by naïve B cells when stimulated with antigen. Due to its pentameric structure, it has a valence of 10, which not only makes it good at fixing complement but very efficient in leading to the lysis of microorganisms.

IgA

In terms of structure, alpha gammaglobulin is a monomer in serum but a dimer in secretions. It is the second most common serum Ig and is the major class of Ig in secretions (i.e., tears, salvia, mucus, and colostrum). Its most important function is as secretory **IgA** in mucosal immunity. It does not fix complement and is capable of binding to a few cells.

IgD

Delta gammaglobulin is found in very low levels in serum, so its function there is uncertain. It is found primarily on B cell surfaces where it functions as a receptor for antigen. Its structure is as a monomer and it does not bind complement.

IgE

Epsilon gammaglobulin, with a monomer structure, is the least common serum Ig because it binds very tightly to Fc receptors on basophils and mast cells before interacting with antigen. As a result of this tight binding, it is involved in allergic reactions. The binding of an allergen to IgE on the cells results in the release of pharmacological mediators that result in allergic symptoms. It does not bind complement. IgE does play a role in parasitic helminth diseases. Since serum IgE levels rise in parasitic diseases, measuring IgE levels is helpful in diagnosing parasitic infections. Eosinophils have Fc receptors for IgE, and binding of eosinophils to IgE-coated helminths results in the death of the parasite.

Allergens can trigger an overwhelming response in the immune system. An allergen is generally a small particle that can be carried in the air and into an individual's respiratory track. The size of the allergen may determine the type of allergy; e.g., grass pollen is large and remains in the upper respiratory track to cause hay fever. Allergens from dust mites, cat dander, and cockroaches, however, are small enough to infiltrate the lungs to trigger asthma. Both humoral and cellular immunity take part in an allergic response. The antibody IgE binds to mast cells, sending signals that cause them to open and release allergy mediators such as histamine and heparin. Allergy mediators also cause inflammation with additional symptoms that could cause narrowed pathways, rashes, or the overwhelming bodywide reaction of anaphylactic shock.

Idiotype determinants were previously mentioned as located in the variable part of the antibody associated with the hypervariable regions that form the antigen-combining sites. An additional antigenic determinant is referred to as the isotype determinant, which is the dominant type found on the immunoglobulins of all animals of a species. Last is the allotype determinant, which is a genetically determined variation representing the presence of allelic genes at a single locus within a species—e.g., a marker on IgG referred to as Gm. An additional phenomenon that can occur with immunoglobulins is termed **class switching**. Immunoglobulin class switching (isotype switching) is a biological mechanism that changes a B cell's production of antibody from one class to another—for example, from an isotype called IgM to an isotype called IgG. During this process, the constant region portion of the antibody heavy chain is changed, but the variable region of the heavy chain stays the same.

Lymphocyte Recirculation

Lymphocytes continuously move through the blood stream and lymphatics, from one peripheral lymphoid tissue to another and then to peripheral inflammatory sites as needed. If they do not encounter an antigen in any of the lymph nodes, they leave via the lymphatics and return to the blood via the thoracic duct. It is estimated that 1%–2% of lymphocytes recirculate every hour, and it is probable that each lymphocyte goes through a node once a day on average. The recirculation and migration of lymphocytes to particular tissues are facilitated by adhesion molecules on lymphocytes, endothelial cells, and extracellular matrix and chemokines produced in the endothelium and in tissues. Adhesion to and detachment from extracellular matrix components within the tissues determine how long lymphocytes are retained at a particular site. The adhesion molecules expressed by the lymphocytes are called homing receptors, and the ligands expressed on the vascular endothelium are called addressins. The homing receptors on lymphocytes include three families of molecules: the **selectins**, the **integrins**, and the Ig superfamily. Different populations of lymphocytes exhibit distinct patterns of homing: Naïve T cells migrate preferentially to lymph nodes, and the activated T cells prefer the peripheral tissue sites.

If the lymphocytes in the lymph nodes encounter an antigen, which has been transported to the lymph node via the lymphatics, the cells become activated, and divide and differentiate to become a plasma cell, Th cell, or Tc cell. After several days, the effector cells can leave the lymph nodes via the lymphatics, return to the blood via the thoracic duct, and then make their way to the infected tissue site. Homing receptors on naive lymphocytes direct them to **high endothelial venules (HEV)**, where they can then enter the lymph nodes from the blood. In the lymph nodes, antigen-specific receptor lymphocytes encounter antigens, which have been transported to the lymph nodes by dendritic cells or macrophages. After activation, the lymphocytes express new receptors that allow the cells to leave the lymph nodes and reenter the circulation. Receptors on the activated lymphocytes recognize cell adhesion molecules expressed on endothelial cells near the site of an infection, and chemokines produced at the infection site help attract the activated cells. Thus the process keeps repeating to ensure that specific subsets of lymphocytes encounter certain tissue microenvironments where they are needed for adaptive immune responses.

SECTION THREE REVIEW

1. A function of the cell-mediated immune response NOT associated with humoral immunity is
   A. defense against viral and bacterial infection.
   B. initiation of rejection of foreign tissues and tumors.
   C. defense against fungal and bacterial infection.
   D. antibody production.
2. The primary or central lymphoid organs in humans are the
   A. bursa of Fabricius and thymus.
   B. lymph nodes and thymus.
   C. bone marrow and thymus.
   D. lymph nodes and spleen.
3. All of the following are a function of T cells EXCEPT
   A. mediation of delayed-hypersensitivity reactions.
   B. mediation of cytolytic reactions.
   C. regulation of the immune response.
   D. synthesis of antibody.
4. The major clinical manifestation of a B-cell deficiency is
   A. impaired phagocytosis.
   B. diminished complement levels.
   C. increased susceptibility to bacterial infections.
   D. increased susceptibility to parasitic infections.
5. Most diseases associated with a primary defect are ____________ disorders.
   A. T-cell
   B. B-cell
   C. complement
   D. phagocytic

Answers: 1. B; 2. C; 3. D; 4. C; 5. B

SECTION FOUR: Immunogenetics

With the completion of the finished human genome sequence in 2003, a partnership of scientists and funding agencies from Canada, China, Japan, Nigeria, the United Kingdom, and the United States was founded to cultivate a public resource to help researchers find genes associated with human disease and their response to pharmaceuticals. This organization, named the International HapMap Project, has provided a rich resource for understanding the nature and extent of human genetic diversity (International HapMap Project, 2011). Subsequently, many new genes responsible for the immune response have been discovered along with their functions and interactions.

One of the first discoveries with the innate immune system response was the family of Toll-like receptors, which was named after a cell-surface receptor, Toll, first described in fruit flies. The genes that encode the human and fruit-fly versions of Toll-like receptors have a remarkable similarity to one another, which implies its necessity in maintaining an innate immune response in a variety of organisms. In fact, all multicellular organisms are thought to possess innate immune systems. If, however, as the first responder, the innate immune system is incapable of overpowering the infection, a more specific and effective immune response is needed (i.e., the adaptive immune system). It is speculated that the adaptive immune system is a more recent evolutionary development than the innate immune system and is found only in vertebrates.

As the term *adaptive* denotes, this immune system must alter its population of immune cells in response to various stimulators as they are encountered. A major element of the adaptive immune response begins when specialized types of phagocytes, part of the innate system, engulf invading microbes and then present peptides derived from these microbes on their cell surfaces. These foreign microbe peptides, or antigens, are presented on antigen-presenting cells (APCs), which can be macrophages, dendritic cells, or B cells.

The APCs alert the adaptive immune system to the presence of pathogens in two ways. First, the antigen was transported to the surface of the APC by a class II major histocompatibility complex (MHC) molecule. When the APCs initially meet a pathogen, they display costimulatory molecules on their cell surface to signal the encounter. This signal, together with the MHC complex, which projects into the extracellular environment, is recognized by T lymphocytes cell receptors (TCR). The T lymphocytes now become activated and secrete cytokines to help stimulate the subset of B lymphocyte cell receptors (BCR) to provided immunoglobulins that will bind to the invading microorganism's peptides. The immunoglobulin's capacity to bind a specific foreign peptide—i.e., its affinity for the peptide—is determined by its shape and other characteristics.

It is estimated that upon initial exposure to a microbe, as few as 1 in every 1 million B lymphocytes happen to produce cell surface receptors capable of binding to the microbe (Jorde, Carey, & Banshad, 2010). This number is too small to fight an infection, and its binding affinity is thought to be relatively poor at this stage. Once stimulated, however, they begin an adaptive process in which additional DNA sequence variation is generated. These DNA mutations, which are confined to the genes that encode the cell-surface receptors, in turn produce alterations in the receptors' binding characteristics; i.e., the shape of the protein. Many of these variant receptors will possess a higher level of binding affinity for the microbe. The B cells that produce these variant receptors are favorably selected because they bind the antigen for a longer period of time and they proliferate rapidly. These B cells have now become plasma cells, which secrete their immunoglobulins into the blood stream.

The immune system cannot plan in advance for what types of microbes it will encounter; therefore, the system contains a huge reservoir of structurally diverse immune cells so that at least a few cells can respond to any invading microbe. The humoral immune system is capable of generating at least 10 billion structurally distinct antibodies (Jorde et al., 2010). Since the human genome has only 20,000 to 25,000 genes, it becomes evident that each antibody cannot be encoded by a different gene.

Antibody Structure

There is considerable diversity among the different classes of antibodies (Ig), which implies that they perform different functions in addition to their primary function of antigen binding. Essentially, each Ig molecule is bifunctional; one region of the molecule involves binding to antigen, and a different region mediates binding of the Ig to host tissues, including cells of the immune system and the first component (C1q) of the classic complement system.

The primary core of an antibody consists of a sequence of amino acid residues linked by peptide bonds. All antibodies have a common, basic polypeptide structure with a three-dimensional configuration. The polypeptide chains are linked by covalent and noncovalent bonds to produce a unit composed of a four-chain structure based on pairs of identical heavy and light chains. The basic unit of an antibody structure is the homology unit or **domain**. A typical molecule has 12 domains, arranged in 2 heavy (H) and 2 light (L) chains, linked through cysteine residues by disulfide bonds such that the domains lie in pairs (Figure 15–7 ■). The antigen-binding portion of the molecule demonstrates tremendous heterogeneity, thus it is known as the variable (V) region. The remaining section contains relatively constant (C) amino acid sequences.

The IgG molecule represents a characteristic model of antibody structure, appearing Y shaped as a monomer chain. If the molecule is chemically treated to break the sulfide bonds, it separates into four polypeptide chains. The light (L) chains are small chains common to all Ig classes and are of two subtypes, kappa (κ) and lambda (λ), which have different amino acid sequences and are antigenically different. The larger heavy chains (H) extend the full length of the molecule (Figure 15–8 ■). The first 110 to 120 amino acids of both L and H chains have a variable sequence and form the V region; the remainder of the L chains represents the C region, with a similar amino acid sequence for each type and subtype. The remaining portion of the H chain is also constant for each type and has a hinge region. The class and subclass of an Ig molecule are determined by its H-chain type. This hinge region in IgG links three globular regions: two Fab fragments and one Fc fragment. The Fab fragments are antigen binding and can swing freely around the center (hinge) of the molecule. The hinge contains a group of about 15 amino acids, which is variable and unique for each Ig class and subclass.

The heavy and light chains with both constant (C) and variable (V) regions of the antibody molecules and B cell receptors are encoded by genes on three loci. Chromosome 14 contains genes for the Ig heavy chains; chromosome 2 contains genes for the Ig kappa light chains; and chromosome 22 contains genes for the Ig lambda light chains. Multiple genes for the variable regions are encoded in the human genome to contain three distinct types of segments. For example, Ig heavy chain regions can contain Variable (V) genes plus Diversity (D) and Joining (J) genes. The light chains possess numerous V and J genes but do not have D genes. This process of DNA rearrangement for these regional genes with the VDJ combination creates the opportunity to generate a vast antibody selection. Thus, there are several mechanisms responsible for generating antibody diversity in the human body.

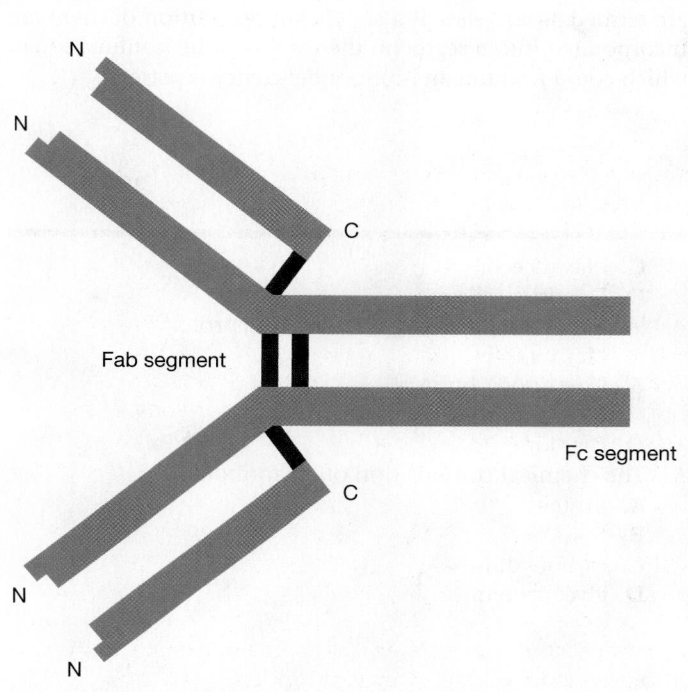

Figure 15–7 ■ Basic immunoglobulin configuration

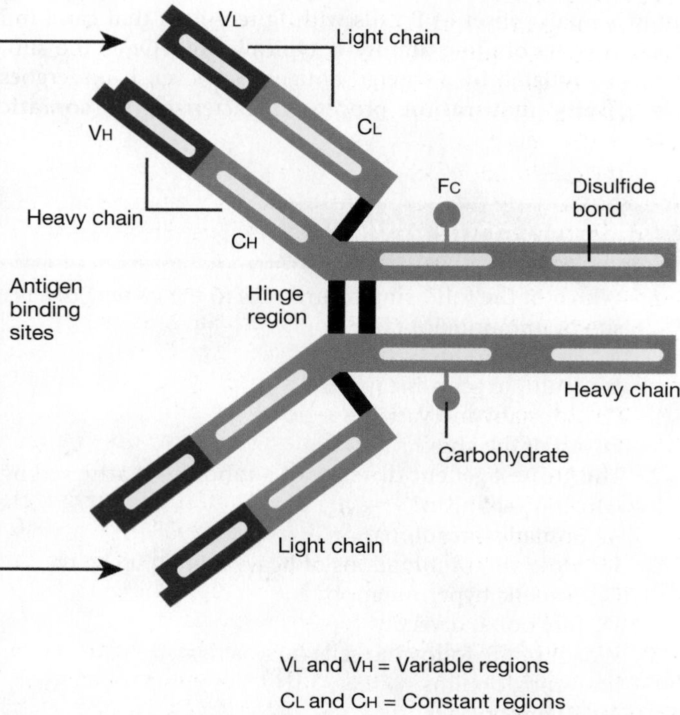

Figure 15–8 ■ Basic structure of IgG

Multiple Germline Immunoglobulin Genes

Molecular genetic studies, such as cloning and DNA sequencing, have demonstrated that one individual can have more than 80 different V segments located in a germline, 6 different J segments, and at least 30 D segments present in the heavy chain.

Somatic Recombination (VDJ)

A process involving the deletion of DNA sequences that separate single V, J, D segments before they are transcribed into mRNA is carried out by VDJ recombinase enzymes. Following the deletion of all but one V, D, and J segment, the nondeleted segments are joined by **ligases**. This process is termed *somatic recombination,* and it can generate approximately 100,000 to 1,000,000 different types of antibody molecules (Jorde et al., 2010).

Junctional Diversity

During the reassembling of the V, D, and J regions, slight variations can occur in the position at which they are joined, and small numbers of nucleotides may be deleted or inserted at the junctions joining the regions. This creates greater variation in antibody amino acid sequence.

Somatic Hypermutation

Upon initial contact with a foreign antigen, there is typically only a small subset of B cells with Ig receptors that can bind to it, and its binding affinity is typically low. Once the subset is stimulated by a foreign antigen, however, it undergoes an **affinity maturation** process characterized by **somatic hypermutation** of the V segments of immunoglobulin genes. The hypermutation is achieved by a deaminase enzyme causing cytosine bases to be replaced with uracil within DNA. Subsequently, error-prone DNA polymerases are recruited and DNA repair processes are modified so that mutations can persist in the DNA sequence. This creates a mutation rate increase of almost 10^6 gene segments per base pair per generation. This causes considerable additional variation in immunoglobulin-encoding DNA sequences, and thus in the antigen-binding properties of the encoded immunoglobulins. Since mutation is such a random process, however, many of the new receptors have poor binding affinity and are not selected. Eventually, a subset of immunoglobulins are produced that do have a high affinity binding to the foreign antigen, and those B cells that possess these Igs are selected to proliferate extensively. The end result is a population of mature plasma cells that secrete antibodies highly specific to the invading antigen.

Multiple Combinations of Heavy and Light Chains

The random combination of different heavy and light chains during the assembly of the immunoglobulin molecule creates further diversity of the antibodies. Each of these mechanisms, when considered together, could potentially produce as many as 10^{10} to 10^{14} distinct antibodies. The genetic basis for antibody diversity as presented through these mechanisms creates the potential for an infinite response to foreign substances. It could also simultaneously create many problems if any of the mutations became damaging; for example, not all gene segments are functional and have accumulated mutations that prevent them from encoding a functional protein. These gene segments are termed *pseudogenes;* if a significant proportion of them are incorporated into a segment, the result will be nonfunctional, which could result in an immunodeficiency disease.

SECTION FOUR REVIEW

1. Which of the following contributes to the genetic diversity of immunoglobulins?
   A. Heavy and light chains
   B. Multiple germline genes
   C. Constant and variable regions
   D. All of the above
2. The greatest genetic diversity of antibodies is achieved by which mechanism?
   A. Somatic recombination
   B. Multiple combinations of heavy and light chains
   C. Somatic hypermutation
   D. Junctional diversity
3. Which of the following cells carry activated immunoglobulins?
   A. T lymphocytes
   B. B lymphocytes
   C. Plasma cells
   D. Dendrite cells
4. Which of the following is a signaling protein?
   A. Plasma cells
   B. Immunoglobulin
   C. T lymphocytes
   D. Cytokine
5. The chemical composition of an antibody is
   A. protein.
   B. lipid.
   C. carbohydrate.
   D. glycoprotein.

Answers: 1. D; 2. C; 3. C; 4. D; 5. D.

SECTION FIVE: Immune Diseases

Remarkable advances in the field of human genetics over the past few years have disseminated an explosion of information that can be applied to genetic immunity. Many of the recent discoveries are the result of the application of genome-wide association (**GWA**) scans as promoted through various international research organizations and the Internet.

Gregersen and Olsson (2009) described three basic approaches to identifying genetic variations that might contribute to any human phenotype, including autoimmune disorders. The first was candidate gene association studies, the mainstay for human genetic studies for decades. Secondly was a linkage analysis in multiplex families. Both of these approaches were lacking in statistical power owing to inadequate sample cases. Lastly was the GWA scanning approach, which coincides with the HapMap Project. A realization from this project was that to define most of the common variations among individuals, it is not necessary to genotype all 3 million single nucleotide polymorphism (SNP) differences among them, but only a subset of these—around 300,000 to 500,000 SNPs. The reason for this was that SNP alleles are distributed nonrandomly among individuals to form a **linkage disequilibrium** (**LD**) that could extend to thousands or more base pairs. This creates a distinct pattern that can be used to define common genetic variation across the genome of an individual. A single SNP could be tagged to a block of LD formed by many other SNPs, which would permit the analysis of a large section of a genome with a single marker.

Prior to GWA scans, a number of genetic diseases showed significant associations with specific major histocompatibility complex (MHC) alleles; i.e., individuals with the allele were much more likely to develop a particular disease than those who lack it. The MHC complex plays a major role in the recognition of self from nonself in the immune system response. In **autoimmune diseases**, the body's immune system attacks its own normal cells, which appears to be a breakdown in self-tolerance—i.e., genes associated with the MHC complex. Other autoimmune diseases may involve molecular mimicry, where a peptide that stimulates an immune response is so similar to the body's own peptides that the immune system begins to attack the body's own cells. Autoimmunity can also be caused by specific defects in the regulation of immune system components as with the T regulatory cells, which help prevent the formation of self-reactive immune cells. A mutation in a gene for these cells or a missing gene would cause a deficiency of regulatory T cells and a resultant autoimmune disease. Other common diseases that involve autoimmunity include rheumatoid arthritis, systemic lupus erythematosus, psoriasis, and multiple sclerosis. It is estimated the approximately 5% of the general population worldwide suffer from autoimmune diseases.

From GWA scans Gregersen and Olsson (2009) noted that the most replicated and broadly relevant association with autoimmune disorders was with the allele for intracellular tyrosine phosphatase, PTPN22, which had previously been reported as associated with Type 1 diabetes, rheumatoid arthritis, Graves' disease, Hashimoto thyroiditis, myasthenia gravis, systemic sclerosis, Addison's disease, and others. These patterns of association between an allele and autoimmunity support previous knowledge that common susceptibility genes underlie diverse autoimmune phenotypes. In terms of strength of association, PTPN22 is second in importance only to the MHC for autoimmune diseases.

Immunodeficiency diseases result when one or more components of the immune system (e.g., T cells, B cells, MHC, complement proteins) are missing or fail to function normally. Primary immunodeficiency diseases are caused by abnormalities in cells of the immune system and are generally caused by genetic alterations. To date, more than 100 different primary immunodeficiency syndromes have been described, and it is estimated that approximately 1 in 10,000 persons are affected. Secondary immunodeficiency results when components of the immune system are altered or destroyed by other factors, i.e., radiation, infection or drugs. The human immunodeficiency virus (HIV), which causes acquired immunodeficiency syndrome (AIDS), attacks macrophages and helper T lymphocytes—central components of the immune system. The result of this infection is increased susceptibility to a multitude of opportunisitic infections.

Use of the GWA scans for genetic research has already produced considerable insight into a variety of genetic diseases and will, no doubt, serve to identify new risk genes for many others. Autoimmune diseases in particular have been found to have a complex genetic basis with multiple genes contributing to disease risk. Analyzing for SNPs through the GWA scans will only serve to exponentially increase what is known and what can be done. An additional venue to research would relate to environmental triggers and the epigenome, which would also include ancestor history.

SECTION FIVE REVIEW

1. Autoimmune diseases have a complex genetic basis.
   A. True
   B. False
2. Which of the following describes the essential cause of autoimmunity?
   A. Too many antigenic determinants
   B. Lack of antibody formation
   C. Breakdown in self-tolerance
   D. Lack of macrophages
3. Which of the following provides the most information for genetic disease research?
   A. Study of individual candidate gene history
   B. Study of linkages in multiple families
   C. Reviewing medical genetic research
   D. Performing GWA scans for SNPs
4. HIV is a primary immunodeficiency disease.
   A. True
   B. False
5. Which of the following are typically autoimmune diseases?
   1. Lupus
   2. Graves' disease
   3. Type 1 diabetes
   4. Rheumatoid arthritis

   A. 1, 2, 4
   B. 3, 2, 4
   C. 1, 3, 4
   D. 1, 2, 3, 4

Answers: 1. A; 2. C; 3. D; 4. B; 5. D

POSTTEST

1. The strength of a bond between a single antigenic determinant and an individual combining site is called
   A. specificity.
   B. affinity.
   C. avidity.
   D. immune complex.
2. The ability of an antibody to combine with one antigen instead of another is referred to as
   A. immune complex.
   B. affinity.
   C. specificity.
   D. avidity.
3. Antigens are characterized by all of the following EXCEPT
   A. they are usually large organic molecules.
   B. they are usually lipids.
   C. they can be glycolipids or glycoproteins.
   D. they are also called immunogens.
4. Antibodies are also referred to as
   A. immunoglobulins.
   B. haptens.
   C. epitopes.
   D. gamma globulins.
5. The strongest bond of antigen and antibody chiefly results from the
   A. type of bonding.
   B. goodness of fit.
   C. antibody type.
   D. quantity of antibody.
6. Immediate hypersensitivity consists of the reactions primarily mediated by the ________________ class of immunoglobulins.
   A. IgM
   B. IgG
   C. IgE
   D. IgA
7. This immunoglobulin is found in tears, saliva, colostrum, milk, and intestinal secretions.
   A. IgM
   B. IgG
   C. IgE
   D. IgA
8. Antigen presenting cells are typically ________________.
   A. T cells
   B. macrophages
   C. B cells
   D. mast cells
9. The identification proteins on the surface of cells belong to a class of molecules called the
   A. cytokines.
   B. major histocompatibility complex.
   C. interleukins.
   D. interferons.
10. ________________ are cytokines that cause fever, temporarily maintaining a higher body temperature.
    A. Interferons
    B. Interleukins
    C. Tumor necrosis factors
    D. Collectins

Posttest answers are located in the Appendix.

CHAPTER SUMMARY

A comprehensive grasp of the immune system is vital to fully understand the full extent of infectious diseases and pathological malfunctions within individuals. The innate immune system and the adaptive immune system work separately and together to prevent the invasion of pathogens into a host's body.

- Nursing practice can influence a patient's response for healing through stress reduction.
- Social genomics and nutrigenomics play an essential role in the development of health and disease.
- The immune system consists of cells and biochemicals that distinguish self from nonself antigens.
- The innate system is primed and ready for a response once a foreign entity breaches the first line of defense. If the innate response becomes overwhelmed, the adaptive system induces the cellular mediated immunity system and the humoral system to respond. The adaptive immune system differs from the innate in terms of specificity and memory.
- The adaptive immune system possesses an enormous amount of genetic diversity through the structure of the immunoglobulins in order to respond to the vast array of microbes and pathogens within the environment.
- An understanding of immunogenetics provides a broader background for the health care professional to contribute not only to the care of an individual but to greater insight of phenotypical characteristics.
- Genetic research and knowledge is expanding at an enormous rate due to the resources available to researchers through partnerships such as the HapMap Project.

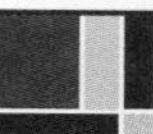

CRITICAL THINKING CHECKPOINT

CL, a 40-year-old Caucasian female, has been experiencing episodes of fatigue and excessive sleepiness at the end of the day, especially after dinner. She states, "I can barely stay awake to get the kids to bed." She loves her job as a programmer because she can sometimes telecommute from home if she needs to stay home with a sick child. She is 5'4" tall, weighs 120 pounds, and routinely jogs three miles every day in the morning before breakfast. She adds to this information that she has also been extremely hungry and thirsty after her run, which is unusual because "running usually curbs my appetite." When questioned about her health recently, she remembers that she did have a 24-hour bug about a month ago that "knocked me off my feet. I had a high fever and everything!" She adds that it was at a particularly stressful time because she had a deadline for a work project. She then remembers that this fatigue in the evening started after that episode. She has a family history of maternal late-onset diabetes, but that "was because my mother was fat and I vowed I'd never let myself get that bad."

1. What are the significant points in CL's history that could indicate a problem?
2. What lab tests would you want to run immediately?
3. What other questions could provide important information?
4. What would you advise her to do for follow-up?

Answers are provided in the Appendix

Pearson Nursing Student Resources

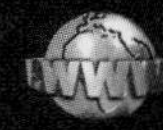

Find additional review materials at nursing.pearsonhighered.com

Prepare for success with additional NCLEX®-style practice questions, interactive assignments and activities, web links, animations, videos, and more!

ONLINE RESOURCES

International HapMap Project: http://hapmap.ncbi.nlm.nih.gov

National Cancer Institute Understand Cancer Series – The Immune System: http://www.cancer.gov/cancertopics/understandingcancer/immunesystem/page1

REFERENCES

Abbas, A. K., Lichtman, A. H., & Pillai, S. (2010). *Cellular and molecular immunology* (3rd ed.). Philadelphia, PA: Saunders Elsevier.

Azar, B. (2011). The psychology of cells. *American Psychological Association, 42*(5), 32.

Bambrick, G. (2011). The DNA diet. *Tufts Nutrition Magazine,* Summer Issue. July 25, 2011. Retrived July 5, 2012, from http://now.tufts.edu/articles/dna-diet

Chen, J. Y., Lin, C. Y., Wang, C. M., Lin, Y. T., Kuo, S. N., Shiu, C. F., et al. (2011). IL28B genetic variations are associated with high sustained virological response (SVR) of interferon-α plus ribavirin therapy in Taiwanese chronic HCV infection. *Genes and Immunity, 12,* 300–309. doi:10.1038/gene.2011.1

Cousins Center for Psychoneuroimmunology. (2011). http://www.semel.ucla.edu/cousinsi/research

Genetic Science Learning Center. (2012). http://learn.genetics.utah.edu

Gregersen, P. K., & Olsson, L. M. (2009). Recent advances in the genetics of autoimmune disease. *Annual Review of Immunology, 27,* 363–391. doi:10.1146/annurev.immunol.021908,132653

Hasan, H., & Hasan, T. F. (2009). Laugh yourself into a healthier person: A cross cultural analysis of the effects of varying levels of laughter on health. *International Journal of Medical Science, 6*(4), 200–211.

Hui-Ling, L., Yin-Ming L., & Li-Hua, L. (2012). Effects of music intervention with nursing presence and recorded music on psycho-physiological indices of cancer patient caregivers. *Journal of Clinical Nursing, 21*(5–6), 745–756.

Ifill, G., & Johnson, J. (2012, 27 February). The power of music therapy. *PBS Newshour.* Retrieved July 4, 2012, from http://www.pbs.org/newshour/bb/health/jan-june12/musictherapy_02-27.html

Jirtle, R. L., & Skinner, M. K. (2007). Environmental epigenomics and disease susceptibility. *Nature Reviews Genetics 8,* 253–262. doi:10.1038/nrg2045

Jorde, L. B., Carey, J. C., & Banshad, M. J. (2010). *Medical genetics* (4th ed.). Philadelphia, PA: Mosby Elsevier.

Kiecolt-Glaser, J. K., McGuire, L., Robles, T. F., & Glaser, R. (2002). Emotions, morbidity, and mortality: New perspectives from psychoneuroimmunology. *Annual Review of Psychology,* 83–107.

Martin, R. A. (2002). Is laughter the best medicine? Humor, laughter, and physical health. *Current Directions in Psychological Science, 11*(6), 216–218.

Mayer, G. (2011). *Microbiology and immunology on-line.* University of South Carolina School of Medicine. Retrieved July 4, 2012, from: http://pathmicro.med.sc.edu/ghaffar/innate.htm

Mayer, G., & Nyland, J. (2011). *Microbiology and immunology on-line.* University of South Carolina School of Medicine. Retrieved July 4, 2012, from http://pathmicro.med.sc.edu/bowers/mhc.htm

Nightingale, F. (1863). *Notes on hospitals.* London: Longman, Green, Longman, Roberts, and Green.

Nightingale, F. (1859). *Notes on nursing: What it is, and what it is not.* London: Harrison, 59, Pall Mall, Bookseller to the Queen.

Overton, J. P., Al-Lazikani, B., & Hopkins, A. L. (2006). How many drug targets are there? *Nature Reviews Drug Discovery, 5,* 993–996. doi:10.1038/nrd2199

Pembrey, M. E., Bygren, L. O., Kaati, G., Edvinsson, S., Northstone, K., Sjöström, M., et al. (2006). Sex-specific, male-line transgenerational responses in humans. *European Journal of Human Genetics,14,* 159–166. doi:10.1038/sj.ejhg.5201538

Pert, C. B. (1997). *Molecules of emotion: The science behind mind body medicine.* New York, NY: Touchstone.

Turgeon, M. L. (2009). *Immunology and serology in laboratory medicine.* St. Louis, MO: Mosby Elsevier.

Vascular Medicine. (2006). Watching funny movies boosts blood flow to the heart. *Health & Medicine Week,* 1660. Research Library database. (Document ID: 9802266611)

CHAPTER

16 Cancer Genetics

Sharon Olsen

LEARNING OUTCOMES

Following the completion of this chapter, the learner will be able to

1. Describe the hallmarks of cancer development and progression.
2. Relate two theories of cancer development.
3. Define cancer gene.
4. Explain how oncogenes influence cancer development.
5. Relate the significance of tumor suppressor gene mutations.
6. Compare and contrast the role of genomic and epigenomic factors in cancer development.
7. Explain how genetic, genomic, and epigenetic factors contribute to cancer.
8. Relate four examples of how contemporary understanding of the molecular biology of cancer has been translated into clinic practice to improve patient care.
9. Apply concepts previously discussed to two hereditary cancer exemplars.
10. Describe how growth in the science of cancer genetics, genomics, and epigenomics is reframing the professional patient care responsibilities of generalist nurses for the care of persons with or at risk for cancer.
11. Describe how growth in our understanding of the molecular biology of cancer is reframing the patient and professional responsibilities of generalist nurses for the care of persons with or at risk for cancer.

This chapter provides an introduction to contemporary understandings of the molecular biology of cancer, with an extensive description of cancer genes. The clinical applications of cancer genomics lend themselves to a personalized approach to the course of cancer treatment through targeted therapies. The practical applications of some genetic concepts that were explored earlier in the book are considered in relation to the genetics of cancer.

PRETEST

1. Which of the following best describes the cause(s) of cancer?
   A. A critical gene mutation
   B. The accumulation of DNA mutations as well as changes in epigenetic processes
   C. An inherited genetic condition
   D. A complex, multistep process
2. Which of the following is NOT a hallmark capability of cancer according to Hanahan and Weinstein (2011)?
   A. Ability to sustain chronic proliferation
   B. Ability to evade growth suppressors
   C. Ability to generate germ line mutations
   D. Ability to resist cell death
   E. Ability to activate invasion and metastasis
3. Which of the following best describes a proto oncogene?
   A. A subset of tumor suppressor genes.
   B. A gene that when mutated can become an oncogene.
   C. A gene with a point mutation that is common in many cancers.
   D. A gene that makes proteins that inhibit normal cell division.
   E. A major cause of chronic myelogenous leukemia.
4. Which of the following best describes why viruses like Epstein Barr and hepatitis B can contribute to cancer development?
   A. Infection with these viruses leads to clonal expansion of infected cells with loss of normal function.
   B. Infection with these viruses can activate invasion and metastasis.
   C. Viral DNA are inserted into cellular DNA during replication.
5. The development of drugs that targets angiogenesis are a promising new model for treating cancer.
   A. True
   B. False

6. Which of the following has NOT been described as an effect of epigenetics?
   A. Epigenetics has the ability to chemically program cellular behavior.
   B. Epigenetic changes in tumor cells are potentially reversible.
   C. Epigenetic functions are heritable.
   D. Epigenetics can turn a particular gene *on* as well as *off*.
   E. Cancer drugs do not influence epigenetic function.
7. How will an improved understanding of the molecular genetics of a particular type of cancer contribute to personalized medicine?
   A. Treatment can be targeted to the particular gene, gene product, or molecular pathway that triggers a cancer.
   B. The genetic signature of a cancer can be used to predict prognosis.
   C. Biomarkers can monitor the effect(s) of cancer treatment.
   D. All of the above
8. Nurses must understand cancer genetics because
   A. They make up the largest number of direct care providers.
   B. There are insufficient genetic experts to translate cancer genetic information to patients and the public.
   C. They are the case finders for cancer predisposition.
   D. All of the above
9. Red flags that suggest inherited predisposition for cancer include all of the following EXCEPT
   A. multifocal or bilateral disease.
   B. early age of cancer onset, typically before age 50 years.
   C. multiple affected family members.
   D. evidence for rapid metastasis among multiple individuals with cancer.
   E. occurrence of similar cancers across multiple generations.
10. Cancer treatment is evolving and new drugs are being developed to target very specific gene functions and or cancer development pathways. Which of the following skills or competencies is most important for a nurse?
    A. History taking and physical assessment skills
    B. Initiation and participation in systems processes that enable continuous monitoring for and recording of adverse events.
    C. Collaboration with other providers to develop patient care guidelines for the management and prevention of unanticipated events.
    D. Patient education about the drug effects, interactions, and the need to report unexpected drug effects.
    E. All of the above

Pretest answers are located in the Appendix.

SECTION ONE: Introduction to Cancer Genetics

Cancer is an umbrella term for many diseases and there are at least 200 different types of human cancers (Hanahan & Weinberg, 2011). Unlike classical genetic diseases that are typically caused by a single faulty gene, there is no single gene mutation that triggers all cancers. Cancers are known to arise in response to the accumulation of DNA mutations as well as to changes in epigenetic processes that typically program the behavior of our genetic makeup. Both processes can alter the protein products of the normal genes that regulate cell growth, cell differentiation, cell migration, invasion, or cell death. Mutations can be inherited or triggered by mistakes in DNA replication or exposure to a variety of environmental or behavioral triggers (e.g., benzene and arsenic in tobacco, ultraviolet radiation in sunlight, or certain viruses). Some of these triggers lead to a process known as methylation, a chemical epigenetic response to external, as well as, host-related (endogenous) factors (e.g., aging, hormones, obesity, etc.) that facilitate DNA-associated changes with malignant potential. Occasionally, mutations will occur in a critical "cancer gene" that gives a selective growth advantage to a cell leading to the clonal expansions of a set of abnormal cells (a tumor). Over time, these cells accumulate additional mutations, rendering the tumor increasingly unstable genetically. This process accounts for **carcinogenesis**, which is the evolution of tumors from being benign lesions to malignant and then metastatic cancers.

During the past two decades, our understanding of the pathogenesis of cancer has grown tremendously and it is now clear that **tumorigenesis** represents a complex, multistep process wherein cells progressively acquire a common set of features that underlie their malignancy. In 2000, Hanahan and Weinstein first described a set of six hallmark capabilities of cancer. These hallmarks are part of the multistep process that supports tumor growth, cancer development, and metastasis. Eleven years of published research later, the authors updated this list and posited two additional hallmarks. Experts believe these hallmarks are essential for cancer development and metastasis. Each is briefly described in the list that follows (Hanahan & Weinstein, 2011).

- *Ability to sustain chronic proliferation.* Cancer cells are able to deregulate growth factor signals that in a normal cell carefully control the production and release of growth-promoting signals. These signals may also influence cell survival and energy metabolism. As a result, cancer cells assume the capacity for unrestrained growth and proliferation (Hanahan & Weinstein, 2011).
- *Ability to evade growth suppressors.* This is achieved through the inactivation of tumor suppressor genes whose normal function is to suppress aberrant cell growth. For example, mutations in the *TP53* and the *RB* genes produce proteins that encourage cancer cell growth instead of activating pathways that promote cell senescence or apoptosis (Hanahan & Weinstein, 2011).

- *Ability to resist cell death.* As just noted, the loss of normal *TP53* function to recognize cell damage disengages the normal apoptosis response. Another example is demonstrated by the growth advantage that is triggered by necrotic cell death. Research suggests that when necrotic cells break down, they actually recruit tumor promoting inflammatory cells from the immune system. These cells are capable of fostering **angiogenesis**, cancer cell proliferation, and metastasis (Hanahan & Weinstein, 2011).
- *Ability to support replication immortality.* In the normal aging process, cells are hardwired for a selective number of doublings in response to the gradual shortening of telomeres. Cancer cells have the ability to produce DNA polymerase, an enzyme that adds telomere segments to the ends of DNA thereby producing immortalized cancer cells (Hanahan & Weinstein, 2011).
- *Ability to induce angiogenesis.* In cancer cells, an "angiogenic switch" is turned on very early in tumor growth to support the development of new blood vessels. In the face of hypoxia, cancer cells are able to upregulate vascular endothelial growth factor (***VEGF***) to promote vessel growth. It has been demonstrated that the blood vessels produced in tumor tissue appear abnormal including "excessive capillary sprouting, convoluted and excessive vessel branching, distorted and enlarged vessels, erratic blood flow, microhemorrhaging, leakiness, and abnormal levels of endothelial cell proliferation and apoptosis" (Hanahan & Weinstein, 2011, p. 653).
- *Ability to activate invasion and metastasis.* Two examples are instructive. Typically, E-cadherin (a cell adhesion molecule) controls tissue architecture and integrity via cell-to-cell adhesion. If this function is lost, cancer cells can invade surrounding tissues. In a second example, it has been observed that macrophages located at the edges of a tumor are able to support local tissue invasion by releasing enzymes that break down the walls of cells, lymph tissue, and blood vessels to allow micrometastasis. Today, researchers are actively investigating a recently described "invasion-metastasis cascade" that might provide greater understanding of the biology of this process. It is also thought that the potential for invasion and metastasis will be proven to be tumor specific (Hanahan & Weinstein, 2011).
- *Ability to reprogram energy metabolism.* Research suggests that glucose metabolism is reprogrammed in cancer cells to support the need for unregulated cell growth and proliferation. In a fascinating example, Hanahan and Weinstein describe research that supports this process in two subpopulations of cancer cells. Both "appear to function symbiotically: the hypoxic cancer cells depend on glucose for fuel and secrete lactate as waste, which is imported and preferentially used as fuel by their better-oxygenated brethren" (Hanahan & Weinstein, 2011, p. 660).
- *Ability to evade destruction by the immune system.* The immune system (made up of white blood cells including B cells and T cells, natural killer cells, macrophages, and dendritic cells) typically seeks to destroy abnormal bacteria or viruses. But cancer cells often evade this fate because they resemble normal, healthy cells in enough ways to obstruct immune responses from being directed against them. In addition, even as tumors grow and their cells develop more and more genetic mutations—in effect becoming more "foreign" to the body—they are able to suppress the immune-modulating function of normal cells in their microenvironment to further thwart the immune system's ability to attack and destroy cancer cells (Hanahan & Weinstein, 2011; National Cancer Institute [NCI], 2012).

Models of Cancer Development

Some of our earliest understandings of cancer causation came from epidemiological studies of specific groups of individuals. For example, during the late 1700s, high rates of scrotal cancers were found in men who worked in youth as chimney sweeps. This finding suggested a relationship between cancer and coal soot. In the 1970s, Dr. Bruce Ames furthered our understanding of the relationship between exposure to specific carcinogens, their induction of DNA mutations, and the development of cancer. His research, as well as the publication of a comprehensive list of carcinogens enhanced our understanding of the need to reduce or prevent carcinogen exposure as part of cancer prevention.

Two-Hit Theory

During the 1970s, Alfred Knudson, MD, PhD, was exploring a clinical puzzle that he observed in children with retinoblastoma. He noted that when retinoblastoma was inherited, children frequently exhibited early onset, bilateral disease that was often characterized by multifocal tumors in each eye (Chial, 2008). Alternatively, in children without a family history of retinoblastoma, cancer developed in only one eye and often at a later age. Knudson correctly discerned that retinoblastoma occurred in both sporadic and inherited forms, and hypothesized that two gene-driven mutations were necessary for retinoblastoma to develop—the Knudson Two-Hit Hypothesis. He proposed that the first hit was inherited via the germ line, making a mutated allele present at birth in every cell. And a second hit, randomly acquired later in life, would account for the somatic loss of the second (nonmutated or wild type) allele. Together, these steps accounted for the increased likelihood of bilateral disease, the multifocal presentation (remember, **germ line mutations** are expressed in every cell of the body), and the earlier age of onset common with inherited cancers.

Alternatively, in sporadic cases of retinoblastoma, two randomly acquired "hits" are necessary to cause disease, accounting for cancer presentation as a single lesion in one eye and a later age of onset. The "two-hit" theory continues to have relevance today to explain mutations in tumor suppressor genes, whereby germ line mutations present as heterozygous mutations in normal cells, but both alleles must be missing or mutated in the tumor genome.

Cancer Stem Cell Theory

In the last 10 years, scientists have begun to explore a stem cell theory of cancer (Frank, Schatton, & Frank, 2010; Hanahan & Weinstein, 2011; Soltanian & Matin, 2011). **Cancer stem cells (CSCs)**, also referred to as tumor-initiating cells or tumorigenic cancer cells, have been documented in acute myelogenous leukemia as well as solid tumors (breast, brain, lung, prostate, ovary, colon, skin, liver, and pancreas cancers). Although the attributes of these cells are only beginning to be uncovered, they are believed to be very long-lived, which allows them to acquire mutations along the course of an individual's lifetime. CSCs appear to be able to proliferate and initiate tumor growth. They may also have a role in cancer relapse and metastasis as well as in treatment resistance. CSCs are believed to exist in tumors as a distinct population. Scientists believe that if they can differentiate CSCs from normal stem cells in various tissues then they may be able to develop novel treatments to target the destruction of CSCs without adversely affecting normal stem cells.

Cancer Genes

The identification and cataloging of **somatic mutations** that are known to drive the development of cancer (referred to as *cancer genes*) is the goal of COSMIC (Catalogue of Somatic Mutations in Cancer), a project supported by the Welcome Trust organization. To date, 465 cancer genes have been cataloged. Inheritance patterns for these genes have been analyzed, and approximately 90% of cancers have been shown to exhibit somatic mutations, 20% demonstrate germ line mutations that predispose to cancer, and 10% show both somatic and germ line mutations.

Germ line mutations are inherited and contribute a single, defective copy of a gene to every cell in an individual. They play a significant role in perhaps 3%–10% of all cancers. Because genes come in pairs (one inherited from each parent), an inherited defect in one copy (one allele) predisposes a person to cancer but generally does not lead to it because the second normal allele is still functional. If, however, the second allele undergoes somatic mutation, cancer may develop because there is no longer any functional copy of the gene. Because the rate of somatic loss of a single allele is more common than the random mutation of two alleles, the incidence of specific cancers in mutation carriers is dramatically increased over that of the general population. Mutated genes typically associated with germ line inheritance and increased risk for cancer include, but are not limited to, ***BRCA1*** and ***BRCA2*** (breast and ovarian cancers), ***APC*** (familial adenomatous polyposis colon cancer), and ***RB1*** (retinoblastoma).

The majority of cancers occur randomly and in somatic cells (normal as well as cancerous cells), resulting in the clonal expansion of unrepaired DNA mistakes that occurred during DNA replication. Somatic cells can also acquire completely new DNA sequences, notably those of viruses such as human papillomavirus, Epstein Barr, hepatitis B, human T lymphotropic virus 1, and human herpes virus 8. Each of these is known to contribute to the development of one or more types of cancer (Stratton, Campbell, & Futreal, 2009). In these instances, viruses can completely inactivate a host cell or overactivate it.

The actual transformation from a single, genetically altered cell to a malignant cancer with the capability of invading surrounding tissue and metastasizing to distant tissues can extend over a period of decades and give rise to a diverse number of somatic mutations that ultimately contribute to clonal expansions of mutated cells. In fact, today we know that there can be 1,000 to 10,000 somatic mutations in the genomes of most adult cancers, including breast, ovary, colorectal, pancreas, and glioma (Stratton, 2011). Scientists have observed fewer mutations in medulloblastomas, testicular germ cell tumors, acute leukemias, and more mutations in lung cancers and melanomas. Mutated cells must be able to confer a growth advantage to the tumor over the surrounding normal tissue for its continued growth. The study of changes in genes and their expression in whole **cancer genomes** is the work of The Cancer Genome Atlas (**TCGA**) project sponsored by the National Cancer Institute (**NCI**) and the National Human Genome Research Institute (**NHGRI**). Scientists are working to differentiate between the critical somatic mutations that may actually drive cancer development (known as *driver mutations*) and any random "passenger mutations" that accumulate in specific tumor cells but do not contribute to cancer development (Bunz, 2008; Greenman et al., 2007; Stratton, Campbell, & Futreal, 2009). Passenger mutations are known to exist in cancer cells because somatic mutations without functional consequences commonly occur during cell division. It is anticipated that the identification of critical driver mutations in specific cancers will enhance tumor classification and lead to targeted cancer treatment and improved clinical outcomes.

Today, scientists understand that human cancers, for the most part, are caused by the activation of **proto-oncogenes** and the loss of tumor suppressor genes. The failure of a subset of these genes, known as DNA repair genes, can lead to DNA instability and increase the risk for mutation of both. Each of these cancer genes is reviewed in the following sections.

Oncogenes

Proto-oncogenes are normal genes whose protein products contribute to fundamental cellular processes such as cell division and differentiation. Mutations in proto-oncogenes result in oncogene formation (see Table 16–1). When oncogenes arise in normal cells, they make proteins that increase the level of proto-oncogene function. Such mutations are called activating mutations, which are known to result in excessive cell growth, inhibition of cellular differentiation, and/or the prevention of cell death (Bunz, 2008). To use a common metaphor, the presence of an oncogene is like having a gas pedal that is stuck to the floorboard, causing cells to continually grow and divide.

Oncogene activations can, in turn, be generated from chromosomal translocations that result in the fusion of genes and production of a fusion protein with cancer-causing activity (Vogelstein, 2004). For example, the translocation fusion of the *BCR* and *ABL* genes is associated with chronic myelogenous leukemia, and fusion of the *EWS* and *FLI1*

TABLE 16–1: Select Cancer Genes

Gene Symbol (Official Name)	Location	Classification and Known DNA Damage	Normal Protein Function	Associated Cancer(s)
BCR-ABL (Philadelphia chromosome)	A reciprocal translocation between chromosomes 22 and 9	*Classification:* Oncogene *Known DNA damage:* translocation	Encodes a protein that activates other proteins involved in cell cycle regulation and cell division.	Chronic myelogenous leukemia; acute myelogenous leukemia (T cell type)
EGFR (epidermal growth factor receptor)	7p12	*Classification:* Oncogene *Known DNA damage:* deletions; insertions	Encodes a growth factor receptor involved in cell proliferation, differentiation, motility, survival, and tissue development.	Glioblastoma; non–small cell lung cancer
ERBB2 (v-erb-b2 erythroblastic leukemia viral oncogene homolog 2, neuro/glioblastoma derived oncogene homolog [avian]); also known as *HER2* and *Her-2/neu*	17q11.2-q12	*Classification:* Oncogene *Known DNA damage:* amplification	Encodes the ErbB2 growth factor receptor that promotes cell growth, cell adhesion, cell specialization, and cell movement.	Breast cancer (found in ~25% of cases and associated with aggressive tumors that are more likely to metastasize); ovarian cancer; cervical cancer; non–small cell lung cancer; stomach cancer; glioblastoma; medulloblastoma
KRAS (v-Ki-ras2 Kirsten rat sarcoma viral oncogene homolog)	12p12.1	*Classification:* Oncogene	Codes the K-Ras cell-signaling protein that regulates cell growth, division, maturation, and differentiation.	Cancers of the pancreas, lung, colon, and rectum
MET (met proto-oncogene [hepatocyte growth factor receptor])	7q31.2	*Classification:* Oncogene *Known DNA damage:* amplification; missense mutations	Encodes HGF-receptor tyrosine kinase that regulates cell proliferation, morphogenesis, and survival. During embryonic development, MET signaling plays a role in gastrulation, development, migration of muscles, neuronal precursors, angiogenesis, and kidney formation. In adults, it assists in wound healing, organ regeneration, and tissue remodeling.	Cancers of the esophagus, stomach, kidney, liver, and lung; medulloblastoma
MYC, also known as *c-Myc* (v-myc myelocytomatosis viral oncogene homolog)	8q24.21	*Classification:* Oncogene *Known DNA damage:* amplification, DNA rearrangement, and translocation	Encodes a protein that activates different growth-promoting genes that play a role in cell cycle progression, apoptosis, and cellular transformation.	Cancers of the breast, prostate, stomach, ovary, and colon; leukemias; lymphomas, including Burkitt's lymphoma
RET (ret proto-oncogene)	10q11.2	*Classification:* Oncogene (identified as a gatekeeper gene)	Encodes a cell-signaling protein. One end of the protein is inside the cell; the other projects to the outer surface of the cell. When growth factors attach to the RET protein, it triggers a complex cascade of chemical reactions inside the cell. These reactions instruct the cell to undergo certain changes, such as dividing or maturing. This protein appears to be essential for normal kidney development, spermatogenesis, and the normal development of nerves in the intestine (enteric neurons) and the autonomic nervous system.	Multiple endocrine neoplasia Type 2; medullary thyroid cancer Type 2A; Pheochromocytoma

(Continues)

TABLE 16–1: Select Cancer Genes *(Continued)*

Gene Symbol (Official Name)	Location	Classification and Known DNA Damage	Normal Protein Function	Associated Cancer(s)
VEGF or *VEGFA* (vascular endothelial growth factor A)	6p12	*Classification:* Oncogene	Encodes a growth factor protein that acts on endothelial cells to mediate increased vascular permeability; induce angiogenesis, vasculogenesis, and endothelial cell growth; promote cell migration; and inhibit apoptosis.	Breast, colorectal, and kidney cancers
APC (adenomatous polyposis coli)	5q21-q22	*Classification:* tumor suppressor gene	Encodes the APC protein. Helps control cell division, adhesion, and mobility. Also helps ensure that the number of chromosomes in a cell is correct following cell division.	Classic and attenuated types of familial adenomatous polyposis (FAP); found in 80% of colon tumors; some cancers of thyroid, stomach, and brain
BRCA1 (breast cancer 1, early onset)	17q21	*Classification:* tumor suppressor gene (identified as both a DNA repair gene and a caretaker gene) *Known DNA Damage:* more than 1,000 mutations identified	Codes for a protein involved in DNA repair, cell cycle checkpoint control, chromatin remodeling, and estrogen responsiveness.	Hereditary breast and ovarian cancers, fallopian tube cancer, and pancreatic cancer
BRCA2 (breast cancer 2, early onset)	13q12.3	*Classification:* tumor suppressor gene (identified as both a DNA repair gene and a caretaker gene) *Known DNA Damage:* more than 800 mutations identified	Codes for a protein involved in DNA repair, cell cycle checkpoint control, chromatin remodeling, and estrogen responsiveness.	Mutations associated with cancers of the breast, ovary, prostate, pancreas, and fallopian tube as well as melanoma, Falconi anemia, and male breast cancer
CDKN2A (cyclin-dependent kinase inhibitor 2A)	9p21	*Classification:* tumor suppressor gene (identified as a gatekeeper gene) *Known DNA Damage:* mutations associated with methalation of promoter region; point mutations.	An antioncogene that antagonizes the growth-promoting activities of certain oncogenes. Able to block the cell cycle in G_1 phase. Can cause accumulation of tumor protein p53.	Melanoma; familial atypical multiple mole melanoma-pancreatic cancer syndrome (FAMMMPC); melanoma-astrocytoma syndrome (MASTS); cancers of the pancreas, breast, bladder, prostate, colon, and esophagus; glioblastoma; mesothelioma
MLH1 (mutL homolog 1)	3p21.3	*Classification:* Tumor suppressor gene (identified as both a caretaker gene and a DNA mismatch repair [MMR] gene) *Known DNA Damage:* nonsense mutations	Encodes the MLH1 protein that joins with the PMS2 protein to form a protein complex that coordinates the activities of other proteins to repair mistakes made during DNA replication.	Lynch syndrome; hereditary nonpolyposis colon cancer (HNPCC); neurofibromatosis; CoLoN syndrome; lymphoma; skin cancer sarcoma

Gene Symbol (Official Name)	Location	Classification and Known DNA Damage	Normal Protein Function	Associated Cancer(s)
MSH2 (mutS homolog 2)	2p22-p21	*Classification:* tumor suppressor gene (identified as both a caretaker gene and a DNA MMR gene) *Known DNA Damage:* nonsense mutations	Encodes the MSH2 protein that helps fix mistakes made when DNA is copied prior to cell division.	Lynch syndrome; HNPCC; Lymphoma; skin cancers; sarcomas; neurofibromatosis; CoLoN syndrome
MSH6 (mutS homolog 6)		*Classification:* tumor suppressor gene (identified as both a caretaker gene and a DNA MMR gene)	Encodes the MSH6 protein that helps fix mistakes made when DNA is copied during replication.	Lynch syndrome; neurofibromatosis; CoLoN syndrome
NF1 (neurofibromin 1)	17q11.2	*Classification:* tumor suppressor gene	Codes for a protein that prevents cell overgrowth by turning off another protein (called Ras) that stimulates cell growth and division.	Neurofibromatosis Type 1; neurofibroma; sarcoma; Glioblastoma; juvenile myelomonocytic leukemia
NF2 (neurofibromin 2 [merlin])	22q12.2	*Classification:* tumor suppressor gene	Encodes the merlin. Believed to play a role in controlling cell shape, cell movement, and communication between cells. Prevents cells from growing and dividing too fast or in an uncontrolled way.	Neurofibromatosis; meningioma; mesothelioma
PMS2 (postmeiotic segregation increased 2)	7p22.2	*Classification:* tumor suppressor gene (identified as both a caretaker gene and a DNA MMR gene)	The PMS2 protein joins with the MLH1 protein to coordinate the activities of other proteins to remove errors in DNA and replace them with the corrected DNA sequence.	Lynch syndrome; Turcot syndrome; glioblastoma
PTEN (phosphatase and tensin homologue)	10q23.3	*Classification:* tumor suppressor gene	The **PTEN** enzyme acts as part of a chemical pathway that signals cells to stop dividing and triggers apoptosis. Also helps control cell migration, adhesion, and angiogenesis.	Cowden's syndrome; cancers of the prostate and endometrium; glioblastoma
RB1 (retinoblastoma 1)	13q14.2	*Classification:* tumor suppressor gene (identified as a gatekeeper gene) *DNA Damage:* point mutation.	Codes for a protein that stops other proteins from triggering DNA replication, thereby influencing apoptosis and differentiation.	Responsible for 60% of non-hereditary retinoblastomas and 40% of hereditary forms; cancers of the breast, bladder, and lung; osteosarcoma; glioblastoma
TGFBR2 (transforming growth factor, beta receptor II)	3p22	*Classification:* tumor suppressor gene *DNA Damage:* frameshift mutation	Encodes the transforming growth factor (TGF)-beta Type II receptor, which helps control cell differentiation. Also participates in forming the extracellular matrix, an intricate lattice of proteins and other molecules that forms in the spaces between cells.	Cancers of the colon, rectum, and esophagus

(Continues)

TABLE 16–1: Select Cancer Genes *(Continued)*

Gene Symbol (Official Name)	Location	Classification and Known DNA Damage	Normal Protein Function	Associated Cancer(s)
TP53 (tumor protein p53; also known as the "guardian of the genome" because it is essential for cell division and tumor prevention)	17p13.1	*Classification:* tumor suppressor gene (identified as both a gatekeeper gene and a caretaker gene) *DNA Damage:* point mutation; missense mutations	The p53 protein regulates nucleotide excision repair (NER) by activating other genes to repair DNA damage, or it promotes apoptosis if damage cannot be repaired. Loss of p53 function results in deficient global genomic repair, which targets and removes lesions from the whole genome.	Occur in about half of all cancers and coincide with the transition of large adenomas into invasive carcinomas; cancers of the breast, bladder, brain, colon, rectum, esophagus, liver lung, prostate and ovary; Li-Fraumeni syndrome; sarcomas; leukemia; lymphomas
WT1 (Wilms tumor 1)	11p13	*Classification:* tumor suppressor gene (identified as gatekeeper gene)	The WT1 protein plays a role in cell differentiation and apoptosis.	Wilms tumor;cancers of the lung, prostate, breast, and ovary; leukemia
XPA (xeroderma pigmentosum, complementation group A)	9q22.3	*Classification:* tumor suppressor gene	The XPA protein facilitates NER. It verifies DNA damage, binds to damaged DNA, and interacts with other proteins to unwind the damaged section of DNA, snip it out, and replace it with the correct DNA.	Xeroderma pigmentosum

Source: Ellisen & Haber (2010); Hanahan & Weinberg (2011); Markowitz & Bertagnollil (2009); Negrini, Gorgoulis, & Halazonetis (2010); Russo et al., (2005); Stricker, Catenacci, & Seiwert (2011); Genetics Home Reference: http://ghr.nlm.nih.gov; Online Mendelian Inheritance in Man (OMIM): http://omim.org

genes produces a translocation that is associated with Ewing's sarcoma. **Oncogenes** can also result from gene amplifications that result in extra chromosomal copies of a proto oncogene (e.g., *C-MYC* **amplification** in breast and ovarian cancers). Or, oncogenes can be caused by intragenic mutations such as point mutations, deletions, or insertions.

Nearly all of the mutations that convert proto-oncogenes to oncogenes are acquired by somatic mutation (Ellisen & Haber, 2010). Approximately 90% of the known somatically, mutated cancer genes act in an autosomal dominant fashion, wherein mutation in just one allele is sufficient to contribute to cancer development (Stratton, Campbell, & Futreal, 2009). "Oncogene addiction" has been observed by some researchers and suggests that the growth and survival of some cancers is strongly dependent on the activation of a very specific or a small number of oncogenes (Weinstein & Joe, 2008). This concept came about as the result of recognition that some cancers can regress when antibodies or drugs target specific oncogenes. For example, the monoclonal antibody, trastuzumab (Herceptin®), targets the *HER2*/neu receptor that is overexpressed in some patients with breast cancer; Imatinib (Gleevec®) targets protein kinases in the *BCR-ABL* oncogene in chronic myeloid leukemia; gefitinib (Iressa®) and erlotinib (Tarceva®) target the epidermal growth factor receptor (***EGFR***) in non–small cell lung carcinoma (NSCLC), pancreatic cancer, and glioblastoma (Weinstein & Joe, 2008).

There is also research that suggests tumors within a particular organ share a set of affected pathways instead of individual mutated genes. This concept has come to be described as *pathway addiction*, and understanding this process might be an important target for cancer treatment. For example, Jones and colleagues (2008) examined mutations in pancreatic cancers and found genetic alterations of a large number of genes that functioned through a relatively small number of biological pathways. Currently, two large research groups (TCGA and the International Cancer Genome Consortium) are targeting comprehensive cancer genome sequencing and molecular pathway mapping. Such research has the potential to highlight new and novel treatment options and targets.

Tumor Suppressor Genes

Tumor suppressor genes (see Table 16–1) are a family of normal genes that encode proteins with a number of different functions that inhibit cell growth and cell survival. These proteins have the ability to slow or inhibit progression through a specific stage of the cell cycle, arrest the cell cycle if DNA is damaged or chromosomes are abnormal, promote apoptosis, directly inhibit cell proliferation, and promote DNA repair (Bunz, 2008; Foulkes, 2008; Vogelstein, 2004). Tumor suppressor genes typically function like the brake pedal of an automobile. For example, *TP53* normally codes for the p53 protein that triggers cell suicide (apoptosis). In cells that have undergone DNA damage, the p53 protein acts like a brake pedal to halt cell growth and division. If the damage cannot be repaired, the p53 protein will initiate cell suicide to prevent the genetically damaged cell from growing out of control. Loss

Emerging Evidence

Standards of practice

- NCCN Guidelines Panel. (2011a). *Genetic/familial high-risk assessment: Breast and ovarian. Version 1.2011*. National Comprehensive Cancer Network, Inc.
- NCCN Guidelines Panel. (2011b). *Colorectal cancer screening. Version 2.2011*. National Comprehensive Cancer Network, Inc.

Standards for cancer risk assessment

- Riley, B. D., Culver, J. O., Skrzynia, C., Senter, L. A., Peters, J. A., Costalas, J. W., et al. (2012). Essential elements of genetic cancer risk assessment, counseling, and testing: Updated recommendations for the National Society of Genetic Counselors. *Journal of Genetic Counseling, 21*(2), pp. 151–161. doi:10.1007/s10897-011-9462-x

of normal tumor suppressor gene function is like having a dysfunctional brake pedal, whereby the abnormal cell is allowed to grow and divide continually. Mutations in tumor suppressor genes can be caused by missense mutations, mutations that result in a truncated protein, deletions or insertions of various sizes, or epigenetic silencing. They generally inactivate or abolish the gene product. In most cases, a single tumor suppressor gene allele suffices to control normal cell proliferation; however, both alleles of a tumor suppressor gene must be lost or inactivated (a process recognized as loss of heterogeneity) to promote cancer development. Thus, cancer-promoting, loss-of-function mutations in tumor suppressor genes act recessively. Most of the genes associated with hereditary cancer are tumor suppressor genes, but most mutations in tumor suppressor genes are not inherited. Tumor suppressor genes have been divided into three categories: 1) caretaker, 2) gatekeeper, and 3) landscaper genes.

Caretaker Genes

Caretaker genes function to stabilize cell processes by directly participating in DNA repair (Bunz, 2008; Kinzler & Vogelstein, 1998; Russo, et al., 2005; Vogelstein, 2004). They are involved in detecting DNA damage and activating repair machinery, directly repairing damaged DNA and inactivating or intercepting mutagenic molecules (e.g., carcinogens) before they can damage the DNA (Hanahan & Weinstein, 2011). When caretaker genes are inactivated, the overall rate of mutations increases. This includes an increased tendency to activate oncogenes and inactivate other tumor suppressor genes. Some of the best-studied caretaker genes include *MLH1*, *MSH2*, *MSH6*, and *PMS2*. These genes, also known as mismatch repair genes, code for proteins that fix mistakes that are made when DNA is copied during replication. Mutations in these four genes greatly increase the rate of **point mutations** in genes (Bunz, 2008). They are associated with about 10% to 50% of Lynch syndrome cases, as well as Turcot syndrome and CoLoN syndrome. (CoLoN syndrome includes colon cancer, leukemia or lymphoma, and neurofibromatosis.) Persons with mutations in the *MSH6* gene also have an increased risk of developing cancers of the ovary, stomach, small intestine, liver, gallbladder duct, upper urinary tract, brain, and skin.

Gatekeeper Genes

Gatekeeper genes normally control cell growth by inhibiting proliferation through apoptosis and/or promoting terminal differentiation. They are able to inhibit cell division or promote cell death when there is a need to eliminate damaged cells from the population. This is important because damaged cells will continue to multiply, thereby creating more and more cells that are similarly damaged. Vogelstein (2004) concluded that gatekeepers "absolutely must be inactivated before a cell can become cancerous." Gatekeepers also tend to be tissue specific (Russo et al., 2005). For example, mutations in the *APC* gatekeeper gene have been found in the majority of colon tumors (benign and malignant) whether they are of a sporadic or germ line origin. In its most lethal form, *APC* mutations lead to the development of hundreds to thousands of polyps on the lining of the colon and the certainty that colon cancer will develop by the early 30s for most germ line–affected individuals.

Landscaper Genes

Landscaper genes act by adapting the microenvironment in which cells exist (Bunz, 2008). For example, germ line mutations in the *SMAD4* gene appear to alter the growth of stromal cells in the colon mucosa. Complete *SMAD4* inactivation alters the colon mucosa, setting up an abnormal microenvironment that promotes the outgrowth of epithelial neoplasia. Defects in tissue landscapes can also be caused by chronic inflammation (Bunz, 2008). This is thought to be the basis of an increased risk for colorectal cancer associated with ulcerative colitis, a premalignant condition characterized by inflammation of the colon. We now know that inflammation simultaneously produces mutations and creates an environment where mutated cells will tend to proliferate.

Genomic Instability and DNA Repair

Genomic instability is a characteristic of most cancers. It is expressed as a high rate of abnormal chromosome structures and numbers, **microsatellite instability**, and increased frequency of base-pair mutations (Negrini, Gorgoulis, & Halazonetis, 2010). DNA repair genes, a subset of oncogenes and tumor suppressor genes, trigger processes that are responsible for detecting DNA damage and activating pathways that lead to cell cycle arrest to allow for repair, or if the damage is too great, to induce apoptosis. Damage to repair pathways does not typically lead directly to cancer but can result in genetic instabilities that increase opportunities for mutations in proto-oncogenes and tumor suppressor genes (Kinzler & Vogelstein, 1997). Two major types of DNA repair exist (Lahtz & Pfeifer, 2011). The first repairs DNA damage that arises from external sources such as UV and ionizing rays, chemical mutagens, fungal, and bacterial toxins. This includes the base excision repair (**BER**) pathway and the nucleotide excision repair (**NER**) pathway. The second type of damage repairs the mistakes made during DNA replication and includes the mismatch repair (**MMR**) pathway.

BER involves the excision and repair of an altered base. It is the major DNA repair pathway for most spontaneous, alkylative, and oxidative DNA damage (Wilson, Kim, Berquist, & Sigurdson, 2011). Defects in BER have been linked to cancer predisposition in the autosomal recessive form of familial adenomatous polyposis (FAP) commonly referred to as MYH-associated polyposis (MAP). Mutations to the *MGMT* gene lead to DNA alkylation damage and have been associated with glioblastoma, colon cancer, non–small cell lung cancer, gastric cancer, and head and neck squamous cell carcinoma (Lahtz & Pfeifer, 2011).

NER is the most versatile and best-studied DNA repair system in humans, and it repairs DNA damage due to UV-light exposures (Friedberg, 2001). NER is defective in the xeroderma pigmentosum group C (*XPC*) gene that causes xeroderma pigmentosum, an autosomal recessive hereditary disease characterized by a severe predisposition to squamous and basal cell skin cancers (Lahtz & Pfeifer, 2011).

Finally, the DNA mismatch repair (MMR) system is responsible for identification, removal, and repair of mismatched bases during DNA replication. It corrects replication errors introduced in microsatellites, which are stretches of DNA distributed throughout the human genome in which a short run of usually one to five nucleotides is repeated multiple times (Pino & Chung, 2011). The repetitive nature of microsatellites results in a susceptibility to replication errors that lead to the insertion or deletion of loops of DNA. This process is known as microsatellite instability (**MSI**) and is caused by the slippage of DNA polymerases over the tandem repeats. MSI is a common molecular finding in hereditary nonpolyposis colorectal cancer (HNPCC).

Cancer Progression

As cancer progresses, there is evidence that the cancer genome evolves. Tumor progression and metastasis require additional genetic and genomic actions that target changes in the surrounding normal tissue and tumor environment (Bunz, 2005; Ellisen & Haber, 2010; Nguyen & Massague, 2007). Cancer cells lose receptors that normally respond to triggers that call for the cessation of abnormal growth and they will amplify growth processes that insure cancer cell immortality over time. For example, cancer cells may activate *VEGF* to insure blood vessel development and access to an adequate supply of oxygen and nutrients via angiogenesis. They may also inundate adjoining cells and tissues with cytokines and proteases to promote invasion of local lymph nodes or the development of pathologically leaky blood vessels to facilitate entry into the circulation.

Scientists have identified a class of genes known as metastasis-suppressor genes (*MSG*) whose normal function is to suppress processes or pathways that promote metastasis. Shoushtari, Szmulewitz, and Rinker-Schaeffer (2011) define metastasis genes as "those in which gain or loss of function specifically enables tumour [sic] cells to circulate, home to, penetrate, or colonize distant organs" (p. 333). Insights into MSG function show that upregulation of the metastasis gene metadherin (*MTDH*) promotes chemo-resistance, as well as metastasis, in 30% to 40% of breast cancers (Hu et al., 2009). Research suggests that *MTDH* is a poor prognostic marker for glioma, melanoma, neuroblastoma, liver cancer, and prostate cancer (Wei, Hu, & Kang, 2009). Work with MSGs has led to the development of novel, antimetastatic treatment strategies designed to increase metastasis suppressor expression or pathway activation and subsequently inhibit the metastatic process (Shoushtari, Szmulewitz, Rinker-Schaeffer, 2011).

Epigenetics, Methylation, and Cancer

Up to now, this chapter has focused on DNA mutation in the genome as the major driving force in cancer development and progression. An evolving understanding of the epigenome suggests epigenetic influence is also a critical contributor to cancer development. The epigenome is a normal cellular constituent that metaphorically sits on top of the genome, just as the Greek prefix *epi* suggests. It has a fundamental role in gene regulation (Martens, 2011). Just as genes provide the same basic code for producing proteins in every cell of the body, what makes cells, tissues, and organs different is that chemicals called epigenetic marks sit on top of the genes and offer instructions to tailor cellular behavior (see Figure 16–1 ■). Epigenetic marks alter how genes interact with a cell's transcribing machinery by turning genes on or off, allowing or preventing a gene from being used to make a protein.

The epigenetic state of a cell represents the sum of its developmental, environmental, and physiological influences (Milosavljevic, 2011). As such, the epigenome provides an important interface between the environment and the genome. Indeed, factors such as nutrition, lifestyle practices, drugs, infection, disease state, and exposure to toxic agents are known to affect both DNA and epigenetic modifications (Martens, 2011). More specifically, it is via changes to the epigenetic marks that these factors influence genes. These effects can be passed on from one generation to the next as cells divide.

The relevance of epigenetics in cancer is that nonmutational changes to DNA can lead to alterations in gene expression. At least two types of epigenetic changes are thought to play a role in tumor progression: DNA methylation and post-translational modifications of histone tails.

DNA Methylation

DNA methylation is associated with a large number of human malignancies and occurs in two forms: hypermethylation and hypomethylation (Bunz, 2008; Ellisen & Haber, 2010; Stricker et al., 2011). Methylation results when a methyl group (one carbon atom attached to three hydrogen atoms) attaches to a specific spot on a gene—most commonly a cytosine/guanine-rich region of the genome—known as a CpG island and located in the promoter section (the regulatory region) of a gene. This process interferes with normal transcription and effectively turns the associated gene off or on. In normal cells, gene promoters are not methylated and transcription proceeds normally. In cancer cells, many promoters are hypermethylated and their corresponding genes are transcriptionally

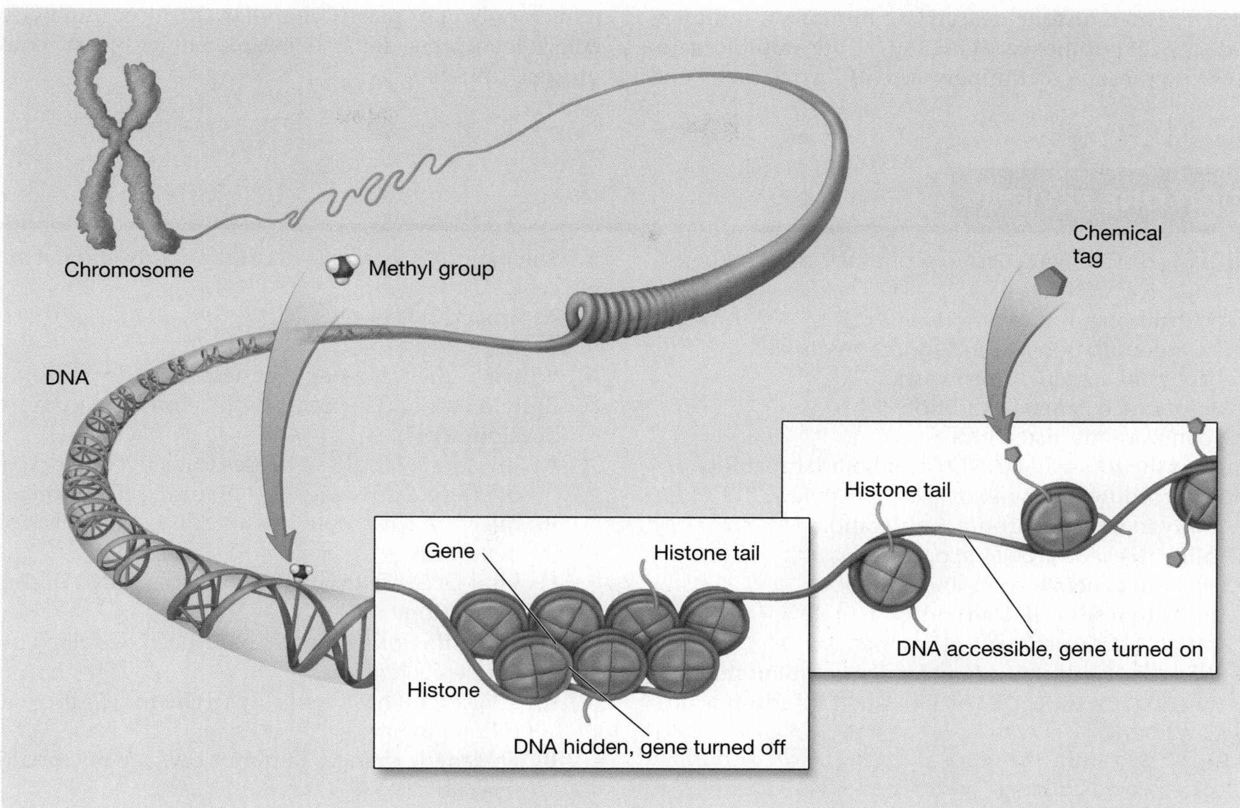

Figure 16–1 ■ Epigenetic marks

Source: Courtesy of National Human Genome Research Institute (http://www.genome.gov/27532724)

downregulated, resulting in the phenomenon known as gene silencing. DNA methylation and gene silencing is one way to achieve loss of a tumor suppressor allele. Stricker and colleagues (2011) note that tumor suppressors (such as ***TP53***, ***CDKN2A***, ***MLH1***, and ***RB1***), cell cycle genes, DNA repair genes, nuclear hormone receptors, and cell adhesion molecules have all been shown to be silenced by DNA methylation in cancer. DNA promoter, hypermethylation, is found in all types of cancer and is believed to be as common a method of deactivating tumor suppressors as mutation. About 50% of the genes that cause familial cancer have been shown to be silenced in sporadic cancers (Stricker et al., 2011).

Research has further demonstrated that in addition to the presence of localized hypermethylation at CpG islands, tumors are also characterized by a phenomenon known as global hypomethylation (Jin, 2011). Global genomic hypomethylation affects repetitive sequences, imprinted genes, tissue-specific genes, and genes associated with invasion and metastases. It leads to genomic instability and oncogene activation, which contribute to tumor progression.

Histone Methylation

A second mechanism for epigenetic gene silencing involves posttranslational modifications to histone tails (Bunz, 2008; Ellisen & Haber, 2010). Histones are small proteins that form spools for wrapping DNA into nucleosomes. Methylation and acetylation are chemical actions that target specific amino acids in histone tails and alter the histone's ability to tighten or loosen coils of genes. In cancer, these actions more commonly cause histones to tighten, which effectively prevents a gene from being exposed for translation—the gene is essentially silenced.

Relevance for Practice–Epigenetic Therapy

Recent research suggests that epigenetic changes may not necessarily be permanent and, if the offending trigger can be removed, the epigenetic marks will eventually fade and the DNA code will revert to its original programming over time (Bunz, 2008; Ellisen & Haber, 2010). The fact that epigenetic changes in tumor cells are potentially reversible opens the door to new therapeutic opportunities. DNA methylation inhibitors have demonstrated the ability to inhibit hypermethylation, restore suppressor gene expression, and exert antitumor effects for in-vitro and in-vivo laboratory models (Gore, 2005). Epigenetic therapeutic approaches involving DNA methylation inhibition and histone deacetylase inhibition are being used to treat cancer. For example, two DNA methyltransferase inhibitors, azacitidine (Vidaza®) and decitabine (Dacogen®), have shown significant activity in the treatment of myelodysplastic syndromes, and early use in acute myeloid leukemia has been positive. Three histone deacetylase inhibitors, romidepsin (Istodax®), panobinostat (LBH589), and valproic acid, have shown significant preliminary activity in recurrent and refractory lymphomas (Cabanillas, 2011). A number of other epigenetic agents are being explored in breast, colon, and prostate cancers.

SECTION ONE REVIEW

1. Which of the following best describes the cause(s) of cancer?
   A. A critical gene mutation
   B. The accumulation of DNA mutations as well as changes in epigenetic processes
   C. An inherited genetic condition
   D. A complex, multistep process
2. Which of the following is NOT a hallmark capability of cancer according to Hanahan and Weinstein (2011)?
   A. Ability to sustain chronic proliferation
   B. Ability to evade growth suppressors
   C. Ability to generate germ line mutations
   D. Ability to resist cell death
   E. Ability to activate invasion and metastasis
3. The Two-Hit Hypothesis of cancer development that was described in the 1970s by Dr. Alfred Knudson is no longer relevant.
   A. True
   B. False
4. Which of the following best describes a proto oncogene?
   A. A subset of tumor suppressor genes
   B. A gene that, when mutated, can become an oncogene
   C. A gene with a point mutation that is common in many cancers
   D. A gene that makes proteins that inhibit normal cell division
   E. A major cause of chronic myelogenous leukemia
5. The majority of cancers occur randomly and in somatic cells.
   A. True
   B. False
6. Which of the following best describes why viruses like Epstein Barr and hepatitis B can contribute to cancer development?
   A. Infection with these viruses leads to clonal expansion of infected cells with loss of normal function.
   B. Infection with these viruses can activate invasion and metastasis.
   C. Viral DNA are inserted into cellular DNA during replication.
7. Which of the following has NOT been described as an effect of epigenetics?
   A. Epigenetics has the ability to chemically program cellular behavior.
   B. Epigenetic changes in tumor cells are potentially reversible.
   C. Epigenetic functions are heritable.
   D. Epigenetics can turn a particular gene *on* as well as *off*.
   E. Cancer drugs do not influence epigenetic function.

Answers: 1. B; 2. C; 3. B; 4. B; 5. A; 6. C; 7. E

SECTION TWO: Personalized Medicine and the Clinical Application of Cancer Genomics

At its most basic level, understanding the molecular biology of cancer holds the promise of tailoring treatment that targets select genes, gene products, and/or pathways that trigger cancer. From a clinical perspective this should provide clinicians and patients with strategic information to facilitate decision making on a course of cancer treatment that would be informed by the patient's unique genetic, genomic, and epigenomic information. Such health care would allow accurate predictions about susceptibility for cancer (perhaps through genetic testing), expectations for disease progression, and response to treatment.

Building the Science

International researchers with two large research cooperatives are building the scientific foundation that is expected to drive targeted cancer therapies. In 2008, the International Cancer Genome Consortium (**ICGC**) brought together leading cancer researchers from around the world to catalogue the genetic alterations in 50 common cancers. They will analyze 500 genomes from each cancer type and make the results freely available on the Internet. Systematic analysis of the more than 25,000 cancer genomes at the genomic, epigenomic, and transcriptomic levels is expected to reveal the range of cancer-causing mutations, define clinically relevant cancer subtypes for prognosis and treatment, and enable the development of new cancer therapies. American scientists are collaborating with the ICGC through TCGA on the analysis of a number of cancers including bladder, brain, breast, cervical, colorectal, endometrial, gastric, head and neck, liver, lung, ovarian, prostate renal, skin, and blood-related cancers. Recently, TCGA researchers published an analysis of the genomic changes in ovarian cancer (The Cancer Genome Atlas Research Network, 2011). They found that mutations in *TP53* were present in 96% of ovarian serous adenocarcinoma tumors (the most common ovarian tumor type) and that approximately 21% of the tumors showed mutations in *BRCA1* and *BRCA2*, which confers a survival benefit over disease due to other mutations. Additionally, two genetic signature patterns were identified; one associated 108 genes with poor survival and the other correlated 85 genes with better survival. These scientists also identified one particular type of drug, a poly ADP ribose polymerase (**PARP**) inhibitor that could potentially counteract the effects of some of the genetic damage observed in about half of the ovarian tumors studied. Although these are exciting findings, their application in the clinical setting has yet to be rigorously tested in clinical trials.

Predisposition Genetic Testing

The basic rationale for genetic testing is to identify individuals at risk for cancer due to an inherited or genetic predisposition for cancer (Foulkes, 2008). In hereditary cancer syndromes, one abnormal copy of a gene is inherited in the germ line from either parent and the other copy must be inactivated in a somatic cell. This occurs typically by random processes in which genes, chromosomes, or both are rearranged, deleted, or replaced.

The identification of carriers of inherited germ line cancer genes serves both as an early warning of increased lifetime risk for disease and an indication for the need for close lifelong surveillance (IOM, 2012). Predisposition genetic testing is currently available to assess the risk of breast (*BRCA1* and *BRCA2* gene mutations) and select colorectal cancers (*MLH1* and *MLH2*). Nationally recognized guidelines for prevention and screening are available for select high-risk individuals (National Comprehensive Cancer Network [**NCCN**] Guidelines Panel, 2011a & 2011b). Genetic testing of biological relatives of patients newly diagnosed with cancers of germ line origins is recommended. However, mass screening for mutations that suggest increased risk for cancer is not useful due to the relatively low prevalence of deleterious mutations in the general population. Typically, a blood sample is required for these tests and genetic counseling is recommended before and after testing. Most gene tests look for DNA changes in the gene(s) of interest; however, some will assess expression of the protein products produced by the gene(s) of interest. Both can be important, as the expression of the gene product (absence, overexpression, underexpression) can have implications for physiologic compensation, or the lack thereof, by the gene on its parallel allele.

Direct to Consumer Testing

Direct to consumer (DTC) genetic tests are increasingly being marketed and sold online directly to consumers without a doctor's order or a consultation with a genetic counselor. As online accessibility increases and the cost of such testing drops, the market for DTC genetic testing is expected to grow. However, the reliability, validity, and interpretation of test results have been questioned (Kutz, 2010). Concern has also been voiced over the lack of integration with traditional forms of health care that would allow for meaningful interpretation of results and discussion around recommendations (American Society of Human Genetics, 2007).

Biomarkers for Diagnosis, Prognosis, and Treatment

Today, most applications of innovative genomics-based diagnostics are used for cancer (President's Council of Advisors on Science and Technology, 2008). In-vitro molecular diagnostics are laboratory tests that can be used on blood, tissue, or other biological samples to identify the presence of specific biomarkers. Most molecular diagnostic testing uses microarray technology. A **microarray** is a very small glass chip that has been spotted at fixed locations with thousands of biologic molecules such as DNA, RNA, or protein fragments that correspond to various genes of interest. **Biomarkers** can be used to screen patients for early cancers, to diagnose disease and predict survival, to determine tumor aggressiveness, to predict and monitor drug or other treatment effectiveness, and to identify molecular targets for particular cancer therapy (Manne, Srivastava, & Srivastava, 2005). Although scientists are actively pursuing the development of reliable biomarkers, the number of molecular tests and cancer biomarkers in clinical use is quite small.

Diagnosis

Biomarker analysis for cancer screening is possible but most **tumor markers** are not sensitive or specific enough to be used for diagnosis. For example, **PSA** (prostate-specific antigen) levels are often used to screen men for prostate cancer, but this is controversial. Data suggest that elevated PSA levels can be caused by prostate cancer or benign conditions, and most men with elevated PSA levels turn out not to have prostate cancer (Chou et al., 2011). Moreover, it is not clear if the benefits of PSA screening outweigh the risks of follow-up diagnostic tests and cancer treatments. Another tumor marker, **CA-125** (cancer antigen-125), is sometimes used to screen women who have an increased risk for ovarian cancer. CA-125 is a protein that is overexpressed in most ovarian cancer cells. To date, CA-125 measurement is not sensitive or specific enough to be used to screen all women for ovarian cancer. Mostly, CA-125 is used to monitor response to treatment and check for recurrence in women with ovarian cancer.

Prognosis

Molecular markers have been useful predictors of prognosis; for example, when overproduced, epidermal growth factor receptors (*EGFR*) are associated with poor prognosis for breast, bladder, colon, lung, and esophageal cancers. In breast cancer, overexpression of the ***HER2*** growth factor receptor is associated with poor prognosis for breast and ovarian cancers. For women with early stage breast cancer, Oncotype DX®, a 21-gene molecular signature test (also called a gene-expression profile or a multiparameter genomic test), can be used to predict the likelihood of disease recurrence. This test is recommended in the 2007 guidelines of the American Society of Clinical Oncology for the evaluation of patients with node-negative, **ER**-positive disease. It can be used to identify those who may obtain the most benefit from adjuvant tamoxifen and who may not require chemotherapy (McDermott, Downing, & Stratton, 2011).

Multiparameter genomic tests are also used to predict prognosis in colon cancer, **AML**, and **DLBCL**.

Treatment

Knowledge of cancer mutations has led to the development of specific new drugs or biologic agents (known as inhibitors) that can target proteins that are encoded by mutated cancer genes (McDermott, Downing, & Stratton, 2011). Many of these are known as small molecule drugs—drugs that can pass through cell membranes and reach targets inside the cell. One example is imatinib mesylate (Gleevec®), which targets *BCR-ABL* tyrosine kinase for the treatment of chronic myeloid leukemia (CML) (The International Cancer Consortium, 2010). This drug helped to boost the 5-year survival rate of patients with CML to 89%. The sequencing of genes encoding kinases also led to the discovery of a *BRAF* mutation in melanoma. This in turn led to the development of PLX4032, a Phase I drug with demonstrated ability to inhibit the mutant BRAF protein and cause tumor regression (Hudson et al., 2011).

In breast cancer, expression of the estrogen receptor (ER) is a biomarker for prognosis and identifies women who are likely to benefit from a class of antiestrogen drugs known as aromatase inhibitors. These drugs work by blocking the enzyme aromatase, which turns the hormone androgen into small amounts of estrogen in the body. Similarly, the overexpression of the *HER2* protein in breast cancer (common in 25%–30% of breast cancer patients) serves as a biomarker for treatment with trastuzumab (Herceptin®), a laboratory developed monoclonal antibody that targets *HER2* receptor function (Nass & Moses, 2007; President's Council of Advisors on Science and Technology, 2008). Drugs have also been developed to disrupt tumor angiogenesis. For example, bevacizumab (Avastin®), a monoclonal antibody, binds to *VEGF* and prevents it from interacting with receptors on endothelial cells, blocking a step that is necessary for the initiation of new blood vessel growth (Wu, Huang, & Chang, 2008).

Biomarker analysis can identify patients who may selectively experience adverse or no effects from a given drug or dosage. One example tests for genetic variation in the activity of an enzyme called thiopurine methyltransferase (**TPMT**), which affects the level of bone marrow toxicity experienced by patients receiving purine drugs for acute lymphocytic leukemia. Another example is the test to detect a gene variant that elevates the risk for white blood cell depletion from irinotecan (Camptosar®), an agent used in the treatment of colorectal cancer (President's Council of Advisors on Science and Technology, 2008). It is also known that patients with colorectal cancers with select somatic mutations in *KRAS* do not respond to drugs, such as cetuximab (Erbitux™) and panitumumab (Vectibix®) (Hudson et al., 2011). Large scale biomarker analysis has recently been applied in a new program known as PG4KDS (pharmacogenetics for kids) at St. Jude Children's Research Hospital (IOM, 2012). There, clinicians and scientists are using the Affymetrix DMET-plus array to test for more than 1,900 polymorphisms in 225 genes. The primary objective is to estimate the proportion of patients with high-risk or actionable pharmacogenetic results. These results are entered in the patient's electronic medical record (EMR), which is programmed with decision support (automated information alerts to assist health care providers in making decisions about a patient's care). The secondary objectives are to use systematic procedures for prioritizing and migrating pharmacogenomic test results to the EMR, to link test results to medication use, and to assess the attitudes and concerns of research participants and clinicians.

SECTION TWO REVIEW

1. The development of drugs that target angiogenesis are a promising new model for treating cancer.
   A. True
   B. False
2. How will an improved understanding of the molecular genetics of a particular type of cancer contribute to personalized medicine?
   A. Treatment can be targeted to the particular gene, gene product, or molecular pathway that triggers a cancer.
   B. The genetic signature of a cancer can be used to predict prognosis.
   C. Biomarkers can monitor the effect(s) of cancer treatment.
   D. All of the above
3. Your patient has elected to pursue online direct-to-consumer genetic testing for breast cancer. Which of the following would you want to make her aware of?
   A. The reliability, validity, and interpretation of online gene test results have been questioned.
   B. Online gene test results are highly reliable and valid.
4. The number of molecular tests and biomarkers in clinical use is small and most commonly used for cancer.
   A. True
   B. False

Answers: 1. A; 2. D; 3. A; 4. A

SECTION THREE: Cancer Exemplars

This section provides examples of the practical application of genetic concepts previously discussed. Scientists are continuing to develop a strong and ever expanding body of knowledge about the molecular genetics of cancer and have used this information to develop evidence-based and standardized recommendations for prevention, screening, and highly targeted molecular treatment strategies.

Hereditary Breast and Ovarian Cancer Syndrome (HBOC)

There are at least 10 known genes associated with an increased risk of breast cancer. Inheritance of an autosomal dominant breast cancer gene mutation occurs in about 10% to 15% of all breast or ovarian cancers. Mutations in *BRCA1* and *BRCA2* are primarily associated with hereditary breast and ovarian cancer syndrome (HBOC) (Clark & Domchek, 2011). These genes contribute to a 5- to 20-fold increase risk of developing breast or ovarian cancer compared with the general population. Although breast and ovarian cancer frequently occur in this syndrome, different cancers can be expected to develop depending on which gene is inherited. For example, *BRCA1* mutation carriers are at increased risk for cervical, uterine, pancreatic, and colon cancer (NCI, 2009). *BRCA2* mutation carriers are at increased risk of male breast cancer, pancreatic, stomach, gallbladder and bile duct cancers, and melanoma (Clark & Domchek, 2011; NCI, 2009).

Genetic testing for *BRCA1* or *BRCA2* mutations is available. Referral for genetic testing is recommended when specific criteria are identified in a three-generation pedigree (NCCN, 2011a). Persons at risk for HBOC may elect to undergo bilateral prophylactic mastectomy and prophylactic salpingo-oophorectomy (removal of healthy fallopian tubes and ovaries) for primary prevention and/or lifelong surveillance that may include more frequent breast imaging, transvaginal ultrasound, blood tests for CA-125 antigen, and selective screening for other high risk cancers (e.g., skin examinations and GI tests). In high-risk women, tamoxifen (Nolvadex®) and raloxifene (Evista®) have been shown to reduce the risk of invasive breast cancer and oral contraceptive use has been shown to reduce the risk of ovarian cancer (Clark & Domchek 2011).

Our understanding of the molecular genetics of breast cancer has greatly expanded treatment options, should a man or woman develop the disease. Extensive molecular testing of tumor tissue at the time of diagnosis to assess prognosis and sensitivity to certain hormonal therapy or chemotherapy is standard of care and includes ER, progesterone receptor (PR), and *HER2* status. More recently, targeted molecular therapy has been developed for the treatment of breast or ovarian cancers specifically in carriers of a *BRCA1* or *BRCA2* mutation. A class of new agents known as PARP inhibitors has shown promise in recent clinical trials, and their action is an example of the application of a phenomenon known as synthetic lethality, in which two molecular lesions combine to have a lethal effect on the cell (Calvert & Azzariti, 2011):

> . . . this hypothesis has been applied to cells deficient in *BRCA1* and *BRCA2* (resulting in defective homologous DNA repair recombination [HR]) that should be extremely sensitive to drugs that inhibit PARP, an essential component for the repair of single-strand breaks through the base excision repair pathways. In fact, exposure of the cells to a PARP inhibitor led to the accumulation of spontaneously occurring single-strand breaks in DNA, since these cannot be repaired. When the cell divides and DNA replication takes place, these single-strand breaks are converted to double-strand breaks in one of the daughter strands. In cells that have functional HR these double strand breaks are repaired without errors, explaining the lack of toxicity of the PARP inhibitors towards the heterozygote and wild-type cell lines. However, if HR is deficient, as it is in the BRCA-negative cell lines, these double-strand breaks cannot be repaired, leading to collapse of the replication fork and cell death (p. i54).

Colorectal Cancer (CRC)

A number of authors have described the molecular basis of colorectal cancer in depth (Bedeir & Krasinskas, 2011; Gala & Chung, 2011; Markowitz & Bertagnolli, 2009; Pino & Chang, 2011). CRC is one of the most common cancers in the U.S. and both oncogenes and tumor suppressor genes are associated with tumor initiation and progression in this disease. The majority of CRCs are characterized by chromosomal instability. Approximately 15% are specifically due to microsatellite instability (MSI), which is caused by alterations in the DNA mismatch repair (MMR) system whose responsibility is to recognize and repair mismatched nucleotides and insertion/deletion loops caused by slippage of DNA polymerase (Pino & Chung, 2011). About 25% of CRC is associated with a family history of the disease (Gala & Chung, 2011). There are many types of CRC. Two commonly inherited examples are discussed here.

Familial Adenomatous Polyposis (FAP)

FAP is associated with an inherited germ line mutation in the *APC* tumor suppressor gene and carries an 80% to 100% lifetime risk of colorectal cancer (Markowitz et al., 2009). The presence of greater than 100 adenomatous polyps in the colon is pathoneumonic for FAP, and colorectal cancer is typically assured by age 40. More commonly, the colon is carpeted with polyps necessitating prophylactic colectomy.

Lynch Syndrome/Hereditary Nonpolyposis Colorectal Cancer (HNPCC)

Lynch syndrome, also referred to as HNPCC, is associated with an inactivating germ line mutation in any one of four tumor suppressor genes (*MLH1*, ***MSH2***, ***MSH6***, ***PMS2***). These genes are involved in DNA mismatch repair, with *MLH1* and *MSH2* accounting for about 60% of all diagnosed Lynch syndrome cases (Reeves et al., 2011). Although colorectal cancer (CRC) is the predominant cancer, women with this syndrome have about a 50% risk of developing uterine cancer and a 10% risk of developing ovarian cancer. The lifetime risk for CRC among persons with Lynch syndrome has historically been estimated at 80%; however, recent data suggest men and women have a lifetime risk of 47% and 34% (respectively) of developing CRC (Alarcon et al., 2007). Persons with this syndrome also have an increased risk of gastric, small intestinal, hepatic, pancreaticobiliary, ureteral, and brain tumors. Colorectal cancers associated with HNPCC exhibit microsatellite instability (MSI) and sequencing technology has made it routinely possible to test directly for DNA repeats. Immunohistochemistry (**IHC**) testing is a way of indirectly testing for gene mutation. It is used to stain tumor tissue for protein expression of the four MMR genes mutated in this syndrome. MSI analysis is useful for colorectal cancer diagnosis, prognosis, and prediction of response to chemotherapeutic agents. An extensive algorithm for risk assessment, genetic testing, and lifelong surveillance has been published by the National Comprehensive Cancer Network (NCCN, 2011b).

SECTION THREE REVIEW

1. Mutations in which of the following autosomal dominant genes are commonly associated with breast cancer in men?
   A. *BRCA1*
   B. *BRCA2*
2. The presence of more than 100 adenomatous polyps in the colon is pathoneumonic for familial adenomatous polyposis (FAP).
   A. True
   B. False
3. *MLH1*, *MSH2*, *MSH6*, and *PMS2* are known as mismatch repair genes. This is a subclassification of which of the following?
   A. Tumor suppressor genes
   B. Oncogenes
   C. None of the above
4. Risk assessment and long-term surveillance and screening guidelines have been published for most cancers.
   A. True
   B. False

Answers: 1. B; 2. A; 3. A; 4. B

SECTION FOUR: Role of the Nurse

Nurses are on the front lines of translating cancer genetics, genomics, and epigenomic research into clinical practice for two reasons: (1) They make up the largest group of direct care providers, and with such visibility must be able to respond to the rapidly evolving targeted treatment needs of this population; and (2) there are only about 1,000 medical geneticists and 3,000 genetic counselors in the United States (IOM, 2012). Therefore, nurses must be able to respond to the genetic information needs of patients and the public. The Oncology Nursing Society and the American Nurses Association strongly support the integration of genetic and genomic information into practice (Consensus Panel on Genetic/Genomic Nursing Competencies, 2009; ONS 2009a; ONS 2009b). In the United States, cancer accounts for one in four deaths (ACS, 2011), our aging population is rapidly growing (the source of two-thirds of all cancers), our understanding of cancer genetics and epigenomics is rapidly evolving, and the relevance of this knowledge for clinical practice is growing. Today and in the future, nurses must be adequately prepared to identify, refer, educate, and provide direct care for patients and their family members with, or at risk for, cancer (Frazier, Calzone, & Jenkins 2010). The following section addresses genetically relevant clinical competencies that would be expected of all nurses caring for persons with cancer and that are consistent with nationally recognized standards for nurses in all aspects of health care (Consensus Panel on Genetic/Genomic Nursing Competencies, 2009).

Prevention

Nurses must use every possible opportunity to educate and empower patients and the public about how to prevent cancer if we are to substantially reduce the incidence of this major disease. By understanding that cancer is the result of a complex interplay between inherited genetic predisposition and environmental and lifestyle exposures that can trigger chemical changes in the epigenome, nurses can educate and support patient and family efforts to take an active role in reducing exposures to cancer-causing agents, adopting healthy lifestyles, and exploring family history of cancer at opportune moments.

Case Finding

Nurses must recognize red flags that suggest inherited predisposition for cancer (early age of onset—generally under age 50, known family history, multiple-affected family members, similar cancers occurring across generations, multifocal or bilateral disease), elicit a three-generation family health history, construct a pedigree using standardized symbols and terminology (Riley et al., 2011), collaborate with appropriate providers regarding need for referral, and facilitate referral for genetic counseling and testing as appropriate (see NCI's Cancer Genetics Services Directory online). It is also important to support high-risk patients and family members who must comply with more frequent, lifelong screening and surveillance requirements and to advocate for insurance reimbursement for such testing.

Education

Nurses are obligated to regularly participate in activities that enhance clinical knowledge. Personal knowledge of cancer genetics, genomics, and epigenomics is critical given the rapid growth in this specialty field. An ideal way of linking everyday patient care responsibilities with cutting-edge research would be to actively participate in regular patient rounds and grand rounds. Traditional education efforts should include attending relevant professional CME/CE activities, joining professional organizations and groups that support nursing education in genetics (e.g., Oncology Nursing Society, International Society of Nurses in Genetics), and seeking the counsel of genetic nurse experts in local and regional cancer centers. Patients, families, the public, and other nursing staff will need credible, accurate, appropriate, and current cancer genetic, genomic, and epigenomic information and resources for informed decision making. Patients and families will need clarification about direct-to-consumer gene-testing options, assistance in evaluating the validity of claims made in promotional materials, recommendations for appropriate resources for the interpretation of test results, and advice concerning possible privacy limitations on genomic information (Evans et al., 2010).

Certification

Professional certification recognizes specialized knowledge, skills, and expertise, and demonstrates competency in a defined area. The Oncology Nursing Society identifies three levels of expertise for nurses engaged in genetic practice: (1) the general oncology nurse who has basic genetic knowledge; (2) the advanced practice oncology nurse who, through education and experience, has attained advanced expertise in general oncology and genetics; and (3) the Advanced Practice Nurse-Certified in Genetics (ONS 2009b).

The Genetic Nursing Credentialing Commission (GNCC) has established criteria by which RNs can obtain certification for specialty knowledge in genetics. An RN with a bachelor's degree in nursing who works in a genetic setting may apply to the GNCC and, upon meeting specific criteria, attain the credential of genetic clinical nurse. Masters preparation and experience in genetics, including extensive case experience and continuing education credits in genetics, are needed for advanced certification. Credentialing requirements are described on the GNCC website.

Direct Patient Care

Nurses can help patients understand how genetic information informs diagnosis, prognosis, and treatment so they can become informed, active participants in their own care. Targeted therapy will demand attention to patient safety and quality of care. Drugs that target specific cancer proteins and pathways should have fewer safety issues and side effects, compared with older cytotoxic drugs that kill normal as well as abnormal cells, a factor that nurses intuitively recognize. However, there is growing evidence that this may not be so. For example, in a drug study that resulted in improved overall survival among patients with melanoma (n = 540), the drug ipilimumab (Yervoy™) was associated with a number of serious side effects, including seven drug-related deaths associated with autoimmune reactivity in the skin, gastrointestinal tract, and endocrine system (Hodi et al., 2010). In another example, patients with CML who cannot take or do not respond to imatinib may be prescribed the newer medication, nilotinib (Tasigna®), a kinase inhibitor. However, this drug can cause QT prolongation. Nurses must also know that persons taking this drug should avoid certain food and medications, such as grapefruit juice, ciprofloxin, fluconazole, and some HIV medications that inhibit the CYP3A4 pathway, as these can increase side effects. In a final example, use of the drug Bevacizumab in patients with *HER2* negative metastatic breast cancer was recently revoked by the U.S. Food and Drug Administration (FDA News Release, November 18, 2011). This drug is known to impede the growth of endothelial cells (***VEGF***) and was approved for use in metastatic breast cancer in 2008. Side effects of concern included severe high blood pressure; bleeding and hemorrhaging; heart attack or heart failure; and the development of perforations in the nose, stomach, or intestines.

The preceding examples highlight the critical importance of professional competency in a number of areas: history taking and physical assessment skills; initiation and participation in systems processes that enable continuous monitoring for and recording of adverse events; collaboration with other providers to develop patient care guidelines for the management and prevention of these unanticipated events; and patient education about the drugs being taken, in particular, potential side effects, drug and food interactions, and the need to report any unexpected drug effects.

Finally, publishing case studies and interventions will inform practice for the discipline as a whole. An important example is presented by Bryce, Bauer, and Hadji (2011). They describe management guidelines for the treatment of bone loss and elevated fracture risk among patients receiving aromatase inhibitors for postmenopausal breast cancer.

SECTION FOUR REVIEW

1. Nurses must understand cancer genetics because
   A. they make up the largest number of direct care providers.
   B. there are insufficient genetic experts to translate cancer genetic information to patients and the public.
   C. they are the case finders for cancer predisposition.
   D. All of the above
2. A pedigree is a standardized pictorial representation of family data collected during a health history.
   A. True
   B. False
3. Red flags that suggest inherited predisposition for cancer include all of the following EXCEPT
   A. multifocal or bilateral disease.
   B. early age of cancer onset, typically before age 50 years.
   C. multiple affected family members.
   D. evidence for rapid metastasis among multiple individuals with cancer.
   E. occurrence of similar cancers across multiple generations.
4. Certification in oncology nursing as well as genetic nursing is possible.
   A. True
   B. False
5. Cancer treatment is evolving and new drugs are being developed to target very specific gene functions and/or cancer development pathways. Which of the following skills or competencies is most important for a nurse to possess?
   A. History taking and physical assessment skills
   B. Initiation and participation in system processes that enable continuous monitoring for and recording of adverse events
   C. Collaboration with other providers to develop patient care guidelines for the management and prevention of unanticipated events
   D. Patient education about the drug effects, interactions, and the need to report unexpected drug effects
   E. All of the above

Answers: 1. D; 2. A; 3. D; 4. A; 5. E

POSTTEST

1. Which of the following best describes the cause(s) of cancer?
   A. A "critical gene" mutation
   B. The accumulation of DNA mutations as well as changes in epigenetic processes
   C. An inherited genetic condition
   D. A complex, multistep process
2. Which of the following is NOT a hallmark capability of cancer according to Hanahan & Weinstein (2011)?
   A. Ability to sustain chronic proliferation
   B. Ability to evade growth suppressors
   C. Ability to generate germline mutations
   D. Ability to resist cell death
   E. Ability to activate invasion and metastasis
3. Which of the following best describes a proto oncogene?
   A. A subset of tumor suppressor genes
   B. A gene that when mutated can become an oncogene
   C. A gene with a point mutation that is common in many cancers
   D. A gene that makes proteins that inhibit normal cell division
   E. A major cause of chronic myelogenous leukemia
4. Which of the following best describes why viruses like Epstein Barr and hepatitis B can contribute to cancer development?
   A. Infection with these viruses leads to clonal expansion of infected cells with loss of normal function.
   B. Infection with these viruses can activate invasion and metastasis.
   C. Viral DNA are inserted into cellular DNA during replication.
5. The development of drugs that target angiogenesis are a promising new model for treating cancer.
   A. True
   B. False
6. Which of the following has NOT been described as an effect of epigenetics?
   A. Epigenetics has the ability to chemically program cellular behavior.
   B. Epigenetic changes in tumor cells are potentially reversible.
   C. Epigenetic functions are heritable.
   D. Epigenetics can turn a particular gene *on* as well as *off*.
   E. Cancer drugs do not influence epigenetic function.

7. How will an improved understanding of the molecular genetics of a particular type of cancer contribute to personalized medicine?
   A. Treatment can be targeted to the particular gene, gene product, or molecular pathway that triggers a cancer.
   B. The genetic signature of a cancer can be used to predict prognosis.
   C. Biomarkers can monitor the effect(s) of cancer treatment.
   D. All of the above
8. Nurses must understand cancer genetics because
   A. they make up the largest number of direct care providers.
   B. there are insufficient genetic experts to translate cancer genetic information to patients and the public.
   C. they are the case finders for cancer predisposition.
   D. All of the above
9. Red flags that suggest inherited predisposition for cancer include all of the following EXCEPT
   A. multifocal or bilateral disease.
   B. early age of cancer onset, typically before age 50 years.
   C. multiple, affected family members.
   D. evidence for rapid metastasis among multiple individuals with cancer.
   E. occurrence of similar cancers across multiple generations.
10. Cancer treatment is evolving and new drugs are being developed to target very specific gene functions and or cancer development pathways. Which of the following skills or competencies is most important for a nurse?
   A. History taking and physical assessment skills
   B. Initiation and participation in systems processes that enable continuous monitoring for and recording of adverse events
   C. Collaboration with other providers to develop patient care guidelines for the management and prevention of unanticipated events
   D. Patient education about the drug effects, interactions, and the need to report unexpected drug effects
   E. All of the above

Posttest answers are located in the Appendix.

CHAPTER SUMMARY

Cancers generally arise in response to an accumulation of DNA mutations that alter the protein products of normal genes typically responsible for the regulation of cell growth, cell differentiation, cell migration and invasion, and/or apoptosis. Cancer is many diseases, and each type of cancer may be uniquely defined by personal exposures to cancer-causing agents as well as our unique genetic makeup.

Eight "hallmarks" of cancer development and progression have been identified and include the ability to sustain chronic proliferation, evade growth suppressors, resist cell death, support replication immortality, induce angiogenesis, activate invasion and metastasis processes, reprogram energy metabolism, and evade immune destruction.

Our understanding of the molecular genetics of cancer is rapidly evolving and has led to the development of evidence-based and standardized recommendations for prevention, screening, and highly targeted molecular treatment strategies for select cancers.

The generalist nurse will increasingly be confronted with the need to understand, interpret, and apply genetic knowledge and principles in the care of persons with or at risk for cancer.

CRITICAL THINKING CHECKPOINT

Adrian is a 26-year-old Caucasian woman who is admitted to your unit for surgical care following a mastectomy for Stage II breast cancer. She tells you she is very scared because her paternal grandmother, paternal aunt, and her father have all had breast cancer.

1. What red flags tell you that there is a need to collect a comprehensive three-generation family history?
2. What can you tell her about the relationship between breast cancer and genetics that might be relevant in her case?
3. Given the brief information in this case, what gene mutation might be common in her family? Why do you say this?
4. Is a genetic counseling referral relevant in this case? Why?

Answers are provided in the Appendix

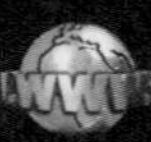

Pearson Nursing Student Resources

Find additional review materials at nursing.pearsonhighered.com

Prepare for success with additional NCLEX®-style practice questions, interactive assignments and activities, web links, animations, videos, and more!

ONLINE RESOURCES

Genetics Home Reference: http://ghr.nlm.nih.gov

GNCC website: http://geneticnurse.org/home.html

National Cancer Institute Understanding Cancer Series: http://www.cancer.gov/cancertopics/understandingcancer

National Toxicology Program: http://ntp.niehs.nih.gov/?objectid=03C9AF75-E1BF-FF40-DBA-9EC0928DF8B15

NCI Cancer Fact Sheets:

- Angiogenesis Inhibitors Therapy: http://www.cancer.gov/cancertopics/factsheet/Therapy/angiogenesis-inhibitors
- BRCA1 and BRCA2: Cancer Risk and Genetic Testing: http://www.cancer.gov/cancertopics/factsheet/Risk/BRCA
- Epigenomics Fact Sheet: http://www.genome.gov/27532724
- Targeted Cancer Therapies: http://www.cancer.gov/cancertopics/factsheet/Therapy/targeted

NCI's Cancer Genetics Services Directory: http://www.cancer.gov/cancertopics/genetics/directory

Welcome Trust organization: http://www.sanger.ac.uk/genetics/CGP/cosmic/

REFERENCES

Alarcon, F., Lasset, C., Carayol, J., Bonadona, V., Perdry, H., Desseigne, F., et al. (2007). Estimating cancer risk in HNPCC by the GRL method. *European Journal of Human Genetics, 15*(8), 831–836.

American Cancer Society. (2011). *Cancer facts & figures 2011*. Atlanta: American Cancer Society.

American Society of Human Genetics. (2007). ASHG statement on direct-to-consumer genetic testing in the United States. *American Journal of Human Genetics, 81*, 635–637.

American Society of Health System Pharmacists. (2008). *Nilotinib*. Retrieved November, 22, 2011, from http://www.ncbi.nlm.nih.gov/pubmedhealth/PMH0000429/#

Bedir, A., & Krasinskas, A. M. (2011). Molecular diagnostics of colorectal cancer. *Archives of Pathology in Laboratory Medicine, 135*, 578–587.

Bryce, J., Bauer, M., & Hadji, P. (2011). Aromatase inhibitor-associated bone loss. *Oncology Nursing Forum, 38*(3), 273–276.

Bunz, F. (2008). *Principles of cancer genetics*. Springer, New York.

Cabanillas, F. (2011). Non-hodgkin's lymphoma: The old and the new. *Clinical Lymphoma, Myeloma & Leukemia, 11*(Supplement 1), S87–90.

Calvert, H., & Azzariti, A. (2011). The clinical development of inhibitors of poly(ADP-ribose) polymerase. *Annals of Oncology, 22*(Supplement 1), i53–i59. doi:10.1093/annonc/mdq667

Chau, B. N., & Wang, J. Y. (2003). Coordinated regulation of life and death by RB. *Nature Reviews Cancer 3*, 130–138. doi:10.1038/nrc993

Chial, H. (2008). Tumor suppressor (TS) genes and the two-hit hypothesis. *Nature Education, 1*(1). Retrieved February 24, 2012, from http://www.nature.com/scitable/topicpage/tumor-suppressor-ts-genes-and-the-two-887

Chou, R., Croswell, J. M., Dana, T., Bougatsos, C., Blazina, I., Fu, R., et al. (2011). *Screening for prostate cancer: A review of the evidence for the U.S. Preventive Services Task Force.* Retrieved November 22, 2011, from http://www.uspreventiveservicestaskforce.org/uspstf12/prostate/prostateart.htm

Clark, A. S., & Domchek, S. M. (2011). Clinical management of hereditary breast cancer syndromes. *Journal of Mammary Gland, Biology and Neoplasia, 16*, 17–25. doi:10.1007/s10911-011-9200-x

Clarke, M. F., et al. (2006). Cancer stem cells–perspectives on current status and future directions: AACR Workshop on cancer stem cells. *Cancer Research, 66*(19), 9339–9344.

Consensus Panel on Genetic/Genomic Nursing Competencies. (2009). *Essentials of genetic and genomic nursing: Competencies, curricula guidelines, and outcome indicators* (2nd ed.). Silver Spring, MD: American Nurses Association.

Durbecq, V., & Larsimont, D. (2010). Tumor biology and pathology. In M. W. Reed & R. A. Audisio (Eds.). *Management of breast cancer in older women*. Springer-Verlag London Limited 2010, pp. 21–35. doi:10.1007/978-1-84800-265-4_2

Ellisen, L. W., & Haber, D. A. (2010). Basic principles of cancer genetics. In D. C. Chung, & D. A. Haber (Eds.). *Principles of clinical cancer genetics. A handbook from the Massachusetts General Hospital*. New York: Springer.

Esteller, M. (2011). Cancer epigenetics for the 21st century. *Genes & Cancer, 2*(6), 604–606.

Food and Drug Administration [FDA]. (2011). *FDA commissioner announces Avastin decision*. Retrieved November 18, 2011, from http://www.fda.gov/NewsEvents/Newsroom/PressAnnouncements/ucm280536.htm

Foulkes, W. D. (2008). Inherited susceptibility to common cancers. *New England Journal of Medicine, 359*(20), 2143–2153.

Frank, N. Y., Schatton, T., & Frank, M. H. (2010). The therapeutic promise of the cancer stem cell concept. *The Journal of Clinical Investigation, 120*(1), 41–50.

Frazier, L, Calzone, K. A., & Jenkins, J (2010). Genetic/genomic competencies and recommendations for education. In K.A. Calzone, A. Masney, & J. Jenkins (Eds.). *Genetics and genomics in oncology nursing practice*. Oncology Nursing Society, pp. 287–296.

Friedberg, E. C. (2001). How nucleotide excision repair protects against cancer. *Nature Reviews Cancer, 1*, 22–33. doi:10.1038/35094000

Gore, S. D. (2005). Combination therapy with DNA methyltransferase inhibitors in hematologic malignancies. *Nature Clinical Practice Oncology, 2*, S30–S35. doi:10.1038/ncponc0346

Greenman, C., Stephens, P., Smith, R, Dalgliesh, G. L., Hunter, C., Bignell, G., et al. (2007). Patterns of somatic mutation in human cancer genomes. *Nature, 446*, 153–158.

Hanahan, D., & Weinberg, R. A. (2000). Hallmarks of cancer: The next generation. *Cell, 144*, 646–674.

Hanahan, D., & Weinberg R. A. (2011). Hallmarks of cancer: The next generation. *Cell, 144*, 646–674.

Hodi, F. S., O'Day, S. J., McDermott, D. F., Weber, R. W., Sosman, J. A., Haanen, J. B., et al. (2010). Improved survival with ipilimumab in patients with metastatic melanoma. *New England Journal of Medicine, 363*, 711–723.

Hu, G., Chong, R. A., Yang, Q., Wei, Y., Blanco, M. A., Li, F., et al. (2009). MTDH activation by 8q22 genomic gain promotes chemoresistance and metastasis of poor-prognosis breast cancer. *Cancer Cell, 15*(1), 9–20.

IOM (Institute of Medicine). (2012). *Integrating large-scale genomic information into clinical practice: Workshop summary.* Washington, DC: The National Academies Press.

Jin, B., Li, Y., & Robertson, K. D. (2011). DNA methylation: Superior or subordinate in the epigenetic hierarchy? *Genes & Cancer, 2*(6), 607–617.

Jones, S., Zhang, X., Parsons, D. W., Lin, J. C., Leary, R. J., Angenendt, P., et al. (2008). Core signaling pathways in human pancreatic cancers revealed by global genomic analyses. *Science, 321*, 1801–1806. doi:10.1126/science.1164368

Kinzler, K. W., & Vogelstein, B. (1997). Gatekeepers and caretakers. *Nature, 386*, 761–762.

Kinzler, K. W., & Vogelstein, B. (1998). Landscaping the cancer terrain. *Science, 280*(5366), 1036–1037.

Lahtz, C., & Pfeifer, G. P. (2011). Epigenetic changes of CNS repair genes in cancer. *Journal of Molecular Cell Biology, 3*, 51–58. doi:10.1093/jmcb/mjq053

Levine, A. J. (2011). The changing directions of p53 research. *Genes & Cancer, 2*(4), 382–384.

Manne, U., Srivastava, R. G., & Srivastava, S. (2005). Recent advances in biomarkers for cancer diagnosis and treatment. *Drug Discovery Today, 10*(14), 965–976.

Markowitz, S. D., & Bertagnolli, M. M. (2009). Molecularbasis of colorectal cancer. *The New England Journal of Medicine, 361*, 2449–2460.

Martens, J. H. A., Stunnenbert, H. G., & Logie, C. (2011). The decade of the epigenomes? *Genes & Cancer, 2*(6), 680–687.

Milosavljevic, A. (2011). Emerging patterns of epigenomic variation. *Trends in Genetics, 27*(6), 242–250.

Nass, S. J., & Moses, H. L. (2007). *Cancer biomarkers: The promises and challenges of improving detection and treatment*. Washington, DC: National Academies Press.

National Cancer Institute [NCI]. (n.d.). *NCI dictionary of genetics terms*. Retrieved November 16, 2011, from http://www.cancer.gov/cancertopics/genetics/genetics-terms-alphalist/a-e

National Cancer Institute [NCI]. (2009). *Genome-wide profiling.* Retrieved November 16, 2011, from http://www.cancer.gov/cancertopics/understandingcancer/genomewideprofiling

National Cancer Institute [NCI]. (2012). *Cancer, changing the conversation: The nation's investment in cancer research: An annual plan and budget proposal for fiscal year 2012*. NIH Publication No. 11-7760.

NCCN Guidelines Panel. (2011a). *Genetic/familial high-risk assessment: Breast and ovarian*. Version 1.2011. National Comprehensive Cancer Network, Inc.

NCCN Guidelines Panel. (2011b). *Colorectal cancer screening.* Version 2.2011. National Comprehensive Cancer Network, Inc.

Negrini, S., Gorgoulis, V. G., & Halazonetis, T. D. (2010). *Nature Reviews Molecular Cell Biology, 11*, 220–228.

Nguyen, D. X., & Massague, J. (2007). Genetic determinants of cancer metastasis. *Nature Reviews Genetics, 8*, 341–352. doi:10.1038/nrg2101

Oncology Nursing Society. (2009a). *Cancer predisposition genetic testing and risk assessment counseling*. Retrieved November 22, 2011, from http://www.ons.org/Publications/Positions/Predisposition

Oncology Nursing Society. (2009b). *The role of the oncology nurse in cancer genetic counseling*. Retrieved November 22, 2011, from http://www.ons.org/Publications/Positions/GeneticCounseling

Pino, M. S., & Chung, D. C. (2011). Microsatelite instability in the management of colorectal cancer. *Expert Reviews Gastroenterology Hepatology, 5*(3), 385–399. doi:10.1586/EGH.11.25

President's Council of Advisors on Science and Technology. (2008). *Priorities for personalized medicine*. Retrieved November 1, 2011, from http://www.ostp.gov

Reeves, S. G., Meldrum, C., Groombridge, C., Spigelman, A., Suchy, J., Kurzawski, G., et al. (2011). DNA repair gene polymorphisms and risk of early onset colorectal cancer in Lynch syndrome. *Cancer Epidemiology, 2012, 36*(2), pp. 183–189. doi:10.1016/j.canep.2011.09.003

Riley, B. D., Culver, J. O., Skrzynia, C., Senter, L. A., Peters, J. A., Costalas, J. W., et al. (2011). Essential elements of genetic cancer risk assessment, counseling, and testing: Updated recommendations for the National Society of Genetic Counselors. *Journal of Genetic Counseling, 21*(2), pp. 151–161. doi:10.1007/s10897-011-9462-x

Russo, A., Migliavacca, M., Zanna, I., Macaluso, M., Gebbia, N. and Bazan, V. (2005). Caretakers and gatekeepers. *Encyclopedia of life sciences*. Hoboken, NJ: John Wiley & Sons, Ltd., pp. 1–9. Retrieved November 7, 2011, from http://onlinelibrary.wiley.com/doi/10.1038/npg.els.0006048/full

Shoushtari, A. N., Szmulewitz, R. Z., & Rinker-Schaeffer, C. W. (2011). Metastasis-suppressor genes in clinical practice: Lost in translation? *Nature Reviews/Clinical Oncology, 8*, 333–342. doi:10.1038/nrclinonc.2011.65

Stratton, M. R. (2011). Exploring the genomes of cancer cells: Progress and promise. *Science, 331*, 1553–1558. doi:10.1126/science.1204040

Stratton, M. R., Campbell, P. J., & Futreal, P. A. (2009). The cancer genome. *Nature, 458*, 719–724.

Stricker, T., Catenacci, D. V. T., & Seiwert, T. Y. (2011). Molecular profiling of cancer–the future of personalized cancer medicine: A primer on cancer biology and the tools necessary to bring molecular testing to the clinic. *Seminars in Oncology, 38*(2), 173–185.

Soltanian, S., & Matin, M. M. (2011). Cancer stem cells and cancer therapy. *Tumor Biology, 32*, 425–440.

The Cancer Genome Atlas Research Network. (2011). Integrated genomic analyses of ovarian carcinoma. *Nature, 474*, 609–615. doi:10.1038/nature10166

The International Cancer Consortium. (2010). International network of cancer genome projects. *Nature, 464*, 993–998. doi:10.1038/nature08987

Vogelstein, B., & Kinzler, K. W. (2004). Cancer genes and the pathways they control. *Nature Medicine, 10*(8), 789–799.

Walk, E. L., & Weed, S. A. (2011). Recently identified biomarkers that promote lymph node metastasis in head and neck squamous cell carcinoma. *Cancers, 3*, 747–772.

Wei, Y., Hu, G, & Kang, Y. (2009). Metadherin as a link between metastasis and chemoresistance. *Cell Cycle, 8*(14), 2131–2132.

Weinstein, I. B., & Joe, A. (2008). Oncogene addiction. *Cancer Research, 68*(9), 3077–3080.

Wilson, D. M., Kim, D., Berquist, B. R., & Sigurdson, A. J. (2011).Variation in base excision repair capacity. *Mutation Research, 711*, 100–112.

Wu, H. C., Huang, C. T., & Chang, D. K. (2008). Anti-angiogenic therapeutic drugs for treatment of human cancer. *Journal of Cancer Molecules, 4*(2), 37–45.

PART 6

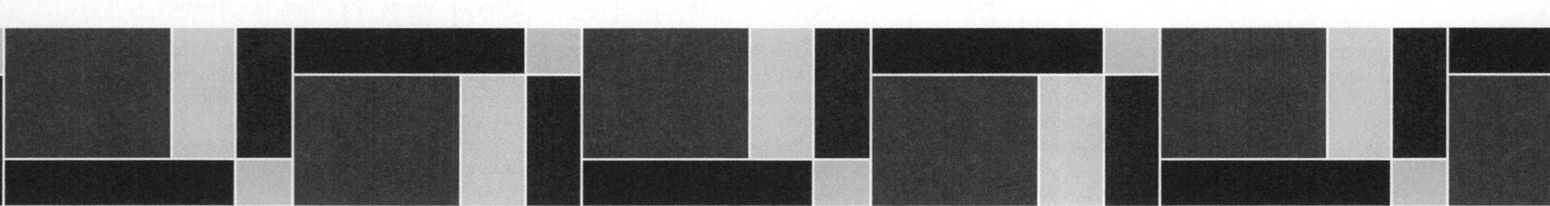

Public Health Genetics

CHAPTER

17 Impact of Environment on Health: Interaction with Genes

Robert M. Fineman

LEARNING OUTCOMES

Following the completion of this chapter, the learner will be able to

1. Outline basic concepts of genetic susceptibility.
2. Outline basic concepts of environmental perturbations.
3. Explain the multifactorial interactions involving genetic, environmental, and behavioral risk factors that cause ill health and disease, with a special emphasis on gout.
4. Identify intervention/management strategies that promote health and/or prevent disease in individuals and populations at high risk for developing chronic diseases, with a special emphasis on gout.

Since a significant amount of premature death and disability in the United States is preventable (Danaei et al., 2009), this chapter uses gout (a common, adult-onset, metabolic condition) as a springboard for understanding how genetic, environmental, behavioral, and other risk factors cause multifactorial diseases; how and why different individuals respond differently to external/environmental perturbations; and what lifestyle changes and other interventions can be used to promote health and prevent common complex diseases in individuals and populations (Khoury, Burke, & Thomson, 2000; Khoury, 2003; Parrish, 2010; "Healthy People 2020," 2011; WHO, 2011).

Genetic susceptibility is a predisposition to disease at the genetic level that may be activated under certain conditions. Single nucleotide polymorphisms (SNP) are single bases within a gene sequence; these differ from the consensus sequence and are present in a subset of the population. SNPs broadly range in effect: they may not have any effect on gene expression, or they can completely change the function of a gene. In some cases the resulting gene expression changes can result in disease, or in susceptibility to disease (e.g., bacterial or viral infection).

As a result of genetic susceptibility assessment, some people will gain assurance through their expanded knowledge of familial genes or history. For others who already have a disease, assessment of their genetic susceptibility may lead them to seek medicines or therapies. Still others may discover that they are susceptible to a disease that has no cure, offering the foreknowledge to make choices to prevent or delay the on-set of that disease through increased health education, in making lifestyle changes, through finding preventive therapies or identifying by environmental triggers of the disease.

The implementation of genetic susceptibility screening for a whole populations and the historical promotion of genetic prediction and prevention rests on a number of biological assumptions, some implausible or improbable. Genetic variants are poor predictors of most diseases in most people and biology is complex. A process of independent assessment of the benefits of assessing population genetic susceptibility as a health strategy is overdue, as is regulation of clinical validity.

However, population-based newborn screening has been available for decades and is a widely accepted clinical practice. Population-based prenatal screening for conditions such as cystic fibrosis, Trisomy 21, and neural tube defects also has become the standard of care.

The term **public health genetics** applies to advances in human genetics, genomics, and molecular biotechnology concentrating on improving public health and preventing disease. It focuses on increasing knowledge of genetic inheritance in order to better understand common health conditions and how to slow their spread. (www.genome.gov) Population-based screening of seemingly healthy adults for genetic susceptibility depends on factors such as risk assessment, cost-effective testing mechanisms, sensitivity and specificity of tests, provider education, cultural relevance, consumer acceptance, reimbursement for services, and public policy initiatives. Until the cadre of primary health care providers, including advanced practice nurses and physicians, increases their genetic literacy to be able to effectively explain and interpret test results, this will not happen.

Environmental perturbations are environmental factors or agents that can alter the functioning of biologic systems in response not only to the individual characteristics of the factor or agent, but also to the timing, magnitude, frequency and duration of the exposure. These environmental factors are too numerous to explore in depth in this book but may derive from geography, hygiene, life-stressors, pathogens, chemical exposure, drinking water, and nutrition, among other factors. (See chapter 6 for more on environmental factors related to pregnancy).

PRETEST

1. A ______ is a cancer-causing substance or agent.
   A. carcinogen
   B. mutation
   C. vitamin
   D. enzyme
2. A ______ is any internal (e.g., maternal phenylketonuria or diabetes mellitus) or external (e.g., certain infectious, physical, chemical or nutritional agents) perturbation that can disturb the development of an embryo or fetus.
3. Epigenetic is defined as
   A. the study of heritable changes in gene function/expression that occur without a change in the sequence of the DNA.
   B. a change from a normal to an abnormal size and shape secondary to a mechanical force(s).
   C. the abnormal growth or development of a structure, e.g., in cells, tissues, or organs.
   D. None of the above
4. Hyperuricemia and gouty arthritis go hand in hand; i.e., if a person has one then he or she will also have the other.
   A. True
   B. False
5. Which of the following terms refers to an organism's observable characteristics or traits, e.g., structure, functions, or behavior?
   A. Genotype
   B. Phenotype
   C. Alleles
   D. All of the above
   E. None of the above
6. A mutagen is something that can induce a genetic mutation or can increase the rate of mutation, e.g., certain substances, viruses, X-rays, and wave lengths of ultraviolet irradiation.
   A. True
   B. False
7. ______ is a systematic investigation aimed at the discovery of new knowledge including the revision of accepted laws, theories, and facts, and/or the practical application of such new or revised laws, theories, and facts.
8. Multifactorial inheritance is a mode of inheritance in which an attribute or characteristic is controlled by one gene or one of a pair of allelic genes.
   A. True
   B. False
9. Medications used to treat gout include
   A. nonsteroidal anti-inflammatory drugs (NSAIDs).
   B. colchicine.
   C. corticosteroids.
   D. aspirin.
   E. All of the above
10. Standard of care practice refers to the diagnostic and treatment process that a clinician should follow for a certain type of patient, illness, or clinical circumstance. In legal terms, this is the level at which the average prudent provider in a given community would practice.
    A. True
    B. False

Pretest answers are located in the Appendix.

SECTION ONE: Gout

Be temperate in wine, in eating, girls, and sloth; or the gout will seize you and plague you both.

Benjamin Franklin, American statesman and gout sufferer (1706 CE–1790 CE)

Gouty arthritis is one of the oldest and most frequently recognized and recorded diseases in the history of medicine (Nuki and Simkin, 2006). It was first identified as podagra (acute gout in the first metatarsophalangeal joint) by the Egyptians around 2640 BCE. Hippocrates of Cos (ca. 460 BCE–ca. 370 BE) referred to it as the "unwalkable disease." He also noted what he thought was a connection between the disorder and an excessive lifestyle, referring to it as the arthritis of the rich as opposed to rheumatism, an arthritis of the poor. Galen (131 CE–201 CE) recognized the heritable nature of gout, and he also described **tophi**, the crystallized **monosodium urate** deposits that can follow long-standing **hyperuricemia** (i.e., an excess of uric acid in the blood).

Many other luminaries have been associated with the history of gout since ancient times including, but not limited to, Seneca (ca. 4 BCE–65 CE), Thomas Sydenham (1624 CE–1689 CE), Antoni van Leeuwenhoek (1632 CE–1723 CE), Benjamin Franklin, William Pitt, the Elder (1708 CE–1778 CE), Charles Gravier (the Compte de Vergennes, 1717 CE–1787 CE), Thomas Jefferson (1743 CE–1846 CE), Sir Alfred Baring Garrod (1819 CE–1907 CE) and his son, Sir Archibald Garrod (1857 CE–1936 CE). Indeed, gout is not only a disease that has great medical/scientific significance but is also a disease that changed the course of history (Nuki and Simkin, 2006).

Pathophysiology and Prevalence

Gout is an acute and potentially chronic disease caused by hyperuricemia, which can lead to the deposition of monosodium urate crystals in tissue (Richette & Bardin, 2010; Doghramji, 2011). Hyperuricemia is caused by both the overproduction of uric acid in the body and also the underexcretion of uric acid in the urine. Underexcretion is the more common cause of gout, and it is thought to account for 80%–90% of hyperuricemia (Luk & Simkin, 2005). Approximately 60% of affected individuals have a second attack within a year of the initial attack, and 80% have a second attack within 2 years.

The metabolic pathways of purine catabolism in humans are well understood (Voet, Voet, & Pratt, 2008) and will not be reviewed here in detail. Suffice it to say, the final product of purine degradation in humans is uric acid, which is excreted in the urine. The inflammation and pain associated with an acute gout attack appear to be caused by the activation of the *NLRP3* inflammasome by monosodium urate crystals leading to the release of interleukin-1B (Neogi, 2011).

Hyperuricemia is not the same as gout. It is possible to have an elevated serum uric acid level and never develop gout. Therefore, treatment of individuals with asymptomatic hyperuricemia is usually not necessary unless the uric acid level is very high (normal values usually fall between 3.0 and 6.8 mg/dL), or there is a personal or strong family history of multiple individuals with gout or other conditions such as uric acid nephropathy or urolithiasis (Dincer, Dincer, & Levinson, 2002).

The prevalence of gout in U.S. adults in 2007–2008 was about 3.9% (8.3 million): 5.9% among men (6.1 million) and 2.0% (2.2 million) among women (Zhu, Pandva, & Choi, 2011). There is considerable evidence that the prevalence of gout and hyperuricemia may have increased during the past two decades, which is likely related to increasing presence of adiposity and hypertension, and the aging of the population (Lawrence et al., 2008).

Signs and Symptoms

From a clinical perspective, gout is a condition that often occurs in multiple stages, described as follows:

1. The asymptomatic tissue deposition stage, during which time individuals have no signs or symptoms, but do have hyperuricemia and the asymptomatic deposition of monosodium urate crystals in tissues (e.g., joints and kidneys).
2. Acute flares occur when monosodium urate crystals in joints (most frequently in the big toes, but also in the knees, ankles, heels, elbows, wrists, and fingers) cause acute inflammation. During acute flares, which can last days or weeks, the pain is usually sudden in onset and very intense. Affected joints often swell, are both warm and tender to touch, and may take on a deep red or purple hue. Older individuals frequently have more affected joints than younger people. Uric acid levels may be in the normal range during an acute flare.
3. An "interacute" phase or stage can occur after an acute flare has subsided. Although the person may be asymptomatic, hyperuricemia often continues with additional deposition of monosodium urate crystals in tissues resulting in additional damage. The interval/time period between acute flares (days, months, or years) often becomes shorter as the disease progresses.
4. In chronic gout, the arthritic pain is often dull, aching, and persistent due to permanent joint damage. Chronic joint pain and acute flares can occur at the same time in the same joint or in different joints. Nodules known as tophi, caused by accumulations of monosodium urate crystals, often appear in soft tissue under the skin near joints. Permanent kidney damage and other important complications can also occur.

Tests and Diagnosis

An informative personal and family medical history (of at least three generations, if possible), physical findings consistent with the diagnosis, and finding monosodium urate crystals in joint aspiration/synovial fluid or in tophi are important in making a definitive diagnosis of gout.

In the absence of joint/synovial fluid testing, criteria developed by the American College of Rheumatology can be used to diagnose an attack of acute gout. Six of the following 12 criteria must be present in order to confirm a diagnosis (Dore, 2008; Terkeltaub, Edwards, & Wortmann, 2009):

- Asymmetric swelling within joint on X-ray
- Hyperuricemia
- Joint fluid culture negative for organisms during attack
- Maximum inflammation developed within a day
- Monoarthritis
- More than one attack of acute arthritis
- Painful/swollen first MTP joint
- Redness over joints
- Subcortical cysts without erosions on X-ray
- Tophus (proved or suspected)
- Unilateral attack of first MTP joint
- Unilateral attack of tarsal joint

As noted previously, serum uric acid levels are important but they can be misleading. Some individuals with signs and symptoms of gout have normal or even low normal uric acid levels during an attack, and asymptomatic individuals with no history of gout can have hyperuricemia.

The imaging features of gout typically appear 15 or more years after disease onset. The online version of Wheeless' *Textbook of Orthopedics* (2011) provides excellent examples of X-rays of patients with gout. X-rays are not considered useful in confirming the diagnosis of early gout.

Risk Factors

Causal factors that increase the risk of developing gout include but are not limited to the following:

1. Genetic/genomic risk factors: i.e., relatively common, predisposition genes associated with a low to moderate penetrance (Dalbeth & Merriman, 2009; Choi, Zhu, & Mount, 2010; Richette & Bardin, 2010; Merriman & Dalbeth, 2011; also search the **OMIM** database (2011) for the term *gout* for up-to-date information about genetic risk factors associated with gout).
2. A positive family history for the condition.
3. Gender and age: Gout occurs more frequently in men than in women because men have higher serum uric acid levels starting at a younger age. However, after menopause women's uric acid levels approach those of men. Men also are more likely to develop gout earlier, at around 40–50 years of age, while women generally develop signs and symptoms after menopause.
4. Environmental risk factors: e.g., exposure to lead/lead poisoning, and serious infections.
5. Behavioral factors and treatment-related complications (Choi et al., 2004a and 2004b; Choi et al., 2005).

Genome-wide association studies (GWAS) (Dalbeth & Merriman, 2009; Choi, Zhu, & Mount, 2010; Richette & Bardin, 2010; Merriman & Dalbeth, 2011) have identified significant associations between DNA polymorphisms (SNPs), genes,

Emerging Evidence

Genetic variation is the underlying cause of genetic susceptibility regarding gout as well as many other multifactorial conditions including but not limited to most forms of cancer, heart disease, diabetes mellitus, hypertension, cerebrovascular diseases, autoimmune disorders, allergies, asthma, and certain forms of mental illness—i.e., a diathesis-stress model. What this means, in essence, is genetics loads the gun and environmental and behavioral factors pull the trigger in common diseases with multifactorial etiologies. With the extraordinary advances that have taken place over the past 20 years in the fields of human, medical, and pharmogenetics and genomics, and the advances which will most likely take place over the next 20 years, it will not be much longer before standard, everyday health care practice will include our need to do the following:

1. Accurately and inexpensively predict the susceptibility of an individual to develop a multifactorial, complex disease based on genetic, genomic, environmental, behavioral, and other risk factors (e.g., have ready access to education and care).
2. Provide useful, inexpensive, affordable, and readily accessible screening and diagnostic tests (e.g., DNA, protein, and metabolite based), as well as other tools aimed at the early identification of high risk/asymptomatic individuals, diagnosis, and improved personalized treatment, and a prognosis and the prediction of a recurrence risk.
3. Better understand and utilize pharmacogenetics/genomics, which will improve individualized medicinal therapies and also decrease complications secondary to the therapies.

There is no doubt nurses have, and will continue to play, an important role in all aspects of human and medical genetics and genomic-environmental-behavioral **research** and related clinical, public health, and education efforts for many years to come.

and an increased risk of developing gout. **Genetic screening** for an increased risk of developing gout could be available in the near future using this kind of association information.

Behavioral and treatment-associated risk factors include being overweight or obese, having hypertension, excess alcohol intake (beer and spirits more than wine), and a diet rich in meat and seafood. As noted previously, uric acid comes from the degradation of purines, a subclass of proteins that are abundant in a variety of foods noted in the later section "Lifestyle Management."

Also, a number of medications/supplements/perturbations can increase blood uric acid levels and form irritating crystals in joints. These include salicylates (the active component of aspirin), vitamin B3 (niacin), excess vitamin C, and diuretics (e.g., thiazides) that may be prescribed for high blood pressure, edema, or cardiovascular disease. Others are cyclosporine used to prevent rejection of transplanted organs, levodopa for Parkinson disease, and pyrazinamide used to treat tuberculosis. Additional risk factors include dehydration and conditions that acidify the blood: e.g., uncontrolled diabetes, renal insufficiency, serious infections, surgery, or ketogenic weight loss diets such as the Atkins diet (Choi et al., 2004a and 2004b; Choi et al., 2005).

Differential Diagnosis

A differential diagnosis for gout could include but is not limited to the following conditions: pseudo-gout (when calcium pyrophosphate dehydrate crystals are deposited in a joint), painful osteoarthritis, Lyme disease, psoriatic arthritis, rheumatoid arthritis, septic arthritis, chronic lead poisoning, spondyloarthropathy, Lesch-Nyhan syndrome, and familial juvenile hyperuricemic nephropathy Types 1 and 2 (Terkeltaub, Edwards, & Wortmann, 2009; OMIM, 2011).

Treatment

The medications most commonly used to treat acute gout attacks and/or prevent additional attacks from occurring in the future include the following:

1. Nonsteroidal anti-inflammatory drugs (NSAIDs) that decrease inflammation and pain. NSAIDs include ibuprofen (Advil, Motrin, and others) and naproxen (Aleve and others), as well as the more powerful prescription NSAIDs (e.g., indomethacin [Indocin]). Side effects of NSAIDs include stomach pain, bleeding, and ulcers. Higher doses of NSAIDs are frequently used to treat an acute attack, followed by a lower daily dose to prevent future attacks.
2. Colchicine reduces gout inflammation and pain, especially if it is started shortly after symptoms first appear. Side effects of colchicine therapy include nausea, vomiting, and diarrhea. Higher doses of this medication are frequently used to treat an acute attack, followed by a lower daily dose to prevent future attacks.
3. Corticosteroids, like prednisone, that are either injected into an affected joint or taken by mouth can be used to control inflammation and pain. Side effects of corticosteroid therapy include osteopenia (thinning bones), poor wound healing, and a decreased ability to fight infection. As with NSAID and colchicine therapy, use of the lowest dose for the shortest period of time decreases the risk of side effects with corticosteroid therapy.
4. Xanthine oxidase inhibitors that block or limit the amount of uric acid produced in the body: e.g., allopurinol (Zyloprim, Aloprim, Lopurin) and febuxostat (Uloric). As the blood uric acid level is decreased over time with the use of these medications, the risk of developing attacks over time also decreases. Side effects of allopurinol include but are not limited to nausea, diarrhea, headache, hives, and (rarely) two life-threatening dermatological conditions: Stevens-Johnson syndrome and toxic epidermal necrolysis (PubMed Health/Allopurinol, 2010). The side effects of febuxostat include but are not limited to rash, nausea, and elevated liver enzymes in the blood and reduced liver function (PubMed Health/Fubuxostat, 2009). Xanthine oxidase inhibitors can cause an acute attack if they are taken before a recent attack has totally resolved. A short therapeutic course of low-dose colchicine before starting xanthine oxidase inhibitor therapy can significantly reduce this risk.

5. Probenecid (Probalan, Benemid, Benuryl) improves the kidneys ability to remove uric acid from the body. As the blood uric acid level is decreased over time with the use of these medications, the risk of developing attacks over time also decreases. However, the level of uric acid in urine is increased. Side effects include but are not limited to a rash, stomach pain, vomiting, and kidney stones (PubMed Health/Probenecid, 2008).

Lifestyle Management

Individuals who suffer from gout or who are at high risk of developing it need to know and understand the importance of the following preventive information. Those who do not may cause themselves increased physical and other types of distress (Reach, 2011).

1. Maintain a high fluid intake. Drink at least eight 8-ounce glasses of water daily to flush uric acid from the system and also to prevent monosodium urate crystal deposition in the joints and kidneys.
2. Maintain a healthy body weight. Being overweight increases the risk of gout attacks, and losing weight slowly to a desirable body weight lowers the risk (Cunningham, 2004; Hayman & Marcason, 2009).
3. Maintain a healthy diet. Paying close attention to foods and/or drinks that are purine rich and result in an increase in the production of uric acid and also to foods/liquids that reduce uric acid elimination in the urine lowers the chances (Hayman & Marcason, 2009; Mayo Clinic, 2011):
   - Reduce to up to 4–6 ounces daily or eliminate from the diet animal protein (meat, fish, shellfish, and poultry) and also asparagus and mushrooms.
   - Reduce or eliminate the intake of alcohol (especially beer and liquor), coffee, and other sources of caffeine because they promote dehydration.
   - Eat plant-based protein sources (e.g., beans and legumes), and fruits, vegetables, whole grains, and low-fat milk products.

There are no known adverse side effects to this diet. Actually, with the addition of moderate exercise, this type of lifestyle is recommended to prevent not only gout but also other serious chronic diseases including hypertension and cardiovascular disease.

SECTION ONE REVIEW

1. In humans, uric acid is the final product of
   A. purine degradation.
   B. pyrimidine degradation.
   C. A and B, above
2. A differential diagnosis for a person with gout could include which of the following conditions?
   A. Pseudo-gout
   B. Osteoarthritis
   C. Psoriatic arthritis
   D. Lyme disease
3. Individuals who suffer from gout or who are at high risk of developing gout should drink lots of water: i.e., at least eight 8-ounce glasses per day.
   A. True
   B. False
4. The prevalence of people with gout in the United States in 2007–2008 was approximately
   A. 1 million.
   B. 5 million.
   C. 8 million.
   D. 12 million.

Answers: 1. A; 2. E; 3. A; 4. C

POSTTEST

1. Which term refers to the variation seen as a result of genetic mutation(s) in the genomes of individuals in a species or between different species?
   A. Deformations
   B. Dysplasias
   C. Malformations
   D. All of the above
   E. None of the above
2. A genome-wide association study is the analysis of most or all of the genetic markers in the genomes of different individuals in a particular species—or between species—to determine how much genetic variation exists and to understand how the variation could contribute to different traits (including diseases), the strategies that could be used to detect, treat, and prevent diseases, and also to determine the prognoses and recurrence risks.
   A. True
   B. False

3. Genetic factors account for approximately what percent of the risk for developing gout?
   A. 20%
   B. 40%
   C. 60%
   D. 80%
4. The diet and exercise regimens used to reduce the risk of future/recurrent gout attacks are also useful in preventing other serious chronic conditions including hypertension and cardiovascular disease.
   A. True
   B. False
5. Causal factors that increase the risk of developing gout include
   A. biologic factors.
   B. gender and age.
   C. environmental factors.
   D. behavioral and treatment-related factors.
   E. All of the above
6. Gouty arthritis is one of the oldest and most frequently recognized and recorded diseases in the history of medicine.
   A. True
   B. False
7. Nature versus nurture refers to the relative importance of the sum of genetic factors (nature) versus the sum of environmental factors (nurture) in the development and/or functioning of living things and, most often, in the causation of human behavior.
   A. True
   B. False
8. Gout occurs more frequently in women than men.
   A. True
   B. False
9. Which of the following statements is correct?
   A. Gout is caused by an overproduction of uric acid in the body.
   B. Gout is caused by the underelimination of uric acid in the urine.
   C. Gout is caused by both an overproduction of uric acid in the body and an underexcretion of uric acid in the urine.
10. Which of the following can increase the risk of having a gout attack?
    A. Salicylates (the active component in aspirin)
    B. Vitamin B3 (niacin)
    C. Diuretics (e.g., thiazides)
    D. All of the above

Posttest answers are located in the Appendix.

CHAPTER SUMMARY

Gout is an acute and potentially chronic disease caused by hyperuricemia, which can lead to the deposition of monosodium urate crystals in tissue. Hyperuricemia is caused by both the overproduction of uric acid in the body and also the underexcretion of uric acid in the urine. Underexcretion is the more common cause of gout, and it is thought to account for 80%–90% of hyperuricemia. The inflammation and pain associated with an acute gout attack appear to be caused by the activation of the *NLRP3* inflammasome by monosodium urate crystals leading to the release of interleukin-1B.

Hyperuricemia is not the same as gout. It is possible to have an elevated serum uric acid level and never develop gout. Therefore, treatment of individuals with asymptomatic hyperuricemia is usually not necessary unless the uric acid level in the blood is elevated markedly (normal values usually fall between 3.0 and 6.8 mg/dL), or there is a personal or strong family history of multiple individuals with gout or other conditions such as uric acid nephropathy or urolithiasis.

The prevalence of gout in U.S. adults in 2007–2008 was about 3.9% (8.3 million): 5.9% among men (6.1 million) and 2.0% (2.2 million) among women. There is considerable evidence that the prevalence of gout and hyperuricemia may have increased during the past two decades, which is likely related to increasing presence of adiposity and hypertension and the aging of the population.

The multifactorial/causal factors that increase one's risk of developing gout include but are not limited to genetic and genomic risk factors (for the most part relatively common predisposition genes associated with a low-to-moderate penetrance), a positive family history for the condition, older age and maleness, environmental risk factors such as marked exposure to lead/lead poisoning, and behavioral factors and treatment-related complications. Additional risk factors include dehydration and conditions that acidify the blood: e.g., uncontrolled diabetes, serious infections, surgery, or ketogenic weight loss diets such as the Atkins diet.

From a clinical perspective, gout is a condition that often occurs in multiple stages: i.e., the asymptomatic tissue deposition stage, during which time individuals have no signs or symptoms but do have hyperuricemia and the asymptomatic deposition of monosodium urate crystals in tissues; the acute flare stage when monosodium urate crystals in joints (most frequently in the big toes, but also in the knees, ankles, heels, elbows, wrists, and fingers) cause acute inflammation; an "interacute" phase or stage that can occur after an acute flare has subsided; and a chronic stage in which the arthritic pain is usually dull, aching, and persistent due to permanent joint damage. Nodules known as tophi, caused by accumulations of monosodium urate crystals, often appear in chronic gout in soft tissues under the skin near joints. Permanent kidney damage can also occur.

A differential diagnosis for gout could include but is not limited to the following conditions: pseudo-gout (when calcium pyrophosphate dehydrate crystals are deposited in a joint), painful osteoarthritis, Lyme disease, psoriatic arthritis, rheumatoid arthritis, septic arthritis, chronic lead poisoning, spondyloarthropathy, Lesch-Nyhan syndrome, and familial juvenile hyperuricemic nephropathy Types 1 and 2.

An informative personal and family medical history (of at least three generations, if possible), physical findings consistent with the diagnosis, and finding monosodium urate crystals in joint aspiration/synovial fluid or in tophi are important in making a definitive diagnosis of gout. In the absence of joint/synovial fluid testing, clinical criteria developed by the American College of Rheumatology can be used to diagnose an acute gout attack.

The medications most commonly used to treat acute gout attacks and/or prevent future attacks include NSAIDs, colchicine, corticosteroids, and xanthine oxidase inhibitors. In addition, individuals who suffer from gout or who are at high risk of developing gout need to know and understand the importance of maintaining a high fluid intake, a healthy body weight, and a low-purine diet with a reduced intake of beer and spirits. Finally, there are certain medications like high doses of aspirin, niacin, diuretics, and others that should be avoided, if possible.

Disclaimer: This information in this chapter is for educational purposes only. Readers should consult a physician regarding the applicability of this information to their patients and others.

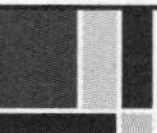

CRITICAL THINKING CHECKPOINT

A 55-year old upper middle class male presented in the emergency department of a local hospital with mild chest pain radiating to the left shoulder and arm. He was 74 inches tall and weighed 235 pounds (BMI approximately 30). He ate very little meat except for fish (no shellfish) and drank approximately 32 ounces of fluid including 2 cups of coffee daily and 1–2 glasses of wine per week. Exercise consisted mostly of walking in a local park, three miles 3–4 times per week. He took no medications, and the findings at his regular annual physical examinations (the last one was 2 months earlier) were essentially unremarkable except for borderline hypertension (i.e., 130–135/80). He had no history of arthritis or psoriasis. His three-generation family history was significant in that several individuals were diagnosed with diabetes, usually between 35–45 years of age. There was no family history of gout. Subsequent testing at the hospital revealed no heart muscle damage, but on angiography he had a 90+% occlusion in his right coronary artery that was successfully treated with stent therapy.

Upon discharge from the hospital the patient was placed on a statin medication and low-dose aspirin therapy. He was also advised to lose weight and exercise more often. A few months later his family physician prescribed daily low-dose diuretic (thiazide) therapy for the borderline hypertension and niacin to boast his HDL cholesterol level.

Several months later the patient developed an acute onset of pain and minimal swelling in the first MTP joint in his right foot. There was no history of trauma or infection of any kind. Physical examination was consistent with the diagnosis of gout. No joint fluid analysis was performed. A serum uric acid level was 9.2 mg/Dl. The patient was told to discontinue taking niacin, drink at least 64 ounces of fluid daily while avoiding beer and spirits, lose more weight, and exercise more often. Within a week the pain in his right foot was gone, and over the next 10 years it never returned. Subsequent uric acid levels were in the 6–7 mg/Dl range.

1. Was genetic testing appropriate for this man?
2. What are the risk factors for developing gout and how many of them did he have?
3. Would an X-ray of his right foot have helped in making the diagnosis of gout?

Answers are provided in the Appendix

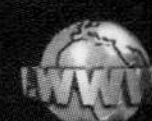

ONLINE RESOURCES

American Academy of Family Physicians CME Bulletin: http://www.aafp.org/online/etc/medialib/aafp_org/documents/cme/selfstudy/bulletins/gout-hyperuricemia.Par.0001.File.dat/Gout.pdf

American College of Rheumatology - Gout: http://www.rheumatology.org/practice/clinical/patients/diseases_and_conditions/gout.asp

Centers for Disease Control and Prevention - Arthritis: http://www.cdc.gov/arthritis/basics/gout.htm

Gene Tests: http://www.ncbi.nlm.nih.gov/sites/GeneTests/?db=GeneTests

Johns Hopkins Arthritis Center – Biochemical causes of gout: http://www.hopkins-arthritis.org/ask-the-expert/gout-pseudogout-other-009/biochemical-causes-of-gout-928.html

Mayo Clinic - Gout: http://www.mayoclinic.com/health/gout/DS00090

Medline Plus: http://www.nlm.nih.gov/medlineplus/ency/article/003476.htm; http://www.nlm.nih.gov/medlineplus/gout.html; and http://vsearch.nlm.nih.gov/vivisimo/cgi-bin/query-meta?v%3Aproject=medlineplus&query=gout&x=11&y=13

National Human Genome Research Institute: http://www.genome.gov; http://www.genome.gov/search.cfm?keyword=GWAS;http://www.genome.gov/19518663; and http://www.genome.gov/10000464

National Institute of Arthritis and Musculoskeletal and Skin Diseases: http://nihseniorhealth.gov/gout/toc.html;http://www.niams.nih.gov/Health_Info/Gout/default.asp; and http://www.niams.nih.gov/Health_Info/Gout/gout_ff.asp

National Institute of Environmental Health Sciences – National Institutes of Health: http://www.niehs.nih.gov/health/topics/science/gene-env/index.cfm

National Institutes of Health - Genes, Environment and Health Initiative (GEI) Program: http://www.nhlbi.nih.gov/resources/geneticsgenomics/programs/gei.htm

Online Mendelian Inheritance in Man (OMIM): http://www.ncbi.nlm.nih.gov/omim

Pub Med Health: http://www.ncbi.nlm.nih.gov/pubmedhealth/PMH0001459/

REFERENCES

Choi, H. K., Atkinson, K., Karlson, E. W., Willet, W., & Curhan, G. (2004a). Alcohol intake and risk of incident gout in men: A prospective study. *Lancet*, 363, 1277–1278.

Choi, H. K., Atkinson, K., Karlson, E. W., Willet, W., & Curhan, G. (2004b). Purine-rich foods, dairy and protein intake, and the risk of gout in men. *New England Journal of Medicine, 350*, 1093–1103.

Choi, H. K., Atkinson, K., Karlson, E. W., & Curhan, G. (2005). Obesity, weight change, hypertension, diuretic use, and risk of gout in men. *Archives of Internal Medicine, 165*, 742–748.

Choi, H. K., Zhu, Y., & Mount, D. B. (2010). Genetics of gout. *Current Opinion in Rheumatology, 22*, 144–151.

Cunningham, E. (2004). What nutritional factors affect the risk of gout? *Journal of the American Dietetic Association, 104*, 1737.

Dalbeth, N., & Merriman, T. (2009). Crystal ball gazing: New therapeutic targets for hyperuricaemia and gout. *Rheumatology, 48*, 222–226.

Danaei, G., Ding, E. L., Mozaffarian, D., Taylor, B., Rehm, J., Murray, C. J. L., et al. (2009). The preventable causes of death in the United States: Comparative risk assessment of dietary, lifestyle, and metabolic risk factors. *PLoS Medicine, 6*(4), e1000058. Retrieved August, 2011, from http://www.plosmedicine.org/article/info:doi/10.1371/journal.pmed.1000058

Dincer, H. E., Dincer, A. P., & Levinson, D. J. (2002). Asymptomatic hyperuricemia: To treat or not to treat. *Cleveland Clinic Journal of Medicine, 69*(8), 594–608. Retrieved August, 2011, from http://www.ccjm.org/content/69/8/594.full.pdf+html

Doghramji, P. P. (2011). Managing you patient with gout: A review of treatment options. *Postgraduate Medicine, 123*, 56–71.

Dore, R. K. (2008). Gout: What primary care physicians want to know. *Journal of Clinical Rheumatology, 14*(5 Suppl), S47–S54.

Hayman, S., & Marcason, W. (2009). Gout: Is a purine-restricted diet still recommended? *Journal of the American Dietetic Association, 109*, 1652.

HealthyPeople2020. (2011). *Determinants of Health.* Retrieved August, 2011, from http://www.healthypeople.gov/2020/about/DOHAbout.aspx

Khoury, M. J. (2003). Genetics and genomics in practice: The continuum from genetic disease to genetic information in health and disease. *Genetics in Medicine, 5*(4), 261–268.

Khoury, M. J., Burke W., & Thomson E. J. (2000). *Genetics and public health in the 21st century: Using genetic information to improve health and prevent disease.* Oxford University Press, Inc.

Lawrence, R. C., Felson, D. T., Helmick, C. G., et al. (2008). Estimates of the prevalence of arthritis and other rheumatic conditions in the United States. Part II. *Arthritis and Rheumatism, 58*(1), 26–35.

Luk, A. J., & Simkin, P. A. (2005). Epidemiology of hyperuricemia and gout. *American Journal of Managed Care., 11*, (15 Suppl), S435–S442.

Mayo Clinic. (2011). *Gout Diet.* Retrieved August, 2011, from http://www.mayoclinic.com/health/gout-diet/MY01137

Merriman, T. R., & Dalbeth, N. (2011). The genetic basis of hyperuricaemia and gout. *Joint Bone Spine, 78*, 35–40.

Neogi, T. (2011). Gout. *New England Journal of Medicine, 364*, 443–452.

Nuki, G., & Simkin, P. A. (2006). A concise history of gout and hyperuricemia and their treatment.

Arthritis Research & Therapy, 8(Suppl 1), S1, Retrieved August, 2011, from http://arthritis-research.com/content/8/S1/S1.

OMIM. (2011). Available at www.ncbi.nlm.nih.gov/omim. Search this data base for: gout, statistics, and genes and disease. Accessed August 2011.

Parrish, R. G. (2010). Measuring population health outcomes. *Preventing Chronic Disease, 7*(4). Retrieved August, 2011, from http://www.cdc.gov/pcd/issues/2010/jul/10_0005.htm

Public Health Geneticist, retrieved August 22, 2012, from http://www.genome.gov/GenomicCareers/career.cfm?id=40

PubMed Health/Allopurinol. (2010). Retrieved August, 2011, from http://www.ncbi.nlm.nih.gov/pubmedhealth/PMH0000746/

PubMed Health/Fubuxostat. (2009). Retrieved August, 2011, from http://www.ncbi.nlm.nih.gov/pubmedhealth/PMH0000499/

PubMed Health/Probenecid. (2008). Retrieved August, 2011, from http://www.ncbi.nlm.nih.gov/pubmedhealth/PMH0000669/

Reach, G. (2011). Treatment adherence in patients with gout. *Joint Bone Spine 78*(5) 456–459. doi:10.1016/j.jbspin.2011.05.010

Richette, P., & Bardin, T. (2010). Gout. *Lancet, 375*, 318–328.

Terkeltaub, R. A., Edwards, N. L., & Wortmann, R. L. (2009). *FAQs in the modern management of gout CME/CE.* Retrieved August, 2011, from http://cme.medscape.com/viewarticle/705466

Voet, D., Voet, J. G., & Pratt, C. W. (Eds.). (2008). *Essentials of biochemistry* (3rd ed.). John Wiley & Sons, Inc., pp. 839–844.

Wheeless, C. R., III. (2011). *Wheeless' textbook of orthopedics.* Available at http://www.wheelessonline.com. Retrieved August, 2011, from http://www.wheelessonline.com/ortho/arthritis.

WHO. (1999). *Services for the prevention and management of genetic disorders and birth defects in developing countries.* Retrieved August, 2011, from http://whqlibdoc.who.int/hq/1999/WHO_HGN_GL_WAOPBD_99.1.pdf

WHO. (2011). *The determinants of health.* Retrieved August, 2011, from http://www.who.int/hia/evidence/doh/en/

Zhu, Y., Pandva, B. J., & Choi, H. K. (2011). Prevalence of gout and hyperuricemia in the US general population. *Arthritis & Rheumatism.* July 28. doi: 10.1002/art.30520

CHAPTER

18 Common Diseases with Genetic Linkages

Cindy L. Munro

LEARNING OUTCOMES

Following completion of this chapter, the learner will be able to

1. Describe the role of family history, race, and ethnicity as indicators of genetic factors in common diseases.
2. Discuss the interrelatedness of genetics, epigenetics, and environment on occurrence of common diseases.
3. Evaluate contributions of candidate gene studies and association studies (including genome-wide association studies) on understanding of genetic linkages to common diseases.
4. Relate pathophysiology of common diseases to genes associated with those diseases.
5. Explain implications for clinical practice of increased knowledge of genetic linkages to common diseases.

This chapter focuses on the relationship of genetics to common diseases. It defines common diseases (focusing on cardiovascular disease, Type 2 diabetes mellitus, and chronic pulmonary disease) and reviews the patterns that are clues indicating that a disease has a genetic component. It also examines how heritability varies among different diseases and within variations of the same disease. The interaction of genetics, epigenetics, and environment on etiology and development of disease are discussed. In addition, this chapter examines several examples of current understanding of genetics in common diseases as well as current and potential applications for health care.

PRETEST

1. Which disease consistently accounts for highest mortality in the United States?
   A. HIV infection
   B. Cardiovascular disease
   C. Diabetes mellitus
   D. Cancer
2. Family history can provide information about
   A. shared genetic risks for disease.
   B. shared environmental risks for disease.
   C. both shared genetic and environmental risks for disease.
3. Race is a very good indicator of an individual's genotype.
   A. True
   B. False
4. Candidate gene studies
   A. select a gene for study based on a hypothesis about the gene's role in a disease.
   B. do not require any prior knowledge about the gene.
   C. are done by examining large families.
   D. are no longer useful.
5. Most common diseases are
   A. monogenetic.
   B. polygenetic.
   C. epigenetic
   D. heritable
6. Epigenetic changes
   A. are always permanent.
   B. cannot be identified.
   C. modify DNA to turn genes on or off.
   D. All of the above
7. Most of the genetic linkages to Type 2 diabetes mellitus found in genome-wide association studies have involved genes associated with
   A. insulin resistance.
   B. obesity.
   C. glucose metabolism.
   D. development of pancreatic beta cells.
8. Which of the following common diseases can have a monogenetic cause?
   A. Type 2 diabetes mellitus
   B. Chronic Obstructive Pulmonary Disease
   C. Hyperlipidemia
   D. All of the above
9. In some cases, the same genes are associated with more than one common disease.
   A. True
   B. False

10. Better knowledge about genetic linkages to common diseases could improve care by
    A. identifying ethnic groups with specific disease-associated genes.
    B. improving the ability to tailor interventions.
    C. enabling providers to select which patients to treat.
    D. reducing costs for diagnostic tests.

Pretest answers are located in the Appendix.

SECTION ONE: Common Diseases: High Mortality, High Prevalence

What are common diseases? For this chapter, they are defined as health problems that have high mortality (leading causes of death) and high **prevalence** (many people have the disease). The chapter focuses on three of the most common disease types: cardiovascular disease (**CVD**), malignant neoplasms (cancers), and chronic lower respiratory diseases (including asthma and chronic obstructive pulmonary disease [**COPD**]). The top 10 causes of death in 2009 (the latest year for which the Centers for Disease Control and Prevention has compiled statistics) are presented in Table 18–1 (CDC, 2011). Forty-five percent of Americans live with one or more chronic conditions, with the most prevalent chronic diseases being cancer, diabetes, CVD (including heart disease, hypertension), mental disorders, pulmonary conditions, and stroke (cerebrovascular disease) (Partnership to Fight Chronic Disease, 2009).

In the United States, CVD has consistently been the leading cause of death since 1900 with the exception of 1918, when pandemic influenza caused more deaths. CVD is also very prevalent. It is estimated that one in three Americans have some form of CVD (Lloyd-Jones, 2010). Cardiovascular disease includes problems of the heart and blood vessels, such as coronary artery disease, hypertension (high blood pressure), and hyperlipidemia (elevation of cholesterol and blood lipids).

Diabetes mellitus is a disease that affects metabolism; it is most often thought of as a disease that involves blunting of the effect of insulin on carbohydrate metabolism (insulin resistance) or reduced production of insulin, resulting in elevated blood glucose levels and complications. Diabetes mellitus affects 8% of the U.S. population, but prevalence increases with age and an estimated 27% of adults over age 65 have diabetes (American Diabetes Association [ADA], 2011). While diabetes was the seventh leading cause of death in 2009, it was listed as a contributing factor in an additional 160,022 deaths according to death certificate data (CDC, 2011) (see Table 18–1). T2DM is the most prevalent form of diabetes.

TABLE 18–1: Leading Causes of Death in the United States (CDC, 2011)

Cause of Death*	Number of Deaths in 2009
Cardiovascular disease	599,413
Cancer	567,628
Chronic lower respiratory diseases	137,353
Cerebrovascular diseases	128,842
Unintentional injuries	118,021
Alzheimer disease	79,003
Diabetes	68,705
Influenza and pneumonia	53,692
Renal diseases	48,935
Septicemia	35,639

*Excludes intentional self-harm
Source: CDC, 2011

Two major disorders, asthma and chronic obstructive pulmonary disease (COPD), are the most prevalent forms of chronic pulmonary disease. Asthma is a chronic inflammatory pulmonary disease characterized by episodes of wheezing, coughing, and shortness of breath in response to triggers. Asthma affects 8.2% of adults and 9.4% of children in the United States (CDC, 2011). COPD, including chronic bronchitis and emphysema, affects 6.2% of adults in the United States and is characterized by airflow obstruction. Unlike asthma, in COPD the airflow obstruction is chronic, progressive, and not fully reversible.

Common diseases are most often defined by phenotype, where the disease phenotype is described by pathophysiologic changes or by a specific set of signs, symptoms, and diagnostic tests. In many instances, the definition of phenotypic characteristics for common diseases has been imprecise, and much variability may exist within a single disease classification. Disease definitions have changed significantly as improved diagnostic technologies permit earlier diagnosis of people with less overt signs and symptoms, and permit discrimination between phenotypes that are very similar. Deciphering the role of genetic factors in common diseases has been difficult because similar disease phenotypes may be associated with diverse underlying genetic factors; different genotypes can give rise to the same overall pathologic changes and disease manifestations.

In the past, knowledge of genetics was applied primarily to diseases with a clear Mendelian inheritance pattern—a generally straightforward analysis of dominant and recessive **traits** resulting from a single gene with defined implications for health. However, the application of genetics to clinical practice has expanded far beyond the traditional scope of single gene disorders. The occurrence and the severity of many common health problems are influenced by complex genetic interactions rather than single gene abnormalities, and the interactions among multiple genes and between genes and the environment in development of common diseases are much more complicated than originally envisioned.

Several factors have enabled new understanding of the importance of genetics in common health problems not traditionally thought of as genetic diseases. Perhaps most important was completion of the Human Genome Project. The research base for understanding the role of genetics in common diseases has been substantially advanced by the Human Genome Project. It provided information not only about the sequence of the human genome, but also about genomes of other organisms that are important as model systems in research. Knowledge of physiology, development, and pathophysiology in these model systems has been applied to improve understanding of human health as well. In addition, the Human Genome Project fostered the development of powerful analytic technologies that enabled the examination of multiple genes simultaneously and interactions among genes. Knowledge of the influence of genetics on common diseases and health has increased and continues to be uncovered.

Patterns of Occurrence Indicate Heritability

Many common diseases demonstrate patterns of occurrence that indicate heritability in risk of the disease as well as disease progression. Heritability is the proportion of observed variation in a particular trait that can be attributed to inherited genetic factors rather than environmental factors. One important clue to an underlying genetic influence in disease is a familial pattern of occurrence. Clinicians understand that family history is an important part of assessment. Diseases with a strong family history pattern are likely to have a genetic component because members of a family share a common genetic heritage, which may influence disease susceptibility. For CVD, a positive family history is an independent risk factor, which increases risk even when other risk factors such as hyperlipidemia and hypertension are considered. An early heart attack in either parent doubles the risk of a heart attack in men and increases the risk in women by about 70%, and having a sibling who has heart disease doubles the likelihood of heart disease in both men and women (Roger et al., 2011).

Race and ethnicity are commonly used to group people according to various factors. Ethnic groups are identified based on common culture or background. Racial groupings may be constructed based on ancestral background, visible characteristics, and social identity. Differences in prevalence of specific diseases may be based in part on shared genetic heritage of racial or ethnic groups because of shared ancestral background. These influences have been difficult to understand, because they occur in a complex context of social and environmental factors. The concepts of race and ethnicity are social constructs based on an individual's identity with a group, which may not be a true reflection of shared genetics and are not descriptive of an individual's genotype. People within any racial or ethnic group are heterogeneous, and variation within the group can be extensive. Groups vary widely from one another in how homogenous or heterogeneous their members are based on many factors. Traditions of permissibility of marriage outside the group can influence group homogeneity. Past political and geographic considerations can also affect heterogeneity. For example, African-American ancestry has been impacted by forced migrations and slavery. African-American ancestry is a genetic mixture of African, European, and Native American sources, and there is considerable variation within original African populations contributing further to African-American heterogeneity (Reiner et al., 2005; Stefflova et al., 2011; Yeager et al., 2008). African-American ancestry has been influenced by forced migrations related to slavery.

In examining the effect of family history, race, or ethnicity, the role of shared environmental and social factors must be considered as a potential explanation for shared disease risks as well. Despite these cautions, however, there are differences in disease prevalence for specific groups that do appear to be attributable at least in part to shared genetics. The high prevalence of T2DM in Pima Indians in the United States has been well documented and genetic predisposition is proposed as an important factor, although the importance of environment is demonstrated by the lower risk of T2DM in Pima Indians living in Mexico. In general, Hispanics and African-Americans also have higher prevalence of T2DM than Americans of European descent.

SECTION ONE REVIEW

1. Common diseases have
   A. high prevalence.
   B. high mortality.
   C. either high prevalence or high mortality.
   D. both high prevalence and high mortality.
2. Race and ethnicity
   A. predict an individual's genotype.
   B. reflect shared ancestry.
   C. can be defined genetically.
   D. are well-defined concepts.
3. The amount of variability within a racial or ethnic group may result from
   A. traditions within the group.
   B. geography.
   C. past political factors.
   D. All of the above
4. Technological advances resulting from the Human Genome Project have advanced the understanding of common diseases.
   A. True
   B. False
5. Which of the following is true?
   A. Strong family history is an important risk factor for CVD.
   B. Family history is less important in highly heritable diseases.
   C. Familial risks are determined only by shared genetics.
   D. Family history is not an independent risk factor for CVD, but indicates other problems like hypertension.

Answers: 1. C; 2. B; 3. D; 4. A; 5. A

SECTION TWO: Heritability of Common Diseases

The importance of genetic factors in disease occurrence or progression varies widely among different common diseases. This variation is reflected in different levels of risk associated with family history of common diseases. Positive family history increases risk of both heart attacks and T2DM. In both diseases, the parent's age when diagnosed influences the offspring's risk, with earlier age of onset conferring greater risk. Since early age of onset for disease can be an indicator of genetic etiology, this supports the heritability of CVD and T2DM. However, the strength and the specifics of risk related to family history differ between these two diseases. As noted in Section One, an early heart attack in either parent conveys a twofold risk of a heart attack in men. People who have one parent with early diagnosis of T2DM have a 3.5-fold increased risk of developing T2DM (Fletcher, Gulanick, & Lamendola, 2002). For heart attacks, risk associated with parental history does not appear to depend upon which parent is affected. In contrast, some data suggest that the risk of T2DM is greater if the diabetic parent is one's mother rather than one's father (ADA, 2011).

Heritability Varies Within Variations of the Same Disease

As discussed in Section One, diseases have traditionally been defined by phenotypes; for complex diseases, many different genotypes can result in similar phenotypes. T2DM is a good example of this concept. The diagnosis of T2DM is established by evidence of blood glucose levels exceeding established thresholds. However, T2DM is a complicated metabolic disease, with alterations not only in glucose utilization but also abnormalities in utilization of proteins and lipids.

The pathophysiology of T2DM involves two primary alterations, which ultimately result in diagnostic elevations of blood glucose: insulin resistance by peripheral cells (which is not present in Type 1 diabetes) and defective insulin secretion by pancreatic beta cells. Insulin resistance occurs when muscle, fat, and liver cells are unable to effectively use insulin; this may result from problems with the insulin receptor on the cell's surface, glucose transport, or mitochondrial abnormalities. More than 70 mutations affecting the insulin receptor, as well as other mutations affecting insulin secretion and utilization, have been identified in patients with T2DM. In addition to problems with the insulin receptor, many other genes may contribute to T2DM; these will be further explored in Section Three. Any of these changes can result in a phenotype of T2DM, and the mechanisms of precipitating factors (genetic and environmental) remain largely unexplained.

Interaction of Genetics, Epigenetics, and Environment on Etiology and Development of Disease

Although particular genotypes have been linked to common diseases, DNA sequence provides only partial information about risk and progression of disease. The environment plays a large role that influences not only gene expression, but also available lifestyle choices. Diet and physical activity both contribute to risk of CVD and T2DM, and are highly influenced by environment. American diets have increasingly become higher in calories and fat in part because of the availability and convenience of processed foods. Decreased activity levels may be related to increased availability of sedentary activities and decreased availability of safe and convenient places to walk or exercise.

The environment may also influence phenotype by serving as triggers for epigenetic changes in DNA. Epigenetic changes refer to activation and deactivation of genes without any change in the underlying DNA sequence of the organism. Epigenetic regulation of gene activity occurs through chemical modifications, such as methylation of DNA or histone proteins around which the DNA is wrapped. Epigenetic changes to DNA can occur within genes or in noncoding segments of DNA. These modifications can increase or decrease transcription of specific genes, resulting in more or less gene product (RNA or protein) and differences in phenotype. Environmental factors (such as diet) can serve as triggers for epigenetic changes. Epigenetics has been an important field of study in cancer, and recent evidence has emerged that epigenetic changes play a role in CVD (Shirodkar & Marsden, 2011), glycemic control, and complications in diabetes (Cooper & El-Osta, 2010), and other common diseases.

SECTION TWO REVIEW

1. Many genotypes can result in the same phenotype.
   A. True
   B. False
2. Heritability
   A. may vary within different types of a common disease.
   B. is constant within a particular disease.
   C. is important in monogenetic forms of disease, but not in polygenetic forms.
   D. has primarily determined by factors of race and ethnicity.
3. The environment may influence risk and progression of common diseases by
   A. affecting lifestyle choices.
   B. influencing epigenetic changes in DNA.
   C. having direct effects on DNA.
   D. All of the above
4. Epigenetic modifications
   A. upregulate gene transcription.
   B. downregulate gene transcription.
   C. may either upregulate or downregulate gene transcription.
   D. do not have a direct effect on genetic regulation.
5. Epigenetic changes can occur outside of the coding sequence of a gene.
   A. True
   B. False

Answers: 1. A; 2. A; 3. D; 4. C; 5. A

SECTION THREE: Understanding Selected Complex Common Diseases

Two approaches have been used to identify genes involved in common diseases and to estimate the contribution of specific genes to disease risk. In the first approach, candidate genes are selected for study based on a connection between the gene's function and the hypothesized pathophysiology of the disease. The candidate gene approach has provided insight into the role of selected individual genes in common diseases, but it is generally limited to examination of one gene at a time and has been most useful in rarer monogenetic forms of a disease (for example, COPD due to alpha1-antitrypsin deficiency). The candidate gene approach has been less helpful in understanding the relationships among multiple genes, the environment, and epigenetic factors involved in more prevalent polygenetic forms of common diseases. In the second approach, genetic loci linked to common diseases are identified using association studies by comparing genetic similarities of those with and without disease. This approach is more likely to uncover genes that were not previously suspected to be involved in a particular disease, and newer methods permit examination of epigenetic factors as well. Methods such as linkage analysis, case control studies, and genome-wide association studies (GWAS) are useful ways to find genetic loci involved in risk without targeting a specific gene in advance. GWAS identify variations in small areas of genetic sequence through examination of single nucleotide polymorphisms (SNPs); SNPs may be found in genes or in noncoding DNA. GWAS are a relatively new approach to discovering genes involved in common diseases, with the first GWAS results published in 2007. Association studies may yield potential candidate genes, which can then be confirmed in candidate gene studies.

Diabetes

The importance of a genetic contribution to T2DM is demonstrated by the high risk conferred by family history. Recently, genetic risk for diabetes and its complications has been studied by linkage analysis, meta-analysis, case-control studies, and GWAS. While several genes have been linked to increased risk, variations in these genes occur frequently and the amount of risk conferred by any single gene is very small. It is estimated that together, all of the known diabetes risk genes account for only about 10% of heritable disease risk (Hirschhorn & Gajdos, 2011; Herder & Roden, 2010). This is congruent with the polygenetic nature of T2DM, where the total effect is the result of the interaction among many genes, environment, and epigenetics.

Multiple GWAS to date have linked 40 genes to increased risk for diabetes (McCarthy, 2010; Herder & Roden, 2010; Hirschhorn & Gajdos, 2011). Herder and Roden (2010) summarized available GWAS related to T2DM and concluded that most of the genes identified have roles in the development of beta cells and the pancreas or pancreatic function. Surprisingly, GWAS has uncovered relatively few genes linked to underlying T2DM pathophysiology (insulin resistance, obesity, or glucose metabolism).

Three examples of genes that have been linked to increased risk of development of diabetes (*TCF7L2*, *PPARγ2*, and *Kir6.2*) illustrate the relationships between genes that have been identified by GWAS and pathophysiology. Transcription factor 7–like 2 (encoded by *TCF7L2*) regulates beta cell function. The product of *PPARγ2*, Peroxisome Proliferator-Activated Receptor–γ, is a protein located in the cell nucleus that is important in regulating lipid and glucose metabolism. The *Kir6.2* protein is one subunit of a potassium channel on the membrane of pancreatic beta cells; interestingly, the other subunit of the potassium channel is where sulfonylureas bind to increase insulin production. In each of these examples, the connection between the gene and potential mechanisms underlying T2DM appears clear. In other instances, GWAS have linked T2DM risk to genes with more global activity, such as genes regulating the cell cycle and genes involved in the inflammatory response.

Investigation of epigenetics in T2DM is just beginning. Hyperglycemia appears to act as a trigger for epigenetic changes (Cooper & El-Osta, 2011). The hypothesis that epigenetic changes may be involved in the development of T2DM or in the progression of diabetic complications is intriguing, but to date little supporting evidence is available.

Cardiovascular Disease

The relationship of genetics to CVD has focused in two areas. One focus has been exploration of the influence of genetic factors on risk factors, such as hyperlipidemia and hypertension, that are thought to contribute to the underlying pathophysiology of CVD. Another focus has been on examination of genetic factors related to specific cardiovascular events such as coronary artery disease or myocardial infarction. Candidate gene studies have been useful in determining genetic risks in subsets of CVD such as monogenetic hyperlipidemias. Association studies, including several GWAS, have been conducted. As in diabetes, the effect size of any given factor identified through GWAS has been small.

Risk Factor: Hyperlipidemia

Hyperlipidemia (elevation of blood lipids and cholesterol) is one of five major modifiable risk factors for CVD; the other modifiable risk factors are smoking/tobacco use, physical inactivity, overweight/obesity, and diabetes mellitus (Lloyd-Jones et al., 2009). Low density lipoprotein-cholesterol (LDL cholesterol) is known to be associated with CVD; each 1% decrease in LDL cholesterol concentrations reduces the risk of coronary heart disease by an estimated 1%. While several types of monogenetic hyperlipidemias have been described, the condition more often results from a complex relationship that likely involves many genes, environmental factors, and epigenetic regulation. Alterations in the LDL receptor (*LDLR*), apolipoprotein B (*APOB* genes) and apolipoprotein E (*APOE* genes) can result in dramatic elevations in cholesterol levels and increased incidence of coronary artery disease. Four genes, *PPP1R3B*, *SORT1*, *TTC39B*, and *GALNT2*, have been of particular interest in hyperlipidemia research because of their identified roles in regulating cholesterol levels (Hirschhorn & Gajdos, 2011). Recently, more than 100 genetic loci have been linked to hyperlipidemia by GWAS. The effect of each individual locus is small, but it is estimated that together these loci may account for 25%–30% of the variation in lipid levels (Hirschhorn & Gajdos, 2011). In a recent meta-analysis of three GWAS, 11 of the variants that were linked to increased LDL cholesterol levels were also associated with increased risk for coronary artery disease. In multiple GWAS, *SORT1* is associated not only with elevated LDL levels, but also with coronary artery disease and myocardial infarction. Conversely, an *LDLR* variant was associated with decreased low density lipoprotein cholesterol (LDL-cholesterol) levels and also with a reduced risk of coronary artery disease (Relton & Smith, 2010).

Risk Factor: Hypertension

Hypertension (elevated systolic or diastolic blood pressure) is another important risk factor for CVD. It is prevalent in the United States: Approximately 22% of white Americans and 32% of African-Americans have hypertension (Lloyd-Jones et al., 2008). Hypertension has been the focus of a great deal of physiological research aimed at understanding the regulation of blood pressure by the renin-angiotensin-aldosterone system and corticoid hormones. Candidate gene studies targeted elements of the pathways of blood pressure control discovered in previous physiological research. Using this approach, genes involved with the renin-angiotensin-aldosterone system, genes encoding enzymes and receptors of the mineralo- and glucocorticoid pathways, and genes involved in the structure and/or regulation of vascular tone (endothelins and their receptors) were identified as important contributors to some familial forms of hypertension (Butler, 2010). However, these genes did not appear to be determinants of essential hypertension, which is the most prevalent form and appears to be polygenetic. GWAS studies of hypertension have provided intriguing information; of 14 genetic loci with an association to hypertension, only two (*CYP17A1* and *MTHFR*) were previously identified in candidate gene studies (Ehret, 2010). The other 12 genetic loci had not been previously linked to hypertension. Further examination of these may lead to better understanding of mechanisms underlying the disease.

Cardiovascular Events

Recently, GWAS have been used to examine the importance of specific genetic factors in the occurrence of cardiovascular events rather than on risks contributing to those events. Myocardial infarction is a good example of a discrete event that can be used to define coronary artery disease, and the association of genetics to heart attack has been the focus of several GWAS (Arking & Chakravarti, 2009). While several genetic loci have been linked to coronary artery disease, specific candidate genes have not been confirmed and interpretation is not yet entirely clear. An early study identified genes related to autoimmunity and inflammation as "MI susceptibility genes" (*LTA*, lymphotoxin-A; *LGALS2*, galectin-2; and *BRAP*, *BRCA1*-associated protein). More recently, an interesting locus at 9p21 has been associated with increased risk for coronary artery disease in people of European ancestry. There are two genes in this region (*CDKN2A* and *CDKN2B*), which are known to be important in cell proliferation but had not been previously linked to CVD.

Pulmonary Disease

Asthma and COPD are common chronic pulmonary diseases. While there are examples of monogenetic causes for chronic pulmonary disease (such as alpha1-antitrypsin deficiency as a cause of COPD), in most cases risk of disease and progression are likely to involve multiple genes and epigenetic factors interacting with environmental stimuli. Disease occurrence and progression are highly dependent on environmental exposures. In the United States, exposure to tobacco smoke is a major contributor to development of COPD, and 90% of patients with COPD have a history of exposure to smoke. Tobacco smoke increases severity of both COPD and asthma. However, similar exposures do not lead to disease in all individuals. Not every cigarette smoker develops COPD (only about 10% do), and not every child exposed to the same environmental triggers develops asthma. Genetic susceptibility to these common diseases is an active area of investigation, recently reviewed by several authors (Boezen, 2009; March, Sleiman, & Hakonarson, 2011; Weiss, 2010).

Asthma

Asthma is a chronic inflammatory pulmonary disease characterized by episodes of wheezing, coughing, and shortness of breath in response to triggers. Two underlying problems in asthma are reversible airflow obstruction and airway hyperresponsiveness. More than 100 genes have been examined in candidate gene studies focused on asthma. March, Sleiman, and Hakonarson (2011) categorized the genes linked to asthma into four broad categories: barrier function of epithelial cells, environmental sensing and immune detection, tissue response, and polarization and response of T helper (TH2) cells. Specific genes linked to asthma susceptibility include many related to immune function, such as cytokine genes on chromosome 5q and toll-like receptor genes. Other genes of interest are those involved in airway responsiveness, including *ADAM33* and *PDE4D*. *ADAM33* and *PDE4D* (phosphodiesterase 4D) are each involved in airway smooth muscle response and airway contractility. An entire class of asthma medications used in treating bronchoconstriction (including aminophylline and others) are *PDE4* inhibitors (Boezen, 2009).

Additional asthma susceptibility genes have been suggested by GWAS. As with T2DM and CVD, GWAS analyses have confirmed some genes already linked to asthma (such as *PDE4*), and suggested linkage of novel genes. GWAS linked a variant of *IL1RL1* (interleukin 1 receptor-like 1) to asthma. This receptor is thought to be involved in inflammation and in T helper cell (TH2) function, and these activities fit well with current understanding of asthma pathophysiology. A region on chromosome 17q21 has been linked to asthma susceptibility; *ORMDL3* (encoding a transmembrane protein linked to childhood asthma) and *GSDML* (involved in programmed cell death, or apoptosis) are found in this region.

COPD

COPD is a disease characterized by airflow obstruction, but unlike asthma, in COPD the airflow obstruction is chronic, progressive, and not fully reversible. An abnormal inflammatory pulmonary response to environmental particles or gases, damage to lung tissues from oxidative stress, and imbalances between protease and antiprotease in lung tissues are all part of the pathophysiology of COPD.

Alpha1-antitrypsin deficiency is the only known monogenetic cause of COPD, has an autosomal recessive pattern of inheritance, and accounts for 1% of all COPD cases. Alpha1-antitrypsin inhibits neutrophil elastase in the lung; without inhibition, neutrophil elastase breaks down lung tissues. Alpha1-antitrypsin is encoded by *SERPINA1*. Individuals who are homozygous for the disease allele may develop COPD at an early age even if they never smoke. Heterozygotes are at higher risk for COPD and are particularly at risk if exposed to smoke or pollutants.

In almost all cases, COPD susceptibility, development, and progression are multifactorial. Both single candidate gene studies and GWAS have yielded insights into polygenetic forms of COPD. Some of the earliest candidate gene studies in COPD examined *MMP12* (matrix metalloproteinase 12). *MMP12* affects susceptibility to COPD in individuals exposed to tobacco smoke, with one variant is associated with reduced risk of COPD in smokers. Mice genetically modified to be lacking the gene (*MMP12* knockout mice) are more susceptible to tobacco smoke damage. A gene important in lung development, *serpin E2*, has also been identified as linked to COPD. GWAS have identified 11 novel loci that had not been identified in candidate gene studies. The *CHRNA 3/5* locus (a nicotinic acetylcholine receptor) was known to affect risk for nicotine dependence and lung cancer; it has also been identified as a genetic risk factor for COPD (Boezen, 2009).

Emerging Evidence

- Epigenetic changes play a role in CVD (Shirodkar & Marsden, 2011), as well as glycemic control and complications in diabetes (Cooper & El-Osta, 2010).
- Epigenetic changes that alter gene expression may be started by hyperglycemia, which appears to act as a trigger for epigenetic changes (Cooper & El-Osta, 2011).
- Genome-wide association studies have linked 40 genes to increased risk for diabetes and more than 100 genetic loci to hyperlipidemia (McCarthy, 2010; Herder & Roden, 2010; Hirschhorn & Gajdos, 2011).

Overlap of Genetic Linkages to More than One Disease

In several instances, the same genetic loci have been linked to more than one disease. For example, a SNP variation in *MMP12* associated with a reduced risk of COPD in adult smokers also was linked with a positive effect on lung function in children with asthma. There is overlap among genetic loci linked to risks for T2DM, CVD, and obesity as well. In some instances, the overlaps may be indicative of a shared underlying mechanism for different phenotypes that we view as different diseases. An example of this idea is the "Dutch hypothesis" (proposed by several Dutch pulmonary researchers over the past decades). This is the premise that asthma and COPD are different manifestations of the same underlying pulmonary disease, with presentation influenced by host genetics and environment. It is possible that better knowledge of genetic risks may improve recognition of common mechanisms for common diseases. Alternatively, although the same **genetic locus** may be linked to more than one disease, the specific variants associated with individual diseases may be different. Hirschorn and Gajdos (2011) suggest that these differences may be related to different regulatory effects on genes linked to multiple diseases.

SECTION THREE REVIEW

1. Genes that were not previously suspected to be involved in a particular disease are more likely to be discovered by
   A. candidate gene studies.
   B. association studies.
   C. linkage and meta-analysis.
   D. case-control studies.
2. Candidate genes have been identified in all of the following EXCEPT
   A. hypertension.
   B. hyperlipidemia.
   C. coronary artery disease.
   D. COPD
3. A monogenetic form of COPD is linked to which gene?
   A. *MMP 12*
   B. *SERPINA1*
   C. *CHRNA 3/5*
   D. Any of these genes can cause monogenetic COPD.
4. When the same genetic loci are linked to more than one common disease, it may indicate that
   A. there is an underlying mechanism shared by the diseases.
   B. different variants of the same gene may be important in different diseases.
   C. Both A and B are true.
   D. Neither A nor B are true.

Answers: 1. B; 2. C; 3. B; 4. C

SECTION FOUR: Implications for Health Care

Increased information about genetic linkages may alter our conception of pathophysiology underlying common diseases. Already completed GWAS have expanded candidate genes for risk of CVD, T2DM, and pulmonary diseases; in many cases, the genetic loci linked to these common diseases were previously unsuspected and may suggest new pathways or determinants of disease development. As more instances of shared linkages among diseases are uncovered, pleiotropic mechanisms for risk and disease treatment may emerge. Shared genetic risks among common diseases might also be due to global epigenetic factors, linking genetic susceptibility to environmental factors.

Expansion beyond examination of individual genes to the exploration of gene networks and the interaction of those networks with the environment will further deepen understanding of pathophysiology and lead to better risk prediction, treatments, and prevention strategies (Weiss, 2010).

Diagnostic Implications

In monogenetic forms of common diseases, genetic testing is feasible. For example, alpha1-antitrypsin deficiency can be detected by genotyping of *SERPINA1*. However, monogenetic linkages account for a minority of common disease cases. In most polygenetic diseases, individual genotyping is not currently clinically useful. Although associations between multiple genetic loci have been linked to common diseases, these data are best understood as population data, and predictive value for individuals is very small. Common diseases usually result from a complex interplay of multiple genes and environmental factors that decreases the predictive value of individual genetic testing (Janssens & van Duijn, 2010).

Genetic testing has not yet demonstrated any additional predictive value when added to well-validated risk calculators for common diseases such as the Framingham tools (Framingham Heart Study, 2011). This may be due to the current focus on genes for well-known risk factors where the phenotype already can be easily measured. As an example, adding assessment of genes related to cholesterol, triglycerides, and blood pressure is unlikely to improve the predictive ability of CVD risk tools that already incorporate clinical values of cholesterol, triglycerides, and blood pressure. In the future, as more loci are linked to common diseases and their contributions to risk are documented, evaluation of novel genetic markers may improve risk assessment and diagnosis (Humphries, Yiannakouris, & Talmud, 2008).

Epigenetics may play a role in risk assessment and diagnosis as the science develops (Relton & Smith, 2010). The influence of the environment is critical in many common diseases, and epigenetics may provide predictive models of the interaction of susceptibility genes with environmental factors.

Technical advances may improve diagnostic precision and enhance the role of genetic analysis in common diseases. Whole genome sequencing, which determines every base pair in an individual's genome, is not yet clinically or economically feasible. When it does become widely available, direct testing for a wide catalogue of DNA variations can expand to include additional rare variants of susceptibility genes, copy number variations, and structural variations (Janssens & van Duijn, 2010).

Novel Treatments

There are intriguing hints that better information about genetic linkages to common diseases will improve treatment option for patients. Genotyping could be useful in identifying patients who are more likely to respond well (or poorly) to specific interventions, or in predicting side effects. As an example, variations in *TCF7L2* genotype predict response to sulfonylurea medications in patients with T2DM, although the effect is not large enough to guide treatment decisions (McCarthy, 2010). Multiple susceptibility genes might be combined into treatment profiles with sufficient power to inform clinical decision making. Both patients and health care providers appear receptive to incorporating genetic information into treatment plans. In a survey of T2DM patients and physicians, both groups believed that genetic test results would significantly impact patient motivation in lifestyle modification and in medication adherence (Grant et al., 2009). The survey authors speculated that personal genetic information may be uniquely powerful in changing patient behavior.

Epigenetics is a potential target for novel treatments for common diseases. Some cancer treatments are directed at epigenetic modifications. Azacytidine and decitabine are DNA methyltransferase inhibitors, thought to exert a therapeutic effect by reactivating tumor suppressor genes that have been inactivated by hypermethylation in cancer cells (Stresemann & Lyko, 2008). Caution is necessary. The utility of interventions directed at epigenetic changes in common diseases will depend on how important those changes are to disease occurrence and progression. Epigenetic changes might directly contribute to disease, and in that case would be important targets for intervention. However, if epigenetic changes are instead a reflection of an underlying cause of disease, then altering the epigenetics would not necessarily change the disease process (Relton & Smith, 2010). Epigenetic variations have not yet been linked to specific disease phenotypes.

Prevention

Better understanding of genetic linkages to common disease could lead to earlier and more targeted disease prevention efforts. These efforts may be directed at individuals or at larger populations identified as at risk because of shared ancestry. In many cases, the modifiable risk factors for common diseases are already part of clinical practice, but many recommendations are generic. Enhanced information about genetic susceptibilities could lead to more tailored interventions designed to focus on those risk factors most critical for particular individuals or groups.

SECTION FOUR REVIEW

1. Genetic testing is most feasible for __________ forms of common diseases.
   A. monogenetic
   B. polygenetic
2. Patients are expected to be highly resistant to incorporating genetic risk factors into clinical practice.
   A. True
   B. False
3. An example of an application of epigenetics in therapy is
   A. using *TCF7L2* genotype to predict response to sulfonylurea medications.
   B. adding genes for cholesterol metabolism to CVD risk calculators.
   C. using DNA methyltransferase inhibitors to treat cancer.
   D. All of the above

Answers: 1. A; 2. B; 3. C

POSTTEST

1. Which of the following suggest that genetic linkages are important in common diseases?
   A. There is phenotypic variation within common diseases.
   B. Prevalence of disease does not differ among racial or ethnic groups.
   C. Family history is a strong risk factor.
   D. No candidate genes have been identified.
2. GWAS are a form of
   A. candidate gene studies.
   B. association studies.
   C. novel genetic studies.
   D. linkage analysis.
3. Candidate gene studies
   A. are best suited to identifying novel genetic associations with a disease.
   B. can only be conducted following GWAS.
   C. test hypotheses about the involvement of specific genes in a disease.
   D. can only be done in humans.
4. Having a sibling who suffered from an early heart attack increases the risk of heart attack by
   A. Twofold.
   B. Fourfold.
   C. Tenfold.
   D. The risk is only increased if one's parent had a heart attack also.
5. Monogenetic forms of common diseases are __________ common than polygenetic forms.
   A. less
   B. more
   C. equally
6. Current well-developed risk calculators for common diseases already incorporate genetic testing into risk calculations.
   A. True
   B. False
7. Epigenetic changes
   A. may be influenced by environmental factors.
   B. may directly influence disease occurrence and progression.
   C. may reflect factors causing disease.
   D. All of the above
8. Testing for genotype is most feasible in __________ forms of common diseases.
   A. monogenetic
   B. polygenetic
9. In most cases, risk for common diseases is
   A. inherited in a Mendellian pattern.
   B. increased by genetic susceptibility.
   C. not associated with environmental factors.
   D. unpredictable.
10. Whole genome sequencing of individuals may enable
   A. detection of rare genetic variants in individuals.
   B. determination of epigenetic influences.
   C. refinement in racial and ethnic groupings.
   D. examination of the influences of environment on genetics.

Posttest answers are located in the Appendix.

CHAPTER SUMMARY

Common diseases often have complex etiologies that involve multiple genes, interaction with environmental factors, and epigenetic regulation. Information about genetic linkages important to common diseases is beginning to emerge, and has been fueled by recent GWAS studies. The potential benefit to clinical care is large, but much work remains before information about polygenetic and epigenetic risks can be used to guide care of individuals or groups of patients.

- Common diseases often demonstrate heritability, but are not usually monogenetic.
- Heritability differs among different diseases, and within variations of the same disease.
- Many genotypes can result in the same phenotype.
- The phenotype is determined not only by underlying genotype, but by epigenetics and environmental influences.
- Candidate gene studies are useful in examining the role of genes hypothesized to be involved in a disease.
- Association studies, such as GWAS, are useful in identifying novel genetic loci associated with a disease.
- Genetic linkages have been demonstrated for common forms of CVD, T2DM, and chronic pulmonary disease.
- Better knowledge of genetic linkages to common diseases has potential for improving understanding of pathophysiology, and in the diagnosis, treatment, and prevention of common diseases.

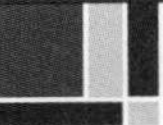

CRITICAL THINKING CHECKPOINT

How might knowledge about genetic linkages to a common disease change nursing interventions for patients with that disease?

ONLINE RESOURCES

American Diabetes Association: http://www.diabetes.org

American Lung Association: http://www.lungusa.org

American Heart Association: http://www.heart.org/HEARTORG/

GeneTests: http://www.ncbi.nlm.nih.gov/sites/GeneTests/?db=GeneTests

Talking Glossary of Genetic Terms: http://www.genome.gov/Glossary/

REFERENCES

American Diabetes Association. (2011). *Genetics of diabetes*. Retrieved July 20, 2012, from http://www.diabetes.org/diabetes-basics/genetics-of-diabetes.html

Arking, D. E., & Chakravarti, A. (2009). Understanding cardiovascular disease through the lens of genome-wide association studies. *Trends in Genetics, 25,* 387–394.

Boezen, H. M. (2009). Genome-wide association studies: What do they teach us about asthma and chronic obstructive pulmonary disease? *Proceedings of the American Thoracic Society, 6,* 701–703.

Butler, M. G. (2010). Genetics of hypertension: Current status. *The Lebanese Medical Journal, 58,* 175–178.

Center for Disease Control and Prevention (CDC). (2011). *Deaths and Mortality*. Retrieved July 20, 2012, from http://www.cdc.gov/nchs/fastats/deaths.htm

Cooper, M. E., & El-Osta, A. (2010) Epigenetics: Mechanisms and implications for diabetic complications. *Circulation Research, 107,* 1403–1413.

Ehret, G. B. (2010). Genome-wide association studies: Contribution of genomics to understanding blood pressure and essential hypertension. *Current Hypertension Reports, 12,* 17–25.

Fletcher, B., Gulanick, M., & Lamendola, C. (2002). Risk factors for type 2 diabetes mellitus. *Journal of Cardiovascular Nursing, 16,* 17–23.

Framingham Heart Study. (2011). *Framingham Study Risk Score Profiles*. Retrieved July 20, 2012, from http://www.framinghamheartstudy.org/risk/index.html

Grant, R. W., Hivert, M., Pandiscio, J. C., Florez, J. C., Nathan, D. M., & Meigs, J. B. (2009). The clinical application of genetic testing in type 2 diabetes: A patient and physician survey. *Diabetologia, 52,* 2299–2305.

Herder, C., & Roden, M. (2010). Genetics of type 2 diabetes: Pathophysiologic and clinical relevance. *European Journal of Clinical Investigation,* [Epub ahead of print] PubMed PMID: 21198561

Hirschhorn, J. N., & Gajdos, Z. K. (2011). Genome-wide association studies: Results from the first few years and potential implications for clinical medicine. *Annual Review of Medicine, 62,* 11–24.

Humphries, S. E., Yiannakouris, N., & Talmud, P. J. (2008). Cardiovascular disease risk prediction using genetic information (gene scores): Is it really informative? *Current Opinions in Lipidology, 19,* 128–132.

Janssens, A. C., & van Duijn, C. M. (2010). An epidemiological perspective on the future of direct-to-consumer personal genome testing. *Investigative Genetics, 1,* 10.

Lloyd-Jones, D., Adams, R., Carnethon, M., De Simone, G., Ferguson, T. B., Flegal, K., et al. (2009). Heart disease and stroke statistics—2009 update: A report from the American Heart Association Statistics Committee and Stroke Statistics Subcommittee. *Circulation, 119,* 480–486.

March, M. E., Sleiman, P. M., & Hakonarson, H. (2011). The genetics of asthma and allergic disorders. *Discovery Medicine, 11*(56), 35–45.

McCarthy, M. I. (2010). Genomics, type 2 diabetes, and obesity. *New England Journal of Medicine, 363,* 2339–2350.

Partnership to Fight Chronic Disease. (2009). Retrieved July 20, 2012, from http://www.fightchronicdisease.org

Reiner, A. P., Ziv, E., Lind, D. L., Nievergelt, C. M., Schork, N. J., Cummings, S. R., et al. (2005). Population structure, admixture, and aging-related phenotypes in African American adults: The Cardiovascular Health Study. *American Journal of Human Genetics, 76,* 463–477.

Relton, C. L., & Davey Smith, G. (2010). Epigenetic epidemiology of common complex disease: Prospects for prediction, prevention, and treatment. *PLoS Medicine, 7,* e1000356. doi:10.1371/journal.pmed.1000356

Roger, V. L., Go, A. S., Lloyd-Jones, D. M., Adams, R. J., Berry, J. D., Brown, T. M., et al. (2011). American Heart Association Statistics Committee and Stroke Statistics Subcommittee. Heart disease and stroke statistics—2011 update: A report from the American Heart Association. *Circulation, 123*(4), e18–e209.

Shirodkar, A. V., & Marsden, P. A. (2011). Epigenetics in cardiovascular disease. *Current Opinions in Cardiology, 26,* 209–215.

Stefflova, K., Dulik, M. C., Barnholtz-Sloan, J. S., Pai, A. A., Walker, A. H., & Rebbeck, T. R. (2011). Dissecting the within-Africa ancestry of populations of African descent in the Americas. *PLoS One, 6,* e14495.

Stresemann, C., & Lyko, F. (2008). Modes of action of the DNA methyltransferase inhibitors azacytidine and decitabine. *International Journal of Cancer, 123,* 8–13.

Weiss, S. T. (2010). What genes tell us about the pathogenesis of asthma and chronic obstructive pulmonary disease. *American Journal of Respiratory and Critical Care Medicine, 181,* 1170–1173.

Yaeger, R., Avila-Bront, A., Abdul, K., Nolan, P. C., Grann, V. R., Birchette, M. G., et al. (2008). Comparing genetic ancestry and self-described race in African Americans born in the United States and in Africa. *Cancer Epidemiology, Biomarkers & Prevention, 17,* 1329–1338.

PART 7

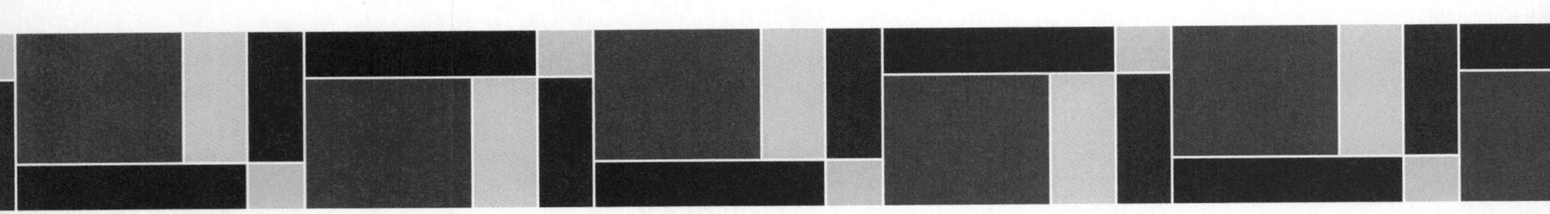

Psychiatric Disorders

CHAPTER

19 Bipolar Disorder and Genetic Linkages

Matthew Sorenson

LEARNING OUTCOMES

Following the completion of this chapter, the learner will be able to

1. Describe the relationship between genetic variables and the symptoms of bipolar disorder.
2. Discuss how genetic variation in circadian rhythm relates to bipolar disorder.
3. Identify the means by which genetic variables influence pharmacologic approaches to the treatment of bipolar disorder.
4. State the role of nursing in providing evidence-based care to individuals with bipolar disorder.

This chapter reviews the connections between genetic variables and bipolar disorder. It provides an overview of bipolar disorder and its characteristics, and reviews the findings from linkage and association studies in relation to bipolar disorder. This chapter also discusses genetic ties with mania, a characteristic symptom of bipolar disorder, and explores how genetic influences can affect mood changes and cycling. In addition, this chapter examines the interaction between pharmacologic therapies for bipolar disorder and genetic pathways and discusses implications for nursing in terms of assessment and intervention.

PRETEST

1. Bipolar disorder is best described as a condition marked by
   A. sustained elevation of mood mixed with periods of depression.
   B. periods of depression that alternate with periods of normal mood.
   C. sustained depression of mood.
   D. social isolation and avoidance of risk taking.
2. Bipolar disorder is thought to be inherited.
   A. True
   B. False
3. The chief symptom of bipolar disorder is mania. This elevation of mood is most likely the result of dysregulation of
   A. cortisol.
   B. *NR3C1*.
   C. the *CLOCK* gene.
   D. sirtuin 3.
4. The circadian cycle is involved in the regulation of
   A. appetite and risk-taking behavior.
   B. sickness behavior.
   C. sleep and alertness.
   D. spatial relations and proprioception.
5. The nurse needs to assess the patient with bipolar disorder for
   A. increased risk taking and participation in pleasurable activities.
   B. decreased risk taking and social exploration.
   C. decreased sleep and increased energy.
   D. increased sleep and decreased appetite.
6. The pharmacologic agents given for the treatment of bipolar disorder, particularly lithium, influence genetic mechanisms through
   A. lengthening of the circadian cycle.
   B. shortening of the circadian cycle.
   C. increasing expression of the *CLOCK* gene.
   D. decreasing expression of the *CLOCK* gene.
7. The *CLOCK* gene is believed to play a role in bipolar disorder through
   A. effects on cortisol secretion.
   B. suppression of cortisol secretion.
   C. prolongation of the circadian rhythm.
   D. shortening of the circadian rhythm.

8. The main catecholamines of interest in those with bipolar disorder are
   A. dopamine and serotonin.
   B. dopamine and cortisol.
   C. dopamine and epinephrine.
   D. dopamine and prolactin.
9. The primary genetic mechanism underlying the effectiveness of pharmacologic agents in the treatment of bipolar disorder is
   A. regulation of histone acetyltransferases.
   B. regulation of histone deacetylases.
   C. regulation of prolactin.
   D. regulation of cortisol.
10. Hyperthymia is a term that best refers to
   A. disrupted thermoregulation.
   B. a sustained low-level mania.
   C. a low level of depression.
   D. a sustained major depression.

Pretest answers are located in the Appendix.

SECTION ONE: Bipolar Disorder

Bipolar disorder is a condition that involves a dysregulation of mood characterized by periods of varying degrees of mania alternating with periods of depression. There are various forms of the disorder, and it may be more appropriate to consider it as a spectrum of several conditions reflecting varying degrees of mania and depression. This diagnostic spectrum encompasses Bipolar I and II, cyclothymic disorder, manic episode, hypomanic episode, and dysthymia. Bipolar disorder is considered one of the most common disorders of mood, with an adult prevalence of up to 2.6% in the United States. Out of those with the disorder in the U.S., approximately 83% are considered to have symptoms that would be classified as severe enough to interfere with daily function (Kessler, Chiu, Demler, Merikangas, & Walters, 2005). Throughout this chapter it is important to maintain awareness that the identification and diagnosis of psychiatric conditions such as bipolar disorder is dependent upon patterns of behavior and the appearance of certain symptoms. There are no pathophysiologic findings that can lead to identification of bipolar disorder.

Bipolar Disorders: Definitions and Criteria

The term *bipolar* reflects the manner in which mood can alternate between two poles: **depression** and **mania**. The various diagnostic categories reflect the degree of mania and duration of symptoms. In Bipolar I Disorder, there has been a clinical course characterized by the presence of one or more manic episodes that may alternate with episodes of major depression. The individual may also display symptoms of psychosis. Psychotic symptomatology manifests as either delusional thinking or the experience of hallucinations. There may also be the presence of a mixed episode during which the individual meets the diagnostic criteria for both **major depression** and mania during the course of one week. In Bipolar II Disorder, the clinical course is characterized by the presence of episodes of major depression along with at least one episode of hypomania. Hypomania is best viewed as a less acute form of mania. Psychosis is not seen in those with Bipolar II Disorder. Cyclothymic disorder can be viewed as a less intense and sustained form of bipolar disorder that lasts for a period of at least 2 years. In that condition, the individual experiences periods of hypomania and depressive symptoms not meeting the diagnostic criteria for major depression. **Dysthymia** is a chronic period of depression that lasts for at least 1 year (American Psychological Association, 2000). A related term is **hyperthymia**, which is not a diagnosable condition but refers to a personality type considered prone to periods of mildly elevated mood or hypomania (Matorin and Ruiz, 2009).

The Nature of Mania

Mania is defined as persistent mood elevation for at least 1 week. This elevation of mood may appear as expansive or irritable, and is characterized by a cluster of symptoms that can include reduced sleep, excessive talking, inflated self-esteem, a feeling of thoughts racing or of many thoughts flitting through the mind, and an increase in either restlessness or goal-directed behaviors. During periods of mania, the individual will often increase participation in pleasurable activities that could result in adverse consequences. This can include risk-taking behaviors, or participation in normal social activities such as shopping to an extreme level, to the point where the individual may place themselves at financial risk due to excessive purchases. All in all, the mood elevation must cause a degree of disruption in social or occupational settings in order to be diagnosed as mania. The term *hypomania* is used to describe elevations of mood that do not interfere with daily function or are of shorter duration (American Psychological Association, 2000).

SECTION ONE REVIEW

1. Mania is a persistent elevation of mood. Characteristics of this elevated mood state include
   A. increased sleep, racing thoughts, and social isolation.
   B. decreased sleep, racing thoughts, and increased risk taking.
   C. racing thoughts, social isolation, and reduced sleep.
   D. racing thoughts, focused thinking, and decreased sleep.
2. Dysthymia is a mood disorder best described as
   A. a chronic state of low-level mania.
   B. a chronic state of psychosis.
   C. a chronic state of low-level depression.
   D. a chronic state of mania.
3. Bipolar disorder is best described as a thought disorder in which there are
   A. periods of low energy and depression mixed with psychosis.
   B. periods of high energy with psychotic features.
   C. periods of high energy.
   D. periods of high energy alternating with periods of depression.
4. Bipolar disorder affects up to what percentage of adults in the United States?
   A. 3
   B. 6
   C. 9
   D. 20
5. Bipolar II disorder differs from Bipolar I in that the degree of mania
   A. is less severe.
   B. is more severe.
   C. displays psychotic features.
   D. presents at the same time as dysthymia.

Answers: 1. B; 2. C; 3. D; 4. A; 5. A

SECTION TWO: Linkage and Association Studies: The Evidence

Bipolar disorder is considered one of the most heritable psychiatric disorders, with symptom onset generally occurring before age 19. For many years, anecdotal evidence supported strong familial association, with several familial clusters of the disease noted around the country. Research has demonstrated that the risk of developing bipolar disorder is approximately 9% among families with first-degree relatives having the condition, a rate significantly higher than the degree of risk in the general population (Smoller & Finn, 2003). Additionally, it appears inheritability risk is even higher for forms of the disorder that develop early in life. Select variants of the bipolar disorder spectrum may be more inheritable than others, although this has not been conclusively demonstrated (Barnett et al., 2010).

Twin and Family Studies

Familial clusters of a disease do not necessarily prove there is a genetic cause. To examine for the presence of genetic variables, twin and adoption studies are often done (Barnett et al., 2010; Barnett & Smoller, 2009). A review of twin studies estimated the heritable risk of bipolar disorder at 85%, which was a higher percentage risk than that of Parkinson disease. Bipolar disorder was then found to be the most heritable disorder (Bienvenu, Davydow, & Kendler, 2011). Twin concordance has been found to range between 40%–45% (Barnett & Smoller, 2009). What remains unclear are the etiologic factors associated with the development of bipolar disorder.

It is possible that select genetic pathways are associated with any disorder of emotional regulation, such as the serotonergic (Canli, Ferri, & Duman, 2009) or dopaminergic pathways. While genetic heritability appears high, the fact that twin concordance is only at 40%–45% indicates that other factors may come into play. The evidence for genetic variables in the etiologic process of bipolar disorder is mixed, with some consistent findings relating to a select few genes.

Another important consideration is the presence of symptomatology that does not meet diagnostic criteria for a disorder. A study of children who had parents with bipolar disorder found a higher risk for the development of bipolar disorder, but also found that those children who did not develop bipolar disorder still displayed elevated mood levels and a degree of psychosocial dysfunction (Findling et al., 2005). Therefore, it is still possible for genetic susceptibility to result in adverse effects without meeting diagnostic criteria for a disorder.

Biologic Significance of Genes Associated With Bipolar Disorder

While the biologic mechanisms underlying bipolar disorder are not fully established, much of the literature has focused on regulation of neurotransmitters (serotonin and dopamine in particular) within the central nervous system. Serotonin and dopamine are neurotransmitters involved in emotional regulation and the reward system (Kranz, Kasper, & Lanzenberger, 2010) and have profound influence on sleep and wakefulness (Ursin, 2008). Both depression and bipolar disorder are associated with the presence of significant sleep disturbance, either hypersomnia or insomnia. In those with bipolar disorder, the presence of a reduced need for sleep, higher levels of energy, and increased risk taking has led researchers to focus on elements of circadian regulation.

The serotonin transporter (5-HTT) moves serotonin from the synaptic cleft into the neuron. This protein is a member of the solute carrier family and is encoded by a gene that is located on chromosome 17 (17q11.1-q12). Referring to this protein as being a member of the solute carrier family means that this protein transports a compound—in this case, serotonin—across the cell membrane. Allelic variation of this gene can then result in reduced transcription and affinity of the receptor in those with bipolar disorder (Mazza et al., 2010). Serotonin is a neurotransmitter known to be expressed to a higher degree in those parts of the brain that regulate responses to risky situations. Obtaining a reward reinforces the expression of serotonin, and serotonergic activity is associated with addictive behavior (Kranz, Kasper, & Lanzenberger, 2010). The behavioral manifestations of bipolar disorder, particularly in terms of increased activity in pleasurable and risk-taking activities, most likely reflect disruptions of serotonergic mechanisms. Dysregulation of the serotonergic receptor would not only affect serotonin expression and biologic function but also the levels of dopamine and other monoamines as well (Bearer, Zhang, Janvelyan, Boulat, & Jacobs, 2009).

The genes discussed next regulate enzymes that in turn influence the presence of dopamine and serotonin. Increased levels of these neurotransmitters are associated with the presence of mania and could be tied to the increased risk taking seen in individuals with bipolar disorder. Genetic variation in the functional ability of these genes could then place individuals at risk for the development of bipolar disorder; these genes represent a fraction of the genetic variables that may be involved in the etiology the disorder (please see Abdolmaleky, Thiagalingam, and Wilcox [2005] for more examples), but have produced the most consistent findings.

Catechol-O-methyltransferase (**COMT**) is an enzyme that degrades catecholamines, such as dopamine, epinephrine, and norepinephrine. The enzyme is produced by a gene of the same name and is the primary substance involved in the catabolism of dopamine within the frontal cortex. Allelic variation of the gene can then influence the involvement of cortisol and dopamine in emotional regulation. Variations in the gene encoding for *COMT* are considered to place individuals at susceptibility for bipolar disorder (Burdick et al., 2007; Zhang et al., 2009). A disruption of this gene could lead to higher levels of dopamine, through a lack of catabolic activity. Higher levels of dopamine are associated with the symptoms of mania (Cousins, Butts, & Young, 2009). Thus, a variation in the *COMT* gene could lead to a reduction in the catabolic degradation of dopamine, which could manifest as mania. Variation in the *COMT* gene also appears to have effects on memory in those with bipolar disorder, through effects on prefrontal concentrations of dopamine (Burdick et al., 2007).

Monoamine oxidase A (MAOA) is another catabolizing enzyme that primarily targets serotonin and is encoded by the *MAO-A* gene. Dysregulation of expression can lead to aggression and emotional lability. A lack of degradation of serotonin and dopamine can then have effects on reward mechanisms in the brain, through the presence of heightened levels of these neurotransmitters.

D-amino acid oxidase activator (DAOA) is a protein that appears throughout the brain and spinal cord. While the biologic action is not completely known, it appears to degrade an activator of glutamate receptors. Several studies have shown that polymorphisms of the gene increase susceptibility to bipolar disorder and schizophrenia (Barnett & Smoller, 2009; Dalvie et al., 2010).

Emerging Evidence

- A new line of research is investigating genetic regulation of the hypothalamic-pituitary-adrenal axis and bipolar disorder. Polymorphisms of the gene regulating the glucocorticoid receptor appear to influence the course of bipolar disorder (Szczepankiewicz et al., 2011).
- Allelic variation in gene promoter sequences influences the expression of proteins produced by a particular gene. A specific variation in a calcium-binding gene primarily expressed in the brain (*S100B*) appears tied to the appearance of those forms of bipolar disorders with psychotic features (Dagdan et al., 2011).
- A gene that regulates cell death (*FOX03A*) appears to confer susceptibility for bipolar disorder, demonstrating the complex regulatory processes that can underlie mood disorders (Magno et al., 2011).
- Epigenetic influences may affect the manifestation of a key gene (*HTR2A*) targeted by antipsychotic medications (Abdolmaleky et al., 2011). It is then possible that genetic and epigenetic mechanisms affect not only the appearance of bipolar disorder, but also responsiveness to pharmacologic treatment.

SECTION TWO REVIEW

1. The risk of developing bipolar disorder among first-degree relatives of those with bipolar disorder is approximately
   A. 3%.
   B. 6%.
   C. 9%.
   D. 18%.
2. Twin concordance for bipolar disorder ranges between
   A. 10%–20%.
   B. 20%–30%.
   C. 40%–50%.
   D. 70%–80%.
3. Catechol-O-methyltransferase is an enzyme that contributes to
   A. increased expression of catecholamines.
   B. the degradation of catecholamines.
   C. selective expression of dopamine.
   D. selective expression of serotonin.
4. Serotonin and dopamine appear to be involved in bipolar disorder through their effects on parts of the brain involved in the processing of
   A. sensory stimuli.
   B. ambient noise.
   C. pain.
   D. risk and reward.
5. Symptom onset in those with bipolar disorder is generally before age
   A. 15.
   B. 19.
   C. 30.
   D. 50.

Answers: 1. C; 2. C; 3. B; 4. D; 5. B

SECTION THREE: Mania and Genetic Links

Mania is a period of mood elevation in which the individual may exhibit grandiosity and inflated self-esteem. This period of heightened energy alternating with periods of depression is the diagnostic hallmark of bipolar disorder. The symptomatology in those with bipolar disorder is thought to result from increased activity of glutamatergic neurons in the frontal cortex. Evidence obtained through proton magnetic resonance spectroscopy has shown elevated glutamate levels in the prefrontal cortex of individuals with mania (Michael et al., 2003). As glutamate is an excitatory neurotransmitter, increased levels would lead to the symptoms of mania, while reduced levels may be associated with periods of depression. Disruptions in circadian regulation of this system could then explain mood cycling in those patients with bipolar disorder. Alternatively, evidence has emerged from work on mouse models of bipolar disorder that proposes an etiologic role for dopamine (Young et al., 2010). Dopamine has several known effectors on behavioral and mood regulation, such that an excess could contribute to mania, with a deficiency contributing to depression (Cousins, Butts, & Young, 2009). It is then possible that genetic variables can contribute to the increased expression of glutamatergic neurons in the frontal cortex.

A combination of genetic variations may need to exist for bipolar disorder susceptibility. Dopamine exerts effects primarily through receptor binding (Beaulieu & Gainetdinov, 2011). A polymorphism of the dopamine receptor has been found to interact with a polymorphism of the receptor for catechol-O-methyltransferase in terms of increasing susceptibility for bipolar disorder (Lee et al., 2011). Another study demonstrated that select polymorphisms of the dopamine transfer gene can differentiate between psychiatric conditions (Pinsonneault et al., 2011). The ability to transport and bind dopamine effectively is necessary for biologic function. Any disruption of these activities could then result in increased dopaminergic expression or availability resulting in increased susceptibility for bipolar disorder.

SECTION THREE REVIEW

1. A diagnostic hallmark of bipolar disorder is
   A. depression.
   B. psychotic features.
   C. mania.
   D. social isolation and withdrawal.
2. Mania is thought to be associated with increased levels of __________ neurotransmitters.
   A. excitatory
   B. inhibitory
   C. dopamine
   D. serotonin
3. The presence of mania may emerge from increased activity of __________ neurons in the frontal cortex.
   A. serotonergic
   B. dopaminergic
   C. glutamatergic
   D. cortisol-sensitive
4. Dopamine has effects primarily through its
   A. actions on cortisol.
   B. influence on glutamate.
   C. glycogen synthase.
   D. receptor binding.
5. Glutamate is an __________ neurotransmitter.
   A. inhibitory
   B. excitatory

Answers: 1. C; 2. A; 3. C; 4. D; 5. B

SECTION FOUR: Cycling of Mood: Circadian Regulation and Genetic Influences

During the manic phase of bipolar disorder, the heightened sense of energy often results in significant sleep disruption. Depressive states and phases are also characterized by sleep disruption, with the individual either sleeping more or less than usual. Sleep patterns, affect, appetite, and other metabolic patterns are under the influence of the circadian system.

The **circadian rhythm** system is a complex process regulated by cells located in the suprachiasmatic nuclei within the hypothalamus. This system regulates several biologic pathways that function in a rhythmical manner across a 24–26 hour cycle, and it is influenced in turn by several neurotransmitters including serotonin and **GABA**. Among the pathways regulated by the circadian system are responses to light and darkness along with sleep regulation. Many of the genes that are involved in wakefulness and alertness appear involved in the process of bipolar disorder. Regulation of the circadian rhythm is under the influence of the ***CLOCK*** gene, which influences the transcription of many of the other genes associated with circadian regulation such as the PER genes along with ***CRY-1*** and *CRY-2*. Genetic variance in the expression of these genes may be associated with the development of bipolar disorder.

Most patients with bipolar disorder can be viewed as having a disrupted circadian rhythm with sleep disturbances that often precede changes in mood and other symptoms. In individuals with bipolar disorder, increased activity of the *CLOCK* gene is associated with decreased sleep and increased time to falling asleep (Benedetti et al., 2007). The pharmacologic agents used in the treatment of bipolar disorder are capable of extending the circadian pattern to an extent.

Biologic Significance of Candidate Genes

The cryptochrome genes (*CRY-1* and *CRY-2*) aid in maintaining the rhymicity and length of the circadian cycle. The proteins transcribed by these genes aid in the transportation of other circadian proteins into the cell nucleus and contribute in circadian pattern stability. In those patients with bipolar disorder, four single nucleotide polymorphisms have been found that result in decreased expression of *CRY-2* messenger RNA, particularly during depressive periods (Sjoholm et al., 2010). This is supported by other research demonstrating that single nucleotide polymorphisms (SNPs) of *CRY-1* and *2* are associated with major depression, and that SNPs of the *CLOCK* gene are significantly associated with bipolar disorder (Soria et al., 2010). Extending the length of aspects of the circadian cycle could contribute to periods of mania or other mood dysregulation.

The *CLOCK* gene is perhaps the major regulatory influence of the circadian system, contributing to transcription of other regulatory proteins involved in diurnal patterning. This gene is also thought to play a role in decision-making processes and other executive functions. SNPs of the *CLOCK* gene appear to significantly influence cognitive tasks and moral judgments (Benedetti et al., 2008). Disruptions of the major regulatory influence could then contribute to the impulsive decision making often seen in those with bipolar disorder.

In animal study of *CLOCK* knockout mice, those mice with the gene removed from a group of cells in the midbrain displayed hyperactivity and higher levels of depression-like behaviors (social isolation and reduced exploration), providing evidence for a mixed type of bipolar disorder (Mukherjee et al., 2010). That study also found changes in the pattern of the circadian rhythm in the mice, providing additional evidence for the role of the circadian pattern in bipolar disorder.

SECTION FOUR REVIEW

1. Select single nucleotide polymorphisms have been found in those with bipolar disorder that result in __________ expression of *CRY-2*.
   A. increased
   B. decreased
   C. cyclic
2. Which of the following genes is most responsible for regulation of the circadian system?
   A. *CLOCK*
   B. *GSK-3*
   C. *FOX 3*
   D. *DAOA*
3. The circadian system is regulated by a group cells located within the
   A. suprachiasmatic nuclei within the hypothalamus.
   B. midbrain raphe.
   C. frontal lobe.
   D. pituitary.
4. In psychiatric conditions, sleep disturbances usually __________ changes in mood.
   A. occur after
   B. precede
   C. improve after
   D. worsen after
5. In an animal study that removed the *CLOCK* gene from mice, the mice displayed
   A. decreased sleep and increased social exploration.
   B. increased sleep and social isolation.
   C. hypoactivity and social isolation.
   D. hyperactivity and social isolation.

Answers: 1. B; 2. A; 3. A; 4. B; 5. D

SECTION FIVE: Pharmacotherapy and Genetics: Implications for Bipolar Disorder

Lithium was the first drug approved for the treatment of bipolar disorder, and it is still one of the primary agents used as monotherapy. Initially, lithium was believed to exert effects by reducing central nervous system response to glutamate and by enhancing beta-receptor activity. Glutamate is one of the main excitatory neurotransmitters. In other words, lithium was seen as making the brain less excitable and decreasing responsiveness to catecholamines. Research with animal populations has since demonstrated that lithium is capable of mediating the circadian system by lengthening the circadian pattern influencing sleep (Serretti & Drago, 2010). One of the potential mechanisms through which bipolar disorder induces symptomatology is the shortening of circadian sleep patterns. The use of a pharmacologic agent that extends the circadian rhythm could then restore a state of circadian balance, helping to alleviate symptoms.

Lithium has also been shown to work synergistically with histone deacetylase HDAC inhibitors perhaps through inhibition of glycogen synthase kinase-3 (**GSK-3**). GSK-3 inactivates a metabolic enzyme (glycogen synthase) that converts glucose into glycogen. The inhibition of GSK-3 by lithium could then lead to an increase in glycogen synthase, providing an increase in glycogen (Li & Jope, 2010) that provides an energy source for neurons. GSK-3 inhibition appears to protect neuron cells from damage, implying that lithium may provide a degree of neuronal protection (Camins et al., 2009; Leng et al., 2008). Lithium also has additional influences on neurotransmitter expression and the movement of calcium within the central nervous system, affecting neuronal transmission and responsiveness.

(For additional detail, the reader is directed to Li, Frye, and Shelton [2012]). Should lithium fail to alleviate the symptoms of bipolar disorders, select anticonvulsant agents may be used.

The primary pharmacologic agents for the treatment of bipolar disorder are listed in Table 19–1. These agents represent various potential pharmacologic mechanisms, with the inclusion of a salt (lithium), several anticonvulsants (carbamazepine, valproate), and select atypical antipsychotics (aripiprazole, olanzapine, quetiapine, reisperidone). The atypical antipsychotics block mesolimbic dopamine receptors and select serotonergic receptors (5-HT Type 2) (Post & Altshuler, 2009), influencing pathways that are associated with the perception and reinforcement of risk and reward.

Several anticonvulsants have been found to be effective in the treatment of bipolar disorder, providing a degree of mood stabilization. The most common of these are carbamazepine (Tegretol) and valproic acid (Depakene). These two agents often seem to be more effective than lithium in treating those who rapidly cycle between mood states. Initially, these anticonvulsants were thought to reduce the amount of neurotransmitters available in the synapse, or to increase the levels of GABA, which serves as an inhibitory neurotransmitter.

Carbamazepine has significant effects on enzymes that catabolize serotonin and dopamine. As demonstrated earlier, several studies have focused on the role of genetic variation in changing the functional ability of these enzymatic pathways. Carbamazepine appears to store some of this catabolic activity, leading to a decrease in levels of serotonin and dopamine. It also appears to lower the action potentials of neurons, leading to a decrease in neuronal responsiveness (Altamura et al., 2011).

Recent research has demonstrated that lithium and valproate (Depakote) in particular influence epigenetic pathways with pronounced effects on signaling. Both lithium and valproate appear to have significant effects on neurotrophin signaling (Gupta et al., 2011). Valproate also appears to inhibit histone deacetylase (HDAC). Histone deacetylases (HDAC) are a group of enzymes that have pronounced effects on gene regulation. These enzymes inhibit gene regulation by reducing gene transcription. The use of valproate could then allow for increased gene expression (Machado-Vieira, Ibrahim, & Zarate, 2010). This has been supported by other research demonstrating that valproate increases the expression of select histone proteins in those with bipolar disorder in a manner that could enhance gene expression (Sharma et al., 2006). There are possible risks tied to the use of these agents in those with bipolar disorder. Animal studies have indicated that valproic acid can disrupt the expression of reproductive hormones with end effects on the responsiveness of the hypothalamus (Lakhanpal, Kataria, & Kaur, 2011). Additional research is required to determine whether these findings extend to humans.

TABLE 19–1: Common Pharmacologic Therapies Used in the Treatment of Bipolar Disorder

Class	Generic Name	Trade Name
Antimania	Lithium	Eskalith
Anticonvulsants	Carbamazepine	Tegretol
	Topiramate	Topamax
	Valproic acid	Depakote
Atypical Antipsychotics	Ariprazole	Abilify
	Clozapine	Clozaril
	Olanzapine	Zyprexa
	Quetiapine	Seroquel
	Risperidone	Risperdal
	Ziprasidone	Geodon

The agents listed here represent the most common pharmacologic agents used in the treatment of bipolar disorder. Several other agents may also be used, including calcium channel blockers, antidepressants, other anticonvulsants not listed, and thyroid mediators.

SECTION FIVE REVIEW

1. Lithium has individual effects on transcription of which of the following genes?
   A. *CRY-1*
   B. *CRY-2*
   C. *GSK-3*
   D. *FOX3*
2. The proposed mechanism of action for anticonvulsants in the treatment of bipolar disorder is through effects on
   A. *CLOCK*.
   B. *CRY-1*.
   C. GSK-3.
   D. HDAC.
3. The administration of lithium could have which of the following effects on the circadian regulation of sleep?
   A. It can shorten the sleep cycle.
   B. It can extend the sleep cycle.
   C. It can prevent the encoding of glycogen synthase.
   D. It can enhance responsiveness to glutamate.
4. Histone deacetylases have relevance in the treatment of bipolar disorder as they
   A. suppress the production of cortisol.
   B. enhance the production of cortisol.
   C. enhance gene expression.
   D. suppress gene expression.
5. Valproate has which of the following effects on HDACs?
   A. inhibitory
   B. excitatory
   C. enhance HDAC production through effects on *FOX3*
   D. inhibit HDAC production through effects on *FOX3*

Answers: 1. C; 2. C; 3. B; 4. D; 5. A

SECTION SIX: Implications for Nursing

While no true opportunity exists as yet to reliably test for susceptibility to bipolar disorder, nurses need to be aware of genetic considerations. Individuals with a familial history may be accessing information from the Internet or other sources and require clarification and assistance with interpreting the meaning of the information for health. In the advent of findings demonstrating the epigenetic effect of existent pharmacologic therapies, new treatment modalities may also be developed.

Many of the neurotransmitters and genetic variables involved in the etiologic pathway of bipolar disorder are activated by psychostimulants. It may ultimately prove beneficial to educate patients about the possible role of psychostimulant medications in bipolar disorder and to encourage the avoidance of illicit agents.

Assessment and Intervention

While the focus of this text is on genetic influences, some brief considerations regarding the bipolar patient include an assessment of safety and symptomatology. Evaluation of the individual with bipolar disorder should focus on mood elevation and sleep pattern. Sleep disruptions often precede disease exacerbation and may serve as a marker for early intervention. Having the individual complete a sleep diary can be helpful, as would the use of a standardized symptom checklist. Such lists should include evaluation for mania, depression, and cognitive function. The nurse should also evaluate for use of caffeine and herbal stimulants including teas and yerba mate. The use of such stimulants may worsen prediagnostic sleep disturbances and adversely influence cognition.

A detailed assessment of stressors and coping strategies would be of benefit to the individual who is at risk for the development of bipolar disorder to enhance functional ability and resilience. Such preventive measures may not inhibit the development of bipolar disorder, but may serve to mitigate severity

Patients should be asked questions regarding medication adherence and the possibility of adverse side effects that could influence adherence. It is also important to provide appropriate mental health referrals for patients and family members. A standardized measure should also be used to assess for the risk of self-harm, or a lack of functional ability so great as to pose a risk of self-harm. While the mainstay of treatment for bipolar disorder is pharmacologic, providing information and education regarding interventions that can influence sleep and appetite could provide a benefit to the patient. Any intervention that influences circadian regulation may be able to provide some relief and reinforce the effects of a pharmacologic intervention. Nursing is a profession that is well positioned to provide such teaching.

SECTION SIX REVIEW

1. The assessment on the part of the nurse should include all of the following EXCEPT
   A. an evaluation of sleep and appetite.
   B. an assessment of familial risk.
   C. encouragement of prenatal testing.
   D. identification of coping strategies.
2. Genetic testing for bipolar disorder
   A. is 9% effective.
   B. is 40% effective.
   C. requires two allelic variations to be present.
   D. is ineffective.

Answers: 1. C; 2. D

POSTTEST

1. The diagnostic criteria for bipolar disorders include which of the following?
   A. Periods of depression that alternate with periods of normal mood
   B. Sustained elevation of mood mixed with periods of depression
   C. Sustained depression of mood
   D. Social isolation and avoidance of risk taking
2. The proposed mechanism of action for anticonvulsants in the treatment of bipolar disorder is through effects on
   A. *CLOCK*.
   B. *CRY-1*.
   C. *GSK-3*.
   D. HDAC.
3. The *CLOCK* gene regulates which homeostatic system?
   A. The circadian system
   B. Thermoregulation
   C. Executive functions
   D. Risk and reward perceptions
4. Lithium inhibits glycogen synthase kinase-3 (GSK-3). The end effect of this inhibition is
   A. an increase in glycogen.
   B. a decrease in glycogen synthase.
   C. an increase in HDACs.
   D. a decrease in HDACs.
5. The cryptochrome genes (1 and 2) are believed to play a role in the pathogenesis of bipolar disorder. What is the biologic significance of these genes?
   A. They aid in transporting other proteins into the cell.
   B. They aid in transporting other proteins out of the cell.
   C. They influence the expression of GSK-3.
   D. They influence the expression of serotonin.

6. Twin studies have demonstrated a degree of support for genetic variables in the development of bipolar disorder. Twin concordance for bipolar disorder ranges between
   A. 70%–80%.
   B. 40%–50%.
   C. 20%–30%.
   D. 10%–20%.
7. The patient with bipolar disorder should be screened for
   A. increased sleep and decreased appetite.
   B. pressured speech and decreased social exploration.
   C. increased sleep and increased energy while awake.
   D. increased risk taking and participation in pleasurable activities.
8. A defect in which of the following genes is most likely associated with the insomnia seen in bipolar disorder?
   A. *GSK-3*
   B. *CLOCK*
   C. *CRY-2*
   D. *MAOA*
9. A patient's family asks you about an article found on the Internet regarding genetic testing and bipolar disorder. The family states the article claimed an ability to identify highly permissive polymorphisms in 20% of the population. Your best response is
   A. the percentage is closer to 9%.
   B. the article is inaccurate. There are no reliable tests.
   C. the percentage is closer to 40%, based on twin studies.
   D. it depends on the number of SNPs in the *CLOCK* gene.
10. Which of the following neurotransmitters is associated with risk and reward perceptions?
   A. Acetylcholine
   B. GABA
   C. Serotonin
   D. Glutamate

Posttest answers are located in the Appendix.

CHAPTER SUMMARY

The circadian system is one of the main regulators of sleep and wakefulness. This homeostatic pattern is regulated by cells located in the suprachiasmatic nucleus (SCN) of the hypothalamus, which are in turn under the influence of serotonergic pathways emerging from the raphe section of the brain. A disruption of gene expression affecting circadian regulation can have profound significance leading to dysregulation of sleep and wakefulness, and ultimately, mania. The manifestation of mania in turn involves other pathways in a complex interactional process of mood dysregulation that ultimately has adverse consequences on the functional capability of the individual. Nursing has the opportunity to contribute to homeostatic balance through a process of careful assessment and the provision of necessary education.

- Bipolar disorder is characterized by the appearance of mania that may be accompanied by cyclical or coexistent depression.
- The appearance of mania appears to be an end product of a disruption of the circadian rhythm.
- There are several genetic regulators of the circadian rhythm, of which the *CLOCK* may be the most significant.
- Pharmacologic therapies are designed to influence the circadian pattern through modification of gene expression and the suppression of gene signaling.
- There are no reliable genetic tests to determine susceptibility to bipolar disorder.

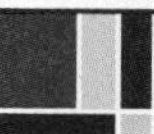

CRITICAL THINKING CHECKPOINT

T. S. is a 24 year old, Caucasian male college student. He presents with a complaint of intermittent, nonrestful sleep for the past 4 days. His sleep has been disrupted by racing thoughts and an intense sense of energy. At this point, he is pacing the room, exhibiting coherent and fluent pressured speech. As well, his vital signs are slightly elevated. As you are interviewing him, he mentions an uncle that is "manic" and expresses concern that this might be happening to him.

1. Which of these signs and symptoms would be consistent with bipolar disorder?
2. Are there links between familial history and bipolar disorder?
3. T. S. asks if there is genetic testing available to determine whether or not he has bipolar disorder. What is the most appropriate response?
4. After discussing his condition, what would be an appropriate follow-up plan for T.S.?
5. What is the role of the nurse in working with this patient?

Answers are provided in the Appendix

ONLINE RESOURCES

National Alliance on Mental Illness: http://www.nami.org

National Institute of Mental Health – Information on Bipolar Disorder: http://www.nimh.nih.gov/health/publications/bipolar-disorder/complete-index.shtml

REFERENCES

Abdolamleky, H. M., Thiagalingam, S., & Wilcox, M. (2005). Genetics and epigenetics in major psychiatric disorders: Dilemmas, achievements, applications, and future scope. *American Journal of Pharmacogenomics, 5*(3), 149–160.

Abdolmaleky, H. M., Yaqubi, S., Papageorgis, P., Lambert, A. W., Ozturk, S., Sivaraman, V., et al. (2011). Epigenetic dysregulation of HTR2A in the brain of patients with schizophrenia and bipolar disorder. *Schizophrenia Research, 129*(2–3), 183–190.

Altamura, C., Lietti, L., Dobrea, C., Benatti, B., Arici, C., & Dell'Osso, B. (2011). Mood stabilizers for patients with bipolar disorder: The state of the art. *Expert Reviews in Neurotherapeutics, 11*(1), 85–99.

American Psychiatric Association. (2000). *Diagnostic and statistical manual of mental disorders* (4th ed., text rev.). Washington, DC: Author.

Barnett, J. H., & Smoller, J. W. (2009). The genetics of bipolar disorder. *Neuroscience, 164*(1), 331–343.

Barnett, J. H., Huang, J., Perlis, R. H., Young, M. M., Rosenbaum, J. F., Nierenberg, A. A., et al. (2010). Personality and bipolar disorder: Dissecting state and trait associations between mood and personality. *Psychology Medicine, 41*(8), 1593–604.

Bearer, E. L., Zhang, X., Janvelyan, D., Boulat, B., & Jacobs, R. E. (2009). Reward circuitry is perturbed in the absence of the serotonin transporter. *NeuroImage, 46*(4), 1091–1104.

Beaulieu, J. M., & Gainetdinov, R. R. (2011). The physiology, signaling, and pharmacology of dopamine receptors. *Pharmacological Reviews, 63*(1), 182–217.

Benedetti, F., Dallaspezia, S., Fulgosi, M. C., Lorenzi, C., Serretti, A., Barbini, B., et al. (2007). Actimetric evidence that CLOCK 3111 T/C SNP influences sleep and activity patterns in patients affected by bipolar depression. *American Journal of Medical Genetics Part B: Neuropsychiatric Genetics, 144B*(5), 631–635.

Benedetti, F., Radaelli, D., Bernasconi, A., Dallaspezia, S., Falini, A., Scotti, G., et al. (2008). Clock genes beyond the clock: CLOCK genotype biases neural correlates of moral valence decision in depressed patients. *Genes, Brain, and Behavior, 7*(1), 20–25.

Bienvenu, O. J., Davydow, D. S., & Kendler, K. S. (2011). Psychiatric 'diseases' versus behavioral disorders and degree of genetic influence. *Psychology Medicine, 41*(1), 33–40.

Burdick, K. E., Funke, B., Goldberg, J. F., Bates, J. A., Jaeger, J., Kucherlapati, R., et al. (2007). COMT genotype increases risk for bipolar I disorder and influences neurocognitive performance. *Bipolar Disorders, 9*(4), 370–376.

Camins, A., Verdaguer, E., Junyent, F., Yeste-Velasco, M., Pelegri, C., Vilaplana, J., et al. (2009). Potential mechanisms involved in the prevention of neurodegenerative diseases by lithium. *CNS Neuroscience & Therapeutics, 15*(4), 333–344.

Canli, T., Ferri, J., & Duman, E. A. (2009). Genetics of emotion regulation. *Neuroscience, 164*(1), 43–54.

Cousins, D. A., Butts, K., & Young, A. H. (2009). The role of dopamine in bipolar disorder. *Bipolar Disorders, 11*(8), 787–806.

Dagdan, E., Morris, D. W., Campbell, M., Hill, M., Rothermundt, M., Kastner, F., et al. (2011). Functional assessment of a promoter polymorphism in S100B, a putative risk variant for bipolar disorder. *American Journal of Medical Genetics Part B: Neuropsychiatric Genetics, 156B*(6), 691–699.

Dalvie, S., Horn, N., Nossek, C., van der Merwe, L., Stein, D. J., & Ramesar, R. (2010). Psychosis and relapse in bipolar disorder are related to GRM3, DAOA, and GRIN2B genotype. *African Journal of Psychiatry (Johannesbg), 13*(4), 297–301.

Findling, R. L., Youngstrom, E. A., McNamara, N. K., Stansbrey, R. J., Demeter, C. A., Bedoya, D., et al. (2005). Early symptoms of mania and the role of parental risk. *Bipolar Disorders, 7*, 623–634.

Gupta, A., Schulze, T. G., Nagarajan, V., Akula, N., Corona, W., Jiang, X. Y., et al. (2011). Interaction networks of lithium and valproate molecular targets reveal a striking enrichment of apoptosis functional clusters and neurotrophin signaling. *The Pharmacogenomics Journal, 12, 328–341*. Retrieved from http://www.nature.com/tpj/journal/v12/n4/full/tpj20119a.html

Kessler, R. C., Chiu, W. T., Demler, O., Merikangas, K. R., & Walters, E. E. (2005). Prevalence, severity, and comorbidity of 12-month DSM-IV disorders in the National Comorbidity Survey Replication. *Archives of General Psychiatry, 62*(6), 617–627.

Kranz, G. S., Kasper, S., & Lanzenberger, R. (2010). Reward and the serotonergic system. *Neuroscience, 166*(4), 1023–1035.

Lakhanpal, D., Kataria, H., & Kaur, G. (2011). Neuroendocrine plasticity in GnRH release is disrupted by valproic acid treatment of cycling rats. *Acta Neurologica Belgica, 111*(2), 121–129.

Lee, S. Y., Chen, S. L., Chen, S. H., Huang, S. Y., Tzeng, N. S., Chang, Y. H., et al. (2011). The COMT and DRD3 genes interacted in bipolar I but not bipolar II disorder. *The World Journal of Biological Psychiatry 12*(5), 385–391.

Leng, Y., Liang, M. H., Ren, M., Marinova, Z., Leeds, P., & Chuang, D. M. (2008). Synergistic neuroprotective effects of lithium and valproic acid or other histone deacetylase inhibitors in neurons: roles of glycogen synthase kinase-3 inhibition. *The Journal of Neuroscience, 28*(10), 2576–2588.

Li, X., Frye, M. A., & Shelton, R. C. (2012). Review of pharmacological treatment in mood disorders and future directions for drug development. *Neuropsychopharmacology Reviews, 37*, 77–101.

Li, X., & Jope, R. S. (2010). Is glycogen synthase kinase-3 a central modulator in mood regulation? *Neuropsychopharmacology, 35*(11), 2143–2154.

Machado-Vieira, R., Ibrahim, L., & Zarate, C. A., Jr. (2010). Histone deacetylases and mood disorders: Epigenetic programming in gene-environment interactions. *CNS Neuroscience & Therapeutics, 17*(6), 699–704.

Magno, L. A., Santana, C. V., Sacramento, E. K., Rezende, V. B., Cardoso, M. V., Mauricio-da-Silva, L., et al. (2011). Genetic variations in FOXO3A are associated with Bipolar Disorder without confering vulnerability for suicidal behavior. *Journal of Affective Disorders, 133*(3), 633–637.

Matorin, A. A., & Ruiz, P. (2009). Clinical manifestations of mood. In B. J. Sadock, V. A. Sadock, and P. R. Ruiz (Eds.), *Kaplan & Sadock's comprehensive textbook of psychiatry* (9th ed.). Philadelphia: Lippincott Williams & Wilkins, pp. 1071–1107.

Mazza, M., Mandelli, L., Martinotti, G., Di Nicola, M., Tavian, D., Negri, G., et al. (2010). Further evidence supporting the association between 5HTR2C gene and bipolar disorder. *Psychiatry Research, 180*(2–3), 151–152.

Michael, N., Erfurth, A., Ohrmann, P., Gossling, M., Arolt, V., Heindel, W., et al. (2003). Acute mania is accompanied by elevated glutamate/glutamine levels within the left dorsolateral prefrontal cortex. *Psychopharmacology, 168*, 344–346.

Mukherjee, S., Coque, L., Cao, J. L., Kumar, J., Chakravarty, S., Asaithamby, A., et al. (2010). Knockdown of Clock in the ventral tegmental area through RNA interference results in a mixed state of mania and depression-like behavior. *Biological Psychiatry, 68*(6), 503–511.

Pinsonneault, J. K., Han, D. D., Burdick, K. E., Kataki, M., Bertolino, A., Malhotra, A. K., et al. (2011). Dopamine transporter gene variant affecting expression in human brain is associated with bipolar disorder. *Neuropsychopharmacology, 36*(8), 1644–1655.

Post, R. M., & Altshuler, L. L. (2009). Mood disorders: Treatment of bipolar disorders. In B. J. Sadock, V. A. Sadock, & P. Ruiz (Eds.), *Kaplan & Sadock's comprehensive textbook of psychiatry*. New York: Lippincott, Williams & Wilkins, pp. 1743–1813.

Serretti, A., & Drago, A. (2010). Pharmacogenetics of lithium long-term treatment: Focus on initiation and adaptation mechanisms. *Neuropsychobiology, 62*(1), 61–71.

Sharma, R. P., Rosen, C., Kartan, S., Guidotti, A., Costa, E., Grayson, D. R., et al. (2006). Valproic acid and chromatin remodeling in schizophrenia and bipolar disorder: Preliminary results from a clinical population. *Schizophrenia Research, 88*(1–3), 227–231.

Sjoholm, L. K., Backlund, L., Cheteh, E. H., Ek, I. R., Frisen, L., Schalling, M., et al. (2010). CRY2 is associated with rapid cycling in bipolar disorder patients. *PLoS One, 5*(9), e12632.

Smoller, J. W., & Finn, C. T. (2003). Family, twin, and adoption studies of bipolar disorder. *American Journal of Medical Genetics Part C: Seminars in Medical Genetics, 123C*(1), 48–58.

Soria, V., Martinez-Amoros, E., Escaramis, G., Valero, J., Perez-Egea, R., Garcia, C., et al. (2010). Differential association of circadian genes with mood disorders: CRY1 and NPAS2 are associated with unipolar major depression and CLOCK and VIP with bipolar disorder. *Neuropsychopharmacology, 35*(6), 1279–1289.

Szczepankiewicz, A., Leszczynska-Rodziewicz, A., Pawlak, J., Rajewska-Rager, A., Dmitrzak-Weglarz, M., Wilkosc, M., et al. (2011). Glucocorticoid receptor polymorphism is associated with major depression and predominance of depression in the course of bipolar disorder. *Journal of Affective Disorders, 134*(1–3), 138–144.

Ursin, R. (2008). Changing concepts on the role of serotonin in the regulation of sleep and waking. In J. M. Monti, S. R. Pandi-Perumal, B. L. Jacobs, & D. J. Nutt (Eds.), *Serotonin and Sleep: Molecular, functional and clinical aspects*. Basel, Switzerland: Birkhauser Verlag, pp. 3–24.

Young, J. W., Goey, A. K., Minassian, A., Perry, W., Paulus, M. P., & Geyer, M. A. (2010). The mania-like exploratory profile in genetic dopamine transporter mouse models is diminished in a familiar environment and reinstated by subthreshold psychostimulant administration. *Pharmacology Biochemistry and Behavior, 96*(1), 7–15.

Zhang, Z., Lindpaintner, K., Che, R., He, Z., Wang, P., Yang, P., et al. (2009). The Val/Met functional polymorphism in COMT confers susceptibility to bipolar disorder: Evidence from an association study and a meta-analysis. *Journal of Neural Transmission, 116*(10), 1193–1200.

CHAPTER

20 Depression and Genetic Linkages

Linda Callahan

LEARNING OUTCOMES

Following the completion of this chapter, the learner will be able to

1. Define the symptomatic differences between major depression, dysthymia, and bipolar disorder.
2. Describe the current understanding about specific brain and transmitter changes that are associated with the development of the depressive disorders.
3. Summarize current genetic knowledge regarding depressive disorders as well as the potential areas of genetic research for the future.
4. Discuss how the continued growth of genetic/genomic information will improve the nurse's ability to not only function effectively in the appropriate care and management of affected patients, but to act as a change agent in educating patients, families, and the community regarding the depressive disorders.

The purpose of this chapter is to discuss the recognized and potential genetic factors that influence or are operant in the development of the complex mood disorders, specifically major depression, dysthymia, and bipolar disorder. The incidence, our current understanding of pathology and treatment, the influence of genetics/genomics, and the implications of depressive disorders for the patient and family will be discussed. The chapter will also explore the role of the nurse and other health care professionals in recognition of the depressive disorders, appropriate referral, the need for effective treatment, and the education of patients, families, and the public.

PRETEST

1. Mood Disorders (MD), such as major depression and bipolar depression, are diagnosed by
   A. utilizing laboratory tests to identify certain proteins.
   B. testing for the presence of specific gene alleles.
   C. utilizing specific symptomatic criteria.
   D. observing individual responses to antidepressant drugs.
2. Major Depressive Disorder (MDD) is a syndrome that is
   A. present in humans across the lifespan.
   B. found most often in children.
   C. seldom found in individuals over 65 years of age.
   D. rarely seen in pregnant patients.
3. Bipolar Disorder (BPD) with rapid cycling between depression and mania
   A. generally onsets later in life.
   B. occurs only in men.
   C. is never found in young children.
   D. occurs more frequently in women than in men.
4. Depression may be caused by a(n)
   A. imbalance of neurotransmitters in several parts of the brain.
   B. imbalance of receptor density on the postsynaptic neuronal membrane.
   C. deficiency in signal transduction between neurons.
   D. All of the above
5. Major Depressive Disorder (MDD) and Bipolar Disorder (BPD), like all complex diseases, are thought to develop
   A. in response to the presence of dominant genes in a family.
   B. as the result of genetic susceptibility plus environmental stressors.
   C. only in individuals who have reached sexual maturity.
   D. as recessive genes in roughly 25% of the population.
6. In general, antidepressant medications work due to their ability to
   A. increase the amount of neurotransmitter in the neuronal synapse.
   B. decrease the amount of neurotransmitter in the neuronal synapse.
   C. increase reuptake of neurotransmitters into the presynaptic neuron.
   D. increase the activity of the enzyme monoamine oxidase (MAO).

7. The son of a mother who has MDD has a _______ risk of developing MDD at some point in his life.
   A. 100%
   B. two- to fourfold greater
   C. tenfold greater
   D. one- to threefold lesser
8. Genetic research in MDD and BPD has
   A. been able to isolate specific causative genes for these disorders.
   B. identified a number of genes that may contribute to increased susceptibility to these disorders.
   C. been successful in identifying specific genes that allow us to predict the success of pharmacologic treatment of MDD or BPD.
   D. focused primarily on case studies involving twins.
9. Given the heritability of MDD, it is important during patient assessment that the nurse
   A. identify depressive symptoms so appropriate laboratory tests can be drawn.
   B. assume that if the patient has MDD other members of the immediate family will also have the disorder.
   C. gather sufficient information from the patient to develop a three-generation pedigree chart.
   D. reassure the patient that the presence of other illnesses has little effect on the degree of MDD that is experienced.
10. At present, genetic counseling about MDs is primarily concerned with
   A. testing for specific genetic markers for depression.
   B. estimating recurrence rate of disorders based on family history.
   C. reassuring the patient that MDDs will not be passed on to future generations.
   D. reassuring the patient that these diseases are primarily environmental in origin.

Pretest answers are located in the Appendix.

SECTION ONE: Overview of Mood Disorders

Mood can be defined as a pervasive or constant internal feeling that influences both our behavior and our perception of the world. An individual's affect is the external expression of his or her mood. Mood can be described as normal, elevated, or depressed. Healthy people normally experience a wide range of moods and are generally in control of the affect they display in response to their mood.

Mood disorders are a group of clinical conditions that are characterized by a loss of control and by subjective feelings of great and unremitting distress. When a mood disorder is present there is almost always impaired interpersonal, social, and occupational functioning (Sadock & Sadock, 2007).

As indicated by the terminology, mood disorders are those disorders in which a disturbance in mood is the major or dominant feature. As with other psychiatric disorders, mood disorders are currently diagnosed utilizing specific symptomatic criteria found in the *Diagnostic and Statistical Manual of Mental Disorders (DSM-IV-TR)* (American Psychological Association, 2000). The mood disorders are divided into the Depressive Disorders, the Bipolar Disorders, and two disorders based on specific causative events: Mood Disorder Due to a General Medical Condition and Substance-Induced Mood Disorder. The focus of this chapter will be the genetics of **Major Depressive Disorder (MDD)** and Bipolar Disorder (**BPD**), since these have been most studied in recent research.

The Depressive Disorders encompass Major Depressive Disorder, Dysthymic Disorder, **Cyclothymic Disorder**, and the Bipolar Disorders, which are further classified as **Bipolar I Disorder** (BPD-I), and **Bipolar II Disorder** (BPD-II). Brief descriptive definitions for each of the named disorders as specified in the *DSM-IV-TR* may be found in the Glossary located at the end of this text. Stahl (2008) notes that mania and depression are poles apart. This imagery generated the use of the terms *unipolar* for patients experiencing only the down or depressed affective pole and *bipolar* for patients who experience both the up affective pole (mania) and the down affective pole. Mood disorders can be visualized in this way in Figure 20–1 ■. The possibilities of the affective spectrum can be seen to range from normal mood or euthymia upward to hypomania and finally to **mania**, and in the opposite direction downward to dysthymia and MDD.

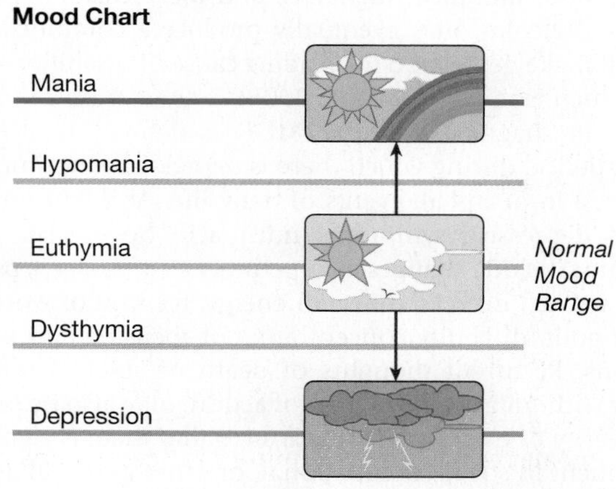

Figure 20–1 ■ Mood chart

Major Depressive Disorder (MDD)

Mood disorders have been recognized as part of the human condition throughout recorded history. Descriptions of depressive syndromes were recounted as part of the Old Testament story of King Saul and in the story of Ajax's suicide in Homer's Iliad. As early as 400 BCE Hippocrates described the opposite affective disturbances he observed with the terms *melancholia* and *mania* (Sadock & Sadock, 2007).

MDD is perhaps the most common psychiatric condition. Approximately 10% to 15% of the total population will experience one period of clinical depression during their lifetime. Statistics from the World Health Organization indicate that 5% of men and 9% of women will have a major depressive event each year (Tsuang, Taylor, & Faraone, 2004; Kessler, Chiu, Demler, Merikanga, & Walter, 2005). The mean age of onset of MDD is 40 years with 50% of patients having onset between 20 and 50 years of age. There is recent evidence of an increased incidence of onset in younger individuals as well as in those over the age of 65. In adolescents and younger adults the increase in incidence of onset may be due to increased utilization of alcohol and recreational drugs. In older patients over 65 years of age the increased incidence may be due to the prospect of greater longevity and coping with loss of peer and family support as well as the need to deal with the chronic nature of coexisting diseases. The ubiquitous nature of these findings across the lifespan points out the universality of MDD as a syndrome present in all ages of humans. *The Global Burden of Disease* (**GBD**) study carried out by the World Health Organization (WHO) and the World Bank calculated that major depression was the fourth leading cause of disability adjusted life years (**DALYs**), after lower respiratory infections, diarrhea diseases, and perinatal illnesses. The calculations of DALYs are based on the years of life that are lost due to premature death plus the years of life lived with disability (**YLDs**). If YLDs alone are counted, depressive disorders become the leading cause of disability (Murray & Lopez, 1997). Results of a later WHO study that included the disease and illness burden of HIV/AIDS estimated that in 2030 the three leading causes of DALYs would be HIV/AIDS, depressive disorders, and ischemic heart disease. It has also been postulated that factors such as the overall decrease in the size of family units, increased urbanization, mobility, migration, and the recreational use of drugs and alcohol may eventually produce a combined effect that will make depression the leading cause of disability and illness burden worldwide (Wood, 2008; Mathers & Lancar, 2006).

By the diagnostic criteria, MDD is defined as at least a 2-week period during which there is depressed mood or a loss of interest in nearly all events of daily life. At least four other defined depressive symptoms must also be present. These symptoms include changes in appetite or weight, sleep, psychomotor activity, decreased overall energy, feelings of worthlessness or guilt, difficulty concentrating or focusing and making decisions. Recurrent thoughts of death or suicidal ideation, with or without a specified plan of action, may also be present. The severity of these symptoms is such that there is significant impairment in social, occupational, or other personal areas of functioning (American Psychological Association, 2000).

Patients suffering from MDD may be sad or discouraged even though they continue to function at a near-normal level, which they admit requires tremendous effort on their part. A lack of feelings with a flat affect or an expression of anxiety may also be present. In addition to these symptoms many patients report physical complaints such as aches and pains in various areas of the body.

Insomnia is the most common sleep disorder associated with MDD. Less frequently, patients may complain of oversleeping (hypersomnia). Decreased energy is common, and an increasing sense of fatigue, unrelated to exercise, is often present. Psychomotor changes may travel the spectrum from agitation to extreme retardation of movement and/or speech.

Dysthymia

The *DSM-IV-TR* defines the symptoms of **dysthymia** as the presence of a depressed mood that is continuous and has seemed to always have been present in the patient's life. Usually this condition begins in childhood or as a young adult. It is defined as a subaffective or subclinical depression that has persisted for at least 2 years. The family histories of individuals with dysthymia often reveal the presence of both depressive and bipolar disorders in other family members.

Dysthymia is found in approximately 5% to 6% of the population. It is noted to affect one-third to one-half of patients encountered in general psychiatric practice (Sadock & Sadock, 2007). Dysthymia may exist with MDD; when this happens there is a decreased likelihood of full recovery between major depressive episodes. In this situation the patient recovers only to the level of dysthymia, or low-level depression, between MDD episodes. This is often referred to as "double depression." The chronicity of the low-level, subclinical depression that defines dysthymia over time impacts the patient's productivity, self-concept, relationships, and overall life satisfaction.

Bipolar Disorder

The Bipolar Disorders (BPD) are divided into Bipolar Disorder I (BPD-I) and Bipolar Disorder II (BPD-II) by the degree of symptoms present. BPD-I is the classic syndrome in which defined mania symptoms occur during the course of the disorder. BPD-II is hallmarked by depressive episodes and the presence of hypomanic symptoms that are not severe enough to meet the diagnostic criteria of full mania (American Psychological Association, 2000).

BPD-I is noted to onset at an earlier age than MDD. Although the onset of BPD-I can occur as early as 5–6 years of age, the mean onset age is around 25–30 years, while the mean onset age for MDD is about 40. Also in contrast to MDD, there is an equal incidence of BPD-I in both men and women. Women tend to more commonly have depressive episodes while men more often experience mania. Women are also more likely to be rapid cyclers, a term that is defined as having four or more manic episodes in one year (Sadock & Sadock, 2007).

The clinical symptoms of BPD-II include those of MDD combined with a hypomanic episode. BPD-II is thought to often onset earlier than BPD-I. An earlier onset may place the patient at greater risk of suicidality than is observed in patients with BPD-I or MDD (Sadock & Sadock, 2007).

SECTION ONE REVIEW

1. MDs are diagnosed primarily by
   A. family history.
   B. laboratory assessment of genetic markers.
   C. symptomatic criteria found in the *DSM-IV-TR*.
   D. observed need for intervention due to social dysfunction.
2. BPD-II differs from BPD-I in that patients with BPD-II
   A. manifest severe manic episodes several times each year.
   B. experience hypomania rather than mania during cycling.
   C. never manifest "rapid cycling" behavior.
   D. have less risk of suicide than those with BPD-I.
3. Individuals with dysthymia
   A. will have a negative family history for MDs.
   B. rarely seek professional help.
   C. report a low-level daily depression that seems to have always been present.
   D. are generally not susceptible to MDD.
4. Recent studies indicate that the incidence of onset of MDD is
   A. increasing in older adults and adolescents.
   B. decreasing in older adults and adolescents.
   C. decreasing overall due to better recognition by society.
   D. unrelated to the presence of chronic coexisting diseases.
5. Patients suffering with MDD
   A. are incapable of functioning at work and want to sleep all the time.
   B. seldom seek medical attention for physical complaints.
   C. rarely commit suicide although they may often speak of doing so.
   D. may continue to function at near normal levels but state they are exhausted by the effort.

Answers: 1. C; 2. B; 3. C; 4. A; 5. D

SECTION TWO: Brain Physiology and Transmission in Mood Disorders

An in-depth discussion of the complexities of neuronal conduction is beyond the scope of this text, but a review of basic concepts is essential to understanding the pathology and treatment of the mood disorders. It will also provide a basis for understanding the developing importance of genetics in both disease development and patient response to treatment.

Although there are hundreds of chemicals that contribute to brain function, three principle monoamine neurotransmitters—norepinephrine, serotonin (**5-HT**), and dopamine—are associated with both the pathology and treatment of mood disorders. All the symptoms associated with mood disorders are thought to be due to dysfunction of combinations of these transmitters in various parts of the brain. All current pharmacologic treatments for mood disorders are predicated on modifying these neurotransmitters to gain control or remission of symptoms.

The biologic cause of depression was initially hypothesized to be a deficiency of a monoamine transmitter, such as norepinephrine, at the synapse between neurons. Currently the functional theory is that all three monoamines, norepinephrine, serotonin, and dopamine, may be unbalanced or malfunctioning at different levels and in different portions of the brain circuitry. The degree of malfunction and the specific transmitters potentially involved are determined based upon the patient's presenting and recurrent symptoms.

Synapses can form on any part of an axon. The purpose of the synapse is to provide communication between neurons by the use of chemical transmitters. The presynaptic membrane that comes before the synaptic cleft contains the neurotransmitter, necessary enzymes, reuptake transporters, ion channels, and specialized proteins necessary for neurotransmitter release. The postsynaptic portion of the synapse or the membrane on the neuron that comes after the synaptic cleft contains postsynaptic receptors structured to bind with the neurotransmitter, signal cascade molecules, and specialized proteins that produce the postsynaptic density required to recognize signals from the presynaptic neuron. Synapses undergo continuous revision in response to changing environmental conditions and the frequency with which they are used. Changing amounts of neurotransmitter can alter the number and the density of both pre- and postsynaptic receptors at the synapse. Many neurons utilize more than one neurotransmitter at a single synapse; therefore, the input to each neuron may involve a number of different transmitters. In order to influence abnormal or altered neurotransmission, it may be necessary to pharmacologically target neurons in several specific circuits by administering multiple drugs with multiple transmitter actions for treatment.

Neurotransmitters are synthesized both in the soma (cell body) with transport to the axonal terminal and at the axonal terminal by enzymes that are present there. Once manufactured, neurotransmitters are stored in presynaptic vesicles. Also present in the presynaptic membrane are enzymatic transporter pumps that function to recapture released transmitter molecules, returning them to the presynaptic cell for reuse in transmission.

In the classic neurotransmission sequence, one neuron releases the neurotransmitter, which diffuses across the synaptic cleft to interact with the receptors of the target neuron. An electrical impulse, or depolarization wave, is converted to a chemical signal at the synapse, which then produces excitation at the second neuron. This happens because the electrical impulses of depolarization produce opening of the Na+ channels in the axonal membranes. The impulse then progresses to the presynaptic nerve terminal opening the Ca++ channels to allow ionic flow. This change in membrane permeability causes the synaptic vesicles to spill the transmitters into the synapse. This is the process by which the electrical impulse resulting from membrane depolarization is changed into a chemical event, the release of the transmitters. Once released the transmitter molecules move by diffusion to interact with the appropriate receptors on the postsynaptic membrane. Occupation of the receptor initiates the process of excitatory response by that neuronal body.

Once sufficient postsynaptic receptor occupation by the neurotransmitter has occurred, 60%–80% of the free transmitter in the synaptic cleft is returned to the presynaptic cell by the membrane transporter proteins. This process is known as reuptake. The remaining excess transmitter is removed from the synaptic area by interaction with the extracellular enzyme, Catechol-O-methyltransferase (**COMT**). Monoamine oxidase (**MAO**), found within the cells, metabolizes excess monoamines within the cellular cytoplasm (see Figure 20–2 ■).

The monoamine hypothesis that states that depression is the result of depletion or loss of a specific transmitter is appealing since the administration of antidepressant medication that increases brain levels of neurotransmitters often improves or produces remission of depressive symptoms. However, conclusive research data providing direct biologic evidence for this hypothesis have been sought, but have not yet been found. The large amount of research completed on this subject since the 1960s has produced mixed and often confusing results. Clinically, therapeutic blood levels of most antidepressant drugs are present within 72 to 96 hours, yet in most instances, symptom improvement is delayed for 3 to 6 weeks. While increasing the amount of transmitter in the synapse is important, it is obvious that there are other processes necessary for pharmacologic effect and change in function. The focus of research has broadened from trying to understand the role of the neurotransmitters to include the study of the receptors that respond to these transmitters and the events that receptor occupation triggers postsynaptically at the molecular level. Downstream activities following receptor activation by a neurotransmitter can include impulse conduction, blockade, and regulation of gene expression. These understandings have resulted in development of the neurotransmitter receptor hypothesis of depression that states that decreased amounts of neurotransmitter at the synapse lead to a compensatory upregulation (increase) in postsynaptic neurotransmitter receptors. This change in the number of receptors can have a negative effect on the production of important postsynaptic proteins and may produce a disease state. Increases in the neurotransmitter or the use of drugs that mimic the neurotransmitter produce downregulation or a decrease in the number of receptors to a more normal functional level. Both these processes take weeks, thereby helping to account for the longer period of time required to see significant symptom remission in depressed patients being treated with antidepressant medications. At this point in time there continues to be a lack of conclusive direct physical evidence verifying these events, although from a clinical standpoint, it is widely accepted that modification of both pre- and postsynaptic events is involved in the treatment of the mood disorders.

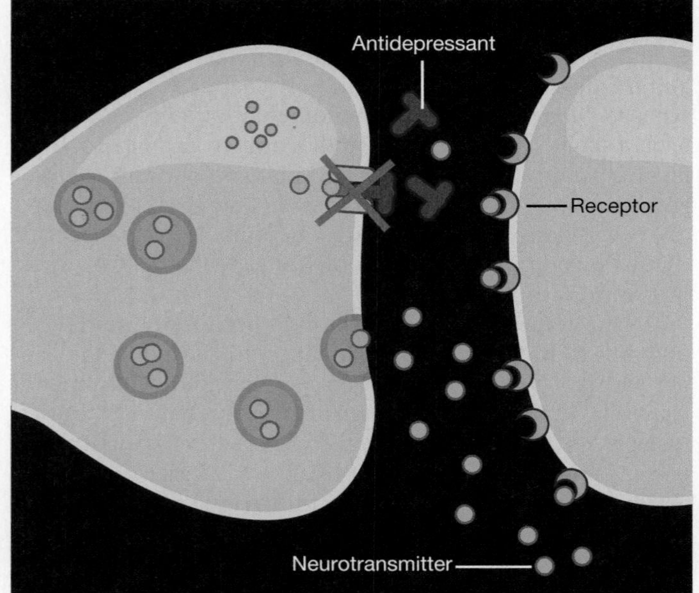

(a) Antidepressant blocks the reuptake pump, causing more neurotransmitter to accumulate in the synapse.

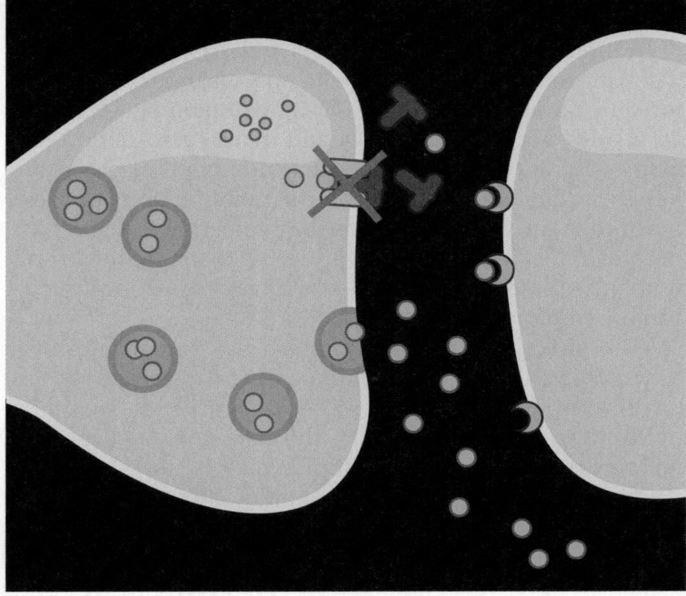

(b) An increase in neurotransmitters causes receptors to downregulate.

Figure 20–2 ■ Neurotransmitter receptor hypothesis of antidepressant action

There also remains the possibility that the defect resulting in depression may be a deficiency in downstream **signal transduction** of the neurotransmitter and the postsynaptic neuron. Therefore, the problem could be the result of disturbances in molecular events distal to the receptor, in the signal conduction cascade system, or in expression of the necessary functional genes in the postsynaptic neuron. The overall number of genes necessary for normal neuronal function appears to be less important than when, how often, and under what circumstances the genes are expressed and become operational (Stahl, 2008).

As an example, the target gene for brain-derived neutrophilic factor (**BDNF**) has been explored as the site for a flaw in signal transduction from the monoamine receptors. Normally, BDNF expression contributes to neuron survival but if repressed, cellular atrophy and the potential death of vulnerable cells in the hippocampus of the brain may occur. The loss of these cells is thought to produce depression, often with recurrent episodes that over time become less responsive to treatment. Data from clinical imaging studies have demonstrated the presence of decreased brain volume in related structures, thereby supporting the hypothesis that decreased size and impaired functionality of the hippocampal neurons may be present in patients suffering from depression and anxiety disorders. This is consistent with development of a pathology that occurs after the receptor and involves gene expression that is abnormal. As previously mentioned, neutrophilic factors like BDNF are essential for neuronal function and survival. Extreme stress is thought to increase vulnerability to depression by decreasing expression of the genes that code for these neutrophilic factors (Stahl, 2008).

The continuous development and exploration of the present hypotheses reflects our growing knowledge of the intricate mechanisms by which the brain functions. Studies of the overall impact of gene expression or repression on brain activity are increasing the knowledge base daily. The hypotheses put forth, while not biologically proven, have led to an increased understanding of the physiological activities of the three primary neurotransmitters. They have also provided the foundation for the growing body of research defining the various mechanisms by which all the psychotropic drugs in current clinical use act to improve neuronal activity.

Treatment of the Depressive Disorders

The use of antidepressant medication has increased in the adult population from 5.8% to10.12% over the past 10 years. This represents approximately 27 million people in the United States alone who take these medications daily. The lowest rates of use of antidepressants are found among African-American and Hispanic populations. The use of antipsychotic drugs also increased over the same time period, from 5.46% to 8.86% in the United States. Meanwhile, the use of psychotherapy declined from 31.5% to 19.87%, possibly due to the increased development and use of psychotropic medications (Lohoff, 2010; Mathers & Loncar, 2006).

Complaints of depressive symptoms are the third most common reason for visits to a doctor's office. Antidepressants

TABLE 20–1: The First Wave of Antidepressant Agents

Tricyclic Antidepressant Agents	MAO Inhibitor Antidepressants
■ Amitriptyline (Elavil®)	■ Phenelzine (Nardil®)
■ Clomipramine (Anafranil®)	■ Isocarboxazid (Marplan®)
■ Doxepin (Sinequan®)	■ Tranylcypromine (Parnate®)
■ Imipramine (Tofranil®)	
■ Nortriptyline (Pamelor®)	
■ Trazodone (Trittico®)	
■ Trimipramine (Surmontil®)	

are the third most common type of medication prescribed, with the selective serotonin reuptake inhibitors (**SSRI**) being most often chosen for use. There has also been increased utilization of the newer atypical antipsychotic medications as adjuncts to treatment of incomplete remission of depression and to control some aspects of the symptoms of bipolar disorder.

There have been three developmental "waves" of antidepressant medications. The first wave, in the 1950s, included the tricyclic antidepressant drugs and the MAO inhibitors. Tricyclic antidepressant agents act to prevent the reuptake of the neurotransmitter into the presynaptic neuron. Normally, reuptake of the transmitter allows excess transmitter to be replaced in presynaptic vesicles and released again when the neuronal membrane is depolarized. Reduction of reuptake leaves more neurotransmitter in the synapse, hypothetically decreasing receptor upregulation, improving overall conduction, and alleviating the symptoms of depression. Different members of the tricyclic antidepressant group affect the three primary neurotransmitters (norepinephrine, serotonin, and dopamine) individually, and often, collectively, to varying degrees. Representative tricyclic antidepressants are listed in Table 20–1.

Psychotropic medications as a group are not selectively active only in brain tissue. There are also symptoms associated with interactions in other peripheral tissues of the body. Side effects associated with tricyclic antidepressant drugs include orthostatic hypotension, tachycardia, and anticholinergic effects such as dry mouth, blurred vision, photophobia, constipation, urinary retention, cardiac toxicity, and sedation. These side effects most often become less over time but can be extremely problematic in the elderly or in individuals receiving other medications that have anticholinergic side effects, such as antihistamines or over-the-counter sleep aids. A number of tricyclic antidepressants are either inducers or inhibitors of the actions of the **cytochrome P450 enzymes** responsible for phase one metabolism of the antidepressants, as well as other drugs that are present. Enzyme induction or inhibition can produce unexpected and untoward drug interactions. The tricyclic antidepressants have, however, stood the test of time and continue to be used in specific situations, including treatment of chronic pain syndromes.

Monoamine oxidase inhibitors (**MAOI**) were developed during the same time period as the tricyclic antidepressants but possessed a different mechanism of action. MAOIs act to increase the amount of neurotransmitter at the synapse by inhibiting the activity of the enzyme, MAO, which is responsible for breaking down the excess neurotransmitters within the cell. Less breakdown allows for more buildup of the transmitter in the synapse, thereby improving depressive symptoms. Again, the peripheral effects produced by MAOIs were problematic. MAO exists in many areas of the body, most specifically of interest to this discussion, in the liver. In the liver, MAO functions to break down vasoactive amines ingested in food before they can reach the general circulation and have an effect on the blood pressure and other circulatory dynamics. The blockade of peripheral MAO activity in the liver by the MAOIs made it necessary for the patient to follow a diet that restricted a large number of foods rich in naturally occurring vasoactive amines. Certain drugs, such as meperidine and vasoconstrictive nasal sprays also had to be avoided. Failure to do so could result in development of a severe hypertensive crisis. Lack of patient compliance with these restrictions, as well as the development of agents with improved side effect profiles, have virtually negated the use of MAOIs in the treatment of depression, except in cases of atypical or refractory depression.

The second wave of antidepressant agents began with the development of the selective serotonin reuptake inhibitors (SSRI). These agents have a mechanism of action that targets and inhibits the reuptake of serotonin (5-HT) into the presynaptic neuron. The mechanism of action is similar to that of the tricyclic antidepressants but is more selective in largely impeding the reuptake of a single transmitter. Members of the SSRI group are listed in Table 20-2. The peripheral effects associated with these agents most often involve the gastrointestinal system. Other side effects associated with this group of drugs include somnolence or insomnia, initial agitation or nervousness, and sexual dysfunction. Most of these side effects diminish over time. In addition to the treatment of depression, several of the SSRI drugs are useful for treatment of other disorders such as obsessive-compulsive disorder (OCD), panic disorder, eating disorders, social phobia, and posttraumatic stress disorder (PTSD). The selectivity and overall positive therapeutic profile of these agents has made them the most prescribed antidepressants by today's clinician.

Development of the third wave of antidepressant drugs has revolved around selective combinations of transmitters to be affected by reuptake inhibition. The overall mechanism of action is the same as that of the SSRI drugs. These combination drugs are classified as serotonin norepinephrine reuptake inhibitors (**SNRI**) and norepinephrine dopamine reuptake inhibitors (**NDRI**). Examples of these drugs can be found in Table 20–2. Greater selectivity for effects in specific brain regions is possible with the use of these drugs and is reflective of our increasing knowledge of the function of these areas in the production of certain defined symptoms.

Antidepressants may be prescribed for patients with BPD when they are experiencing a phase of depression but great care must be taken to avoid producing mania as the depression improves. Most often patients with BPD are managed primarily with agents that are classified as mood stabilizers. The hallmark drug in this category is lithium. Other drugs used to treat BPD include anticonvulsant and antipsychotic agents.

While the mechanism of action of lithium is not fully understood, it has been postulated that it may act by reduction of catecholamine neurotransmitter concentration, or possibly by affecting the Na+ATPase pump, thereby improving membrane transport of Na+ ions. It is also thought that lithium may act at signal transduction sites beyond the receptors. A proposed example may be the ability of lithium to decrease the concentration of the second messenger, cyclic adenyl monophosphate (CAMP), which is responsible for controlling intracellular processes that determine cellular activity in response to a specific transmitter. Lithium is approved for use in both acute and maintenance management phases of mania. It can also be used as an adjunctive agent with an antidepressant for treatment of the BPD patient experiencing depression. Chronic use has been demonstrated to reduce overall suicide risk and mortality rates (Stahl, 2008). A disadvantage of lithium is its narrow therapeutic range. This narrow range creates a situation in which the therapeutically effective serum concentration is very close to the concentration at which toxicity begins to be present. The serum blood levels of lithium are carefully monitored in treated patients as are any other changes in drug therapies or coexisting diseases that might have an effect on the metabolism of lithium in the body. Side effects associated with lithium therapy include early dose–related effects such as gastrointestinal distress, weight gain, muscle weakness, sedation, polyuria, tremor, and impaired cognition. Late adverse effects include psoriasis, nephrogenic diabetes insipidus, hypothyroidism, cardiac conduction problems, and leukocytosis. Tolerance may develop to lithium, but approximately 70% of patients report a lessening of their mania when treated with this agent (Sadock & Sadock, 2007; Virana, Bezchlibnyk-Butler, & Jeffries, 2009).

TABLE 20–2: Representative Antidepressants That Have Greater Selectivity

The Second Wave of Antidepressant Agents	The Third Wave of Antidepressant Agents
Selective Serotonin Reuptake Inhibitors	Selective Serotonin Norepinephrine Reuptake Inhibitors
■ Fluoxetine (Prozac®)	■ Duloxetine (Cymbalta®)
■ Fluvoxamine (Lovox®)	■ Venlafaxine (Effexor®, Effexor XR®)
■ Paroxetine (Paxil®)	Selective Norepinephrine Dopamine Reuptake Inhibitors
■ Sertraline (Zoloft®)	■ Bupropion (Wellbutrin SR®)
■ Citalopram (Celexa®)	Mixed Serotonin-Norepinephrine Effects
■ Escitalopram (Lexapro®)	■ Mirtazapine (Mirtazon®, Remeron®, Remeron SolTab®)

There are a number of drugs that were originally developed for and continue to be utilized to control seizure activity that also have a role in the treatment of BPD. Valproate, carbamazepine, and lamotrigine are three of the anticonvulsant agents commonly used in the treatment of BPD. The mechanisms of action of the anticonvulsant drugs are multiple and not well understood. Among the hypotheses that have been offered for the activity of valproate and carbamazepine are the ability to inhibit voltage-sensitive sodium channels, increase the activity of the inhibitory neurotransmitter known as gamma-aminobutyric acid (**GABA**), or regulate the signal conduction cascades that are downstream from the receptors (Stahl, 2008). Lamotrigine is thought to perhaps reduce the release of the excitatory transmitter, glutamate. Anticonvulsants are often used as adjunctive medications if response to lithium alone has been poor. These agents may be effective in producing stabilization in both manic and depressive phases. As a class of drugs, the members of this group have the capacity to produce a large number of interactions with other drugs based upon their ability to either induce or inhibit the activity of the CYP450 enzymes responsible for phase one drug metabolism.

The antipsychotic agents, particularly the atypical agents developed in the 1990s, have a role in the management of acute mania with or without psychotic features and as adjunctive agents when antidepressant agents are unsuccessful in producing sufficient remission of the symptoms of MDD. The older typical antipsychotic agents act by blocking the dopamine$_2$ (D_2) receptor. Such blockade is a complex event and addresses only part of the dopamine dysfunction or imbalance thought to be causative of psychosis. The atypical antipsychotic agents act a bit more broadly through antagonism of both the D_2 and 5-HT$_2$a (serotonin) receptors. The atypical antipsychotic agents are preferred over the older typical antipsychotic agents primarily because of their improved side effect profile and greater patient tolerance. Although less likely to produce the neurological and extrapyramidal effects associated with the typical antipsychotic medications, the atypical drugs carry a greater risk of weight gain with subsequent development of the metabolic syndrome and diabetes mellitus Type 2 (Stahl, 2008). A list of these agents may be found in Table 20–3.

Another factor of importance in understanding the treatment of mood disorders is the role of pharmacogenetics. The word *pharmacogenetics* was first coined in 1959 and to define the factors in drug metabolism that were influenced by the specific genotypes of individuals (Weinshilboum & Wang, 2004).

TABLE 20–3: Representative Antipsychotic Medications

Typical or Conventional Agents	Atypical, Newer Agents
■ Chlorpromazine (Thorazine)	■ Quetiapine (Seroquel®)
■ Haloperidol (Haldol®)	■ Ziprasidone (Geodon)
■ Thioridazine (Melleril®)	■ Risperidone (Risperdal®)
■ Trifluoperazine (Stelazine®)	■ Olanzapine (Zyprexa®)
■ Thiothixene (Navane®)	■ Clozapine (Clozaril®)
	■ Aripiprazole (Abilify®)

Genetic variations that produce differences in protein expression affect the structure of receptors, transporters, and enzymes necessary for drug activity, metabolism, and clearance. The terms *pharmacogenetic* and *pharmacogenomics* are often used interchangeably. Both words refer to the study of how drug efficacy or tolerability can be changed due to the influence of genetic variability (Zandi & Judy, 2010).

Presently, it is estimated that 75%–98% of observed individual variability in drug-metabolizing enzyme activity is under genetic control. Some variations in drug-metabolizing enzymes are due to rare mutations while many other variations are common and polymorphic. The impact of genetic changes can result in several different scenarios. If changes in genetic coding result in a complete lack of the required enzyme for metabolism, increased plasma levels with a longer than expected duration of the drug may occur, potentially leading to toxicity. Other genetic coding changes may result in production of a partially functional enzyme such that metabolism occurs but with a much slower rate, thereby again producing a longer duration of drug activity. Finally, gene duplications may occur that lead to an increased metabolism with drug duration that may be so short as to negate any therapeutic effect. These processes are of great importance in the treatment of mood disorders because changes in the concentration, duration, and overall activity of psychotropic agents used in treatment are currently difficult, if not impossible, to ascertain prior to introduction of a specific drug. This creates a situation in which trials of several different drugs may be necessary to obtain the best therapeutic response. Prediction of response based upon genetic testing is in its infancy but is growing rapidly as a tool that clinicians may use to optimize drug choices. Only one pharmacogenetic test currently has approval by the Food and Drug Administration (FDA) for clinical use in psychiatry. The Roche Amplichip CYP450 test for CYP2D6 and CYP2C19 can predict phenotypes associated with specifically identified common alleles. Although the metabolism of at least 15 antidepressants and antipsychotic drugs are affected by these two common cytochrome enzymes (Mrazek, 2010), this diagnostic test was developed for global use in management of any of the drugs metabolized by CYP2D6 and/or CYP2C19 and is not specific for use only in psychiatry. The Evaluation of Genomic Applications in Practice and Prevention (EGAPP) panel was established by the Centers for Disease Control and Prevention in 2005 and charged to develop a process for assessing the overall validity and usefulness of genetic tests for clinical practice. The panel assessed all available evidence on the clinical use of CYP genotyping in the management of SSRI selection. The panel determined there was insufficient evidence to make a decision for or against clinical use of the tests, but, at present, the routine use of CYP testing in patients prior to beginning SSRI treatment is discouraged pending completion of further validating clinical trials (Zandi & Judy, 2010; Thakur, Grossman, McCrory, et al., 2007). Another factor delaying the addition of pharmacogenomic testing to psychiatric treatment algorithms is lack of information about cost effectiveness. Each CYP test currently costs approximately $300 to $500; however, over the past 5 years, pharmacogenomic testing costs have decreased substantially and are expected to continue to do so as utilization increases (Mrazek, 2010).

While CYP testing in psychiatry may not be commonly performed outside of academic and tertiary medical centers (Hall-Flavin, Schneekloth, & Allen, 2010), drug labels have long contained information about genomic biomarkers. Many psychiatric drug labels contain information pertaining to the effect of polymorphisms in *CYP450* genes on metabolism and duration of effect. It is hoped that eventually genetic profiles will be developed that will lead to simple tests capable of accurately and economically predicting a patient's response to different psychotropic drugs before they are begun. The eventual ability to utilize predictive genetic testing will contribute to the development of truly personalized medical care for patients in the future.

The use of psychotropic drugs has become a mainstay of therapy but there are also nonpharmacologic therapies that are effective and are often either used alone or in conjunction with drug therapy to treat mood disorders. Short-term psychosocial therapy approaches include cognitive therapy, interpersonal therapy, and behavioral therapy. These approaches assist the patient in dealing with cognitive distortions or specific interpersonal problems or behaviors associated with depression. Long-term psychoanalysis, while effective in treating depression, seeks to change a person's character or personality and foster the development of better coping skills and reality-based interpersonal relationships. Several years of therapy may be required to foster these changes. The cost of such long-term, expensive therapy limits the number of patients for whom this is an option.

SECTION TWO REVIEW

1. Neurotransmitters are initially released into the synaptic cleft as a result of
   A. presynaptic membrane depolarization causing release from storage vacuoles.
   B. postsynaptic membrane stimulation with increased vacuole storage.
   C. suppression of the reuptake pumps.
   D. stimulation from decreasing volume in the synaptic cleft.
2. Once released into the synaptic cleft, excess amounts of neurotransmitters may be taken back into the presynaptic neuron for reuse. This is accomplished by
   A. simple diffusion into the presynaptic neuron.
   B. the activity of COMT at the presynaptic neuron.
   C. the activity of MAO at the postsynaptic neuron.
   D. the activity of enzymatic transport pumps in the presynaptic membrane.
3. The neurotransmitter-receptor hypothesis of depression
   A. explains the side effects often observed with antidepressant medications.
   B. explains the longer time period needed for therapeutic effects to be observed in patients receiving antidepressant medications.
   C. states that the symptoms of depression may be related to the process of excessive downregulation of postsynaptic receptors.
   D. suggests that upstream signal transduction difficulties may be the cause of depression.
4. The action of antidepressant medications such as SSRI and tricyclic agents is based upon the ability of these drugs to
   A. increase the speed of reuptake of the transmitters into the presynaptic neuron.
   B. prevent the reuptake of neurotransmitter, thereby leaving more in the synaptic cleft.
   C. decrease the destruction of the transmitters by MAO.
   D. delay initial depolarization of the presynaptic neuron, thereby strengthening the impulse.
5. Chronic treatment of BPD patients with lithium has been shown to
   A. always result in tolerance that decreases effectiveness in controlling symptoms.
   B. always require the coadministration of antidepressants to control symptoms.
   C. reduce overall suicide and mortality rates.
   D. always require boosting with antipsychotic drugs to control manic episodes.

Answers: 1. A; 2. D; 3. B; 4. B; 5. C

SECTION THREE: The Genetics of Mood Disorders

In discussing the genetics/genomics of complex disorders, the concept of heritability, or the amount of variation for any given trait in a population that can be attributed to genetic influences must be determined. As an example, the heritability for major depression has been calculated at 38% with a 95% confidence interval of 31% to 42 % (Sullivan, Neale, & Kendler, 2000). There are variations in presentation that define particular presenting characteristics of MDD, such as early-onset, severe, and recurrent. When present, these characteristics are thought to be indicative of a higher degree of heritability than other presentations of depression (Belmaker & Agam, 2008). Ascertaining the degree of genetic susceptibility allows us to understand something about the potential for expression of the disorder but the actual symptoms that are observed presently form the basis for diagnosis and are the result of the individual's response to internal or external environmental stressors (Sullivan, Neale, & Kendler, 2000).

Genetic studies of mood disorders began more than 70 years ago. At that time these studies focused on identifying the concordance rates of incidence of these disorders between monozygotic (identical) twins and dizygotic (nonidentical) twins. This research path was chosen because familial aggregation was noted to be present in MDD. Evidence found indicated that the concordance rate for development of mood disorders in monozygotic (identical) twins was 70%–90%. In dizygotic (fraternal) twins the rate of concordance ranged from 16%–35% (Sadock & Sadock, 2007). When these early studies began, MDD and BPD were not segregated as separate disorders, which made the gathered data not as useful in estimating the importance of kinship in the development of each specific disorder (Lohoff & Berrettini, 2008). In more recent twin studies in which recurrent unipolar MDD alone was studied, the estimated heritability was found to be 37% with recognition that the role of environmental risk was unique to each individual. There is also a two- to fourfold increased risk of developing recurrent unipolar MDD in the first-degree relatives of an individual with this disorder (Sullivan, Neale, & Kendler, 2000). If MDD occurs early in life (before the age of 30) and there are a significant number of recurrences, then, the degree of a heritable phenotype appears to be greater.

MDD and BPD are complex disorders that develop in response to both genetic and environmental interactions. The research into these disorders is as complex as the spectrum of disorders themselves. Because a fairly high rate of heritability was demonstrated within families and in twin studies, it was hoped early on that one or a discrete number of causative genes could be identified. Unfortunately the presence of no single gene has proven sufficient to produce MDD. As many as 32 potential candidate genes have been identified at present. Complicating matters further, each of these genes may have several allelic forms located at the same loci on the chromosome. Each identified gene that might confer susceptibility to the disorder has been found to contribute varying small amounts to the overall genetic risk. Also, the great complexity of multiple, partially overlapping sets of susceptibility genes capable of interacting with the environment can predispose patients to other clinical syndromes with similar symptoms, thus complicating diagnosis. Gene localization and identification has proven to be a very laborious task, but even so, progress continues to be made. Some information that has been gained has current usefulness, but some of the information must wait for the growth of technology in order for full understanding of its importance to be realized.

Initial twin and family studies have given way to several other research approaches that take advantage of the rapid growth in genetic knowledge and techniques for exploration resulting from mapping of the human genome in 2003. Research into the genetics of MDD and BPD has been actively pursued, utilizing linkage studies, candidate gene studies, and genome-wide association studies.

Linkage Studies

Initial epidemiological evidence that was found in the earlier twin and family studies seemed to indicate the presence of a genetic component for MDD. Linkage studies have been useful in identifying genetic risk factors for some single gene disorders, so this approach was first utilized to search for specific candidate genes for the complex mood disorders. "Linkage" is defined as the observation that two genetic loci found close to each other on the same chromosome usually are inherited together in families at a rate greater than would be expected by chance. When this occurs, the two separate loci are considered to be linked. This technique is considered useful due to the thought that the parts of the chromosome harboring susceptibility genes for a disease, such as MDD, would be inherited within families at a rate greater than chance (Weissman et al., 1993; Lohoff, 2010).

Unfortunately, even though some of the resulting studies suggested areas of interest in the genome, most findings so far have been inconsistent. At present, no identified genetic risk factor or causative gene for MDD has been identified by this method. Linkage studies have pointed out the complexity of the genetic and environmental interactions responsible for the development of MDD and BPD. The mechanism of inheritance more than likely involves multiple genes, each contributing a small effect, which taken together with significant environmental stressors results in the development of MDD and/or BPD.

As an example, Holmans et al. (2004) reported on the first phase of a multisite collaborative study using a sample of 297 families. These families consisted of 685 affected relative pairs, 555 sibling pairs, and 130 other pair types. Families were excluded from the study if a first- or second-degree relative had BPD. Nonsex specific linkage was observed to be present on chromosome 15q. In a secondary analysis that took sex into account, linkage was found to be present on chromosomes 17p and 8p. Further mapping of the identified region on chromosome 15q produced more evidence of positive linkage (Holmans et al., 2004). Since often there are only a small number of participants from which data may be gathered, carrying out human research can be difficult. The data from this study were particularly robust due to the large number of participating subjects.

Other researchers have demonstrated linkage signals at chromosome 12q23 for MDD. This linkage site had previously been identified as important in the risk for BPD. The overlap in findings indicates that this locus probably increases risk for both BPD and MDD. (Abkevich et al., 2003) In another study that included subjects with early onset MDD, with and without the presence of anxiety, potential linkage was found on chromosomes 3centr, 7p, and 18q. The region on chromosome 18q that was identified in individuals with MDD and anxiety was already well known as a linkage finding in BPD. A recent genome-wide linkage scan of sibling pairs with recurrent MDD found suggestive evidence of linkage on chromosomes 1p36, 12q23.3-q24.11, and 13q31.1-q31.3. The chromosome 13 peak was previously linked strongly to panic disorder (McGuffin et al., 2005). Other genome-wide scans with different MDD populations have identified regions of linkage on chromosome 17 and chromosome 8. In a recent study (Breen et al., 2011), a locus associated with severe recurrent depression was identified at 3p.25-26. The emerging data from these and other ongoing studies have failed to identify a set of universally accepted risk genes for MDD. However, analysis of the ever increasing amount of data has provided insight into which regions of the genome might harbor the sought susceptibility genes.

Candidate Gene Studies

Several candidate genes have shown promise in having a role in the development of depression. Candidate gene studies are usually conducted using a case-control association study design. The basic premise in these association studies is that a specific genetic variant is looked for in a group of cases and a group of control subjects. By determining how frequently a specific variant allele is present when comparing the study cases to the control cases, the supposition can be tested that a selected genetic polymorphism is present more often in one group than the other. From this data, further research is developed based on the concept that the presence of a specific identified polymorphism either increases or decreases the risk for development of a specific phenotype, such as MDD or BPD.

For example, many antidepressant medications act on the serotonin transporter system at the synapse, so the gene (*SLC6A4*) that encodes the serotonin transporter as well as other genes involved in the serotonergic system has been implicated in MDD. A 44bp repeat polymorphism in the promoter region of the *5-HTTLPR* gene has been shown in laboratory experiments to have an effect on the expression of the serotonin transporter. Caspi et al. (2003) studied the *5-HTTLPR* polymorphism in a longitudinal birth cohort of 874 subjects. Analysis of the data collected indicated that the presence of a short allele variant for the transporter rather than the longer allele was associated with risk for MDD, depressive symptoms, and suicidality in subjects who suffered significant environmental stress. Earlier studies indicated that subjects with the longer polymorphic allele for the serotonin transporter were more responsive to treatment with SSRI drugs than those subjects possessing the shorter allele for the transporter. Presently, this polymorphism has been studied more than any other in psychiatric genetics, but unfortunately the results of these studies have produced both positive and negative findings for this effect (Lohoff, 2010).

Brain-derived neutrotrophic factor (BDNF), which is necessary for neurogenesis, has been found to be decreased in the hippocampus of chronically stressed animals (Roceri et al., 2004). In a previous animal study, the administration of an antidepressant drug resulted in an increase in hippocampal BDNF (Nibuya, Morinobu, & Duman, 1995). Although an association has been established between the Val66Met polymorphism in the *BDNF* gene and BPD, the results of research on the effect of this polymorphism on the risk for MDD have been mixed (Schumacher et al., 2005; Surtees et al., 2007). It is important to recognize that the Val66Met polymorphism represents only one small portion of the complex sequence of the *BDNF* gene. It is very possible that continuing research as well as the development of improved study techniques will reveal other variations in this gene that may influence susceptibility to depression (Hashimoto, 2010).

Tryptophan hydroxylase is an enzyme that controls the rate of production of serotonin in the brain. A brain specific gene for this enzyme, THP2, has been located on chromosome 12q. In previous linkage studies, this gene has been associated with increased risk for development of BPD. While no conclusive studies are available, some researchers have demonstrated an association of variants within the *THP2* gene with susceptibility for MDD (Zill et al., 2004). The presence of a functional Arg441His polymorphism in this gene has been shown to result in an 80% reduction in serotonin production in cell cultures. Although this is a rare mutation in humans, Zhang et al. (2005) found it to be present in 9 out of 87 subjects with MDD. Because serotonin is a major neurotransmitter of interest in the study of mood disorders, continued research into genetic causes of decreased serotonin synthesis may eventually reveal any number of variations in the *THP2* gene to be significant factors for unipolar depression.

Genome-Wide Association Studies

Advances in genetic technology have now made possible the genotyping of 500,000 to 1 million SNPs from across the genomes of affected and control groups of subjects. Although this is an expensive and complex process, **genome-wide association studies (GWAS)** GWAS allows the researchers to preselect the genes to be studied. Also, due to the large number of samples analyzed, the robust nature of the findings may predict and verify new avenues of study that will finally provide a conclusive understanding of the genetics factors leading to increased risk of mood disorder development.

While GWAS holds great promise, the five major GWAS dealing with depression that have been completed yielded negative or inconclusive results. Analysis of the data did suggest interesting candidate genes for further study but none of the findings reached genome-wide significance levels. Candidate genes of interest that were identified included 11 SNPs associated with MDD that overlapped the *PCLO* gene, a protein important in monoamine neurotransmission in the brain. Some evidence of association was observed on chromosome 18q22.1 in an area that was previously demonstrated to be linked to increased risk of development of BPD. Another identified SNP of interest in the *ATP6V1B2* gene was found to lie adjacent to the vesicular monoamine transporter gene (*VMAT1*), which had also been previously linked to BPD susceptibility (Sullivan et al., 2000; Lewis et al., 2010; Muglia et al., 2010; Shi et al., 2010; Shyn et al., 2009).

It seems clear that since individual genetic susceptibility factors probably contribute very small effects (Mitchell PB, Meiser B, Wilde A, et.al., 2010, Goldstein, 2009), analysis of very large pooled samples of affected subjects and controls will be necessary to identify and eventually get a cohesive picture of the many genetic players in increased susceptibility to mood disorders. As an example, using data from the largest GWAS study completed to date, a meta-analysis was completed by McMahon et al. (2010). GWAS data were analyzed from BPD and MDD cohorts totaling over 13,600 subjects. The analysis identified 6 SNPs at chromosome 3p21.1 associated with major mood disorders. Considering the population from which the samples were gathered, this finding demonstrates the probability of a shared genetic susceptibility locus at this site for both BPD and MDD. This again points out the great complexity and difficulty in teasing out specific causative genes for the individual mood disorders as they are defined by current diagnostic criteria.

Even though significant research efforts continue and the robustness of the data continue to be enhanced by the use of meta-analysis techniques across multiple data sets, no strong susceptibility gene or set of genetic markers for MDD has yet to be identified. More than 50 studies on BPD have also been completed but few significant results have yet emerged. It is important to remember that genetics is only one aspect of the complex interactions causative of the mood disorders. Well-being or mental illnesses are states that are representative of the sum of all the complex interactions, both internal and external, that make up an individual's life experiences.

Factors that produce difficulties in finding common gene variants with large effects on the development of mood disorders include the overall complexity of the presenting phenotypes, generally smaller study cohorts, an overall inability to replicate findings, and difficulty in being able to fully quantify the impact of lifestyle and environmental stressors on mood disorder development. In spite of these problems, genetic research in the mood disorders, as well as in other complex psychiatric illnesses, is growing rapidly. New technologies, such as whole genome sequencing, hold promise for the development of the large scale studies that will be required to understand the role of genetic factors in the development of complex diseases such as MDD and/or BPD.

SECTION THREE REVIEW

1. The symptoms of major depression are the result of
   A. the presence of increased genetic susceptibility.
   B. response to internal and external environmental stresses.
   C. inherited personality disorders and lack of discipline.
   D. Both A and B
2. Susceptibility genes for development of mood disorders have been found to
   A. be numerous, with each contributing small amounts to overall risk.
   B. be present in only a limited number of chromosomes.
   C. not aggregate in families.
   D. be predictive of disease onset.
3. The degree of heritability of MDD appears to be greatly increased if
   A. there is no identified relative with MDD in the previous generation.
   B. there has been a suicide attempt by the patient.
   C. there is early onset with a number of recurrences.
   D. there is very late onset with dementia.
4. The portions of chromosomes containing susceptibility genes for MDs are thought to be heritable at a rate greater than chance. Completed linkage studies that identify these areas of "linkage" have
   A. allowed identification of specific causative genes for MDD.
   B. isolated a number of genes that make small contributions to overall effect in MDD development.
   C. established MDD as due to inheritance of a dominant gene with 100% penetrance.
   D. failed to demonstrate any heritable linkage sites for MDD.
5. It appears that analysis of very large pooled samples of affected subjects and controls will be necessary to identify fully the role of genetics in the development of mood disorders. This may best be achieved by the use of
   A. analysis of individual family histories.
   B. primary linkage studies.
   C. GWAS and whole genome sequencing.
   D. continued twin studies.

Answers: 1. D; 2. A; 3. C; 4. B; 5. C

SECTION FOUR: Incorporating Genetics into the Care of Patients with Mood Disorders

Currently there are no definitive genomic tests for diagnosis of specific mood disorders, and the use of pharmacogenomic testing for medication management is not common practice in most clinical psychiatric settings. The role of the nurse incorporating genetic concepts into the care of psychiatric patients includes assessment, education, and counseling about both current and future possibilities that genomic research may provide for understanding the pathology, heritability, and treatment of mood disorders.

Nurses have a professional responsibility to develop self-awareness regarding their own personal values and feelings, as well as those of the patients they encounter, about mental disorders and the role that developing genetic science may have in identifying those at risk. Educating patients and the public to the incidence of mood disorders as complex diseases, not character or personality defects remains an important goal. The education of patients and the public at large requires tailoring information on genetics within the reality of specific mood disorders with regard for differences in culture, religion, level of literacy, preexisting knowledge and beliefs, and individual language use.

Given the heritability of mood disorders, an important skill for the nurse to develop is the ability to adequately assess patients to identify those at risk. This requires that the nurse elicit, at a minimum, a three-generation family history from which a pedigree chart can be drawn. Information gathered about each relative should include any history of psychiatric illness, significant medical illnesses, mental retardation, or developmental delays. For each relative that is identified as having had a mood disorder, it is important to record the age of onset, the level and duration of functional impairment, any history of admission to a psychiatric hospital, and any suicide attempts that were made (Finn & Smaller, 2006).

While conducting an assessment, the nurse should continuously analyze gained information for potential genetic or environmental influences that may indicate increased risk of development of a mood disorder. It is also important to be able to recognize the symptoms of depression that are associated with the presence of a chronic illness or that develop following a major illness or surgery. As an example, it is estimated that upwards of 30% of patients experience some degree of depression following coronary artery bypass graft surgery. These patients have been shown to benefit from the act of the nurse recognizing their depression and helping them to understand and reframe their interpretations of the events that have transpired and what will happen during recovery and healing (Martin, 2006). If the symptoms of depression are severe, early recognition and reporting by the nurse allows treatment to be begun quickly.

Educational efforts and active advocacy are important to increase individual and public understanding of the scope and importance of mood disorders. As genetic testing for risk assessment and medication management becomes more available, the nurse should strive to be sufficiently knowledgeable to identify patients who would benefit from genetic testing and to complete the appropriate referral process for further testing, diagnosis, or treatment. At present, the role of a physician geneticist, genetic counselor, or a well-prepared nurse is primarily concerned with educating the patient about the importance of known genetic factors, such as some single gene and chromosomal abnormalities in the development of certain psychiatric disorders, in estimating the recurrence risk of a specific psychiatric disorder based on the family history, and in discussing the complex nature of the genetics of mood disorders.

Although not specific solely to psychiatric genetics, it is important for the nurse to always be aware that genetic information may predict the future health of the patient and that there may be serious psychosocial consequences to learning genomic information. Such information has importance, not only to the individual patient with a mood disorder, but also to his family members. Being given genetic information that may impact future health can produce emotions such as relief, a sense of reduced uncertainty, and an improved ability to plan for the future. It can also result in anxiety, embarrassment, increasing depression, and a sense of hopelessness. Recognition of these emotions and provision of support and appropriate counseling are important nursing actions (Hoop, 2008).

Because the development of mood disorders is the result of the interaction of susceptibility genes with environmental stressors, the nurse should assist the patient to understand and make effective lifestyle changes to decrease the likelihood of disease development. At present we cannot change the patient's genome, but the environmental factors that would produce expression of those genes, thereby leading to development of a mood disorder, may be controllable with knowledge and support. The role of the nurse in health promotion is to educate and motivate, as well as to develop interventions that will equip the patient with the necessary skills and support to institute changes in behavior (Wood, 2008). Health promotion and wellness techniques that promote stress reduction have proven effective in assisting patients deal with the symptoms of mood disorders. At this individual level, interventions should be planned that enhance self-esteem, develop social and coping skills, and increase resourcefulness (Naido & Wills, 2000). The nurse should also focus on the development and provision of interventions for patients at risk that lead to increased social and community participation and that emphasize the individual's ability to positively deal with issues affecting health. The role of the nurse in active advocacy at the societal level includes seeking active participation in the development of institutional, local, and/or national mental health policy designed to reduce inequality and discrimination in access to education for the public about the genetic basis of psychiatric disorders, the availability and usefulness of genetic testing and genetic counseling for individuals at risk, and the need to provide adequate care and treatment for patients suffering from mood disorders (Friedli, 2000). There is also a continuing need to advocate for the right of each individual to receive sufficient education in order to be able to make an informed decision regarding the use of genetic testing for diagnosis, risk assessment, and/or treatment.

SECTION FOUR REVIEW

1. Genetic counselors asked to assess individuals with Mood Disorders will
   A. explain the results of genetic screening tests for the specific disorder to the patient.
   B. discuss appropriate treatment of the specific disorder.
   C. estimate the rate of recurrence using the family history.
   D. counsel the individual about not having children due to the heritability of Mood Disorders.
2. Some degree of depression is estimated to be present in ______ of patient following coronary artery bypass graft procedures.
   A. 10%
   B. 30%
   C. 60%
   D. 75%
3. In order to be effective in educating patients with Mood Disorders, the nurse must
   A. be aware of cultural and language differences that may be present.
   B. be aware of any preexisting knowledge the patient may have.
   C. respect religious beliefs the patient may hold.
   D. All of the above
4. The most important tool the nurse may have in assessing a patient for the risk of development of a Mood Disorder is
   A. a completed three-generation pedigree chart.
   B. a written mood assessment survey completed by the patient.
   C. genetic screening tests for chromosomal defects.
   D. early immunization records.

Answers: 1. C; 2. B; 3. D; 4. A

POSTTEST

1. You are considering referral of a patient diagnosed with MDD to a genetic counselor. You expect that the counselor would
   A. estimate the risk of recurrence by evaluation of the family history.
   B. test the patient for specific chromosomal abnormalities known to be associated with psychiatric disorders.
   C. discourage the patient from having children due to the heritability of MDD.
   D. suggest testing of all offspring for MDD risk factors.
2. MDD is unipolar because
   A. the mood is consistently depressed with lack of interest in the events of daily living for more than 2 weeks.
   B. mania is present only once every few months.
   C. hypomania is present but insufficient to meet the criteria for mania.
   D. there is no improvement following treatment with an antidepressant agent.
3. Mood disorders are currently diagnosed using
   A. genetic screening laboratory tests for chromosomal abnormalities.
   B. symptomatic description in the *DSM-IV-TR*.
   C. response to trial administration of antidepressant medications.
   D. by SPECT or PET scanning of the hippocampus.
4. All current pharmacologic treatments for mood disorders are predicated on
   A. modification of the amount of functional neurotransmitter in the neuronal synapse.
   B. producing hyperpolarization of the presynaptic membrane.
   C. expression of genes responsible for appropriate protein synthesis at the synapse.
   D. presence of specific genetic polymorphisms that enhance drug activity.
5. Your assessment of the patient indicates that he most likely has MDD. This disorder is the result of
   A. clearly identified patterns of inheritance from his parents.
   B. decreased neurotransmitter at the synapse with resultant upregulation of receptors.
   C. downregulation of postsynaptic receptors due to excess neurotransmitter.
   D. overactive transporter systems at the postsynaptic membrane.
6. The heritability of MDD is estimated to be _____ in the general population.
   A. 75%
   B. 68%
   C. 45%
   D. 38%
7. The primary reason for the use of twins to study the rate of incidence of MDD is
   A. twin pairs have a higher incidence of MDD overall.
   B. BPD-I is more common in twin pairs.
   C. study of concordance rates for MDD in twins is useful in establishing incidence because of the presence of familial aggregation.
   D. they are more likely to have variant alleles for MDD.
8. The results of linkage studies, candidate gene studies, and GWAS have
   A. identified important genes that are major contributors to the development of MDD.
   B. confirmed our understanding that there are multiple genes making small individual contributions to susceptibility for MDD.
   C. allowed development of improved treatment modalities for MDD.
   D. produced selective genetic tests for specific types of Mood Disorders.

9. Mood Disorders are complex diseases that are the result of
   A. interaction of susceptibility genes with environmental stressors.
   B. inherited personality traits.
   C. modification of personality due to genetic mutations.
   D. consanguinity with resultant genetic mutation.
10. During the nurse's assessment, the patient states, "You know I have MDD so I guess I just got lousy genes from my mom, who also had MDD." Which of the following actions by the nurse would be most appropriate at this time?
   A. Immediately referring of the patient to a genetic counselor
   B. Discussing the role of stress in development of MDD and assisting the patient to identify stress reduction techniques
   C. Agreeing that genetics can be a problem and suggesting an antidepressant
   D. Recommending discussion of his feelings about his illness with a counselor or minister.

Posttest answers are located in the Appendix.

CHAPTER SUMMARY

Mood disorders are pervasive, complex pathologies that are perhaps the most common psychiatric conditions affecting the lives of humans across the entire lifespan. As complex diseases, the mood disorders are recognized to be the result of genetic susceptibility plus the individual's response to both internal and external environmental stressors. Genetic susceptibility for mood disorder development appears to be conferred by the expression of a number of genes, each contributing in varying small amounts to the overall risk. At present we cannot change an individual's genotype, but identification and verification of the total genetic contribution predisposing humans to the mood disorders would enable better risk assessment, diagnosis, and development of more effective preventative interventions, treatment therapies, and medications.

- Currently, Mood Disorders are diagnosed utilizing recognized symptoms codified in the *DSM-IV-TR*. No specific genetics tests are available for definitive diagnosis of mood disorders.
- Presynaptic neuronal imbalance of neurotransmitters leading to postsynaptic neuronal changes in receptor density is hypothesized to be a pathological mechanism in the development of mood disorders. Much of pharmacologic treatment for mood disorder is predicated on modification of the amount of neurotransmitters present and/or efficiency of transmission in affected areas of the brain.
- Linkage studies, candidate gene studies, and GWAS have led to the identification of at least 32 potential candidate genes that increase susceptibility to development of mood disorders. Each identified gene contributes varying small amounts to the overall genetic risk for mood disorders.
- At present there are no specific genetics tests for identifying absolute risk, exact inheritance patterns, or diagnosis of specific mood disorders. The data gathered so far have provided valuable insight into where in the genome susceptibility genes might be found.
- Pharmacogenetic testing for drug management in psychiatry is currently in its infancy and, at present, is not common in general psychiatric practice.
- New and developing technologies such as GWAS and whole genome sequencing are capable of selection and analysis of millions of polymorphic alleles at a time. The ability to analyze such large amounts of data may, in the near future, provide conclusive evidence of the role of specific genetic factors in the development of the mood disorders.

CRITICAL THINKING CHECKPOINT

Mr. RS, a 24-year-old college student, was found walking on the freeway, shouting obscenities at the oncoming traffic. He is agitated and states "Leave me alone, I am the perfect physical specimen." His mother and wife arrive as you are completing your assessment. His mother states that he has been taking lithium carbonate 600 mg t.i.d. for Bipolar Disorder II for the past 6 years, with good results until several weeks ago. His wife reports that he has been "up all night" for the past few days and has a "harebrained scheme to win the Nobel Prize". RS's mother reveals that she suffers from chronic depression and that she is worried because RS and his wife are expecting their first child in a few weeks. She says, "I know we just have bad genes but is there anything that can be done to make sure my grandchild will not be born with bipolar disorder?"

1. Is family history important in this situation?
2. What are the risk factors for development of Bipolar Disorder in the baby?
3. What is the role of the nurse in education of the patient and family about the etiology and management of bipolar disorder?
4. What interventions might the nurse consider to assist this patient and his family to cope with his bipolar disorder?

Answers are provided in the Appendix

Pearson Nursing Student Resources

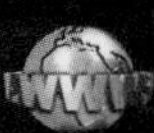

Find additional review materials at nursing.pearsonhighered.com

Prepare for success with additional NCLEX®-style practice questions, interactive assignments and activities, web links, animations, videos, and more!

REFERENCES

Abkevich V., Camp, N. J., Hensel, C. H., Neff, C. D., Russell, D. L., Hughes, D. C., et al. (2003). Predisposition locus for major depression at chromosome 12q22-12q23.2. *American Journal of Human Genetics*, 73, 1271–1281.

American Psychological Association. (2000). *Diagnostic and statistical manual of mental disorders* (4th ed., text rev.). Washington, DC: Author.

Belmaker, R. H., & Agam, G. (2008). Major depressive disorder. *New England Journal of Medicine*, 358(1), 55–68.

Breen, G., Upmanyu, R., Webb, B. T., Craig, I., Butler, A. W., Lewis, C. M., et al. (2011). A genome-wide significant linkage for severe depression on chromosome 3: The depression network study. *American Journal of Psychiatry, 168*, 840–847.

Caspi, A., Sugden, K., Moffitt, T. E., Taylor, A., Craig, I. W., Harrington, H., et al. (2003). Influence of life stress on depression: moderation by a polymorphism in the 5-HTT gene. *Science, 301*, 386–389.

Evaluation of Genomic Applications in Practice and Prevention (EGAPP) Working Group. (2007). Recommendations from the EGAPP Working Group: Testing for cytochrome P450 polymorphisms in adults with nonpsychotic depression treated with selective serotonin reuptake inhibitors. *Genetic Medicine, 9*, 819–825.

Finn, C. T., & Smaller, J. W. (2006). Genetic counseling in psychiatry. *The Harvard Review of Psychiatry, 14*, 109–121.

Friedli, L. (2000). From the margins to the mainstream: The public health potential of mental health promotion - what works? In M. Murray, & C. Reed (Eds.), *Promotion of Mental Health*. Aldershot, UK: Ashgate, p. 77–88.

Goldstein, D. B. (2009). Common genetic variation and human traits. *New England Journal of Medicine, 360*(17), 1696–1698.

Hall-Flavin, D. K., Schneekloth, T. D., & Allen, J. D. (2010). Translational psychiatry: Bringing pharmacogenomic testing into clinical practice. *Primary Psychiatry, 17*(5), 39–44.

Hashimoto, K. U. (2010). Brain-derived neutrotrophic factor as a biomarker for mood disorders: An historical overview and future directions. *Psychiatry and Clinical Neurosciences, 64*, 341–357.

Holmans, P., Zubenko, G. S., Crowe, R. R., DePaulo, J. R., Jr., Scheftner, W. A., Weissman, M. M., et al. (2004). Genome-wide significant linkage to recurrent, early-onset major depressive disorder on chromosome 15q. *American Journal of Human Genetics. 74*, 1154–1167.

Hoop, J. G. (2008). Ethical considerations in psychiatric genetics. *Harvard Review of Psychiatry. 16*, 322–338.

Kessler. R. C., Chiu, W. T., Demler, O., Merikanga, K. R., & Walter, E. E. (2005). Prevalence, severity, and co-morbidity of 12-month DSM-IV disorders in the National Co-morbidity Survey Replication. *Archives of General Psychiatry, 62*, 617–627.

Lewis, C. M., Ng, M. Y., Butler, A. W., Cohen-Woods, S., Uhu, R., Pirlo, K., et al. (2010). Genome-wide association study of major recurrent depression in the U.K. population. *American Journal of Psychiatry, 167*, 949–957.

Lohoff, F. W., & Berrettini, W. H. (2008). Genetics of mood disorders. In D. S. Charney (Ed.), *Neurobiology of mental illness*. New York: Oxford University Press, p. 1504.

Martin, F. (2006). Recognizing depression after coronary artery bypass graft. *British Journal of Nursing, 15*(13), 703–706.

Mathers, C., & Loncar, D. (2006). Projections of global mortality and burden of disease from 2002 to 2030. *PLOS Medicine, 3*, 2011–2030.

McGuffin, P., Knight, J., Breen, G., Brewster, S., Boyd, P. R., Craddock, N., et al. (2005). Whole genome linkage scan of recurrent depressive disorder from the Depression Network Study. *Human Molecular Genetics, 14*, 3337–3345.

McMahon, F. J., Akula, N., Schulze, T. G., Mugha, P., Tozzi, F., Detera-Wadleigh, S. D., et al. (2010). Bipolar Disorder Genome Study (BiGS) Consortium: Meta-analysis of genome-wide data identified a risk locus for major mood disorders on 3p21.1. *Nature Genetics, 42*, 128–131.

Mitchell, P. B., Meiser, B., Wilde, A., Fullerton, J., Donald, J., Wilhelm, K., et al. (2010). Predictive and diagnostic genetic testing in psychiatry. *Psychiatric Clinics of North America, 33*, 225–243.

Mrazek, D. A. (2010). Individualized molecular psychiatry. *Primary Psychiatry, 17*(5), 29–30.

Muglia, P., Tozzi, F., Galwey, N. W., Francks, C., Upmanyu, R., Kong, X. Q., et al. (2010). Genome-wide association study of recurrent major depressive disorder in two European case-control cohorts. *Molecular Psychiatry, 15*, 589–601.

Naido, J., & Wills, J. (2000). *Health promotion: Foundations for practice*. Edinburgh: Bailliero Tindall.

Nibuya, M., Morinobu, S., & Duman, R. S. (1995). Regulation of BDNF and trk B mRNA in rat brain by chronic electroconvulsive seizure and antidepressant drug treatments. *Journal of Neuroscience,15*, 7539–7547.

Roceri, M., Cirulli, F., Pessina, C., Peretto, P., Racagni, G., & Riva, M. A. (2004). Postnatal repeated maternal deprivation produces age-dependent changes in brain-derived neutrotrophic factor expression in selected rat brain regions. *Biological Psychiatry, 55,* 708–714.

Sadock, B. J., & Sadock, V. A. (2007). *Kaplan and Sadock's synopsis of psychiatry* (10th ed.). Lippincott Williams and Wilkins: Philadelphia, PA, pp. 527–569.

Schumacher, J., Jamva, R. A., Becker, T., Ohlraun, S., Klopp, N., Binder, E. B., et al. (2005). Evidence for a relationship between gene variants at the brain-derived neutrotrophic factor (BDNF) locus and major depression. *Biological Psychiatry, 58,* 307–314.

Shi, J., Potash, J. B., Knowles, J. A., Weissman, M. M., Coryell, W., Scheftner, W. A., et al. (2010). Genome-wide association study of recurrent early-onset major depressive disorder. *Molecular Psychiatry, 16*(2), 193–201.

Shyn, S. J., Shi, J., Kraft, J. B., Potash, J. B., Knowles, J. A., Weissman, M. M., et al. (2009). Novel loci for major depression identified by genome-wide association study of sequenced treatment alternatives to relieve depression and meta-analysis of three studies. *Molecular Psychiatry, 16*(2), 202–215.

Stahl, S. M. (2008). *Stahl's essential psychopharmacology: Neuroscientific basis and practical applications* (3rd ed.). Cambridge University Press: New York, NY, pp. 51–90, 453–720.

Sullivan, P. F., Neale, M. C., & Kendler, K. S. (2000) Genetic epidemiology of major depression: Review and meta-analysis. *American Journal of Psychiatry, 157,* 1552–1562.

Sullivan, P. F., deGeus, E. J., Willemsen, G., James, M. R., Smit, J. H., Zandbelt, T., et al. (2000). Genome-wide association for major depressive disorder: A possible role for the presynaptic protein piccolo. *Molecular Psychiatry, 14,* 359–375.

Surtees, P. G., Wainswright, N. W., Willis-Owen, S. A., Sandhu, M. S., Luben, R., Day, N. E., & Flint, J. (2007). No association between the BDNF Val66Met polymorphisms and mood status in a non-clinical community sample of 7389 older adults. *Journal of. Psychiatric Research, 41,* 404–409.

Thakur, M., Grossman, I., McCrory, D. C., et al. (2007). Review of evidence for genetic testing for CYP450 polymorphisms in management of patients with nonpsychotic depression with selective serotonin reuptake inhibitors. *Genetic Medicine, 9,* 826–835.

Tsuang, M. T., Taylor, L., & Faraone, S. V. (2004). An overview of the genetics of psychotic mood disorders. *Journal of Psychiatric Research, 38,* 3–15.

Virani, A. S., Bezchlibnyk-Butler, K. Z., & Jeffries, J. J. (2009). *Clinical handbook of psychotropic drugs* (18th ed.). Ashland, OH: Hogrefe and Huber Publishers, pp. 186–214.

Weinshilboum, R., & Wang, L. (2004). Pharmacogenomics: Bench to bedside. *National Review of Drug Discovery, 3,* 739–748.

Weissman, M. M., Wickramaratne, P., Adams, P. B., Lish, J. D., Horwath, E., Charney, D., et al. (1993). The relationship between panic disorder and major depression. A new family study. *Archives of General Psychiatry, 50,* 767–780.

Wood, S. (2008). The contribution of nursing to public health practice in the prevention of depression. *Nursing and Health Science, 10,* 241–247.

Zandi, P. P., & Judy, J. T. (2010). The promise and reality of pharmacogenetics in psychiatry. *Psychiatric Clinics of North America, 33,* 181–224.

Zhang, X., Gainetdinov, R. R., Beaulieu, J. M., Sotnikova, T. D., Burch, L. H., Williams, R. B., et al. (2005). Loss of function mutations in tryptophan hydroxylase-2 identified in unipolar major depression. *Neuron, 45,* 11–16.

Zill, P., Baghai, T. C., Zwanzger, P., Schüle, C., Eser, D., Rupprecht, R., et al. (2004). SNP and haplotype analysis of a novel tryptophan hydroxylase isofrom (TPH2) gene provides evidence for association with major depression. *Molecular Psychiatry, 9,* 1030–1036.

CHAPTER

21 Addictive Behaviors and Genetic Linkages

Eileen Trigoboff

LEARNING OUTCOMES

Following the completion of this chapter, the learner will be able to

1. Classify genetic factors considered contributory to inherited addictive behaviors.
2. Integrate the implications of clinical interviews in testing and screening for clients and their families.
3. Evaluate the diagnostic procedures used to identify substance dependence disorders.
4. Illustrate how genetic linkages are reported to be involved in addictive behaviors in the literature.
5. Design an informational plan for a client and involved family about genetic implications of substance disorders.

This chapter discusses the relationship between certain genetic variables and the behaviors involved in substance dependence and addictive behaviors. It defines substance abuse and intoxication, as well as what substance dependence and substance withdrawal means. It also covers the genetic links to substance issues available to date. In addition, this chapter examines the practical application of the genetic information we have thus far, and incorporates genetics into treatment for substance disorders. Finally, this chapter looks at the implications for nursing interventions and what direction nurses can take in the future.

PRETEST

1. In assessing a client for a substance related disorder, a nurse would
   A. consider only possible use of illegal substances.
   B. assess the client for medication-related side effects.
   C. assess the client for toxin exposure only if there is no close relative who also has a diagnosed substance use disorder.
   D. assess the client for tolerance only if substances were used in the immediately preceding 24 hours.
2. People who are drug dependent
   A. do not recognize costs of the dependency.
   B. are often able to stop using on their own.
   C. keep using despite recognizing associated difficulties and costs.
   D. often have no specific associated behavior or cognitive disturbances or decline.
3. If a person is alcohol dependent
   A. this can change the genotype of the alcohol-dependent person.
   B. it is possible that the genotype has rendered him or her vulnerable to alcoholism.
   C. he or she is not likely to have relatives with alcohol problems.
   D. it is certain that if an alcohol-dependent person has children, those children will have problems with alcohol.
4. Genetics associated with alcohol problems are
   A. simple.
   B. completely understood.
   C. always going to involve specific genetic variations on one part of the genome.
   D. complex.
5. Substance abuse results from
   A. nature.
   B. nurture.
   C. nature, nurture, and genetic modifications due to substance ingestion.
   D. nature and nurture.
6. If a person has a genetic predisposition to substance dependency
   A. no interventions will prevent full expression of vulnerability.
   B. only medications will prevent full expression of vulnerability.

C. an array of psychotherapies can prevent full expression of vulnerability.
D. he or she will manifest specific intoxication and withdrawal symptoms.

7. Findings of genetics studies of substance abuse and dependence
   A. can influence pharmacological and behavioral interventions.
   B. can influence only pharmacological interventions.
   C. can influence only behavioral interventions.
   D. improve our understanding of heritability of these problems but are not relevant to treatment.
8. Defining phenotypes is
   A. not helpful for treatment.
   B. helpful for treatment.
   C. unrelated to assessing the client's metabolic functioning.
   D. helpful when considering the client's possible responses to psychotropic prescribed medication only.
9. Genetic research
   A. has helped to develop pharmacologic treatments for some substance-related disorders.
   B. has helped to develop pharmacologic treatments for all substance-related disorders.
   C. has helped to develop pharmacologic treatments for substance-related disorders associated only with single nucleotide polymorphisms.
   D. has helped to develop pharmacologic treatments for substance-related disorders associated only with variations in the GABA receptor gene.
10. If a client has a blood relative who is alcohol dependent
    A. the client has no presumed genetic predisposition to alcoholism.
    B. the client will develop alcoholism.
    C. the client will be relatively less likely to have medication side effects.
    D. there is a presumed genetic predisposition to alcoholism.

Pretest answers are located in the Appendix.

SECTION ONE: Behaviors Related to Substance Abuse and Dependence

According to the *DSM-IV-TR* (American Psychiatric Association [APA], 2000), substance-related disorders result from abusing a drug (such as alcohol), are side effects of a medication (such as antihistamines), or are related to being exposed to a toxin (such as fuel). Substance-related disorders are divided into the following two groups:

1. Substance use disorders, including substance dependence and substance abuse
2. Substance-induced disorders, including substance intoxication and substance withdrawal as well as other substance-induced disorders such as substance-induced cognitive disorders and mood disorders

The definition of **substance abuse** is repeated use of substances that is maladaptive in that significant adverse consequences occur. Examples include recurrent social and relationship problems. **Substance dependence** is a maladaptive pattern of substance use leading to clinically significant impairment or distress. The hallmarks of this pattern are as follows:

- Tolerance—the state of needing increased amounts of a substance to achieve its desired effect
- **Withdrawal**—the uncomfortable physiological and cognitive behavioral changes associated with lowered blood or tissue concentrations of a substance after an individual has been a heavy user

When people depend on substances, they display these common characteristics—the compulsive use of that substance and unsuccessful efforts to cut down or schedule their use. Someone with this problem spends a great deal of time trying to obtain the substance and either use it or recover from its effects. Dependence involves continuing to use the substance despite the recognition that there are difficulties and costs (physical, financial, and emotional).

Substance intoxication refers to a reversible syndrome of maladaptive physiologic and behavioral changes from the effects of a substance on a person's central nervous system (CNS). Intoxication includes disturbances of mood (such as belligerence), perception, the sleep–wake cycle, attention, thinking, judgment, and psychomotor as well as interpersonal behavior.

Substance withdrawal involves developing maladaptive physiological, behavioral, and cognitive changes as a result of reducing or stopping the heavy and regular use of a substance.

SECTION ONE REVIEW

1. A substance-related disorder can result from all of the following, EXCEPT
   A. abusing a drug such as hydrocodone.
   B. dose alterations such as using prescription strength of a medication alternating with over-the-counter strength.
   C. being exposed to a toxic chemical such as monomethyl hydrazine, which is found in false morels.
   D. experiencing side effects of a medication such as an anticonvulasant.
2. Substance-use disorders include substance-induced cognitive disorders and mood disorders.
   A. True
   B. False
3. When problematic physical changes occur when a substance is reduced or stopped, it is called
   A. heavy and regular use of a substance.
   B. maladaptive physiological changes.
   C. withdrawal.
   D. tolerance.
4. Which of the following are the typical sequelae of repeated substance use?
   A. Recurrent social and relationship problems
   B. Immediate and delayed physiological impacts
   C. Otherwise unexplained changes in academic performance
   D. Changes in occupational and vocational experiences
   E. All of the above
5. Needing increased amounts of a substance in order to obtain euphoria is called
   A. intoxication.
   B. substance dependence.
   C. substance abuse.
   D. tolerance.

Answers: 1. B; 2. A; 3. C; 4. D; 5. D

SECTION TWO: Genetic Links to Substance Issues

When someone uses substances to the point of dependence, it is sufficient to diagnose and to treat simply the behavior of substance dependence. The genetic underpinnings of substance issues have only recently become an active therapeutic concern. The thinking became, "If we knew whether someone had a chromosome or gene that created a vulnerability to abusing a substance, or interfered with that individual developing the skills to reduce or eliminate the problem, then we could make use of that information in treatment." This is a fairly new posture in the science of treating people with substance dependence.

Further genetic information about a potential vulnerability could be used to predict substance-using behavior and therefore anticipate, and possibly prevent, the clinical issue of substance dependence. Keeping in mind that drug abuse is a complex set of behaviors; the likelihood that there would be a simple, single genetic explanation is remote. Our current level of useful information in this regard is low; however, it is growing in a meaningful way.

One of the pressing clinical issues around substance abuse and substance dependence is whether there is genetic evidence for pathology with the most common substance of abuse—alcohol. Can genetics dictate alcohol consumption as well as alcohol problems? Is the genetics explanation simple or complex? The answers have implications for future generations and can guide clinical psychopharmacological practice.

Kimura and Higuchi's study (2011) continues a growing search into the genetic factors that play an important role in the pathogenesis of alcohol dependence. We know from a number of twin studies, family research, and adoption studies with alcohol abuse that genetic factors play a role, in addition to behavioral learning (Agrawal, Lynskey, Heath, & Chassin, 2011; Anstee, Daly, & Day, 2011; Dick, Meyers, Rose, Kaprio, & Kendler, 2011). Complex genetic architecture is involved in both the consumption of alcohol and problems that develop in alcohol use. People who develop liver disease as a result of alcohol consumption have genetic variations that seem to interact with the environment to determine progression of the disease. While additive factors between family genetics and the environment are significant, genetic factors remain the largest and most powerful influence on alcoholism.

When a pregnant woman ingests alcohol, the fetus is placed at risk for a number of problems. These may not be genetic in origin, but may cause genetic damage such that a genetic disorder is created and passed to subsequent generations. Nurses need to be aware of the harmful effects of alcohol on pregnant women and unborn children. Fetal alcohol syndrome (FAS) occurs in children of women who engage in heavy alcohol ingestion during pregnancy. Approximately 1% to 3.5% of babies are born with FAS (Watson, Finkelstein, Gurewich, & Morse, 2011). It is considered the most common nonhereditary form of intellectual disorders. Physical and mental defects of FAS include severe growth deficiency, heart defects, malformed facial features, intellectual disorder, low birth weight, learning problems, and hyperactivity. If a child has one or two of these characteristics, the condition is called fetal alcohol effects (FAE).

Children of alcoholics, aged from adolescent to adult, display an enormous variety of personality types and levels of functioning. If there is a genetic link to substance issues, the offspring of people with alcoholism could have a genetic signature. Genetics may play a part in the development of personality traits and to the level of functioning. Highly similar personality subtypes were identified in one study (Hinrich, Defife, & Westen, 2011) including having emotional dysregulation and externalizing control as well as being inhibited and high functioning. Even so, there were significant differences in whether children of alcoholics had a diagnosis on Axis I or Axis II, and whether there were differences in developmental histories. Genetics play a role, but do not appear to be the only factor in someone developing a problem with substances. As a result of studies like this, it is important to address the individual variables in treatment such as the client's interpretation of experiences and the extent of coping skills.

Another common substance of abuse is nicotine. Genetic differences can be found in who smokes and how smoking behaviors are expressed. Uhl, Walther, Behm, and Rose (2011) examined how heavy smokers tend to prefer menthol cigarettes. This group of smokers is of interest because heavy smoking accelerates morbidity and mortality. There is a gene that is different in people who have this characteristic that is not present in those do not have a preference for mentholated cigarettes. Those individuals with specific nucleotide **polymorphisms** (the building block molecules of DNA and the expression of different alleles of a given gene) display a significant association with a preference for mentholated cigarettes. When it is known a gene is active in a problematic behavior, the search for a way to address the problem can commence.

The underlying mechanism of opioid dependence, despite a multitude of genetics studies, remains unclear (Wu et al., 2011). It is believed to be correlated with the adaptive changes the central nervous system makes at the cellular level following chronic opioid use. These cellular changes are thought to be the main cause for an addict's relapse to drug-taking behavior. The ability to treat an opioid addiction with a pharmaceutical compound targeting damaged cells, even once a particular cellular pathway problem is known to exist, is impeded by the variety and depth of these cellular changes.

Research on polysubstance abuse examines vulnerabilities such as poor coping, distractibility, conduct disorder, and being ill-prepared for adult role success (Sihvola et al., 2011). Each of these creates a disadvantage; having multiple disadvantages places individuals at significant risk for addictive behaviors. There are continued efforts to attempt to unravel the numerous contributing factors that exist in the fabric of substance use. Any headway made toward sorting out the difficulties faced by individuals for whom alcoholism and other substance dependencies is a problem can positively affect their quality of life. It may be that there is no simple genetic pathway that can be identified and thereafter treated with a compound designed to address the genetic problem. Metabolic and genetic changes create disease states that are quite complex (Joenje, 2011). In the meantime, or if no clear genetic pathway is identified, cognitive and behavioral approaches offer considerable promise.

SECTION TWO REVIEW

1. Genetic factors
   A. completely determine the pathogenesis of substance abuse.
   B. are the only known factors that influence the pathogenesis of substance abuse.
   C. play no role in the pathogenesis of substance abuse.
   D. play a role, in addition to behavioral learning, in the pathogenesis of substance abuse.
2. If a pregnant woman ingests alcohol
   A. there is no risk of genetic damage to the fetus.
   B. there is risk of genetic damage to the fetus that can be passed on to subsequent generations.
   C. there is no risk of genetic damage to the fetus that can be passed on to subsequent generations.
   D. it is certain that the baby will have fetal alcohol syndrome.
3. Children of alcoholics
   A. display an enormous variety of personality types and levels of functioning.
   B. have a similar personality type.
   C. will very likely develop Axis I disorders.
   D. will very likely develop Axis II disorders.
4. Nicotine abusers who prefer mentholated cigarettes
   A. have specific nucleotide polymorphisms.
   B. have no specific genetic characteristics.
   C. have nonspecific nucleotide polymorphisms.
   D. have a specific psychological orientation.
5. The underlying mechanism of opioid dependence is clearly understood.
   A. True
   B. False

Answers: 1. D; 2. B; A; 4. A; 5. B

SECTION THREE: Practical Applications of Genetics

So many substances are destructive not only to the substance user's health, but also to the integrity of families and communities. Exploring this area to its greatest extent is necessary to promote public health. When we look at the genetic underpinnings of substance use, we move toward that goal.

Is substance abuse the result of a genetic profile (nature), an environment rife with problematic behaviors (nurture), or some combination of the two? If substance abuse were solely genetic we would be able to identify those who have the genetic profile, counsel against having children, screen out donated eggs and sperm, and consider suspect cell lines used for cloning or regeneration to be off limits. If that were the scientific structure of the problem, without an accessible gene pool the problem of substance abuse would wither and disappear. However, we know that people who abuse substances do not have to be biologically related to their substance-abusing guardians to eventually demonstrate problematic substance behaviors. Infants adopted by couples who could not have their own biological children sometimes reflect, as adults, the substance abuse that existed in the environment.

If substance abuse were specific only to those who had been behaviorally taught and therefore nurtured by an environment of substance abuse, then every child of a substance abuser would become one also. Or a child born to those who had a problem with substance abuse who was then adopted as an infant by a nonsubstance-abusing family would never have a problem with substance abuse. A therapeutic environment would be completely successful in teaching someone with an addiction to be substance free. But we know this is not the case: Rehabilitation is only partially effective in helping an individual remain substance free.

A neurobiological perspective states that inhibition, a fundamental property for responding flexibly to circumstances, can be genetically determined and behaviorally demonstrated. Without the efficient operation of inhibitory mechanisms, behavior can become maladaptive, as seen in a large range of disorders where impulsive responses are common, such as chronic substance abuse (Humby & Wilkinson, 2011). Someone with addictive genetics may need an excess of reward experiences in order to feel satisfied or euphoric. This individual responds to a higher level of reward activation of his or her brain circuitry. How would someone behave when there is a neurobiological need to have a lot of stimulation in order to feel good? Very likely there would be behavior that involve risk, such as gambling or substance abuse, and it would take a significant amount of activity in those areas in order for the individual to feel that life was satisfying and gratifying. If a client knew he or she was genetically predisposed in this direction, efforts to acknowledge this difference could be made. Psychotherapy would focus on the individual's need to validate specific urges while providing adaptive and healthy alternatives to achieve satisfaction. Treatment would consist of acknowledging the neurobiological reality, as well as determining how to provide satisfactory stimulation that does not jeopardize function.

The chances of developing a problem with substance abuse or dependence cannot be definitively quantified. If an individual has a genetic predisposition to substance dependency, there is a risk; however, interventions such as an array of psychotherapies can enhance abilities and prevent full expression of vulnerabilities. While genetics may predispose a client to problem behavior, genetics do not guarantee a problem or prevent learning how to cope and function effectively.

Crystal and associates (2010) examined a particular genotype of the mu opiate receptor gene called TT. From the African-American women studied, the researchers found that the presence of the TT genotype may increase the risk of substance use and abuse. If a client knew she had this particular genotype she would be able to anticipate the difficulties that could arise and take steps to address them. A genetically vulnerable woman would have the information necessary to know the value of minimizing stress and maximizing coping skills.

We do know that those individuals who are most susceptible to having difficulties with substances have genetic predispositions as well as environmental stressors. These clients have living situations where there is widespread substances abuse by others in the setting. People are victimized physically and sexually much more easily in environments where people are disinhibited from substance abuse. Chaos can create a great deal of stress. If coping skills are inadequate, stress can be responded to with even more substance abuse.

The combination of substance abuse (or substance dependence) and another psychiatric problem are common and complicate the picture. Someone who has a mental illness and is a substance abuser experiences much more than just two problems. The characteristics of one illness meld with the features of another, resulting in a deepening of a difficult situation from which few effectively extricate themselves. Substances of abuse cause psychiatric symptoms, interfere with the body's ability to effectively use psychiatric medication for symptom reduction, and interrupt a client's efforts for competent behavior and recovery.

So many factors contribute to a substance abuse problem that treatment focusing on a single factor is unlikely to be effective. Psychiatric care settings that address multifactorial contributions to this problem are better equipped to improve outcomes for these clients.

Emerging Evidence

- Genome-wide association (GWA) is a method of choice for identifying genes whose variants influence vulnerability to complex disorders. It is an easier process when similar genotyping platforms are used that assess allele frequencies. Vulnerability to heavy use and development of dependence on alcohol and/or an illegal abused substance ("addiction vulnerability") appears to be a complex trait. The substantial genetic influences on addiction vulnerability are documented by data from family, adoption, and twin studies. Twin studies also document shared heritable influences on vulnerability to dependence on addictive substances from different pharmacological classes, including alcohol and illegal drugs from several pharmacological classes. Combined data studies suggest that much of the genetic influence on vulnerability to substance dependence is likely to be polygenic. There is strong evidence for involvement of variants in several individual genes. The ongoing understanding of genetic underpinnings of human addiction, as for many complex disorders, requires a great deal of data to develop relevant personalized prevention and treatment strategies (Johnson, Drgon, Walther, & Uhl, 2011).
- Genetic research on cocaine dependence may help clarify our understanding of the disorder as well as provide insights for effective treatment. The cannabinoid receptor 1 protein regulates both the endocannabinoid and dopaminergic neurobiological systems, and polymorphisms in the cannabinoid receptor gene, *CNR1*, have been associated previously with substance dependence. Further work brings closer the day when a test may be available to determine cocaine addiction vulnerability. There is an association in a large study as well as a meta-analysis that a specific alteration in a gene is present in those who demonstrate cocaine addiction (Clarke et al., 2011).

SECTION THREE REVIEW

1. Substance abuse is the result of
   A. a genetic profile.
   B. a specific environment.
   C. a specific combination of genes and environment.
   D. unspecified combinations of genetics and environmental factors.
2. Substance abuse
   A. may be mediated by a problem with inhibitory mechanisms.
   B. may be mediated by problems with inhibitory mechanisms and with reward activation.
   C. may be mediated by a problem with reward activation.
   D. is not mediated by inhibitory or reward activation mechanism dysfunction.
3. The risk of developing a substance abuse disorder
   A. can be quantified using our present understanding of genetic factors.
   B. can be quantified using our present understanding of genetic and environmental factors.
   C. cannot be quantified at present.
   D. is inherently unquantifiable.
4. Substance abuse and psychiatric problems
   A. do not coexist.
   B. rarely coexist.
   C. often coexist.
   D. are associated with a specific genetic marker when they coexist.
5. Vulnerability to substance abuse problems may be associated with specifc types of opiate receptors.
   A. True
   B. False

Answers: 1. D; 2. B; 3. C; 4. C; 5. A

SECTION FOUR: How Genetics Influence Treatment

Technology enables researchers to modify DNA so that both the messages and the expression of the messages can be manipulated. The single nucleotide polymorphism (SNP) technology has been used for many years in genetics, but now is considered nearly obsolete. The lessons learned from its use over the years have been invaluable; however, this procedure allowed only a limited view into an individual's genetic makeup and is being replaced by full sequencing of the human genome. The more we know about how a client's chromosomes affect his or her metabolism, the more likely we can contribute effective pharmacology to treat a problem. We need the full exploration of chromosomes in order to determine the type of metabolism an individual has, and thus the likely most effective direction to take in treatment.

DNA markers from fragments of DNA (restriction fragment length polymorphisms or **RFLPs**) are making it possible to identify and localize the genes involved in a disease process. RFLPs represent a direct reflection of the DNA sequence and can be used to determine accuracy on kinship and group relationships. RFLP separation has led to a large library of DNA sequence markers and a human mutation database. This information assists researchers in determining the probability that a mutation can take place at any specific area of the genome and can affect metabolism, function, and symptoms (Kareken et al., 2010). The data gathered in the mutation database help us to understand the pathophysiology of a disease and its treatment and possibly, in the future, its prevention.

Defining phenotypes is helpful in treatment as an individual is classified as a metabolizer who is poor, intermediate, extensive, or ultrarapid. The extensive metabolizer is considered normal. In treatment for psychiatric symptoms, the cytochrome P_{450} (abbreviated CYP) 2D6 is the enzyme most involved in metabolizing psychiatric medications. This field is expanding and facilitates the application of **pharmacogenetic** (drugs developed to treat an identified gene problem, abbreviated as PGx) to clinical interventions (Mrazek & Lerman, 2011). There is a growing interest in PGx as a way to make pharmacotheraputics safer and more effective (Stingl & Brockmoller, 2011).

Behavioral interventions can include mapping out how an at-risk person reacts when exposed to a stressor. Is the reaction adaptive and healthy? If you detect less-than-ample adaptive coping skills in an at-risk individual, you would proceed with shoring up the weaker areas to prevent (or at least minimize the possibility of) maladaptive coping such as substance abuse. The following lists some client-centered strategies to promote better coping and more adaptive behaviors:

- Become actively involved in shaping a personal support system.
- Identify stressors such as the following:
  - Timing—time of year, holidays, anniversaries, schedule disruptions, varying work shifts
  - Interpersonal issues—arguments, intimacy, loneliness, crowding, demands from others, financial problems
  - Intrapersonal issues—feelings of anger, incompetence, fatigue, frustration, fear
- Rehearse and practice healthy responses to difficult situations.
- Develop an array of activities or behaviors that minimize or reduce stressful times and situations.

SECTION FOUR REVIEW

1. Single nucleotide polymorphism technology:
   A. made a very limited contribution to our understanding of the genetics of substance abuse.
   B. is considered nearly obsolete given new technologies.
   C. is superior to technology examining restricted fragment length polymorphisms.
   D. allows an unlimited view into an individual's genetic makeup.
2. Disease psychopathology is
   A. related to probability of a mutation in certain areas of the genome.
   B. unrelated to probability of a mutation in any area of the genome.
   C. completely determined by probability of a mutation in certain areas of the genome.
   D. the primary determining factor mediating where mutations can occur in the genome.
3. Individuals classified as extensive metabolizers
   A. are at highest risk for cytochrome P_{450} problems.
   B. are at highest risk for problems metabolizing most psychiatric medications.
   C. need treatments developed with pharmacogenetic methods.
   D. are considered normal.
4. Restricted fragment length polymorphisms
   A. do not reflect DNA sequence.
   B. directly reflect DNA sequence.
   C. are found only in individuals classified as poor metabolizers.
   D. do not permit localization of genes in a disease process.
5. Behavioral interventions cannot help individuals with genetically mediated coping skill deficits.
   A. True
   B. False

Answers: 1. B; 2. A; 3. D; 4. B; 5. B

SECTION FIVE: Nursing Implications

Because 4% to 5% of people in Western societies have difficulty with alcohol dependence and the relapse rate is 50% to 80% in a year, understanding its origins and having a reliable genetic analysis are vital. We know from decades of studies that there is heritability and predisposition to alcohol dependence as well as complex environmental influences. The latest research indicates an association of alcohol dependence with single nucleotide polymorphism in a *GABA* receptor gene, especially in those with a presumed genetic predisposition (Kareken et al., 2010). Identifying the genetic components of the disease helps identify high-risk individuals. Once someone is identified as being high risk, you can intervene as a nurse on an interpersonal basis. Interventions include the following:

- Defining weaknesses in stress responses
- Teaching ways to improve resilience to adversity
- Assisting the individual in developing ways to increase support systems
- Maximizing the client's understanding of the action of medications
- Administering relevant pharmacologic agents

The type of nursing intervention is determined, at this point, in part by the desire of the individual to be involved in a recovery process (Trigoboff, 2013). Gene therapy is not an option to any significant degree and therefore places treatment by nurses in an educative and behavioral counseling realm.

Nursing assessment is a key function when alcohol ingestion and pregnancy co-occur. An infant born to an alcoholic mother may need to be withdrawn gradually from alcohol immediately after birth, as opposed to an abrupt cessation. Even brief exposure to very small amounts of alcohol while the fetus is in utero may kill fetal brain cells and cause peripheral nerve damage as well. The burden of these impacts will be felt by that individual all through his or her life.

Nicotine addiction provides ample opportunity for nursing assessment and intervention. While nicotine addiction does respond to behavioral interventions (such as health care provider encouragement toward cessation and access to hotlines), these are largely underutilized (Carlsten et al., 2011). The practical aspect of genetic testing initially is to identify who is at risk for a problem, then subsequently contribute to or guide interventions. Knowing who is at risk for becoming a heavy smoker due to genetic composition can be an important step; however, nonpharmacologic interventions have proven to be more effective and durable.

Genetic research has helped to develop meaningful and effective pharmacologic treatments for some disorders. Once a gene is recognized to be a problem, it is possible to address the problem with a chemical agent. In the specialty area of treating addictive behaviors, however, there is not the specificity that exists when we discover a genetic basis for a different disease process such as, breast cancer. Genetic problems can be expressed in various ways such as a behavioral impact (requiring more stimulation than typical), being damaged and creating genetic dysfunction (as a result of chromosomal replication or a missing section), or a metabolic difficulty. Because addictive behaviors are multifactorial in origin, it tends to follow that interventions need to be as well. The solution to a genetic contributing factor to addictive behaviors may be one or more of the following:

- Approximate the normal functioning of the affected gene.
- Mimic the distorted genetic response—but in a healthier, more manageable manner.
- Block the dysfunctional gene response.

There are only a few pharmacotherapeutic agents available to assist in treating substance dependence. In time there will be more. As discussed already in this chapter, the origin and expression of problems with substances is complicated, and problems are best addressed by considering all aspects of the individual's life. This holistic view has the opportunity to be effective and durable. Combining pharmacotherapy with improving coping skills provides a complete program that can sustain individuals with substance-dependence challenges throughout their lives.

SECTION FIVE REVIEW

1. In Western society, people with alcohol dependence
   A. have an annual relapse rate of 50% to 80%.
   B. have an annual relapse rate of 95% to 100%.
   C. have an annual relapse rate of 10% to 20%.
   D. generally do not relapse if they achieve sobriety and maintain it for 3 months.
2. Alcohol dependence is
   A. not heritable.
   B. heritable.
   C. not influenced by environmental factors.
   D. influenced by environmental factors but not by genetic factors.
3. An infant born to an alcoholic mother who was actively drinking during the pregnancy
   A. should never be given alcohol.
   B. may need to be quickly withdrawn from alcohol following birth.
   C. is unlikely to have sustained any brain damage as long as the pregnancy was full term.
   D. may need to be withdrawn gradually from alcohol immediately following birth.
4. Someone who has a nicotine addiction
   A. cannot be influenced by environmental factors.
   B. is not influenced by genetic factors.
   C. cannot be treated effectively with behavioral interventions.
   D. cannot depend on sufficient deployment of behavioral interventions.
5. A combination of pharmacotherapy with an effort to improve coping skills can help substance dependent client significantly.
   A. True
   B. False

Answers: 1. A; 2. B; 3. D; 4. D; 5. A

SECTION SIX: Future Directions

When someone is diagnosed with a substance-related disorder such as alcoholism, the nurse's involvement with that client and the family will revolve around teaching. The genetic basis for alcohol dependence includes heritability and a predisposition for offspring to be alcohol dependent as well. While the immediate concern is for the client, a future concern will be the life-impacting ramifications that a substance-related disorder will have for the client's children.

Whether the client's children are biologically related or adopted, there are also complex contributions from environmental conditions. Once a blood relative has been identified as alcohol dependent, there is a presumed genetic predisposition to alcoholism. Genetics can serve as advance notice for people to take action. A proactive environment helps the at-risk individual maximize coping skills without turning to substances to cope, and begins the process of prevention for future generations.

Ongoing research examines in more detail the behavioral patterns around substances. Much of the existing research is dichotomous regarding use—in other words, the individual is either using or not using a substance. This characterization misses the many steps between including modest use, intermittent use, daily use, and multiple daily substance use. Future studies could be more sensitive with more accurate depictions when substance use is staged and quantified.

SECTION SIX REVIEW

1. As a nurse, your involvement with substance-dependent clients and their families will revolve around
   A. medication administration.
   B. assessing vital signs.
   C. teaching.
   D. providing reassurance.
2. If a substance-dependent client has children, those children
   A. are at no elevated risk for problems with substances.
   B. have an elevated risk for problems with substances.
   C. do not benefit from proactive interventions.
   D. are less likely to benefit from proactive and prevention-oriented nursing interventons than the children of non-substance-dependent clients.
3. Research on behavioral patterns associated with substances
   A. would be less useful if substance use patterns were not dichotomously classified as using or not using.
   B. would be more useful if intermittent or occasional substance users were excluded.
   C. would be more useful if quantitative methods were not used.
   D. would be more useful if different levels of substance use were staged and quantified.
4. Substance abuse is usually not associated with specific behavior patterns.
   A. True
   B. False
5. Children who are adopted by people who abuse substances
   A. are at higher risk to develop substance abuse due to environmental factors.
   B. are not at higher risk to develop substance abuse because they are not blood relatives of the people who are substance abusers.
   C. are at lower risk to develop substance abuse due to environmental factors.
   D. are at higher risk to develop substance abuse due to genetic factors.

Answers: 1. C; 2. B; 3. D; 4. B; 5. A

POSTTEST

1. Withdrawal symptoms can occur
   A. only when stopping use of a substance.
   B. when stopping or reducing use of a substance.
   C. only when the client exhibits a clinically significant decrease in diastolic blood pressure.
   D. when the client has been clean and sober for over a year.
2. Antihistamines sold over the counter
   A. can be associated with substance abuse disorders.
   B. provide withdrawal symptoms in clients with a defined mu receptor type.
   C. provoke withdrawal symptoms in clients with a defined nucleotide polymorphism.
   D. cannot be associated with substance abuse disorders.
3. The largest and most powerful influences on alcoholism are
   A. environmental factors.
   B. emotional factors.
   C. behavioral factors.
   D. genetic factors.
4. People who are dependent on opioids
   A. may have adaptive changes affecting cellular functioning in the central nervous system following chronic use.
   B. may have adaptive changes affecting cellular functioning in the nucleus accumbens after chronic use.
   C. may have adaptive changes affecting cellular functioning in the thyroid gland after chronic use.
   D. often have peripheral neuropathies after chronic use.
5. Someone with addictive genetics
   A. needs reduced reward experiences to feel satisfied.
   B. needs the same level of reward experiences as other people to feel satisfied.
   C. may need increased reward experiences to feel satisfied.
   D. is likely to have stronger inhibitory mechanism than someone without addictive genetics.
6. Effective substance abuse treatment
   A. usually needs to focus on a single factor.
   B. usually needs to focus on reducing reward.
   C. usually focuses on reducing inhibitory mechanism activation and functioning.
   D. usually needs to focus on a multiple factors.
7. As compared to SNP technology, RFLP technology is
   A. more useful.
   B. less useful.
   C. obsolete.
   D. more likely to focus on single nucleotide polymorphisms.
8. All of the following are appropriate nursing interventions for a client at high risk for alcoholism EXCEPT
   A. defining weaknesses in stress responses.
   B. teaching ways to improve resilience to adversity.
   C. assisting the client in developing ways to increase support systems.
   D. teaching the client to avoid all pharmacologic agents.

9. The type of nursing intervention appropriate for people with alcohol dependence is determined in part by
   A. the desire of the person to be in a recovery process.
   B. the suitability for gene therapy.
   C. the nurse's preference.
   D. the person's blood type.

10. Addictive behaviors are
   A. multifactorial in origin.
   B. single factorial in origin.
   C. unrelated to genetics.
   D. determined only by the environment.

Posttest answers are located in the Appendix.

CHAPTER SUMMARY

The genetics of substance abuse is a growing field, evolving and adding important components on an ongoing basis. This chapter discusses the latest in this specialty area and how the information gained from knowing one's genetics contributes to the following:

- Discovering genetic links
- Applying the information in a practical manner to help people avoid, minimize, or recover from substance abuse
- Understanding how substance abuse, a behavioral as well as a genetically determined problem, can be anticipated and addressed
- Exploring the complexity of substance use and abuse
- Developing nursing interventions and prevention strategies that are relevant and personalized

CRITICAL THINKING CHECKPOINT

Margerie is a 23-year-old Caucasian woman who has been told by numerous people in her life that she has difficulties with alcohol consumption. Her boyfriend, her boss at her part-time job, and her neighbors have all told Margerie she drinks too much and that she is unpleasant when consuming alcohol. She does not necessarily agree with this input. Her mother had a "drinking problem" and was never able to work or improve her circumstances. She recently died at age 42 from cirrhosis. Margerie's father did not abuse alcohol, although he was a regular cannabis consumer who left the family when Margerie was 10 years old. Margerie does not think this is a cautionary tale that applies to her as she only drinks on her days off, does not use any other substances of abuse, maintains employment, and is physically healthy.

1. Would alcohol screening and testing would be appropriate for Margerie? Why or why not?
2. Is a family history important in this case? Why or why not?
3. Does Margerie have a family history that increases her risk for a genetic contribution to a problem? Why or why not?
4. What is the role of the nurse before and after tests are done?
5. What follow-up care would be necessary?

Answers are provided in the Appendix

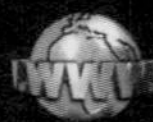

ONLINE RESOURCES

The Center for Collaborative Genomic Studies on Mental Disorders: https://www.nimhgenetics.org

The Substance Abuse & Mental Health Services Administration (SAMHSA): http://www.samhsa.gov

REFERENCES

Agrawal, A., Lynskey, M. T., Heath, A. C., & Chassin, L. (2011). Developing a genetically informative measure of alcohol consumption using past-12-month indices. *Journal of Studies on Alcohol and Drugs, 72*(3) 444–452.

American Psychiatric Association. (2000). *Diagnostic and statistical manual of mental disorders* (4th ed., text rev.). Washington, DC: Author.

Anstee, Q. M., Daly, A. K., & Day, C. P. (2011). Genetics of alcoholic and nonalcoholic fatty liver disease. *Seminars in Liver Disease, 31*(2), 128–146.

Carlsten, C., Halperin, A., Crouch, J., & Burke, W. (2011). Personalized medicine and tobacco-related health disparities: Is there a role for genetics? *Annals of Family Medicine, 9*(4), 366–371.

Chen, T. J., Blum, K., Chen, A. L., Bowirrat, A., Downs, W. B., Madigan, M. A., et al. (2011). Neurogenetics and clinical evidence for the putative activation of the brain reward circuitry by a neuroadaptagen: proposing an addiction candidate gene panel map. *Journal of Psychoactive Drugs, 43*(2), 108–127.

Clarke, T. K., Bloch, P. J., Ambrose-Lanci, L. M., Ferraro, T. N., Berrettini, W. H., Kampman, K. M., et al. (2011). Further evidence for association of polymorphisms in the CNR1 gene with cocaine addiction: Confirmation in an independent sample and meta-analysis. *Addiction Biology*. Epub ahead of print retrieved July 25, 2011. doi: 10.1111/j.1369-1600.2011.00346.x

Crystal, H. A., Hamon, S., Randesi, M., Cook, J., Anastos, K., Lazar, J., et al. (2010). A C17T polymorphism in the mu opiate receptor is associated with quantitative measures of drug use in African American women. *Addictions Biology*. Epub ahead of print retrieved Nov 11, 2011. doi: 10.1111/j.1369-1600.2010.00265.x

Dick, D. M., Meyers, J. L., Rose, R. J., Kaprio, J., & Kendler, K. S. (2011). Measures of current alcohol consumption and problems: Two independent twin studies suggest a complex genetic architecture. *Alcoholism, Clinical and Experimental Research*. Epub ahead of print retrieved June 20, 2011. doi: 10.1111/j.1530-0277.2011.01564.x

Hinrich, J., Defife J., & Westen, D. (2011). Personality subtypes in adolescent and adult children of alcoholics: A two-part study. *Journal of Nervous and Mental Disease, 199*(7), 487–498.

Humby, T., & Wilkinson, L. S. (2011). Assaying dissociable elements of behavioural inhibition and impulsivity: translational utility of animal models. *Current Opinion in Pharmacology*. Epub ahead of print. PMID: 21763200

Joenje, H. (2011). Metabolism: alcohol, DNA and disease. *Nature, 475*(7354), 45–46.

Johnson, C., Drgon, T., Walther, D., & Uhl, G. R. (2011). Genomic regions identified by overlapping clusters of nominally-positive SNPs from genome-wide studies of alcohol and illegal substance dependence. *PLoS One, 6*(7), e19210. Epub July 27, 2011. PMID: 21818250

Kareken, D. A., Liang, T., Wetherill, L., Dzemidzic, M., Bragulat, V., Cox, C., et al. (2010). A polymorphism in GABRA2 is associated with the medial frontal response to alcohol cues in an fMRI study. *Alcoholism: Clinical and Experimental Research, 34*(12), 2169–2178.

Kimura, M., & Higuchi, S. (2011). Genetics of alcohol dependence. *Psychiatry and Clinical Neurosciences, 65*(3), 213–225.

Kirk, M., Calzone, K., Arimori, N., & Tonkin, E. (2011). Genetics-genomics competencies and nursing regulation. *Journal of Nursing Scholarship, 43*(2), 107–116.

Lea, D. H., Skirton, H., Read, C. Y., & Williams, J. K. (2011). Implications for educating the next generation of nurses on genetics and genomics in the 21st century. *Journal of Nursing Scholarship, 43*(1), 3–12.

Mrazek, D. A., & Lerman, C. (2011). Facilitating clinical implementation of pharmacogenomics. *JAMA, 306*(3), 304–305.

Sihvola, E., Rose, R. J., Dick, D. M., Korhonen, T., Pulkkinen, L., Raevuori, A., et al. (2011). Prospective relationships of ADHD symptoms with developing substance use in a population-derived sample. *Psychological Medicine, 20*, 1–9. Epub ahead of print. PMID: 21733216

Stingl, J. C., & Brockmoller, J. (2011). Why, when, and how should pharmacogenetics be applied in clinical studies? Current and future approaches to study designs. *Clinical Pharmacology & Therapeutics, 89*(2), 198–209.

Trigoboff, E. (2013). Recovery and Psychiatric Rehabilitation Strategies. In C. Kneisl, & E. Trigoboff (Eds.), *Contemporary psychiatric-mental health nursing* (3rd ed.). Upper Saddle River, New Jersey: Prentice Hall.

Uhl, G. R., Walther, D., Behm, F. M., & Rose, J. E. (2011). Menthol preference among smokers: Association with TRPA1 variants. *Nicotine & Tobacco Research*, Epub ahead of print retrieved June 30, 2011. PMID: 21719896

Watson, E., Finkelstein, N., Gurewich, D. & Morse, B. (2011). The feasibility of screening for fetal alcohol spectrum disorders risk in early intervention settings: A pilot study of systems change. *Infants & Young Children, 24*(2), 193–206.

Wu, Y., Chen, R., Zhao, X., Li, A., Li, G., & Zhou, J. (2011). JWA regulates chronic morphine dependence via the delta opioid receptor. *Biochemical and Biophysical Research Communications, 409*(3), 520–525.

CHAPTER

22 Autism

Ellen Giarelli

LEARNING OUTCOMES

Following the completion of this chapter, the learner will be able to

1. Describe the core behavioral characteristics, diagnostic criteria, and prevalence of autism spectrum disorder.
2. Summarize the early evidence for the genetic determinants of autism spectrum disorder including findings from twin studies and evidence of a broader autism phenotype among family members.
3. Compare the different approaches to the study of genetics determinants of autism spectrum disorder.
4. Analyze the strength of the scientific evidence for candidate genes for autism spectrum disorder.
5. Describe future directions the research of autism spectrum disorder.
6. Evaluate the role of the nurse in the integrated care of autism spectrum disorders.

This chapter presents basic information on the definition and core behavioral characteristics and proposed etiological determinants of autism spectrum disorders (ASD). It provides an overview of ASD including the core behavioral characteristics, diagnostic criteria, and trends in prevalence. It also describes the early evidence of genetic determinants, including evidence from twin studies and evaluation of the broader autism phenotype. This chapter discusses etiological hypotheses, including an overview of gene/environmental issues, exposure and the prenatal environment, hormonal and immunological issues, and genetic risk factors. In addition, this chapter covers the evidence for genetic determinants of ASD, including descriptions of syndromic disorders associated with ASD such as Fragile X syndrome and tuberous sclerosis. Candidate genes are reviewed. Finally, promising avenues for ASD research is discussed as well as the role of the nurse in ASD care.

PRETEST

1. *Autism spectrum disorder* is the term given to a group of neurodevelopmental disabilities.
   A. True
   B. False
2. The proportion of males to females diagnosed with ASD is approximately
   A. 2:1.
   B. 4:1.
   C. 1:1.
   D. 3:1.
3. Ascertaining the etiology for a child's developmental disability is important because
   A. it helps to establish an accurate diagnosis.
   B. it helps clinicians to predict the course of the disorder.
   C. it helps to establish an accurate recurrence risk within families.
   D. it helps parents to begin to accept the disability.
   E. All of the above
4. Suspected and known genetic causes of ASD are grouped into all of the following categories EXCEPT
   A. structural variation.
   B. Y-linked DNA.
   C. mutated genes.
   D. susceptibility genes.
   E. mitochondrial DNA.
5. What is the pair-wise concordance of ASD among monozygotic twins?
   A. 25%
   B. 31%
   C. 50%
   D. 88%
6. Fragile X syndrome and autism spectrum disorder have which overlapping symptoms?
   A. Infertility and ovarian failure
   B. Intellectual disability in males, only
   C. Impaired communication and avoidance of eye contact
   D. Flexible joints and low muscle tone
   E. None of the above

7. What condition occurs more frequently among families with autism than the general population?
   A. Social phobias
   B. Eating disorders
   C. Sleeping disorders
   D. Bipolar disorder
   E. All of the above
8. Etiologic categories for ASD are
   A. environmental
   B. recognizable syndromes.
   C. diagnosed by molecular cytogenetics.
   D. inherited.
   E. All of the above
9. Homeobox or HOX genes are associated with a higher incidence of autism. On what chromosome are these genes located?
   A. Ch2
   B. Ch5
   C. Ch7
   D. Ch11
10. The dynamic interaction of metabolic pathways (gene mediated) and medications have been implicated in the etiology of ASD. Which pharmaceutical agents have been studied?
   A. Thalidomide
   B. Misoprostol
   C. Valproic acid
   D. Antihistamines
   E. All of the above

Pretest answers are located in the Appendix.

SECTION ONE: Introduction to Autism Spectrum Disorder

Since the passage of the Child Health Act of 2000 (U.S. Congress, 2000), there has been a rising interest in autism spectrum disorders among scientists and clinicians. The National Institutes of Child Health and Human Development (**NICHD**) along with the National Institute for Mental Health (**NIMH**) are two of several federal institutions doing research on the genetics of ASD. In 1997, the NICHD and the National Institutes on Deafness and Other Communication Disorders (**NIDCD**) started the Network on the Neurobiology and Genetics of Autism: Collaborative Programs of Excellence in Autism (CPEA) (National Institute for Child Health and Human Development, 2008). Investigators in this network have developed projects to study and describe how genes might be involved in the etiology of autism and how genes might play a role in the behavioral symptoms (see Box 22–1).

Autism was first recognized in 1943 by Leo Kanner, who labeled it a psychiatric disorder separate from disorders such as schizophrenia, obsessive-compulsive disorder, and mental retardation (Kanner, 1943). It is now considered a genetic disorder, largely due to the efforts of the Autism Genetics Resource Exchange (AGRE), which is an international effort to further understand the genomic structure of ASD (Levine, 2011; Rutter, 2011).

Core Behavioral Characteristics

Autism, also called *autistic disorder*, is a complex neurobiological disorder that is often diagnosed early in childhood and has symptoms that last a lifetime. It is sometimes referred to as a **developmental disability** because symptoms are observed before age 3 (during the period of development) and causes problems or delays in the **development of** many different social and communication skills that arise during the period of infancy to adulthood.

BOX 22–1 Sample of Studies Originating From the CPEA

Study: HOXA gene and autism
Location: University of Pittsburgh and University of Washington
Report:
Devlin, B., Bennett, P., Cook, E. H., Jr., Dawson, G., Gonen, D., Grigorenko, E. L., et al. (2002). No evidence for linkage of liability to autism to HOXA1 in a sample from the CPEA network. *American Journal of Medical Genetics, 114*(6), 667–672.

Study: Genetic sibling linkage study of autism
Location: University of Washington
Report:
Yu, C. E., Dawson, G, Minso, N. J., D'Souza, I., Osterling, J., Estes, A., et al. (2002). Presence of large deletions in kindreds with autism. *American Journal Human Genetics, 71*(1), 100–115.

Study: Reelin gene and autism
Location: University of Pittsburgh and University of Washington
Report:
Devlin, B., Bennett, P., Dawson, G., Figlewicz, D., Grigorenko, E. L., McMahon, W., et al. (2004). Alleles of a reelin CGG repeat do not convey liability to autism in a sample from the CPEA network. *American Journal of Medical Genetics Part B: Neuropsychiatric Genetics, 126B*, 46–50.

Autism spectrum disorders (**ASD**) are a group of developmental disabilities that includes autistic disorder (i.e., autism), **Asperger syndrome** (AS), and **pervasive developmental disability not otherwise specified** (**PDD-NOS**). ASDs are included in a larger group of conditions called pervasive developmental disabilities. The term *spectrum disorder* is used to indicate a range of symptoms and behavioral characteristics that are common to all or most of the individuals who have a diagnosis of one of the three. Also, there is a range in severity of symptoms across individuals and even within the subcategory of diagnosis.

The main signs and symptoms of ASD are called the **core behavioral characteristics** of ASD because they are at the center of the **diagnostic criteria** and central to describing the phenotype. The main symptoms involve language, social behavior, and behaviors related to objects and routines.

According to the *Diagnostic Statistical Manual, Fourth Edition, Text Revised* (***DSM-IV-TR***) there are three main criteria, each with subcriteria. The first is **qualitative impairment** in the use of multiple social skills and social interaction. The second is qualitative impairment in communication. The third is restricted, repetitive, and **stereotyped patterns of behavior**, interest, and activities (American Psychiatric Association, 2000). See Table 22–1 for a list of observations one might make in each of the three main diagnostic criteria.

Clinical signs of ASD are usually present by age 3, but some indicators of ASD can be picked up using screening instruments as early as 6–12 months. There is wide heterogeneity across the ASD **phenotype** with regard to severity and frequency of symptoms, age of recognition, and age of diagnosis (Levy, 2009). Individuals with ASD might also manifest co-occurring medical, psychiatric, and behavioral/developmental problems that are diagnostically separate from ASD (Levy, 2010). For example, 43%–84% of children with ASD have an anxiety disorder, approximately 30% have depression, and approximately 37% have an obsessive-compulsive disorder (Simonoff, 2008). Individuals with ASD are codiagnosed with **seizure disorders** or **epilepsy** (5%–49%) (Rapin, 2008), gastro-esophageal reflux (Nikolov, 2008), and sleep disorders (52%–73%) (Limoges, 2005). Approximately 9%–19% of affected individuals have motor delay, and approximately 50% have hypotonia (Newschaffer, 2007). Each one of these co-occurring conditions might have also has a genetic etiology.

Additionally, according the Fombonne (2002), on average, the rate of **intellectual disability** among people with ASD has been reported to be as high as 70%, with 30% of people scoring in the normal range of mental functioning. More recent reports identify a rate of **cognitive impairment** (IQ < 70) ranging from approximately 29% to 50% (Centers for Disease Control and Prevention, 2009). Cognitive impairment has been associated with genetic disorders, including trisomy 21 (Down syndrome).

TABLE 22–1: Core Characteristics of Autism Spectrum Disorder

Core Characteristics	Observations
Impairment of social interaction	Marked lack of eye contact or eye-to-eye gaze Unusual or impaired facial expressions, body positions Failure to develop peer friendships Lack of spontaneous seeking or sharing with others Lack of showing, bringing or pointing out
Impairment of Language and Communication	Delay in or lack of spoken language Lack of compensation without language, to communicate wants Impaired ability to initiate or sustain conversation with others Stereotyped and repetitive use of words Idiosyncratic language
Stereotypical and repetitive behaviors	Preoccupation with one or more stereotyped behaviors Preoccupation with one or more restricted patterns of interest Abnormal intensity in interest or limited focus Stereotyped or repetitive motor mannerisms, such as hand flapping or spinning Intense or continued preoccupation with parts of objects

Diagnostic Criteria

The *DSM-IV-TR* (American Psychiatric Association, 2000) identified criteria to diagnose individuals on the autism spectrum by three subtypes: autistic disorder, PDD-NOS (including atypical autism), and Asperger disorder or syndrome. At this time, the diagnosis of ASD is based exclusively on developmental patterns and behavioral observations. Several instruments are available to diagnosticians, including tools that are completed by a parent or by a team of professionals. Among these instruments are the Autism Diagnostic Observation Schedule (**ADOS**) and the Autism Diagnostic Inventory-Revised (**ADI-R**). The ADOS is considered the "gold standard." A diagnosis of ASD is most often made by specialists with experience working with patients with ASD including **developmental pediatricians**, psychologists, neurologists, and psychiatrists. To make the diagnosis, criteria described in the *DSM-IV-TR* (American Psychiatric Association, 2000) are applied to the observed and or reported behaviors in the child or the adult. When ASD is diagnosed or highly suspected, genetic testing might be conducted to help specify an etiology or genetic syndrome. However, the highly complex phenotype of ASD complicates the search for the genetic determinants. There are no laboratory tests to diagnose ASD.

Prevalence

In epidemiology, the term *prevalence* is defined as the total number of cases of the risk factor in the population at a given time; or the total number of cases in the population, divided by the number of individuals in the population. It is used as an estimate of how common a disease is within a population over a certain period of time. The prevalence of ASD has been under systematic **surveillance** by the Centers for Disease Control and Prevention (CDC) since the mid-1990s.

Three characteristics of ASD surveillance are important. They are (1) applying a consistent, reliable and valid approach to counting, (2) using a standardized definition of a case, and (3) conducting counts over an extended time to compare unique clusters of cases to confirm trends in rates of the disorder. The most up-to-date statistics on the prevalence of ASD were reported by the Centers for Disease Control and Prevention (CDC) in 2012 (USDHHS/CDC, 2012). According the CDC, the prevalence of ASD among children age 8 years in 2008 across 14 surveillance sites was on average 11.3.0 per 1,000 of children in the population. This converts to approximately 1 in every 88 of the 8-year old children in the population have an ASD (CDC, 2012). This rate is significantly different from what was reported in 2007 (1 in 150). Additionally, ASD is more prevalent among males than females at the proportion of 4.5 to 1 males to females (CI = 95%; $p < 0.001$) (Giarelli, 2010), and varied by race and ethnicity. For example, the CDC reported that the average prevalence among non-Hispanic white children (9.9%; CI = 9.4%–10.4%) was significantly higher ($p < 0.05$) than among non-Hispanic black children (7.2%; CI = 6.6%–7.8%) (Centers for Disease Control and Prevention, 2009).The differences in prevalence by race and sex supports theoretical premises that genetics might be involved in the etiology of ASD.

Rising rates in the prevalence of ASD have alerted health care professionals and researchers to the need to systematically study the causes and develop appropriate treatments to remove or modify causative factors, if possible, and ameliorate symptoms and improve quality of life.

SECTION ONE REVIEW

1. Autism spectrum disorders comprise
   A. Asperger syndrome and autism.
   B. autism, Asperger syndrome, and PDD-NOS.
   C. pervasive developmental disabilities and infantile autism.
   D. autism only.
2. Which health conditions are likely to co-occur with autism spectrum disorder?
   A. Sleep disorders
   B. Anxiety disorders
   C. Depression
   D. Gastro-esophageal reflux
   E. All of the above
3. The CPEA is involved in the study of the genetics of ASD.
   A. True
   B. False
4. ASD was first described by Kanner in
   A. 1943.
   B. 1965.
   C. 1989.
   D. 2000.
5. Nonverbal behavioral impairment is the same as stereotypical patterns of behavior.
   A. True
   B. False

Answers: 1. B; 2. E; 3. A; 4. A; 5. F

SECTION TWO: Early Evidence of Genetic Determinants

Twin Studies

Autism spectrum disorder (ASD) is a complex neurodevelopmental condition. The genetic and environmental origins are not well understood. Only 10% of ASDs have been directly attributed to one or more underlying medical abnormalities (Muhle, 2004). Researchers suspect that most cases of ASD are caused by the interaction of environmental and genetic factors. A major source of information on the potential genetic contribution has been through the study of twins. The earliest twin studies reported the apparent higher incidence of ASD in twin siblings. By the year 2009, there were five epidemiologic studies with twin samples in which at least one autistic proband was described, and all had relatively small samples (less than 50 pairs) (Folstein, 1977; Ritvo, 1985; Bailey, 1995; Steffenburg, 1989; Taniai, 2008). Among these studies, pairwise monozygotic concordance for ASD ranged from 36% to 95%; for dizygotic twins, concordance ranges were from 0% to 23%.

Rosenberg and colleagues (2009) studied patterns of ASD inheritance and other features in twin pairs of by zygosity, sex, and specific ASD diagnosis. After a cross-sectional of 277 twin pairs, they reported pairwise ASD concordance was 31% for dizygotic (DZ) and 88% for monozygotic twins (MZ) (Rosenberg, 2009). In addition, they reported that male and female MZ twins were 100% and 86% concordant, respectively, and affected DZ twins had an earlier age of onset (Rosenberg, 2009). These studies support the assumption that ASD has a genetic etiology.

Broader Autisms Phenotype

Studies have been conducted to quantify the phenotype of ASD. Phenotype is defined as observable characteristics or traits: such as its morphology, development, biochemical or physiological properties, behavior, and products of behavior. Along with twin studies, family studies have provided important information about heritability. In particular, scientists have observed that familial transmission in ASD extends to a range of social and behavioral deficits among family members. These deficits align with, but do not meet the criteria for, a formal diagnosis of ASD. This is referred to as the **broader autism phenotype** (**BAP**). The BAP is characterized by impairments in three core domains of ASD (social behaviors, communications, and repetitive behaviors) that are present in a milder form than required for

BOX 22–2 Steps in the Genetics Analysis of Autism

Step 1 Define and chose phenotypes for analysis.
Consider the rates and distribution of subjects with autism and relative or a control sample.
Assure for sufficient variation and segregation in pedigrees.

Step 2 Choose (a) a candidate gene(s) or (b) a marker set.
Chose candidate genes for an association study.
Chose marker sets for a pedigree linkage study.

Step 3 Check preliminary date and conduct preliminary analysis.
Evaluate genotype for misinheritance, map distance, and allele frequencies.
Evaluate phenotype for outlines and distributions.

Step 4 Conduct (a) linkage analysis or (b) association analysis.
For a linkage analysis do a pedigree study.
For an association analysis do a case-control study.

Step 5 Verify findings.
For a linkage study check that results are robust.
For a candidate study, verify findings with an expression study.
For linkage and candidate verify with independently replicated studies.

Source: Current perspectives on the genetic analysis of autism, Coon, H., American Journal of Medical Genetics Part C, 142C, 24-32. Copyright © 2006 Wiley. Reproduced with permission of Wiley.

a diagnosis. Families with an autistic child show increased rates of BAP among extended family members (Piven, 1987; Folstein, 1999; Bolton, 1994). It is postulated that part of this might be attributed to the environment. Piven and colleagues (1987, 1997) reported that 50% of parents of autistic children manifest the broader phenotype, compared to 2% of parents with a child with Down syndrome. Similar results were reported by Szatmari and colleagues (1995). This strongly suggests a more complex, non-Mendelian mechanism of heritability. Box 22–2 lists steps in the genetic analysis of ASD.

Risk Factors

Family studies combined with larger population-based studies have been mined to uncover factors that are associated with increased risk for ASD. Several risk factors are described in the literature.

Advanced maternal age was associated with several developmental disorders and mental retardation of unknown cause (Croen, 2002. Sanders et al. 2012) as well as with higher risk of damage during pregnancy. Advanced maternal age is defined as the mother's age of 35 years or older. This is the factor most frequently studied for autism and persists as a risk even after controlling for confounding factors.

Advanced paternal age has been associated with autism (Mouridsen, 1993) as have several congenital disorders including Apert's syndrome and neural tube defects (McIntosh, 1995). Advanced paternal age is defined as the father's age of 35 years or older.

Additionally, low birth weight, preterm birth, and fetal grown restrictions have been implicated as risk factors for autism spectrum disorders. Preterm birth and low birth weight are considered markers for newborns who are at risk for later neurological, psychiatric, and neuropsychological problems (Hack, 2005)

Genetic factors are implicated along with these risk factors. Male sex carries greater risk than female sex. The probable mechanism among males is an increased occurrence of spontaneous genomic alterations during spermatogonial stem cell division (Buwe, 2005). The proposed mechanism among females is the accumulated exposure of oocytes to environmental toxin over the life of older mother (Martin, 2008).

SECTION TWO REVIEW

1. Only 10% of ASDs have been directly attributed to one or more underlying medical abnormalities.
   A. True
   B. False
2. In studies of twins, pairwise monozygotic concordance for ASD ranged from 30% to 40%.
   A. True
   B. False
3. Risk factors for autism spectrum disorder are
   A. advanced paternal age.
   B. advanced maternal age.
   C. low birth weight.
   D. genetic predisposition.
   E. All of the above

Answers: 1. A; 2. B; 3. E

SECTION THREE: Etiological Hypotheses

Ascertaining the etiology for a child's developmental disability is important for several reasons that relate directly to patient care. In 2006, in a study of diagnostic yield of pervasive developmental disability among 85 subjects, Battaglia and Carey identify three etiologic categories and four pathogenetic categories. The etiologic categories were environment/acquired, recognizable syndromes, and diagnosed by molecular cytogenetics (Battaglia, 2006). The pathogenetic categories were provisionally unique syndrome, abnormal brain MRI, Landau-Dleffner syndrome, and deafness (Battaglia, 2006). Their work contributed to the systematic study of many possible hypotheses for the etiology of ASD and highlighted the problems as well as the values of this endeavor. The values of a systematic approach are as follows: First, it is essential to establishing an accurate diagnosis and might help clinicians to predict the course of the disorder. Second, it helps to establish an accurate recurrence risk within families. Third, it is important to the process of ongoing monitoring and treatment or when prescribing laboratory and other testing, and when possible. Finally, it is helpful to parents and family members who simply want to understand the nature of their child's disability (Battaglia, 2006).

Evidence from twin, family, and genetic studies supports a role for an inherited predisposition to the development of autism. Also, clinical neuroanatomic, neurophysiologic, and epidemiologic studies suggest that gene penetrance and expression might be influenced by the prenatal and early postnatal environment.

Etiological hypotheses have been proposed for parental and perinatal risk factors, environmental risk factors, oxytocin and social cognition, and genetics/genomics. In explaining symptoms, pathophysiology studies have focused in on serotonin, the GABA and glutamate systems, glucoproteins, neurotrophins, and **neuroligins** and neurexins. All of these systems and organic chemicals are controlled by genetics. Discussion of all these hypotheses is beyond the scope of this chapter.

Gene/Environmental Issues

The environment is defined broadly to include toxic chemical exposure and nutritional, infectious, and other nongenetic factors (National Academy of Sciences, 2000). One might classify the etiology of ASD as from a known disease or idiopathic. If idiopathic, there is no known cause. Presently, the theoretical contribution of environment to ASD is evaluated primarily with respect to idiopathic ASD. **Oligogenic**, polygenic, and mutifactorial mechanisms are being proposed and studied.

BOX 22–3 Known Environmental Causes of Autism

Pharmaceutical Agents:

- Thalidomide
- Misoprostol
- Valproic acid

Infections:

- Rubella

Chemical Exposure:

- Organophosphate insecticides
- Lead
- Methyl mercury
- Polychlorinated biphenyls
- Arsenic
- Manganese

Important clinical and epidemiological features of ASD are not explained by purely genetic hypotheses. One such feature is the discordance of occurrence of autism in monozygotic twins (Daniels, 2006). A portion of the genetic risk is attributed to other factors. Environmental factors, especially in utero exposures, have been implicated in the development of ASD. According to Landrigan (2011), the strongest proof of this comes from evidence that environmental exposures, in early life, are associated with autism. The exposures are pharmaceutical, infectious agents, and organic compounds (see Box 22–3).

Exposure/Environment

Prenatal/Environment

During human development the brain is highly susceptible to injury or damage caused by any assault including traumatic and chemical. The brain is most vulnerable during embryonic and fetal development. The fetal brain must evolve, according to genetic determinants, from a strip of cells along the dorsal ectoderm of the embryo into a complex organ with interconnecting and specialized cells (Grandjean, 2006). Any toxic or environmental exposure that interferes with this developmental process might have a significant effect on intellect, behavior, and sensory function. Moreover, if the developmental process is modified, the effect might be permanent and pervasive. These basic postulates underlie the presumptions among investigators (Voineagu, 2011) that factors in the prenatal and perinatal/postnatal environment might contribute to ASD.

Chemicals Associated With Developmental Neurotoxicity

The National Academy of Sciences concluded in 2000 (National Academy of Sciences, 2000) that 28% of neurodevelopmental disorders in children are the consequence of early environmental exposures. Hundreds of chemicals are known to be neurotoxic (Scorecard, 2011). According to the U.S. Environmental Protection Agency Toxic Release Inventory, over 2 billion pounds of toxic chemicals are released into the environment in the United States each year, and approximately 75% of the top 20 chemicals are known, or suspected developmental neurotoxins (U.S. Environmental Protection Agency, 2008). Theorists reasoned that the combination of a vulnerable brain and exposure to neurotoxins was likely to be associated with ASD; this view was supported by a report from the Institute of Medicine related to the increase in ASD prevalence (Institute of Medicine, 2008).

The CHARGE Study

An important U.S. investigation has been generating data since 2006 regarding the genetic and environmental factors contributing to autism. The underlying conceptual model of CHARGE is that both genetic and environmental factors are likely to contribute the etiology. Reports from this study are in the literature. Some environmental factors that have been associated with autism are residential proximity to freeways (air pollution exposure) (Volk, 2011), blood mercury concentrations (exposure to methyl mercury) (Hertz-Picciotto, 2010), and plasma fatty acid profiles (diet and metabolism) (Weist, 2009).

Another, international investigation is currently studying a more complex paradigm that associates gene, environment, and timing (Stoltenberg, 2010).

SECTION THREE REVIEW

1. A report from the CHARGE Study associated higher prevalence of autism to which of the following?
   A. Freeway driving
   B. Plasma mercury
   C. Protein-rich diet
   D. Interpersonal family dynamics
   E. None of the above
2. Any toxic or environmental exposure that interferes with this developmental process might have a significant effect on intellect, behavior, and sensory function.
   A. True
   B. False
3. Pathogenetic categories of ASD are all EXCEPT
   A. molecular cytogenetics.
   B. provisionally unique syndrome.
   C. abnormal brain MRI.
   D. deafness.
4. Etiological hypotheses have been proposed for
   A. organic exposure to compounds.
   B. oxytocin and social cognition.
   C. glucoprotein metabolism.
   D. neurotrophic activity.
5. The etiology of ASD is described as
   A. from a known cause.
   B. idiopathic.
   C. from a single gene disorder.
   D. linked to maternal bonding.
   E. A and B

Answers: 1. E; 2. A; 3. A; 4. B; 5. E

SECTION FOUR: Genetic Evidence

Studies to collect evidence for the genetic causes of ASD have been reported since the early 2000s as part of a concerted international effort to uncover the etiology. This evidence is grouped below into syndromic disorders and suspected and known genetic causes of ASD.

Syndromic Disorders and ASD

The etiology of ASD is classified as being from a known disease or idiopathic. If idiopathic, there is no known cause. ASD is found in higher proportions among individuals with other genetic disorders.

Several syndromes include autism as a feature. Miles and McCathren (Miles, 2005) estimated that 5%–10 % of cases of ASD are syndromic. Fombonne (2003) stated that a total of 10%–20% of cases of ASD are due to known medical conditions involving chromosomal imbalances, genetic disorders, and environmental factors (valproate and rubella) (Alsdorf, 2005). The other cases remain unexplained. Among these syndromes are Fragile X syndrome, Rett syndrome, tuberous sclerosis, Smith-Magenis syndrome (Laje, 2010), Angelman syndrome, Prader-Willi syndrome (Nurmi, 2001), Smith-Lemli-Opitz syndrome (Opitz, 1994), velocardiofacial syndrome (Shprintzen, 1985), and others. Autism might also coexist with other chromosomal abnormalities and single gene disorders. For example, a chromosomal condition involving duplication of regions on 15q (tetrasomy15q11q13) is associated with autism (Battaglia, 2005). Bishop and colleagues (Bishop, 2010) reported an increased risk of ASD in sex chromosome trisomies (SCT) such as Klinefelter syndrome at a rate substantially above population levels. The authors hypothesized that X- and Y-linked neuroligins might play a role in the etiology. Jacquemont and colleagues (Jacquemont, 2006) reported that 1.7%–4.8% of people with ASD have chromosome abnormalities. In their review of the literature, they summarized that almost all chromosomes have been involved, including unbalanced translocations, inversions, rings, and interstitial or terminal deletions and duplications. A few of major syndromes associated with ASD are described next.

Fragile X Syndrome

Fragile X syndrome (FXS) occurs in 1 in 3,600 males and 1 in 8,000 females It is caused by an excess of CGG trinucleotide repeats on the **FMR1** (Fragile X Mental Retardation-1) gene on Xq27-3 (Cornish, 2007; Devys, 1993). It is a common cause of inherited intellectual disability. Those with FXS are diagnosed with autism at a rate of 15%–30% (Harris, 2011). The Fragile X mutation can cause anxiety and obsessive behavior as well as premature ovarian failure (Goodman, 1987) and infertility in women (Devys, 1993). The maternal grandfathers of children with Fragile X are at risk for Parkinson-like symptoms (Hagerman, 2001). This observation contributes to the theory of the broader autism phenotype. Males are more severely affected than females. In males, intellectual disability (ID) is reported to be mild to severe, but in females the ID is usually mild (Cornish, 2008).

Overlapping features of FXS and ASD include difficulty making eye contact and gaze aversion, communication deficits, and social withdrawal. According to Budimirovic and colleagues (Budimirovic, 2006) the impairments in social interaction observed in individuals with FXS contribute to an individual meeting the criteria for ASD. In contrast, Kaufman and colleagues (Kaufmann, 2004) observed that there can be a general improvement in autistic-like behavior over time in those with FXS. They concluded that the developmental trajectory of ASDs and FXS differ from idiopathic autism and that like FXS, ASD is a distinctive phenotype (Hernandez, 2009).

Rett Syndrome

Rett syndrome is a **degenerative** condition that primarily affects females and has an onset in early childhood. It occurs in 1 in 10,000 to 1 in 15,000 live female births (Hagberg, 1985). It is caused by a mutation on the X-linked gene **MECP2** that produces methyl cytosine binding protein 2 (Amir, 1999). This protein acts to regulate other genes. The protein is present in the normal brain in several kinds of cells including astrocytes, oligodendroctyte progenitor cells, and oligodendrocytes (Harris, 2011). De Bona and colleagues (De Bona, 2000) stated that the preserved speech variant (PSV) of Rett syndrome shares the same course and the stereotypic handwashing activities with classic Rett syndrome, but differs in that patients typically recover some degree of speech and hand use, and usually do not show growth failure. Progressive scoliosis, epilepsy, and other minor handicaps, usually present in Rett syndrome, are rare in the preserved speech variant. The authors reported mutations in the *MECP2* gene in both classic and PSV Rett syndrome, establishing that the two forms are allelic disorders.

Approximately 25%–40% of individuals with Rett syndrome are diagnosed with autism (Harris, 2011). In a study by Krug and colleagues (Krug, 1980), individuals with Rett syndrome scored significantly higher on the Autism Behavior Checklist than individuals with a matched level of ID. The affected individuals appear normal at first. By 6 to 18 months of age they deteriorate and begin to lose language and social skills. The children continue to lose abilities and skills, including motor function. This is manifested as unsteady gait, unusual breathing patterns during sleep, and slowing brain growth. There is a wide range of severity; some individuals retain and develop language skills while others do not (Renieri, 2009). Individuals with Rett syndrome have an atypical profile of autistic-like symptoms compared with idiopathic autism. Therefore, the association between ASD and Rett syndrome is not entirely clear and many differences are apparent.

Tuberous Sclerosis

Tuberous sclerosis (TS) is a multisystem autosomal dominant disorder that results from loss of function in the *TSC1/TSC2* gene that regulates protein synthesis and cell growth. It occurs in 1 in 6,000 live births (O'Callaghan, 1999) and is caused by mutations in the *TSC1* gene on chromosome 9q34 and in the *TSC2* gene on chromosome 16p13.3 (Crino, 2006; Curatolo, 2008). The product of the *TSC1* gene is known as *hamartin*. The product of *TSC2* is *tuberin*. Approximately 10% to 30% of cases of TS are due to mutations in the TSC1 gene; the frequency of cases due to mutations in the *TSC2* gene is consistently higher. According to Crino and colleagues, *TSC2* mutations are associated with more severe disease (Crino, 2006). Approximately 25% to 60% of individuals with TS have autism (Harris, 2011). Evidence for the co-occurrence of ASD and TS was derived from a series of case studies (Winship, 1990; Wiznitzer, 2004). Gene mutations in either of these genes results in the dysregulation of cell development. Abnormal tissue growth leads to benign tumors in the brain, skin, kidneys, and heart (Crino, 2006). Affected individuals suffer from epilepsy, adenoma sebaceum, and intellectual disability. There is wide variability in the phenotype, ranging from mild skin problems to severe organ involvement and profound intellectual disability (Au, 2007). The association between genotype and phenotype is under investigation.

Suspected and Known Genetic Factors

In 1997, the National Institute of Child Health and Human Development (NICHD) and the National Institute of Deafness and Other Communication Disorders (NIDCD) started the Network on the Neurobiology and Genetic of Autism: Collaborative Programs of Excellence in Autism (CPEA) (National Institute of Health, 2001). Investigators in this network have conducted multiple studies to examine mouse and human genomes for evidence of a genetic cause of autism.

Several genome-wide screens for autism and other studies based on genetic linkage analysis have shown autism susceptibility loci on multiple chromosomes. Evidence to date points to chromosomes 1, 2, 3, 5, 6, 7, 8, 13, 16, 17, 18, 19, 22, and X (Autism, 1999; International Molecular Genetic Study of Autism Consortium, 2001; Yonan, 2003; Battaglia, 2006).

Suspected and known genetic causes of ASD are organized by the categories of (a) structural variation, (b) mutated genes, and (c) susceptibility loci. In addition, mitochondrial DNA has been implicated in causation. In the genetics of ASD, causal loci are the known mutations and susceptibility loci are the sites that are associated with an increase risk for the disease.

Structural Variation of Chromosomes in ASD

Structural variation of chromosomes is also known as copy number variants (**CNV**). A copy number variant is defined as a structural variation or alterations of the DNA of a genome that results in the cell having an abnormal number of copies of one or more sections of the DNA compared to the number of copies in the reference human genome. This includes deletions, duplications, translocations, and inversions of segments of DNA. The full role of structural variation is unknown. Microscopic CNVs and *de novo* CNVs might be more common in sporadic forms of ASD (Sebat, 2007). Marshall and colleagues (Marshall, 2008) summarized that cytogenetically detectable chromosome abnormalities are found in 7.4% of ASD cases with a range from 0% to 54%. Balanced translocations and inversions accounted for 17% of rearrangements. The most frequent anomaly appears to be maternally derived duplication of chromosome 15q11-q13 in 1% to 3% of cases (Veenstra-Vanderweele, 2004).

Many structural variants have been identified on multiple chromosomes and many are under investigation.

Example of a CNV in ASD

A CNV (deletion) was identified that occurred in up to 1% of subjects with ASD (Christian, 2008). The structural variation was linked to the 16p11 region. This region was studied by Kumar and colleagues (Kumar, 2008) who found that 12 of 25 genes in this area could be mapped to a network of genes involved in cell-to-cell signaling and interaction (synaptic genes). Another study described additional CNVs in 16p11 that were also mapped to synaptic genes in the SHANK3-NLGN4-NRXN1 pathway (Marshall, 2008).

After structural variants are identified, candidate loci and suspected candidate genes (specific gene mutations) can be explored using expression studies.

Gene Mutations-Causal Loci

Researchers have noted the differences between causal loci, such as mutations and susceptibility loci, that increase the risk for ASD. Specific gene mutations that are causal loci have been identified on chromosomes 2, 3, 7, 15, 22, and X. Most are rare.

Chromosome 2

Areas on chromosome 2 are loci for **homeobox** (or **HOX**) **genes**, which are a group of genes that control early growth and development. There are approximately 38 HOX genes, and each one directs the action of other genes. Expression of the HOX genes are important in brain stem and cerebellum development, two areas of the brain that are affected in ASD (Ingram, 2000; Elsea, 2011).

Chromosome 7

There is a strong link between chromosome 7 and autism. Investigators are focusing on a region called AUT1 and AUTS2. Both are autism susceptibility genes are located on chromosome 7 (Schumann, 2011). There is also evidence that this chromosome is related to speech and language disorders, both of which are characteristics of ASD. Studies of the *FOXP2* gene on chromosome 7 are of interest because of the known association of mutations with severe speech and language disorders (Cecilia, 2001).

Chromosome 15

Genome-wide association screens and cytogenetic studies show that part of chromosome 15 is involved in ASD. Specific errors cause Angelman syndrome and Prader-Willi syndrome, which both have behavioral characteristics like ASD. Errors on chromosome 15 occur in up to 4% of people with ASD (Muhle, 2004).

Chromosome 22

Mutations to chromosome 22 have been linked to psychiatric disorders such as schizophrenia. Itsara and colleagues (2009) compared large CNVs found in their study of 2,500 individuals with published data from affected individuals in nine genome-wide studies of schizophrenia, autism, and mental retardation. They reported evidence in support of an association between a duplication at chromosome 22q11.2 and autism and schizophrenia (Itsara, 2009). Specifically, the SHANK3 on chromosome 22 has been associated with severe cognitive deficits, including language and speech disorder in ASD (Durand, 2007).

X Chromosome

Two specific disorders that have characteristics with ASD are caused by genes on the X chromosome. They are Fragile X syndrome and Rett syndrome (described earlier). The evidence that ASD is four times more prevalent in males supports the idea that genes on the X chromosome are important causative factors.

Equivocal Evidence

Chromosome 16

A frequently reported association has been the presence of recurrent de novo or inherited microdeletions on chromosome 16p11.2. As recently as 2011, a study by (Konyukh, 2011) *did not support* a major role in autism of the candidate gene, SEZ6L2, on chromosome 16p11.2 (Konyukh, 2011). The role of mutations to chromosome 16 remains under review.

Y Chromosome

Due to the sex differences in ASD prevalence, the Y chromosome was considered a possible candidate. Jamain and colleagues (Jamain, 2002) studied Y chromosome haplogroups in autistic subjects and reported no significant difference in Y-haplotype distribution between affected and control subjects. The Y chromosome and epigenetic factors continues to interest researchers.

Susceptibility Loci

Some genes might increase susceptibility to ASD. As of 2011, there were over 100 published association studies. Several kinds of genes are being carefully analyzed. Five of these are *ENS* (Engrailed 2 gene), *GABA* receptor genes, *OXTR* (oxytocin receptor genes), *RELN* (Reelin gene), and *SLC6A4* (serotonin transporter gene) (Sakurai, 2011).

ENS (Engrailed 2 gene) is found on chromosome 7 and is involved in cerebellar development (Brune, 2008). *GABA* receptor genes have a gene product that is a receptor *GABA*, a **neurotransmitter**. Altered GABA receptor genes are associated with Prader-Willi and Angelman syndromes, and ASD. They have a role in anxiety and epilepsy, which are common features of ASD (Cook, 1998). *GABA* receptor genes cluster on chromosome 15q (Hogart, 2007). *OXTR* (oxytocin receptor genes) are involved in social behaviors and have been linked to chromosome 3 (Ylisaukko-Oja, 2006). *RELN* (Reelin gene) is located on chromosome 7q and encodes for a protein that has a role in the development of neural connections (Skaar, 2005). SLC6A4 (serotonin transporter gene) is located on chromosome 17q and is of interest because blood serotonin levels are higher among people with ASDs. **Serotonin** is associated with obsessive-compulsive behaviors, substance abuse, and depression (Devlin, 2005).

Mitochondrial DNA (mtDNA)

Finally, there is increasing evidence that impairment of mitochondrial energy metabolism might play a role in the pathophysiology of ASD. Oliveira and colleagues (Oliveira, 2005) reported that 7% of children in their population-based survey of children with ASD met criteria for mitochondrial respiratory chain disorders, and this feature lead to subsequent analyses of mutations of mitochondrial DNA (**mtDNA**). Alvarez-Iglesias and colleagues (Alvarez-Iglesias, 2011) conducted a case-control study of 148 patients with idiopathic ASD. They assessed for mutations and looked for the most common European haplogroups and their diagnostic single nucleotide polymorphisms by comparing cases to 753 healthy, ethnically matched controls. Contrary to the results reported by Oliveira, Alvarez-Iglesias and colleagues did not find statistical support for an association between mtDNA mutations or polymorphisms and ASD. Due to the equivocal findings, this remains an area of interest.

SECTION FOUR REVIEW

1. The maternal grandfathers of children with Fragile X are at risk for Parkinson-like symptoms.
   A. True
   B. False
2. The RELN gene (Reelin gene) is located on
   A. chromosome 7q.
   B. chromosome 15q.
   C. chromosome 22p.
   D. chromosome X.
3. What percent of cases of ASD are syndromic?
   A. 0%–1%
   B. 5%–10%
   C. 20%–30%
   D. 40%–50%
4. Syndromes associated with ASD are
   A. Fragile X.
   B. Tuberous sclerosis.
   C. Kleinfelter.
   D. A and B above
   E. A, B, and C above
5. Categories of suspected and known genetics causes of ASD are
   A. structural integrity, ribosomal RNA analogs, and molecular genetic determinants.
   B. mitochondrial DNA and copy number variants.
   C. structural variation, mitochondrial DNA, and susceptibility loci.
   D. copy number variants, microscopic loci, and chromosomal linkage.

Answers: 1. A; 2. A; 3. B; 4. D; 5. C

SECTION FIVE: Research Directions

Approach to Research

Autism research has grown considerably in the United States in recent years and most dramatically since the passage of the Child Health Act in 2000 that mandated the study of prevalence and etiology of the disorder (U.S. Congress, 2000), and the Combating Autism Act of 2006 that accelerated the pace of research. Many important questions remain unanswered. At this juncture in research on the genetics of ASD, no definitive genetic mutations leading to autism susceptibility have been established. In 2006, Coon predicted that within the next 5 to 10 years, large consortiums would begin to reveal results on family collections that were larger than previously studied (Coon, 2006). There is a systematic effort across support networks and the Interagency Autism Coordinating Committee in the United States to organize large groups of patients and families and researchers in order to facilitate scientific inquiry. In addition, the National Database for Autism Research (NDAR) has been established to facilitate collaboration and data sharing of genetic and other variables. These collaborative efforts have resulted in large, informative family and population-based studies, and indicate that there might be convergence across regions and different subsets of clinical phenotypes.

Technology is improving exponentially. The research community has access to approximately 9 million single nucleotide polymorphism (SNPS) and to detailed data describing the nonrandom associations of alleles at close genetic markers among populations across the genome.

The genetic mechanisms are complex and involve inherited and de novo changes including mutations, single nucleotide polymorphisms, trinucleotide repeats, copy number variants, and larger chromosomal abnormalities. Multiple interacting risk alleles are involved, but Hollander, Kolevzon, and Coyle remind us that "an increasing proportion of ASD is being recognized as resulting from a single causal locus" (Hollander, 2011, p. 567). The nature of the variants—common or rare—will have an impact on researchers' abilities to define and develop reliable and valid genetic tests. It is apparent that the trend in research leans toward simultaneous analysis of

Emerging Evidence

- Epidemiological studies in different regions of the world indicate that 1 in every 100 people has some form of autism (Klim, 2011).
- New diagnostic criteria for ASD will be released in 2013 and will replace subtypes (autistic disorder, Asperger disorder, and PDD-NOS) with a single category labeled "Autism Spectrum Disorder" (Volkmar, 2009).
- Work is underway to link diagnostic biological markers to behavioral criteria (Walsh, 2011).
- Biomarkers will be developed from gene expression profiles, proteonomic profiles, and metabolic profiles (Walsh, 2011).
- Proponents of neurodiversity might refer to evidence from genome-wide studies to argue that atypical neurological development seen in autism is in fact a normal human variant that should be recognized as an acceptable difference (Glannon, 2007).

Published scientific agreement about the threshold for clinical utility of biomarkers will contribute to improved parental decision making regarding in utero testing for autism, which is already available (Shen, 2010).

multiple genomic mechanisms along with environmental factors. Animal models will play an important role in uncovering etiology as ASD loci are identified. They will be used to examine the function of the gene products before examining the same activity in humans.

Examining the Role of Environment

The Autism Birth Cohort (ABC) (Stoltenberg, 2010) was established to analyze the interaction of genes and environment over time in order to facilitate early diagnosis. This interaction is expressed as "gene X environment X timing." The research approach uses a large birth cohort in which cases are prospectively ascertained through population screening. In this model, cases are compared with a control group. Samples are collected serially through pregnancy and childhood and include parental blood, maternal urine, cord blood, milk teeth, rectal swabs, and questionnaires and surveys. The ABC cohort includes 107,000 children and promises to provide significant data on the relationship among environment and genetics (Stoltenberg, 2010).

Hunting for Susceptibility Genes

Ultimately, researchers and clinicians hope to identify genes that might predispose an individual to ASD. With such information, there is a hope that strategies for prevention of the disease or amelioration of the clinical symptoms might be accomplished.

The hunt for susceptibility genes begins with selecting and defining a phenotype for analysis. Such phenotypes can be used to sort populations of people with ASD into groups that have the same symptoms and other characteristics (phenotypes). The next step is to compare phenotypes across affected subgroups and among relatives who are unaffected. This is followed by the selection of a candidate gene that will become the focus of a study to associate the gene with the clinical presentation. Preliminary analysis of data will hopefully lead to information about the genotype including map distances, allele frequencies, and information about the phenotype. With this preliminary data in hand, linkage, case-control, and family-based association studies can be designed.

The most important direction in ASD genetics research is to ultimately develop a way to predict a relationship among genotype and sets of behavioral and communication characteristics, and medical and psychiatric comorbidities.

SECTION FIVE REVIEW

1. The genetic mechanisms of ASD are complex and involve inherited and de novo changes. These may include
   A. mutations.
   B. single nucleotide polymorphisms.
   C. trinucleotide repeats.
   D. large chromosomal abnormalities.
   E. All of the above
2. Data from large population-based studies suggest that there may be convergence of characteristics by region and population subset.
   A. True
   B. False
3. The hunt for susceptibility genes begins with
   A. selecting a candidate gene.
   B. designing the study.
   C. stratifying the population.
   D. defining the phenotype.

Answers: 1. E; 2. A; 3. D

SECTION SIX: Role for Nurses in ASD Care

Currently, several candidate genes have been identified in family studies. Oligogenic, polygenic, and mutifactorial mechanisms are being proposed and studied. Some subsets of cases might follow a Mendelian mode of inheritance. It is possible that many decades will pass before the genetics of ASD are fully explored and known. Families and affected individuals will seek guidance and information about the genetics of ASD. Nurses will need to understand the multiple theories explaining etiology and will likely find it challenging to communicate explanations and implications reported in research studies.

Biobanking and Informed Consent

Many studies of ASD pose ethical challenges because of the low probability that individuals will directly benefit from the results. These studies are nontherapeutic but have value to the science. Nurses might be involved in the design and implementation of genetic and other studies of children and adults with ASD. They might be asked to collect biosamples such as blood, hair, and buccal cells for biobanking. These samples are likely to be collected from pediatric patients and research participants. Nurses must be able to describe the use and the ultimate disposition of a sample after it is collected. Until the age of majority, parents will be in a position to grant permission for the short- or long-term storage of genetic material taken from their child. With this comes an ethical obligation that is different than that which is applied to oneself. Most importantly, nurses must be able to explain the difference between samples collected for clinical diagnosis versus biomedical research and disclose that biosamples collected for either research or clinical purposes are no longer the property of the donor. Banking of biosamples has become a way to assure that (a) samples are available for study for an extended time, (b) subjects do not have to donate a sample more than once, and (c) genetic materials are available for study when new questions arise.

The nurse's ethical obligation to subjects in biobank research is the same as for clinical practice: Do good or at least do no harm (beneficence/nonmaleficence), respect the autonomy of the individual, and provide just treatment (Beauchamp, 1983).

With regard to patient participation in autism genetics research, a nurse might advocate for the interests of patients by assessing studies for ethical integrity by examining designs for scientific validity, fair subject selection, social or scientific value, favorable risk-to-benefit ratio, and a rigorous process of assuring informed consent. To this list, Chen and colleagues suggest that studies be assessed for the adequacy of independent review and ongoing data monitoring (Chen, 2003).

Finally, for pediatric environmental health studies, federal regulations governing research with human subjects do not directly address ethical issues associated with protection of family members who are not identified as primary subjects (U.S. Department of Health and Human Services, 2005). Data collected on child data about gene–environmental interactions for autism provide probabilistic health information about parents, as well as the child.

Genetic Counseling for ASD

At minimum, nurses should be literate in genetic terminology and inheritance patterns and be prepared to refer clients for genetic counseling. According to McMahon, Baty, and Botkin (2006), the first step in the process is to distinguish idiopathic autism from syndromes that include autism as a feature. Making a correct and exact diagnosis, if possible, will help the family and medical care providers, including nurses, to manage symptoms and accurately provide reproductive counseling. When syndromic autism is ruled out, the diagnosis is "idiopathic autism." Without the benefit of a definitive genetic test to determine loci or mutations, empiric risk analysis remains the main option for counseling.

According to Muhle and colleagues (Muhle, 2004), recurrence risk among children of parents with one child with ASD ranges from 2% to 8%. There is a general risk of 5% for the broader category of pervasive developmental disability (PDD), the overarching category for ASD and other disabilities (Simonoff, 1998).

Counseling for Multifactorial Etiology

The complex picture of multifactorial etiology of ASD complicates the provision of information and counseling to families. This introduces the question of how much information and counseling is needed and reasonable for a family. There are no predictive tests that can be recommended for idiopathic ASD, and diagnosis has relied on clinician expertise in applying evaluation/diagnostic criteria. McMahon and colleagues (2006) advise that the complexity of autism spectrum disorder will likely be a limiting factor in assuring the clinical validity of any genetic test that is developed.

Parents of children with ASD experience great distress during the year or two typically needed to assess all factors and make a diagnosis (Giarelli, 2005). During this time, parents and families would benefit from nursing care that promotes psychological and social adjustment to the threat of living with a chronic, possibly debilitating condition. The best strategy is to develop protocols that incorporate essential information about the genetics of ASD with information about lifelong care. Regardless of the etiology—syndromic or idiopathic—the affected individual will require lifelong behavioral interventions, and medical care plans must accommodate the special needs of the patient.

An additional challenge to nurses is to integrate cultural issues with a plan of genetic care and counseling. The culturally competent nurse might anticipate the need for difference in the content and process of genetic treatment plans.

Family Health History

A major role for nurse is to collect a comprehensive, three- or four-generation health history with respect to the core characteristics, associated features, environmental exposures, and other factors related to ASD. This will assist in making a diagnosis. It will also assist in developing a comprehensive approach to treatment of affected individuals and counseling of parents and other family members. The family history should include assessment and recording of disorders of sleep and eating, cross-generation history of seizures, and gastrointestinal disorder. Idiosyncratic or odd behavioral mannerisms might also be associated with the ASD feature of restricted, repetitive behaviors. Taking a history of the occurrence and intensity of sensory processing issues such as hypersensitivity to textures, sounds, lights, and tastes might be informative.

Consideration of the Broader Autism Phenotype

The autism phenotype has been shown to be familial and includes social, cognitive, and repetitive behavioral features that are increased in number but are of lesser intensity among first- and second-degree relatives of patients.

Familial rates of depression, social phobias, and other psychiatric disorders have been reported more often among families with autism than among the general population (Piven, 1997; Pickles, 2000; Dawson, 2002). These serious psychiatric comorbidities might need to be prioritized in treatment plans as they might significantly impact quality of life and family function.

Informative Results

There is ongoing debate about the clinical value of results from research on the genetics of ASD. Some investigators and parents believe that disclosure of results to individual participants is necessary when findings of a potential genetic association are reported, in aggregate, in the scientific literature (Miller, 2010; Knoppers, 2006). Miller and colleagues (Miller, 2010) studied the opinions of researchers and participants and related that respondents considered genomic research as reportable when results were perceived to explain the cause and answer the question of "why?" It is important to note that only a perceived explanation was a determining factor. This is understandable in the context of the desperation experienced by families who seek an explanation for their child's severe disability. To them, all information is important. Others argue that the meaning of findings from aggregated data cannot be interpreted at the level of the individual patient and family. In the Miller study (Miller, 2010), the researchers believed that disclosure of results to individuals should be justified not only by perceived meaning but also by clarity regarding "appropriate evidentiary standards and attention to the status of epistemological debates regarding the nature and cause of" of autism (p. 867).

Informed consent for enrolled subjects should include an evaluation of the participant's understanding and acceptance that the results might not be offered or be useful.

SECTION SIX REVIEW

1. What is the purpose of the banking of biosamples from children with autism spectrum disorder?
   A. To assure that samples are available for study for an extended period of time
   B. To spare subjects the burden of having to donate a sample more than once
   C. To have genetic materials available for study when new questions arise
   D. To assure that samples are stored systematically using standard procedures
   E. All of the above
2. A nurse's ethical obligation in research involving biobanking of samples from children with ASD is all of the following EXCEPT
   A. beneficience/non-maleficence.
   B. justice.
   C. solidarity.
   D. respect for autonomy.
3. Biosamples collected from a participant in a research study of ASD remain the property of the donor.
   A. True
   B. False
4. Nurses might examine and critique the designs of genetic studies of ASD for
   A. scientific validity.
   B. fair subject selection.
   C. favorable risk to benefit ratio.
   D. methodological rigor
   E. All of the above

Answers: 1. E; 2. C; 3. B; 4. E

POSTTEST

1. The core characteristic(s) of ASD is/are
   A. impairment in communication.
   B. impairment in socialization.
   C. stereotypical patterns of behavior
   D. restricted interests.
   E. All of the above
2. Signs and symptoms of ASD typically appear by the age of
   A. 6 months.
   B. 1 year.
   C. 3 years.
   D. 5 years.
3. The concordance of ASD among dizygotic twins is approximately
   A. 10%.
   B. 30%.
   C. 50%.
   D. 80%.
4. Risk factors known to associate with ASD are
   A. advanced parental ages.
   B. parental psychiatric comorbidity.
   C. fetal alcohol syndrome.
   D. sensory processing dysfunction.
   E. None of the above
5. An etiological category of ASD is
   A. environment
   B. recognizable syndrome.
   C. diagnosed after molecular cytogenetics.
   D. inherited predisposition.
   E. All of the above
6. Which exposure during early life is significantly associated with ASD?
   A. Exposure to organic compounds
   B. Exposure to cleaning products

C. Exposure to antibiotics
D. Exposure to neuropsychiatric medications

7. The syndromic causes of ASD are know to be due to
   A. chromosomal abnormalities.
   B. trisomy 19.
   C. Prader-Willi syndrome.
   D. Angelman syndrome.
   E. All of the above
8. Cases of tuberous sclerosis are more severe when caused by which gene?
   A. TSC1
   B. TSC2
9. Studies have shown that the chromosomes that are involved in ASD are 2, 3, 7, 17, 22 and x.
   A. True
   B. False
10. Examples of copy number variants (CNV) are transmutations and linkages
   A. True
   B. False

Posttest answers are located in the Appendix.

CHAPTER SUMMARY

Autism spectrum disorder is defined and diagnosed through specific behavioral analyses. Epidemiological twin studies demonstrated that ASDs are genetic disorders. ASDs do not follow typical Mendelian patterns of inheritance. De novo mutations, de novo CNVs, X-linked mutations, and other mutations can cause ASDs. Specific CNVs are being identified as causal loci, and the 16p11 deletion is a significant cause as well. A comprehensive screening for known medical genetics conditions in ASDs can lead to a clinically significant finding.

Many medical conditions have been identified that have a clinical picture similar to that of ASD. There is a role for susceptibility loci in the risk for it. New genome-wide association studies will help identify genetic variants with the highest association with ASD.

CRITICAL THINKING CHECKPOINT

Mark is a 24-month-old child with a long history of developmental delays. Mark makes virtually no eye contact and his vocalization is limited to crying. He has an odd fascination with hair; whenever someone comes close or holds him he immediately starts to play with the person's hair by twisting it, smelling it, trying to taste it, and, if it's long, wrapping it around his ears. At age 18 months, Mark was diagnosed with ASD by a child psychiatrist, and his case met the criteria for autism. The family has a history of several paternal uncles with odd mannerisms and behaviors, including one who is a recluse and another who has obsessive-compulsive disorders. His mother brought Mark to the pediatrician's office to discuss next steps in his care and to get some information about the etiology, or cause, because she heard from a neighbor that autism is passed from generation to generation and she and her partner are considering having a second child. Mark's mother has a few questions about what she needs to do.

1. What tests might be done to evaluate for a genetic cause of Mark's autism?
2. The mother asks, "Why should we undergo have genetic testing?" How should you answer?
3. The parents ask, "Can this happen to us again?" How should you answer?

Answers are provided in the Appendix

Pearson Nursing Student Resources

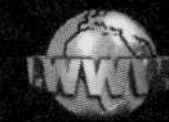

Find additional review materials at nursing.pearsonhighered.com

Prepare for success with additional NCLEX®-style practice questions, interactive assignments and activities, web links, animations, videos, and more!

ONLINE RESOURCES

ABOARD (Advisory Board on Autism & Related Disorders): http://www.aboard.org

Autism National Committee: http://www.autcom.org

Autism Research Institute: http://www.autismresearchinstitute.com

Autism Resources: http://www.autismsource.org

Autism Speaks: http://www.autismspeaks.org

Autism Support Network: http://www.autismsupportnetwork.org

First Signs: http://www.firstsigns.org

Interagency Autism Coordinating Committee: http://iacc.hhs.org

National Autism Association: http://www.nationalautismassociation.org

National Database for Autism Research (NDAR): http://ndar.nih.gov

National Fragile X Foundation: http://www.fragilex.org

National Institute of Child Health and Human Development (NICHD): http://www.nichd.nih.gov

National Institute of Neurological Disorders and Stroke: http://www.ninds.nih.gov

Online Asperger Syndrome Information and Support (OASIS): http://www.asperger.org

Organization for Autism Research: http://www.researchautism.org

S.A.F.E. Inc.: http://www.autismsafe.org

Sibling Support Project: http://www.siblingsupport.org

Unlocking Autism: http://www.unlockingautism.org

US Autism and Asperger Association: http://www.usautism.org

(http://www.ncbi.nlm.nih.gov/SNP)

REFERENCES

Alsdorf, R., & Wyszynski, D. F. (2005). Teratogenicity of sodium valproate. *Expert Opinion on Drug Safety, 4*, 345–353.

Alvarez-Iglesias, V., Mosquera-Miguel, A., Cusco, I., Carracedo, A., Perez-Jurado, L. A., & Salas, A. (2011). Reassessing the role of mitochondrial DNA mutations in autism spectrum disorder. *British Medical Central Medial Genetics, 12*(1–7).

American Psychiatric Association. (2000). *Diagnostic and statistical manual of mental disorders* (4th ed., text rev.). Washington, DC: Author.

Amir, R. E., van den Veyver, I. B., Wan, M., Tran, C. Q., Francke, U., & Zoghbi, H. Y. (1999). Rett syndrome is caused by mutations in X-linked MECP2, encoding methyl-CpG binding protein 2. *Nature Genetics, 23*, 185–188.

Au, K. S., Williams, A. T., Roach, E. S., Batchelor, L., Sparagana, S. P., Delgado, M. R., et al. (2007). Genotype/phenotype correlation in 325 individuals referred for a diagnosis of tuberous sclerosis complex in the United States. *Genetic Medicine, 9*, 88–100.

Bailey, A. J., LeCouteur, A., Gottesman, I., et al. (1995). Autism as a strongly genetic disorder: Evidence from a British twin study. *Psychological Medicine, 25*(1), 63–77.

Bakkaloglu, B., OiRoak, B. J., Louvi, A., et al. (2008). Molecular cytogenetic analysis and resequencing of contactin associated protein-like 2 in autism spectrum disorder. *American Journal of Human Genetics, 82*, 165–173.

Battaglia, A. (2005). The inv dup(15) or idic(15) syndrome: A clinically recognizable neuro-genetic disorder. *Brain Development, 27*, 365–369.

Battaglia, A., & Bonaglia, M. C. (2006). The yield of subtelomeric FISH analysis in the evaluation of autistic spectrum disorders. *American Journal of Medical Genetics Part C Seminars in Medical Genetics, 142C*, 8–12.

Battaglia, A., & Carey, J. C. (2006). Etiologic yield of autistic spectrum disorders: A prospective study. *American Journal of Medical Genetics Part C Seminars in Medical Genetics, 12C*, 3–7.

Beauchamp, T. L., & Childress, J. F. (1983). *Principles of biomedical ethics*. New York: Oxford University Press.

Bishop, D. V. M., Jacobs, P. A., Lachlan, K., Wellesley, D., Barnicoat, A., Boyd, P. A., et al. (2010). Autism, language and communication in children with sex chromosome trisomies. *Archives of Disease in Childhood, 96*(10), pp. 954–959

Bolton, P., Macdonald, H., Pickles, A., Riois, P., Goode, A., Crowson, M., et al. (1994). A case-control family history study of autism. *Journal of Child Psychology & Psychiatry, 35*, 877–900.

Bonaglia, M. C., Giorda, R., Mani, E., et al. (2006). Identification of a recurrent breakpoint within the SHANK3 genetr in the 22q13.3 deletion syndrome. *Journal of Medical Genetics, 43*, 822–828.

Brune, C. W., Korvatska, E., Allen-Brady, K., et al. (2008). Heterogeneous association between engrailed-2 and autism in the CPEA network. *American Journal of Medical Genetics Part B Neuropsychiatric Genetics, 147B*, 187–193.

Budimirovic, D. B., Bukelis, I., Cox, C., et al. (2006). Autism spectrum disorder in Fragile X syndrome: Differential contribution of adaptive socialization and social withdrawal. *American Journal of Medical Genetics A, 140A*, 1814–1826.

Buwe, A., Guttenbach, M., & Schmid, M. (2005). Effect of paternal age on the frequency of cytogenetic abnormalities in human spermatozoa. *Cytogenetics Genome Research, 111*, 213–228.

Buxbaum, J. D., Cai, G., Chaste, P., et al. (2007). Mutation screening of the PTEN gene in patients with autism spectrum disorders and macrocephaly. *American Journal of Medical Genetics Part B Neuropsychiatric Genetics, 144B*, 484–491.

Cecilia, S., Fisher, S. E., Hurst, J. A., Vargh-Khadems, F., & Monaco, A. P. (2001). A forkhead-domain gene is mutated in severe speech and language disorder. *Nature 413*, 519–523s.

Centers for Disease Control and Prevention. (2009). Prevalence of autism spectrum disorder—Autism and Developmental Disabilities Monitoring Network, United States, 2006. *MMWR, 58*(ss-10).

Chen, D. T., Miller, F. A., & Rosenstein, D. L. (2003). Ethical aspects of research into the etiology of autism. *Mental Retardation and Developmental Disabilities, 9*, 48–53.

Christian, S. L., Brune, C. W., Sudi, J., et al. (2008). Novel submicrosopic chromosomal abnormalities detected in autism spectrum disorders. *Biological Psychiatry, 63*(1111–1117).

Collaborative Linkage Study of Autism. (1999). An autosomal genomic screen for autism. *American Journal of Human Genetics, 88*, 609–615.

Cook, E. H., Courchesne, E., Cox, N. J., et al. (1998). Linkage disequilibrium mapping of autistic spectrum disorders, with 15q11-13 markers. *American Journal of Human Genetics, 62*, 1077–1083.

Coon, H. (2006). Current perspectives on the genetic analysis of autism. *American Journal of Medical Genetics Part C, 142C*, 24–32.

Cornish, K., Turk, J., & Hagerman, R. (2008). The Fragile X continuum: New advances and perspectives. *Journal of Intellectual Disability Research, 52*, 469–482.

Cornish, K., Turk, J., & Levitas, A. (2007). Fragile X syndrome and autism: Common developmental pathways? *Current Pediatric Reviews, 3*, 61–68.

Crino, P. B., Nathanson, K. L., & Henske, E. P. (2006). The tuberous sclerosis complex. *New England Journal of Medicine, 355*, 1345–1356.

Croen, L. A., Brether, J. K., & Selvin, S. (2002). Descriptive epidemiology of autism in a California population: Who is at risk? *Journal of Autism & Developmental Disorders, 32*, 217–224.

Curatolo, P., Bombardieri, R., & Jozwiak, S. (2008). Tuberous sclerosis. *Lancet 372*, 657–668.

Daniels, J. (2006). Autism and the environment. *Environmental Health Perspectives, 114*, A396.

Dawson, G., Webb, S., Schellenberg, G., Aylward, E., Richards, T., Dager, S., et al. (2002). Defining the broader phenotype of autism: Genetic, brain, and behavioral perspectives. *Developmental Psycholpathology, 18*(4), 297–321.

De Bona, C., Zappella, M., Hayek, G., Meloni, I., Vitelli, F., Bruttini, M., et al. (2000). Preserved speech variant is allelic of classic Rett syndrome. *Europena Journal of Human Genetics, 8*, 325–330.

Devlin, B., Cook, E. H., Croon, H., et al. (2005). Autism and the serotonin transporter: The long and short of it. *Molecular Psychiatry, 10*, 1110–1116.

Devys, D., Lutz, Y., Rouyer, N., Bellocq, J. P., & Mandel, J. L. (1993). The FMR-1 protein is cytoplasmic, most abundant in neurons and appears normal in carriers of a Fragile X premutation. *Nature Genetics, 4*, 335–340.

Durand, C. M., Betancur, C., Boeckers, T. M., Bockmann, J., Chaste, P., Fauchereau, F., et al. (2007). Mutations in the gene encoding the synaptic scaffolding protein SHANK3 are associated with autism spectrum disorders. *Nature Genetics, 39*, 25–27.

Elsea, S., & Eikler, E. (2011). Deletion on chromosome 2 linked to epilepsy, autism. *American Journal of Human Genetics, 89*, 551–563.

Falk, R. E., & Casas, K. (2007). Chromosome 2q37 deletion: Clinical and molecular aspects. *American Journal of Medical Genetics Part C Seminars in Medical Genetics, 145C*, 357–371.

Folstein, S. E., & Rutter, M. (1977). Infantile autism: A genetic study of 21 twin pairs. *Journal of Child Psychology and Psychiatry, 18*(4), 297–321.

Folstein, S. E., Santangelo, S. L., Gilman, S. E., Piven, J., Landa, R. J., Lainhart, J., et al. (1999). Predictors of cognitive test patterns in autism families. *Journal of Child Psychology and Psychiatry, 40*, 1117–1128.

Fombonne, E. (2002). Epidemiolical trends in rates of autism. *Molecular Psychiatry, 7*, S4–S6.

Fombonne, E. (2003). Epidemiological surveys of autism and other pervasive developmental disorders: An update. *Journal of Autism & Developmental Disorders, 33,* 365–382.

Gauthier, J., Spiegelman, D., Piton, A., et al. (2009). Novel de novo SHANK3 mutation in autistic patients. *American Journal of Medical Genetics Part B Neuropsychiatric Genetics, 150B,* 421–424.

Giarelli, E., Lee, L. C., Levy, S. E., Pinto-Martin, J., Kirby, R. S., & Mandell, D. (2010). Sex difference among 8 year old children. *Disabilities & Health.*

Giarelli, E., Sounders, M., Pinto-Martin, J., Bloch, J., & Levy, S. (2005). Intervention pilot for parents of children with autism spectrum disorder. *Pediatric Nursing, 31*(5), 389–399.

Glannon, W. (2007). Neurodiversity. *Journal of Ethics and Mental Health, 2,* 1–6.

Goodman, R. M., Strauss, S., Friedman, E., & Chaki, R. (1987). Ovarian size in the Fragile X mental retardation syndrome. *American Journal of Medical Genetics, 26,* 17–18.

Grandjean, P., & Landrigan, P. J. (2006). Developmental neurotoxicity of industrial chemicals: A silent epidemic. *Lancet, 368,* 2167–2178.

Hack, M., Taylor, H. G., Drotar, D., et al. (2005). Chronic conditions, functional limitations, and special health care needs of school-aged children born with extremely low-birth-weight in the 1990s. *JAMA, 294,* 318–325.

Hagberg, B. (1985). Rett's sydrome: Prevalence and impact on progressive severe mental retardation in girls. *Acta Paediatrica Scandinavia, 74,* 405–408.

Hagerman, R. J., Leehey, M., Heinrichs, W., Tassone, F., Wilson, R., Hills, J., et al. (2001). Intention tremor, parkinsonism, and generalized brain atrophy in male carriers of Fragile X. *Neurology 57,* 127–130.

Harris, J. C. (2011). Autism spectrum diagnoses in neurogenetic syndromes. In E. Hollander, A. Kolevxzon, & J. T. Coyle (Eds.), *Textbook of autism spectrum disorders.* Washington, DC: American Psychiatric Publishing Co., pp. 223–235.

Hernandez, R. N., Reinberg, R. L., Vaurio, R., et al. (2009). Autism spectrum disorder in Fragile X syndrome: A longitudinal evaluation. *American Journal of Medical Genetics A, 149A,* 1125–1137.

Hertz-Picciotto, I., Green, P. G., Delwiche, L., Hansen, R., Walker, C., & Pessah, I. N. (2010). Blood mercury concentrations in CHARGE Study children with and without autism. *Environmental Health Perspectives, 118*(1), 161–166.

Hogart, A., Nagaranjan, R. P., Patzel, K. A., et al. (2007). 15q11-13 GABAA receptor genes are normally biallelically expressed in brain yet are subject to epigenetics dysregulation in autism spectrum disorders. *Human Molecular Genetics, 16,* 691–703.

Hollander, E., Kolevzon, A., & Coyle, J. T. (2011). Future directions In E. Hollander, A. Kolevzon, & J. T. Coyle (Eds.), *Textbook of autism spectrum disorders.* Washington, DC: American Psychiatric Publishing Co., pp. 567–570.

Ingram, J. L., Stodgell, C. J., Hyman, S. L., Figlewicz, D. A., Weitkamp, L. R., & Rodier, P. M. (2000). Discovery of allelic variants of HOXA1 and HOXB1: Genetic susceptibility to autism spectrum disorders. *Teratology, 62,* 393–405.

Institute of Medicine. (2008). *Autism and the environment: Opportunities and challenges for research.* Washington, DC: National Academies Press.

International Molecular Genetic Study of Autism Consortium. (2001). A genomewide screen for autism: Strong evidence for linkage to chromosomes 2q, 7q, and 16p. *American Journal of Human Genetics, 69,* 570–581.

Itsara, A., Cooper, G. M., Baker, C., Girirajan, S., Li, J., Absher, D., et al. (2009). Population analysis of large copy number variants and hotspots of human genetic disease. *American Journal of Human Genetics, 84,* 148–161.

Jacquemont, M. L., Sanlaville, D., Redon, R., Raoul, O., Cormier-Daire, V., Lyonnet, S., et al. (2006). Array-based comparative genomic hybridisation identifies high frequency of cryptic chromosomal rearrangements in patients with syndromic autism spectrum disorders. *Journal of Medical Genetics, 43,* 843–848.

Jamain, S., Quach, H., Bentancur, C., et al. (2003). Mutations of the X-linked genes encoding neuroligins NLGN3 and NLGN4 are associated with autism. *Nature Genetics, 34,* 27–29.

Jamain, S., Quach, H., Quintana-Murci, L., Betancur, C., Philippe, A., Gillberg, C., et al. (2002). Y chromosome haplogroups in autistic subjects. *Molecular Psychiatry, 7*(2), 217–219.

Kanner, L. (1943). Autistic disturbances of affective contact. *The Nervous Child, 2,* 217–250.

Kaufmann, W. E., Cockerill, R., Kau, A. S., et al. (2004). Autism spectrum disorder in Fragile X syndrome: Communication, social interaction, and specific behaviors. *American Journal of Medical Genetics A, 129A,* 225–234.

Kim, H. G., Kishikawa, S., Higgins, A. W., et al. (2008). Disruption of neurexin 1 associated with autism spectrum disorder. *American Journal of Human Genetics, 82,* 199–207.

Klim, Y. S., et al. (2011). Prevalence of autism spectrum disorders in a total population sample. *American Journal of Psychiatry, 168,* 9-4-9-12.

Knoppers, B., Joly, Y., & Durocher, F. (2006). Emergence of an ethical duty to disclose genetic research results: International perspectives. *European Journal of Human Genetics, 14,* 1170–1178.

Konyukh, M., Delorme, R., Chaste, P., Leblond, C., Lemiere, N., Nygren, G., et al. (2011). Variations of the candidate SEZ6L2 gene on chromosome 16p11.2 in patients with autism spectrum disorders and in human populations. *PLoS ONE, 6*(3), e17298.

Krug, D. A., Arick, J., & Almond, P. (1980). Behavior checklist for identifying severely handicapped individuals with high levels of autistic behavior. *Journal of Child Psychology & Psychiatry, 21,* 221–229.

Kumar, R. A., KaraMohamed, S., & Sudi, J. (2008). Recurrent 16p11.2 microdeletions in autism. *Human Molecular Genetics, 17,* 628–638.

Laje, G., Morse, R., Richter, W., Ball, J., Pao, M., & Smith, A. C. M. (2010). Autism spectrum features in Smith-Magenis syndrome. *American Journal of Medical Genetics Part C, 154C,* 456–462.

Landrigan, P. J. (2011). Environment and autism. In A. J. Hollancer, A. Kolevzon, & J. T. Coyle (Eds.), *Textbook of autism spectrum disorders.* Washington, DC: American Psychiatric Publishing, Inc., pp. 247–264.

Laumonnier, F., Bonnet-Brilhault, F., Gomot, M., et al. (2004). X-linked mental retardation and autism are associated with a mutation in the NLGN4 gene, a member of the neuroligin family. *American Journal of Human Genetics, 74,* 552–557.

Lawrence, S. P., Bright, N. A., Luzio, J .P., & Bowers, K. (2010). The sodium/proton exchanger NHE8 regulates late endosomal morphology and function. *Molecular Biology & Cell, 21*(20), 3540–3551.

Lerer, E., Levi, S., Salomon, S., et al. (2008). Association between the oxytocin receptor (OXTR) gene and autism: Relationship to Vineland Adaptive Behavior Scales and cognition. *Molecular Psychiatry, 13,* 980–988.

Levine, H. E., & Levine, D. D. (2011). Preface: Autism. In E. Hollander, A. Kolevzon, & J. T. Coyle (Eds.), *Textbook of autism spectrum disorders.* Washington, DC: American Psychiatric Publishing, Inc., pp. xxi–xxii.

Levy, S. E., Giarelli, E., Lee, L. C., Schieve, L. S., Kirby, R. S., Cunniff, C., et al. (2010). Autism spectrum disorder and co-occurring developmental, psychiatric, and medical conditions among children in multiple populations in the United States. *Journal of Developmental and Behavioral Problems, 31*(3), 1–9.

Levy, S. E., Mandell, D. S., & Schultz, R. T. (2009). Autism. *Lancet, 374,* 1627–1638.

Limoges, E., Mottron, L., Bolduc, C., Berthiaume, C., & Godbout, R. (2005). Atypical sleep architecture and the autism phenotype. *Brain, 128,* 1049–1061.

Lin, P. I., Vance, J. M., Pericak-Vance, M. A., et al. (2007). No gene is an island: The flip-flop phenomenon. *American Journal of Human Genetics, 80,* 531–538.

Marshall, C. R., Noor, A., Vincent, J. B., et al. (2008). Structural variation of chromosomes in autism spectrum disorder. *American Journal of Human Genetics, 82,* 477–488.

Marshall, C. R., Noor, A., Vincent, J. B., Lionel, A. C., Feuk, L., Skaug, J., et al. (2008). Structural variation of chromosomes in autism spectrum disorder. *American Journal of Human Genetics, 82,* 477–488.

Martin, R. H. (2008). Meitoic errors in human oogenesis and spermatogenesis. *Reproductive Biomedical Online, 16,* 523–531.

McIntosh, G. C., Olshan, A. F., & Baird, P. A. (1995). Paternal age and the risk of birth defects in offspring. *Epidemiology, 6,* 282–288.

McMahon, W. M., Baty, B. J., & Botkin, J. (2006). Genetic counseling and ethical issues for autism. *American Journal of Medical Genetics Part C, 142C,* 52–57.

Miles, J., & Mccathren, R. (2005). Autism overview. *GeneReviews at GeneTests: Medical Genetics Information Resources.*

Miller, F. A., Hayeems, R. Z., & Bytautas, J. P. (2010). What is a meaningful result? Disclosing the results of genomic research in autism to research participants. *European Journal of Human Genetics, 18,* 867–871.

Morrow, E. M., Yoo, S. Y., Flavell, S. W., et al. (2008). Indentifying autism loci and genes by tracing recent shared ancestry. *Science, 321,* 218–223.

Mouridsen, S. D., Rich, B., & Isager, T. (1993). Brief report: Parental age in infantile autism, autistic-like conditions and borderline childhood psychosis. *Journal of Autism & Developmental Disorders, 23,* 387–396.

Muhle, R., Trentacoste, S. V., & Rapin, I. (2004). The genetics of autism. *Pediatrics, 113,* e472–e486.

National Academy of Sciences. (2000). *Scientific frontiers in developmental toxicity and risk assessment.* Washington, DC: National Academy of Sciences Press.

National Database for Autism Research (NDAR). http://ndar.nih.gov

National Institute for Child Health and Human Development. (2008). *The Collaborative Programs of Excellence in Autism (CPEAs).* Retrieved from http://www.nichd.nih.gov/autism/research/cpea.cfm

National Institute of Health. (2001). *The NICHD/NIDCD Network on the Neurobiology and Genetic of Autism: Collaborative Programs of Excellence in Autism (CPEA).* Retrieved from http://www.nichd.nih.gov/autism

Newschaffer, C. J., Croen, L. A., Daniels, J. et al. (2007). The epidemiology of autism spectrum disorders. *Annual Review of Public Health, 28,* 235–258.

Nikolov, R. N., Bearss, K. E., Lettinga, J., et al. (2008). Gastrointestinal symptoms in a sample of children with pervasive developmental disorders. *Journal of Autism & Developmental Disorders, 39,* 405–413.

Nurmi, E. L., Bradford, Y., Chen, Y. H., Hall, J., Arnone, B., Gardiner, M. B., et al. (2001). Linkage disequilibrium at the Angelman syndrome gene UBE3A in autism families. *Genomics, 77*(1–2), 105–113.

O'Callaghan, F. J. (1999). Tuberous sclerosis. *British Medical Journal, 318,* 1019–1020.

Oliveira, G., Diogo, L., Grazina, M., Garcia, P., Ataide, A., Marques, C., et al. (2005). Mitochondrial dysfunction in autism spectrum disorders: A population-based study. *Developmental Medicine & Child Neurology, 47*(3), 185–189.

Opitz, J. M., Penchaszadeh, V. B., Holt, M. C., Spano, L. M., & Smith, V. L. (1994). Smith-Lemli-Opitz (RSH) syndrome bibliography: 1964-1993. *American Journal of Human Genetics, 50*, 339–343.

Pickles, A., Starr, R., Kazak, S., Bolton, P., Papanikolau, K., Bailey, A. J., et al. (2000). Variable expression of the autism broader phenotype: Findings from extended pedigrees. *Journal of Child Psychology, Psychiatry and Alllied Disciplines, 41*(4), 491–502.

Piven, J., Palmer, P., Jacobi, D., Childress, D., & Arndt, S. (1997). Broader autism phenotype: Evidence from a family history study of multiple-incidence autism families. *American Journal of Psychiatry 154*, 185–190.

Piven, J., Palmer, P., Jacobi, D., et al. (1987). Broader autism phenotype: Evidence from a family history study of multipe-incidence autism famimlies. *American Journal of Psychiatry 154*, 185–190.

Piven, J., Palmer, P., Landa, R. J., Santangelo, S. L., Jacobi, D., & Childress, D. (1997). Personality and language characteristics in parents from multiple-incidence autism families. *American Journal of Medical Genetics, 74*, 398–411.

Rapin, I., & Tuchman, R. F. (2008). Autism: Definitions, neurobiology, screening, diagnosis. *Pediatric Clinics of North America, 55*, 1129–1146.

Renieri, A., Mari, F., Mencarelli, M. A., Scala, E., Ariani, F., Longo, I., et al. (2009). Diagnostic criteria for the Zappella variant of Rett syndrome (the preserved speech variant). *Brain Development, 31*, 208–216.

Ritvo, E. R., Freeman, B. J., Mason-Brothers, A., Mo, A., & Ritvo, A. M. (1985). Concordance for the syndrome of autism in 40 pairs of afflicted twins. *American Journal of Psychiatry, 142*(1), 74–77.

Rosenberg, R. E., Law, J. K., Yenokyan, G., McGready, J., Kaufmann, W. E., & Law, P. A. (2009). Characteristics and concordance of autism spectrum disorders among 277 twin pairs. *Archives of Pediatric and Adolescent Medicine, 163*(10), 907–914.

Rutter, M. (2011). A Selective scientific history of autism. In E. Hollander, A. Kolevzon, & J. T. Coyle (Eds.), *Textbook of autism spectrum disorders*. Washington, DC: American Psychiatric Publishing, Inc., pp. 5–23.

Sadakata, T., Washida, M., Iwayama, Y., et al. (2007). Autistic-like phenotypes in Cadps2-knockout mice and aberrent CADPS2 splicing in autistic patients. *Journal of Clinical Investigation, 117*, 931–943.

Sakurai, T., Cai, G., Grice, D. E., & Buxbaum, J. D. (2011). Genomic architecture of autism spectrum disorder. In A. J. Hollancer, A. Kolevzon, & J. T. Coyle (Eds.), *Textbook of autism spectrum disorders*. Washington, DC: American Psychiatric Publishing, Inc., pp. 281–298.

Sanders, S. J., Murtha, M. T., Gupta, A. R., Murdoch, J. D., Raubeson, M. J., Willsey, A. J., et al. (2012). *De novo* mutations revealed by whole-exome sequencing are strongly associated with autism. *Nature*, Apr 4. doi:10.1038/nature10945. [Epub ahead of print]

Schumann, G., Coin, L. J., Lourdusamy, A., Charoen, P., Berger, K. A., Stacey, D., et al. (2011). Genome-wide association and genetic functional studies identify autism susceptibility candidate 2 gene (AUTS2) in the regulation of alcohol consumption. *Procedures of the National Academy of Science, 108*, 7119–7124.

Scorecard. (2011). *Suspected neurotoxicants*. Retrieved December 9, 2011, from http://scorecard.goodguide.com/health-effects/chemicals-2.tcl?short_hazard_name=neuro&all_p=t

Sebat, J., Lakshmik, B., Malhtra, D., Troge, J., Lese-Martin, C., Wash, T., et al. (2007). Strong association of de novo copy number mutations with autism. *Science, 316*, 445–449.

Segurado, R., Conroy, J., Meally, E., et al. (2005). Confirmation of association between autism and the mitochondrial aspartate/glutamate carrier SLC25A12 gene on chromosome 2q31. *American Journal of Psychiatry, 162*, 2182–2184.

Shen, Y. (2010). Clinical genetic testing for parents with autism spectrum disorders. *Pediatrics, 125*, 670–677.

Shprintzen, R. J., Wang, F., Goldberg, R., & Marion, R. (1985). The expanded velo-cardio-facial syndrome (VCF): additional features of the most common clefting syndrome. *American Journal of Human Genetics, 37*, A77.

Simonoff, E. (1998). Genetic counseling in autism and pervasive developmental disorders. *Journal of Child Psychology, Psychiatry and Alllied Disciplines, 28*, 447–456.

Simonoff, E., Pickles, A., Charman, T., Chandler, S., Loucas, T., & Baird, G. (2008). Psychiatric disorders in children with autism spectrum disorders: Prevalence, co-morbidity, and associated features in a population-derived sample. *Journal of American Academy of Child and Adolescent Psychiatry, 47*, 921–929.

Skaar, D. A., Shao, Y., Haines, J. L., et al. (2005). Analysis of the RELN gene as a genetic risk factor for autism. *Molecular Psychiatry, 10*, 563–571.

Steffenburg, S., Gillberg, C., Hellgren, L., et al. (1989). A twin study of autism in Denmark, Finland, Iceland, Norway and Sweden. *Journal of Child Psychology & Psychiatry, 30*(3), 405–416.

Stoltenberg, C., Schjolberg, S., Bresnahan, M. H., M., Hirtz, D., Dahl, C., Lie, K. K., et al. (2010). The autism birth cohort: A paradigm for gene-environment-timing research. *Molecular Psychiatry, 15*, 676–680.

Szatmari, P., Jones, M. B., Fisman, S., Tuff, L., Bartolucci, G., Mahoney, W. J., et al. (1995). Parents and collateral relative sof children with pervasive developmental disorders: A family history study. *American Journal of Medical Genetics 60*(60), 282–289.

Taniai, H., Nishiyama, T., Miyachi, T., Imaeda, M., & Sumi, S. (2008). Genetic influences on the broad spectrum of autism: Study of proband-ascertained twins. *American Journal of Medical Genetics Part B: Neuropsychiatric Genetics, 147B*(6), 844–848.

U.S. Congress. (2000). Children's Health Act of 2000. *106-310, 114 Stat. 1101*.

U.S. Department of Health and Human Services. (2005). Public Welfare: Code of Federal Regulations: Protection of Human Participants. 45CFR46 [Electronic Version]. Retrieved from Http://www.hhs.gov/ohrp/humansubjecs/guidance/45cfr46.htm

USDHHS/Center for Disease Control and Prevention, Autism and Developmental Disabilities Monitoring Network Surveillance Year 2008 Principal Investigators. (2012). Prevalence of autism spectrum disorders—autism and developmental disabilities monitoring network, 14 Sites, United States, 2008. *Morbidity and Mortality Weekly Report (Surveillance Summaries March 30), 61*(3), 1–19.

U.S. Environmental Protection Agency. (2008). *Toxic Release Inventory (TRI)*. Retrieved from http://www.epa.gov/tri/tridata/tri06/index.htm

Ullmann, R., Turner, G., Kirschhoff, M., et al. (2007). Array identifieds reciprocal 16p13.1 duplications and deletions that predispose to autism and/or mental retardation. *Human Mutations, 28*, 674–682.

Veenstra-Vanderweele, J., Christian, S. L., & Cook, E. H. (2004). Autism as a paradigmatic complex genetic disorder. *Annual Review of Genomics and Human Genetics, 5*, 379–405.

Voineagu, I., Wang, X., Johnson, P., Lowe, J. K., Tian, Y., Horvath, S., et al. (2011). Transciptomic analysis of autistic brain reveals convergent molecular pathology. *Nature, 474*, 380–386.

Volk, H. E., Hertz-Picciotto, I., Delwiche, L., Lurmann, F., & McConnell, R. (2011). Residential proximity to freeways and autism in the CHARGE study. *Environmental Health Perspectives, 119*(6), 873–877.

Volkmar, E. R., State, M., & Klin, A. (2009). Autism spectrum disorders: Diagnostic issues for the coming decade. *Journal of Child Psychology and Psychiatry, 50*, 108–115.

Walsh, P. N., Elsabbagh, M., Bolton, P., & Singh, I. (2011). In search of biomarkers for autism: Scientific, social and ethical challenges. *Nature Reviews-Neuroscience, 12*, 603–612.

Weiss, L. A., Shen, Y., Korn, J. M., et al. (2008). Association between microdeletion and microduplicaiton at 16p11.2 and autism. *New England Journal of Medicine, 358*, 667–675.

Weist, M. M., German, J. B., Harey, D. J., Watkins, S. M., & Hertz-Picciotto, I. (2009). Plasma fatty acid profiles in autism: A case-control study. *Prostaglandins Leukotrienes & Essential Fatty Acids, 80*(4).

Winship, I. M., Connor, J. M., & Beighton, P. H. (1990). Genetic heterogeneity in tuberous sclerosis: Phenotypic correlations. *Journal of Medical Genetics, 27*, 418–421.

Wiznitzer, M. (2004). Autism and tuberous sclerosis. *Journal of Child Neurology, 19*, 675–679.

Ylisaukko-Oja, T., Alarcon, M., Cantor, R. M., et al. (2006). Search for autism loci by combining analysis of Autism Genetic Resource Exchange and Finnish families. *Annals of Neurology, 59*, 145–155.

Yonan, A. L., Alarcon, M., Cheng, R., Magnusson, P. K. E., Spence, S. J., Palmer, A. A., et al. (2003). A genomewide screen of 345 families for autism-susceptibililty loci. *American Journal of Human Genetics, 73*, 886–897.

PART 8

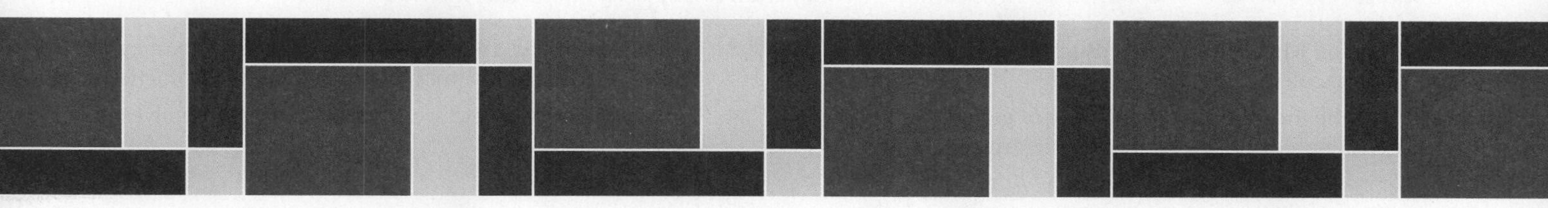

Special Topics

CHAPTER

23 Pharmacogenomics

Cynthia A. Prows, Houry V. Puzantian

LEARNING OUTCOMES

Following the completion of this chapter, the learner will be able to

1. Describe why genomics needs to be considered in pharmacology.
2. Describe the clinical applicability of genetic tests used to identify predispositions to variable drug responses.
3. Describe issues that need to be addressed prior to integration of pharmacogenomics into routine clinical practice.
4. Explain the nurse's role as pharmacogenomics evolves in clinical practice.

This chapter presents an overview of pharmacogenomics and describes the factors that influence clinical utility and clinical acceptance of pharmacogenomic testing. This chapter describes how pharmacogenomics is applied in select clinical settings and discusses evidence gaps and challenges that need to be addressed before medication therapies are routinely informed by pharmacogenomics. It also summarizes the nurse's role within the interdisciplinary team when medication selection and dosing are informed by pharmacogenomics.

PRETEST

1. Clinically important single genes that have been intensively studied in drug response include those that code for
   A. drug absorption.
   B. drug distribution.
   C. drug metabolism.
   D. drug elimination.
2. Pharmacogenetic testing
   A. targets single genes associated with drug response.
   B. uses broad approaches such as microarray.
   C. is only used in drug trials.
   D. is a genetic test ordered by pharmacists.
3. When a drug's effectiveness relies on metabolism it is called
   A. an active drug
   B. a pro-drug.
   C. a reactive drug.
   D. a substrate.
4. Tamoxifen and warfarin are examples of medications for which pharmacogenetic testing is being used in select specialty settings.
   A. True
   B. False
5. A purpose of pharmacogenetic testing is to identify patients who are genetically predisposed to being more sensitive (responsive) or more resistant (less responsive or nonresponsive) to a medication with a narrow therapeutic range.
   A. True
   B. False
6. Nurses need to be able to determine that the patient knows
   A. why a pharmacogenetic test was ordered.
   B. how a pharmacogenetic test result might be used for medication selection or dosing.
   C. the limitations of the test.
   D. the results may be relevant for future medications.
   E. All of the above
7. Nurses can assure patients that once they have had a pharmacogenetic test for one drug they will not need pharmacogenetic testing in the future.
   A. True
   B. False
8. A patient who has a pharmacogenetic test report that states no mutations were found may still have an undetected mutation in the tested gene that could lead to an adverse drug reaction.
   A. True
   B. False

9. Nongenetic factors such as age, weight, and environment do not need to be considered if a pharmacogenetic test was done.
   A. True
   B. False
10. A pharmacogenetic test for a specific medication may indicate
   A. the medication is unlikely to work.
   B. the patient may need a lower dose than routinely used to reduce risk for toxicity.
   C. the patient may need a higher dose than routinely used to experience the intended effect.
   D. the patient may require a different medication.
   E. All of the above
   F. None of the above

Pretest answers are located in the Appendix.

SECTION ONE: What Is Pharmacogenomics?

Pharmacotherapy is the use of medications to prevent or treat disease. It aims at appropriate, safe, and economic use of medications in designated patient populations to prevent deterioration of conditions and promote well-being. Pharmacotherapy consists of the pharmaceutical drug formulation process, **pharmacokinetics** (what the body does to the drug), pharmacodynamics (what the drug does to the body), and the actual therapeutic process of responsiveness (Feucht & Patel, 2011). Multiple factors influence these processes, leading to interindividual variability in drug response.

All drugs (except those given intravenously) delivered to the human body must be absorbed by traveling through cell membranes before reaching the systemic circulation. The formulation of a drug and method of delivery can affect the rate of absorption. The presence of food in the gastrointestinal system and local PH can influence absorption. Medications are absorbed through cell membranes by passive diffusion or by facilitated diffusion requiring carrier proteins, and by active transport. Variations in those proteins can affect absorption. The blood distributes the drug to target tissue as well as to the liver, which is the primary site of drug metabolism. Distribution can be affected by body composition and tissue perfusion status.

Metabolism is the process of changing the structure of a drug; this transformation facilitates a drug's elimination and in some cases is a necessary step to render it active. Different enzymes and nonenzymatic processes are involved in metabolism. If a drug is administered in its active form, and an enzyme involved in biotransformation for elimination purposes is deficient or absent, the patient will be susceptible to toxicity-related **adverse drug reactions (ADRs)**. Some drugs enter the body in an inactive form; they are called **pro-drugs**. Pro-drugs need to be metabolized to release the active component of the drug. If the enzyme necessary for this process is underproduced, inhibited, absent, or nonfunctional, the patient may experience decreased or no effect from the drug. Furthermore, disease processes affecting the liver can interfere with the metabolic process. Kidneys are the primary sites of excretion; some drug components may be eliminated from the body through the bile and intestinal system. Diseases affecting the kidneys can influence the process of elimination.

Other factors affecting response to pharmacotherapy include demographic, environmental, psychological, and lifestyle factors. In children, demographic factors such as age, weight, or body mass index (BMI) are often used to calculate doses. Differences in response associated with sex or race have been reported for some medications. Factors such as pregnancy; complexity/severity of disease being treated; or comorbidity (presence of other diseases) can influence medication selection and dosing. Risk for adverse reactions due to drug–drug interactions can increase as the number of coprescribed medications increases (Edwards & Aronson, 2000). Use of over-the-counter drugs, recreational drugs, alcohol, herbal products, tobacco, and certain drug–food interactions (foods and nutritional supplements) can also increase the risk of a patient experiencing an unintended response to a prescribed medication. Other factors that can influence whether a medication has a therapeutic effect include adherence with prescribed regimen, development of tolerance, or the placebo experience (desirable and undesirable effects related to patient's anticipation of drug results).

In addition to the previously mentioned factors, the role of genes in drug response is beginning to be viewed as an important consideration when selecting and/or dosing medications in clinical settings. As indicated in the brief discussion of pharmacokinetic processes, many different proteins are involved. Variants in genes coding for proteins like drug transporters, metabolizing enzymes, and therapeutic targets can predispose a person to unintended drug responses such as reduced effectiveness or toxicity-related ADRs at therapeutic doses.

Emerging Evidence

The clinical pharmacogenetics implementation consortium (CPIC) of the pharmacogenetics research network is developing, and plans to regularly update evidence-based, freely accessible guidelines for specific drug–gene(s) combinations. Pharmacogenetics guidelines developed by CPIC can be found at the PharmGKB website at http://www.pharmgkb.org.

The Role of Genetics in Pharmacologic Therapy

The fact that the genetic makeup of an individual contributes to an individualized drug-response phenotype has been known for years. However, advancements in the Human Genome Project over the past decade have shed light on broader possibilities in pharmacogenetic and pharmacogenomic applications.

The terms *pharmacogenetics* and *pharmacogenomics* are sometimes used interchangeably in the literature; however, a distinction can be made as follows: **Pharmacogenetics** (PGx) is the study of the role of genetics in observed differences in drug response. It often refers to the effects of single genes (and their variants) on responsiveness to medications. Clinically important single genes that have been intensively studied include those that code for drug-metabolizing enzymes such as TPMT (thiopurine S-methyltransferase) and the superfamily of cytochrome P450 enzymes (Zhou et al., 2008). Cytochrome P450s are the main enzymes responsible for drug metabolism; each isoenzyme within the cytochrome P450 enzyme family is designated by the letters CYP, followed by an Arabic numeral, a letter, and another Arabic numeral (e.g., CYP2D6). A useful site for cytochrome P450 nomenclature is http://www.cypalleles.ki.se. Oftentimes the abbreviation for the gene is the same as the enzyme, with the only difference being genes are italicized and the enzymes are not. Variant alleles may result in poorly functioning or nonfunctioning enzyme; reduced quantities or absent enzyme; increased enzyme quantity or function; or variant function only within the context of a specific medication (Ingelman-Sundberg, Sim, Gomez, & Rodriguez-Antona, 2007). **Pharmacogenomics** provides a more comprehensive outlook on the interconnectedness of pharmacology and genetics, with a wider impact at the population level. It expands on PGx in terms of understanding and relating the functions of multiple genes and their contribution to variability in drug response. The concept of pharmacogenomics springs from technological advances in genetics that enable broader applications of the science. The introduction of high-throughput technology allows for the processing of much larger amounts of data. New approaches like microarray analysis enable the study of DNA expression of a large number of genes. The examination of expression profiles of genes with related functions, in combination with drug response phenotype, can lead to the identification of patterns that can provide for signatures of sensitivity to particular drugs. Certain types of these diagnostic approaches/algorithms may be subject to regulation by the U.S. Food and Drug Administration (FDA) as medical devices (FDA, 2012a). Pharmacogenomic approaches are now employed in new drug discovery and design; moreover, they are used in the reevaluation of existing drugs that were previously put to limited use or taken off the market due to adverse patient outcomes.

In summary, pharmacogenomic tools have the potential to help clinicians identify genetic variations related to drug response and to understand their implications in pharmacotherapeutics. This information enables clinicians to adjust medication regimens with the aim of maximizing therapeutic effectiveness and minimizing adverse effects. Collectively, these developments mark the beginning of a new era of personalized care.

SECTION ONE REVIEW

1. Decreased metabolism of an active drug
   - A. increases the risk for drug toxicity.
   - B. reduces the risk for drug toxicity.
   - C. improves drug efficacy.
   - D. A and C above
   - E. B and C above
2. A poor metabolizer of a pro-drug is at risk for not responding to the medication.
   - A. True.
   - B. False.
3. Drug response of individuals may relate to genetic polymorphisms affecting
   - A. drug transporters.
   - B. metabolizing enzymes.
   - C. drug receptors.
   - D. A and B above
   - E. Any of the above
4. *Pharmacogenomics* refers to a comprehensive outlook to the interplay of genetics and pharmacology due to
   - A. the use of high-throughput technology processing large amounts of data.
   - B. a focus on the individual rather than the population.
   - C. the ability to identify patterns of drug response and develop algorithms.
   - D. A and C above
   - E. All of the above
5. Industry would utilize PGx in
   - A. new drug development.
   - B. reevaluation of existing drugs.
   - C. drug-labeling specifications.
   - D. A and B above
   - E. All of the above

Answers: 1. A; 2. B; 3. E; 4. D; 5. E

SECTION TWO: Clinical Application of Pharmacogenomics

Current technologic advances enable the discovery of a greater number of genes associated with drug response. While the number of laboratories routinely offering PGx testing remains low at the time of this writing, it is expected that availability will become more prevalent. Most prescribing professionals are not aware of pharmacogenomic tests or do not know which genes are relevant for specific medications. As evidence accumulates for a particular gene–drug association, specialists who commonly prescribe the medication are more likely to have heard or read about a genetic test for predicting or explaining unintended responses to the particular medication. However, they may not know how to use the results of the test to modify their routine drug selection and dosing practices. Electronic health records can be built with alerts notifying prescribers when a PGx test is available for a medication or if a relevant test result was obtained in the past. But such systems are rare. Another point of care support being developed is a genetic test report template that includes standard types of information including clinical implications of results to support therapeutic decision making (Lubin, Hilborne, & Scheuner, 2010). The clinical implications section of a PGx test report that uses such a template might suggest dose adjustments or alternative medications based on the result. As the knowledge base of prescribers and the necessary point-of-care supports for decision making improve, nurses will increasingly encounter patients who are having, or have had in the past, genetic testing to individualize their medication therapy. Tamoxifen and warfarin are examples of medications for which genetic testing is being used in select specialty settings.

Tamoxifen, a Pro-drug Exemplar: Drug Efficacy Implications

Tamoxifen is a medication commonly used to treat women who have estrogen receptor positive breast cancer. Although tamoxifen, in its unchanged form, provides some therapeutic effect, two of its metabolites have more potent anticancer effects as estrogen receptor antagonists in breast tissue (Wu et al., 2009). Both metabolites are impacted by the CYP2D6 pathway (see Figure 23–1 ■). Endoxifen is tamoxifen's most abundant metabolite with anticancer properties. Studies consistently demonstrate that women who are CYP2D6 **poor metabolizers (PMs)**, lacking the functional enzyme, have significantly lower plasma concentrations of endoxifen than CYP2D6 **extensive metabolizers** (**EMs**; individuals who have enzyme levels within normal range) (Jin et al., 2005; Kiyotani et al., 2010). Furthermore, **ultra-rapid metabolizers** may be identified who exhibit very high CYP2D6 levels; they thus break down Tamoxifen very fast, producing high plasma concentrations of endoxifen.

CYP2D6 PMs may result from having two nonfunctional variant alleles. Moreover, a person who has two functional alleles for the CYP2D6 may, in turn, have the enzyme inhibited due to drug–drug interactions where a medication inhibits CYP2D6 activity resulting in a decrease in the metabolism of the substrate drug. Examples of medications that inhibit CYP2D6 activity and used to be commonly co-administered with tamoxifen to manage hot flashes or depression are fluoxetine and paroxetine (Jin et al., 2005). What matters to clinicians is, "Do women who are CYP2D6 PMs (by genotype or drug–drug interactions) have a poorer clinical outcome when taking tamoxifen than women who are CYP2D6 EMs?"

In other words, what is the clinical utility of CYP2D6 testing? Unfortunately, this is not easily answered. The vast majority of studies aiming to assess the association of CYP2D6 genotype with tamoxifen treatment outcomes have been small and retrospective with variable consideration of possible confounders and variable outcome measures. A few large studies have been conducted, but those were also retrospective and varied in their consideration of potential confounders and selected outcomes. In some studies, an association between CYP2D6 PMs and poorer outcomes such as reduced time for cancer recurrence or mortality were measured (Goetz et al., 2007; Schroth et al., 2009), but in other studies no differences in outcomes were detected between women taking tamoxifen who were CYP2D6 PMs and those who were CYP2D6 EMs (Seruga & Amir, 2010).

Likewise, results from recent epidemiologic studies considering Selective Serotonin Reuptake Inhibitor (SSRI) association with variable tamoxifen effectiveness have been conflicting. While paroxetine coadministration with tamoxifen was associated with increased risk of death from breast cancer in a cohort study (Kelly et al., 2010), a case-control study did not detect a difference in breast cancer recurrence in women prescribed CYP2D6-inhibitory SSRIs while being treated with tamoxifen (Lash et al., 2011). Again, differences in primary outcomes, design, and measured confounders make it difficult to draw conclusions. Despite equivocal results, at the time of this writing CYP2D6 genotyping prior to prescribing tamoxifen is used in some settings, and the FDA approved a label change for paroxetine noting its reported association with reducing tamoxifen effectiveness (FDA, 2012b).

European and Scandinavian countries have been the leaders in studying and using PGx testing in practice. In 2011, the Pharmacogenetics Working Group of the Royal Dutch Association for the Advancement of Pharmacy (Swen et al., 2011) and the European Science Foundation–University of Barcelona (Becquemont et al., 2011) separately published clinical guidelines for select gene–medication combinations. Both guidelines recommended CYP2D6 testing in women prior to tamoxifen therapy. Both suggested using aromatase inhibitors (a different drug class, interferes with estrogen production) as an alternative in postmenopausal women who have genetic test results consistent with predicted CYP2D6 PM or **intermediate metabolizer (IM)**; the latter exhibiting reduced enzyme activity. In the United States, a Technology Assessment Report funded by the Agency of Healthcare Research and Quality and published in 2010 indicated there was insufficient evidence to recommend CYP2D6 testing prior to prescribing tamoxifen (Terasawa, Dahabreh, Castaldi, & Trikalinos, 2010). The same was concluded in a Blue Cross Blue Shield Association (BBA) Technical Assessment paper (BBA, 2011). Medco, however, offered CYP2D6 testing for tamoxifen as part of its

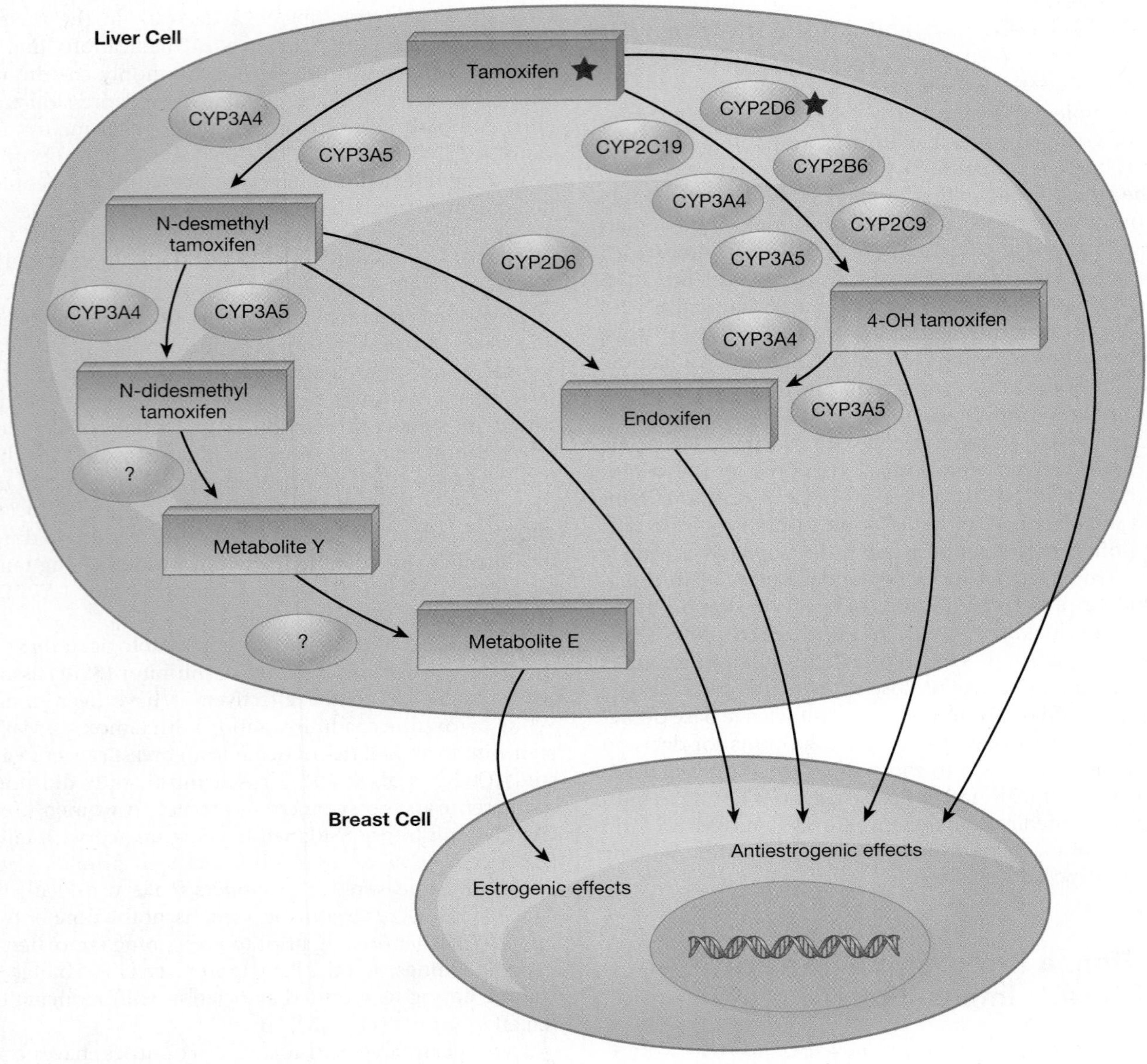

Figure 23–1 ■ Tamoxifen PK. Tamoxifen metabolism in the liver.

Source: E.M. McDonagh, M. Whirl-Carrillo, Y. Garten, R.B. Altman and T.E. Klein. "From pharmacogenomic knowledge acquisition to clinical applications: the PharmGKB as a clinical pharmacogenomic biomarker resource." Biomarkers in Medicine (2011) Dec; 5(6):795–806.

personalized medicine program at the time of this writing (Medcohealth, 2011). In spite of the variable study results, guidelines, and reports, nurses may encounter women who want to know about this test or for whom the test was ordered.

Warfarin, an Active Drug Exemplar: Drug Safety Implications

Warfarin is the most commonly used medication worldwide for oral anticoagulation therapy. It works by interfering with the vitamin K–dependent clotting pathway. Warfarin has a narrow therapeutic range with significant response variability among patients. Rather than measuring actual drug levels, the **international normalized ratio (INR)** is monitored to determine whether warfarin dosing is within therapeutic range. INR is the ratio of a patient's prothrombin time to that of a normal (control) sample. The therapeutic range of INR for people on warfarin is generally 2.0–3.0; however, it may vary with the disease or surgical condition. INR below therapeutic range can result in thromboembolism. Dangerous bleeding is a risk when INRs are above therapeutic range. Adult patients are typically prescribed a standard initial daily dose followed by serial INRs with consequent dose adjustment. Achieving a stable maintenance dose can take weeks, and sometimes months of adjustments. Furthermore, average maintenance warfarin dose requirements have been shown to vary between different ethnic and racial groups, with Asians often requiring lower doses and African-Americans requiring higher doses on average (Dang, Hambleton, & Kayser, 2005). The interest in using pharmacogenetics testing is based on potentially identifying patients who are genetically predisposed to being more sensitive or more resistant to warfarin (Johnson, Horne, Carlquist, & Anderson, 2011).

Warfarin has two main active enantiomers (compounds that have similar molecular formulas and are mirror images of one another, but are not superimposable): S-warfarin and R-warfarin. S-warfarin is the more potent active component. There are many genes that produce proteins contributing to patient response to warfarin. Two of these genes, *CYP2C9* (gene coding for an enzyme that metabolizes warfarin) and *VKORC1* (gene coding for an enzyme that is the therapeutic target of warfarin), have been shown to contribute significantly to the variable responses experienced by patients (Kamali & Wynne, 2010). The *CYP2C9* gene produces the primary enzyme responsible for converting S-warfarin to its less potent metabolites. People who are homozygous or compound heterozygous for two variant *CYP2C9* genes and are either unable to produce enzyme or produce a nonfunctional form of enzyme are considered *CYP2C9* PMs (Lee, Goldstein, & Pieper, 2002). *CYP2C9* PMs can be expected to have longer exposure to the more potent S-warfarin with each dose when compared to people who have fully functioning CYP2C9 enzyme. Patients identified as *CYP2C9* PMs prior to first dose might be started on a lower initial dose. Patients identified within the first week of therapy might have their INRs monitored more frequently in the early period as these patients would be at increased risk for bleeds and might require lower warfarin doses.

The *VKORC1* gene produces an enzyme (vitamin K epoxide reductase **[VKOR]** complex subunit 1) that converts vitamin K–epoxide to activated vitamin K, which in turn activates vitamin K–dependent clotting factors (II, VII, IX, X) involved in thrombin formation (Rieder et al., 2005). Warfarin works by inhibiting this enzyme (see Figure 23–2 ■), thus reducing the amount of vitamin K available for the activation of important clotting factors. Certain variants of the *VKORC1* gene produce lower concentrations of the enzyme, reducing the amount of vitamin K available for activating clotting factors, and lowering the availability of the

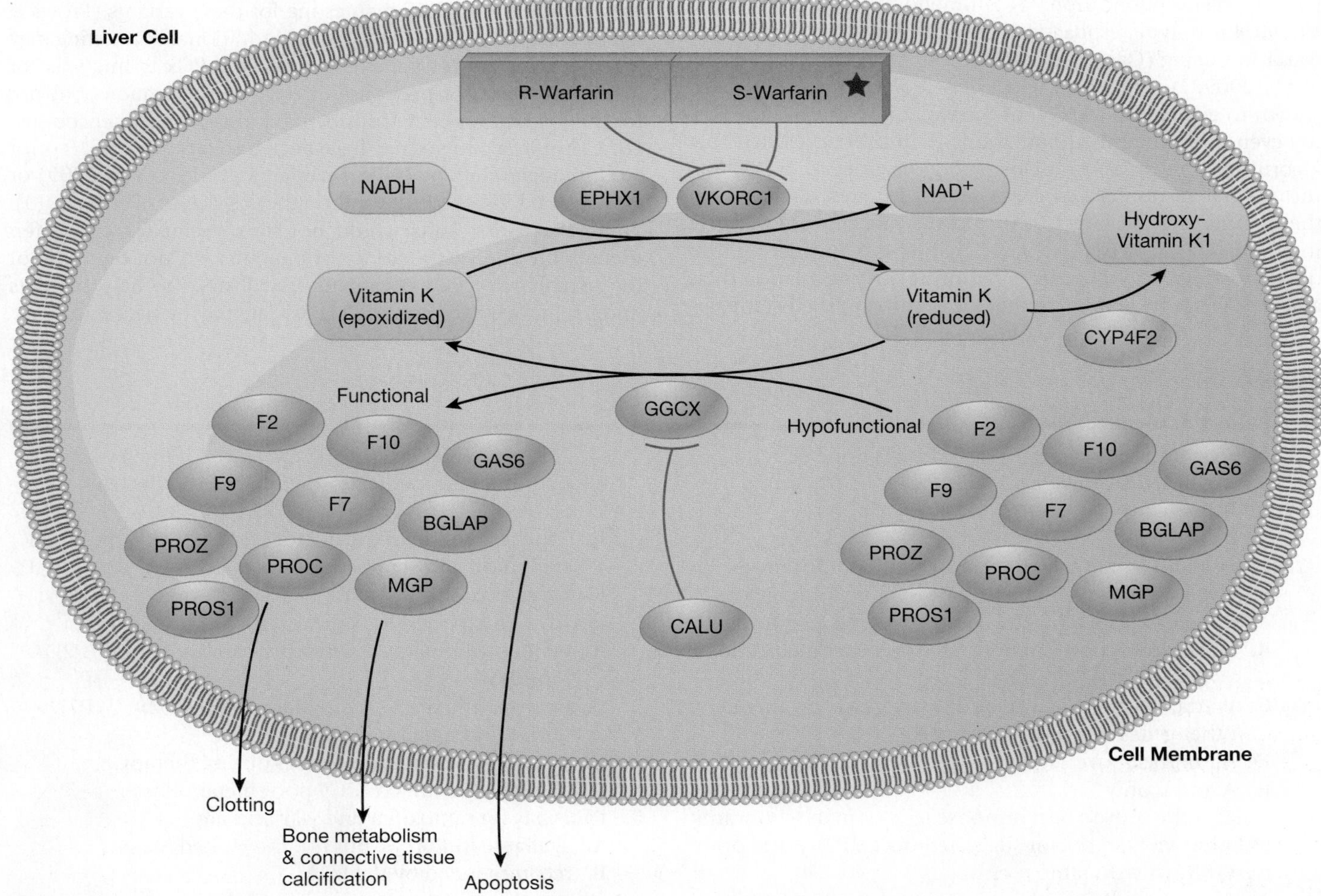

Figure 23–2 ■ Pharmacodynamics. Simplified diagram of the target of warfarin action and downstream genes and effects.

Source: E.M. McDonagh, M. Whirl-Carrillo, Y. Garten, R.B. Altman and T.E. Klein. "From pharmacogenomic knowledge acquisition to clinical applications: the PharmGKB as a clinical pharmacogenomic biomarker resource." Biomarkers in Medicine (2011) Dec; 5(6):795–806.

enzyme (VKORC1) as a warfarin target. These patients would be expected to be more susceptible to warfarin's anticoagulation effect and would require lower warfarin doses.

Patients found to be *CYP2C9* PMs and who have two variant *VKORC1* genes producing less enzyme can be predicted to have a lower warfarin dose requirement (Burmester et al., 2011; Caraco, Blotnick, & Muszkat, 2008; Klein et al., 2009; Lesko, 2008). However, clinical studies have not consistently demonstrated increased risk for bleeding episodes for genetically sensitive patients (Burmester et al., 2011; Flockhart et al., 2008; Klein et al., 2009). Patients who have genotypes consistent with full-functioning *CYP2C9* and full-functioning *VKORC1* will more likely need higher warfarin doses to achieve therapeutic INRs but warfarin dose variability is not limited to differences in genes (Klein et al., 2009).

Warfarin response is also considerably influenced by non-genetic factors such as age, weight, certain foods like green leafy vegetables, disease process, alcohol consumption, tobacco use, and many other medications. Before the availability of genetic testing, dosing algorithms were available that considered many of these clinical factors, including race and ethnicity. A number of recent publications recommend using *CYP2C9* and *VKORC1* genotype results together with clinical factors to guide warfarin dosing (Gage et al., 2008; Johnson et al., 2011; Klein et al., 2009; Lesko, 2008). Gene-based algorithms have been shown to explain up to 55% of the variability in warfarin dosing even in multiethnic populations (Lubitz et al., 2010). Line algorithms such as WarfarinDosing.org (Gage, et al., 2008) that include genetic results are freely available for prescribers to help them anticipate the target dose and the rate of dose titration that may be necessary to achieve ideal INRs. Considering this, nurses who work with patients requiring anticoagulation therapy with warfarin may encounter PGx testing in their settings.

Pharmogenetics Test: Only Needed Once?

It is common knowledge that the genes we inherit from our parents do not typically change, except for occasional spontaneous changes in individual cells. Therefore, people often think that once a genetic test is performed, it will not need to be repeated. This is most often true if the test detected variant genes. To know whether a normal result can be interpreted as the tested genes are free of functional variants, the nurse must determine the type of technology used for the test. At the time of this writing, the vast majority of PGx tests analyze only the most common variants associated with unintended drug responses. If these variants are not identified, then it is assumed that the individual has wild type alleles. In such situations, a negative PGx test result cannot be considered the same as normal. The nurse can only state to the patient that the variants the test analyzed were not present in their genes. However, it is still possible that rare functional variants are present that could influence their response to a medication. As technology is able to identify increasing numbers of variants for each gene in an accurate and less expensive manner, patients may benefit from additional testing for these variants (Prows & Beery, 2008; Prows & Saldana, 2009). Additional PGx testing may also be necessary for patients whose only PGx testing was for genes important for previously prescribed medications but not for the medication being considered during a patient encounter. For example, a patient may have been tested for *CYP2C19* prior to clopidogrel therapy (Ellis, Stouffer, McLeod, & Lee, 2009) or *CYP2C9* and *VKORC1* for warfarin therapy (Lenzini et al., 2010). These PGx test results would not be relevant for tamoxifen therapy but the vast majority of patients will not be aware of the specificity of PGx tests. Nurses will need to help patients understand why additional PGx testing may be necessary.

SECTION TWO REVIEW

1. Genetic testing for warfarin response is done so serial testing of INRs can be avoided.
   A. True
   B. False
2. Why would a patient still be at risk for complications with warfarin even when the starting dose and rate of dose increases are adjusted based on the PGx test?
   A. Warfarin's action can be altered by other medications.
   B. Warfarin's action can be altered by changes in diet.
   C. Warfarin's effectiveness and toxicity risk are altered by other genes that were not tested.
   D. All of the above
   E. A and B only
3. What is the nurse's best response to a woman who wants to know why the doctor suggested the CYP2D6 test prior to starting her on tamoxifen?
   A. "The test will help the doctor know if estrogen stimulates the growth of your breast cancer."
   B. "The test will help the doctor know if your breast cancer is sensitive to tamoxifen."
   C. "The test will help the doctor decide if tamoxifen or a different medication will be most effective for you."
   D. "The test will help the doctor decide if you should be started on a lower dose of tamoxifen."
4. Concentrations of tamoxifen's active metabolite, endoxifen, can be expected to be lower in
   A. women who take an antidepressant that is a CYP2D6 inhibitor.
   B. women who are found by PGx testing to be CYP2D6 ultra-rapid matabolizers.
   C. women who have hot flashes during therapy.
   D. women who are *CYP2C9* poor metabolizers.
5. PGx tests for tamoxifen and warfarin are
   A. available in Europe but not the United States.
   B. recommended by the FDA.
   C. needed once since genes do not change.
   D. used in some specialty clinical settings.

Answers: 1. B; 2. C; 3. D; 4. A; 5. D

SECTION THREE: Before Pharmacogenomics Becomes Common Practice

As more genomics and proteomics data become available, more work is needed to clarify the roles of multiple genes and their interplay. The clinical use of genetic data presents additional challenges. Consequently, the associations of those genes, select drugs, and drug-response phenotypes need to be explored to bridge the gap between the science and practice.

This clinical translation of PGx tests would enable clinicians and patients to make informed decisions regarding choice of therapy, dose adjustment, close monitoring, or change in therapy. With the expected increase in the use of PGx tools in clinical practice, it will also be important to evaluate whether alternative therapy is available for those classified as nonresponders. There needs to be careful consideration about whether genetic testing for predisposition to nonresponse should be performed if alternative therapies do not exist. Knowing that errors can occur and that such testing would rarely be expected to have 100% positive predictive value, patients who could potentially benefit from the medication could have it withheld due to misclassification. Likewise, patients with genotypes indicative of sensitivity to medication could still experience adverse effects if started on a lower than normal dose and if slower titration of increased dosing is used. Adverse effects could be related to reduced or delayed therapeutic response due to the adjustments in dose or due to drug–drug interactions or other environmental factors. For these reasons, it is imperative that clinicians understand that genetic testing will not replace the need to consider all other relevant factors. Diligent monitoring practices for medications with narrow therapeutic ranges or medications treating diseases with high morbidity or mortality will still be essential even when informed by genetic testing.

The completion of the Human Genome Project paved way to the emergence of new medical applications. Additionally, the evolution of high-throughput screening methodologies enabled researchers to conduct a multitude of tests in a short period of time. These high-throughput assays utilize automation to identify large numbers of compounds, proteins, and genes that affect certain biomolecular pathways; moreover, they help assay the biochemical activity of substances. The benefits reside in better understanding the role of biologic substances and providing opportunities for drug design.

These developments, however, are accompanied with a multitude of challenges. One of the major impediments to the clinical implementation of pharmacogenomics is the difficulty of handling large amounts of bioinformatics data resulting from high throughput biological assays. Errors in the processing of this type of pharmacogenomic data can translate into inappropriate pharmacotherapeutic approaches in patient care (Baggerly & Coombes, 2009). A patient falsely identified as a nonresponder to a particular drug might be deprived of necessary treatment. A patient inappropriately classified as responsive to a drug may endure a lengthy series of dose adjustments before switching to an effective medication. Furthermore, patients misclassified as normal metabolizers of a medication that is administered in its active form may experience toxicity with normal doses. Fortunately, scientists increasingly realize the importance of ensuring reproducibility of data resulting from high throughput biological experiments (Baggerly & Coombes, 2011). Emphasis is placed on attention to methodologic precision and accuracy in documentation. Appropriate examination and reporting of pharmacogenomic data requires investigators to generate and comply with written analysis plans, standard operating procedures, documented analytic steps, regular checks for common errors, and validation testing (Baggerly & Coombes, 2009, 2011).

Many studies relating gene variances and drug response have had small sample sizes. In extrapolating results of such studies to the clinical setting as PGx diagnostic tests, clinicians need to take certain considerations into account. It will be important to scrutinize the extent to which a gene variant impacts drug response phenotype, or resort to studies with large sample sizes that would increase validity of a designated test. These measures would improve the appropriateness and cost-effectiveness of PGx screening of patients who are candidates for treatment with a particular drug.

Currently, there is an evidence gap in pragmatic economic consequences of PGx. The determination of economic benefit relies on the availability of more data regarding the clinical effectiveness of specific PGx tests (Deverka, Vernon, & McLeod, 2010). The Centers for Medicare & Medicaid Services (CMS) adopted a "coverage with evidence development" approach (Miller & Pearson, 2008) that relies on technology assessment reports discussing the benefits and harms of specific tests (CMS, 2012). The decision for coverage is made according to criteria such as those developed for warfarin PGx, with *CYP2C9* or *VKORC1* allele testing for previously untested individuals, those who have received less than 5 days of warfarin, and those enrolled in certain randomized controlled studies (CMS, 2012). It will be important to highlight cost containment related to a decrease in the occurrence of adverse events, the reemergence of previously used drugs, and focused drug development in responder groups. This needs to be weighed against the cost of PGx tests as related to the frequency of particular polymorphisms in disease populations.

In addition to economic issues, ethical, social, and legal issues will need to be considered when evaluating the public health implications of PGx (Lee, Ma, & Kuo, 2010). One of the primary ethical issues that is brought up is the potential for ancillary clinical information revealed during a PGx test (Haga, O'Daniel, Tindall, Lipkus, & Agans, 2011). There are concerns that genes associated with drug response may also be associated with disease predisposition, some of which could be stigmatizing (Haga et al., 2011). In a public telephone survey, respondents' interest in PGx testing was high despite being informed about the potential for revealing ancillary information (Haga et al., 2011). Organizational and systems gaps also exist in that there is lack of structured PGx service delivery. Clearer insight is required as to designated personnel and realm of responsibilities regarding PGx testing and interpretation services in health care systems. As a working example, in the first author's institution PGx testing is used for patients admitted to psychiatry inpatient units. A handout about the testing is available for nurses to give to parents and patients. The clinical pharmacist assigned to the unit ensures the treating psychiatrist is aware when a patient's PGx test result comes back abnormal and makes recommendations for dose changes or medication changes based on these results. The psychiatrists and/or nurses explain to patients and/or parents why medications are being adjusted and monitor the effects of the adjustments.

A social consequence of PGx testing and more specifically, ancillary information, is that it requires a genomics informed health care workforce to know how to respond to the information in a way that is beneficial to the person's physical and psychosocial health. Patients are becoming aware of the emergence of PGx tests (Haga et al., 2011). The public expects health providers to explain the impact of the tests on prescribed medication regimens; however, many clinicians are reluctant to initiate PGx services (Haga et al., 2012; Kirk, Tonkin, & Patch, 2006). Increasing numbers of educational programs need to commit to the appropriate training of clinicians in the utilization of PGx applications (Haga et al., 2012).

SECTION THREE REVIEW

1. The challenges of bioinformatics data resulting from high throughput assays include
   A. handling large amounts of data as a result of advanced technology.
   B. dealing with misclassification errors on drug response status.
   C. spending time on regular checks and ensuring reproducibility of data.
   D. A and C above
   E. All of the above
2. PGx testing-related information would improve economic cost effectiveness by which of the following?
   A. Discovering a low frequency of a particular polymorphism in a disease population
   B. Ensuring coverage by the Center for Medicare and Medicaid Services
   C. Decreasing the occurrence of adverse events in susceptible groups
   D. All of the above
   E. None of the above
3. Barriers in implementing PGx testing in clinical practice relate to
   A. whether PGx testing services are available.
   B. whether enough is known to interpret obtained test results.
   C. whether practitioners are trained in PGx.
   D. A and C above
   E. All of the above
4. Issues that require attention for the immediate refinement of clinical PGx include
   A. clarification of roles of multiple genes and their interplay.
   B. whether alternative drugs are present for the non-responder class.
   C. the identification of drug–environment interactions.
   D. A and B above
   E. All of the above
5. Impediment(s) for PGx testing to become widely utilized screening tests include(s)
   A. small sample sizes of PGx studies.
   B. low impact of identified gene on drug-response phenotype.
   C. low frequency of identified polymorphism in a disease population.
   D. A and C above
   E. All of the above

Answers: 1. E; 2. C; 3. E; 4. D; 5. E

SECTION FOUR: The Nurse's Role Within the Interdisciplinary Team

As PGx gradually makes its way into clinical practice, nurses need to acquire a set of competencies to address PGx-related patient care issues. One of the major requirements is acquiring knowledge of genetics (Cashion, 2009; Novak, 2007). This would include but not be limited to the basic genetic concepts and to commonly known genetic polymorphisms (polymorphisms in genes coding for proteins such as enzymes, transporters, receptors, and in signaling pathways) that would confer individual variation in pharmacokinetics and pharmacodynamics. It will be important to understand the relevance of genetic screening tests to personalization of pharmacologic intervention, as pertinent to one's practice (Kirk et al., 2006; Seibert, Edwards, & Maradiegue, 2007). Nurses need to be vigilant in monitoring for drug effect, and in appropriate dose adjustment according to genetic-based algorithms. As patients increasingly get involved in their own care, nurses will need to be prepared for patient education regarding PGx-based approaches to therapy including choice of drug, dose adjustment, and reporting of adverse effects (Fargher et al., 2007).

Nursing Competencies Relevant to Pharmacogenomics

Essential nursing competencies in genetics/genomics were first published in 2006 and a second edition published in 2009. The competency document describes the basic genetic/

genomic competencies for all registered nurses, regardless of level of academic preparation, practice setting, or specialty. Within the professional practice domain, competencies are divided between Nursing Assessment; Identification; Referral Activities; and Provision of Education, Care and Support (Consensus Panel on Genetic/Genomic Nursing Competencies, 2009). In November 2011, a Collaborative Genetic Services Summit was hosted by the National Society of Genetic Counselors to develop a competency-based collaborative model for integrating genetics and genomics services into health care. Pharmacogenomics was one of the service triage models proposed and discussed by leaders from nursing, genetic counseling, medicine, pharmacy, and public health. In the model, nurses, prescribers, and pharmacists were seen as the primary providers in PGx rather than genetic professionals. Relevant competencies when encountering patients for whom PGx testing might be considered or for whom testing was completed are discussed next.

Assess Client Knowledge

Assesses client's knowledge, perceptions, and responses to genetic and genomic information.

(Consensus Panel on Genetic/Genomic Nursing Competencies, 2009)

During the November 2011 Summit, there was general agreement that the informed consent process for PGx testing, ordered at the time of medication decision making or when assessing cause of adverse effects, could be similar to that used prior to other clinical tests. Basic information the patient needs to know is why the test is being ordered, how results might be used, and the limitations of the test. In some settings, handouts are available with this information (Cincinnati Children's Hospital Medical Center, 2011). Nurses must have enough baseline knowledge in PGx to be able to ascertain if a patient's knowledge is accurate and to clarify basic misunderstandings patients might have. The key points nurses need to remember when assessing a patient's knowledge and reinforcing or clarifying their understanding include the following:

> (a) drug response is influenced by many different factors and bodily processes; (b) genetic test results provide a component of the necessary information when prescribers select and dose medications; (c) commercially available PGx tests are not relevant for all medications; (d) genetic test results may be relevant to a patient's future health care because inherited genes, for the most part, do not change; (e) a patient's genetic test result may be relevant to biologic family members since they share inherited genes; (f) depending on the type of analysis performed in the laboratory, a negative or normal test result may be a false negative if all possible variants associated with altered gene function were not analyzed (Prows & Saldana, 2009).

Provide Client With Accurate Information and Resources

Provides client with credible, accurate, appropriate, and current genetic and genomic information, resources, services, and/or technologies that facilitate decision making.

(Consensus Panel on Genetic/Genomic Nursing Competencies, 2009)

Oftentimes the initial explanation about what the PGx test results mean for the patient's plan of care is provided by the advanced practice nurse or physician who ordered the test. However, all nurses should be prepared to make sure patients understand the information that is presented, clarify any misunderstandings, and address any concerns the patients/families express regarding the subsequent plan of care. These responsibilities can seem overwhelming in the rapidly changing field of genetics/genomics.

Clinical nurses typically have patients with similar diagnostic categories that they care for on a routine basis. Therefore, nurses can focus on learning available PGx tests for the medications commonly used to treat patients within their area of specialty. It is recognized that staff nurses are not responsible for ordering laboratory tests as this falls within the scope of practice of advanced practice nurses (**APNs**). Yet, it is within all nurses' roles to share their knowledge about the availability of a PGx test for their patients. And similar to checking allergies prior to administering medications, the nurse will eventually need to check whether a PGx test has already been performed for their patient and assure that the therapeutic implications of the results are considered by those who prescribe the relevant medications.

Evaluate Effectiveness of Interventions

Evaluates impact and effectiveness of genetic and genomic technology, information, interventions, and treatments on clients' outcome.

(Consensus Panel on Genetic/Genomic Nursing Competencies, 2009)

In most clinical settings, it is the nurse who consistently monitors the patient for clinical improvement and closely assesses for early signs of drug toxicity. Nurses can help other health care providers as well as patients realize that PGx testing to inform drug selection and drug dosing does not replace the need to consider nongenetic contributions to drug response nor reduce the need to monitor for early signs of toxicity. The same type and frequency of biochemical and hematologic measures will be necessary to assess for therapeutic effectiveness of medications and detect early signs of potential toxicities. Nurses will need to continue their important teaching role, instructing patients to closely monitor and report any signs of medication allergy and/or adverse drug reactions and to report use of other medications, herbal products, nutritional supplements, tobacco, or alcohol that interfere with medication absorption or are known to alter toxicity risks.

Professional Practice Domain: Referral Activities

Facilitates referrals for specialized genetic and genomic services for clients as needed.

(Consensus Panel on Genetic/Genomic Nursing Competencies, 2009)

As stated earlier, routine PGx testing ordered at the point of care is not expected to require the service of genetics professionals. However, as knowledge of genomics improves and understanding of how genes and proteins interact in ways that contribute toward state of health, clinically relevant ancillary information may be revealed by the PGx test result or by the technology used to identify variant genes in drug response. Ancillary information includes information not related to drug response such as predisposition to a condition for which the patient is not currently seeking treatment or does not manifest symptoms, or prognostic information that does not have bearing on treatment (Haga & Burke, 2008). It will be up to the nurse and prescribing professionals to determine if their genomics knowledge is adequate for discussing PGx test-associated ancillary findings. If not, then a referral to a health professional with specialty training in genetics will be necessary, as a recent survey revealed the public is interested in learning ancillary findings from genetic tests (Haga et al., 2011).

SECTION FOUR REVIEW

1. Concepts nurses need to understand to address PGx-related patient care issues include which of the following? (Select all that apply.)
   A. The gene(s) analyzed in a PGx test may be relevant for more than one medication.
   B. PGx tests usually analyze specific mutations or polymorphisms that have been associated with variability in drug response.
   C. The gene(s) analyzed in a PGx test to determine drug response predisposition for a specific medication may NOT be relevant for a different medication.
   D. There are many different genes that code for many different proteins that influence drug absorption, drug distribution, drug metabolism, and drug elimination.
2. After a medication is selected and dosed based on a PGx test result, the nurse needs to monitor the patient's drug response and consider nongenetic factors that can contribute to drug response variability.
   A. True
   B. False
3. Nurses need to assure that their patients have genetic counseling prior to having their sample obtained for PGx testing.
   A. True
   B. False
4. Genetic/Genomic Nursing Competencies indicate that nurses should be able to do which of the following? (Select all that apply.)
   A. Assess a patient's understanding of the PGx test.
   B. Discuss the reproductive implications of test results.
   C. Clarify patient misunderstandings about the purpose and limitations of the test.
   D. Address any concerns the patients/families express regarding the plan for medications after testing.
5. Ancillary information from a PGx test may include
   A. the type of nutritional supplements expected to interfere with the medication.
   B. medications that are inhibitors and inducers of the enzyme(s) coded for by the genes analyzed in the PGx test.
   C. predispositions to health conditions unrelated to medication response.
   D. A and B only
   E. All of the above

Answers: 1. A, B, C, D; 2. A; 3. B; 4. A, C, D; 5. C

POSTTEST

1. Higher than expected enzyme activity is predicted in
   A. extensive metabolizers.
   B. ultrarapid metabolizers.
   C. immediate metabolizers.
   D. poor metabolizers.
2. A person with a genotype consistent with extensive metabolizers can be expected to function as an intermediate or poor metabolizer when
   A. taking a medication that is an enhancer for the enzyme.
   B. taking a medication that stimulates the immune system to destroy the enzyme.
   C. taking a medication that causes an allergic response.
   D. taking a medication that is an inhibitor for the enzyme.
3. Increased metabolism of a pro-drug
   A. increases the risk for drug toxicity at typical doses.
   B. reduces the risk for drug toxicity at typical doses.
   C. reduces the effectiveness of the drug at typical doses.
   D. increases the effectiveness of the drug if taken at higher doses.
4. Increased metabolism of an active drug
   A. increases the risk for drug toxicity at typical doses.
   B. improves the effectiveness of the drug at typical doses.

C. reduces the effectiveness of the drug at typical doses.
D. has no effect on the drug because it is active.

5. Concentration of tamoxifen's active metabolite endoxifen can be expected to be higher in which of the genotype-predicted metabolizing phenotypes?
   A. Extensive metabolizer
   B. Intermediate metabolizer
   C. Poor metabolizer
   D. Ultra rapid metabolizer
6. When a starting dose for warfarin is based on a PGx test result, repeated blood draws for INR can be avoided.
   A. True
   B. False
7. The utility of PGx can be expected to improve when
   A. prescribers feel knowledgeable enough to use the test and interpret the results.
   B. drug–drug interactions are identified.
   C. when multiple genes can be tested and their interactions measured to predict phenotype.
   D. A and C above
   E. None of the above
8. The results from gene(s) analyzed in a PGx test to predict tamoxifen response can be used later if the patient is prescribed warfarin.
   A. True
   B. False
9. A 50-year-old woman tells you she had a PGx test for CYP2D6 back in 2006 when she started on fluoxetine. The test indicated she was an extensive metabolizer. She wants to know why the CYP2D6 test is being ordered again for tamoxifen since genes don't change. What is the most likely reason?
   A. The current CYP2D6 test analyzes more variant alleles than the previous CYP2D6 test.
   B. Fluoxetine is an antidepressant. Tamoxifen is an anti-cancer medication.
   C. The hormonal imbalances of menopause may reduce tamoxifen's effectiveness.
   D. A test for a gene needs to be repeated with each new medication.
10. A 64-year-old male patient was started on clopidogrel. When his CYP2C19 test came back indicating he was a poor metabolizer, the doctor switched him to warfarin. What is the most likely reason?
   A. Warfarin still works for *CYP2C19* poor metabolizers, but lower doses are needed because the patients are at risk for bleeding.
   B. Clopidogrel is a pro-drug and metabolized by *CYP2C19* as a pro-drug. Therefore, clopidogrel is unlikely to work in poor metabolizers.
   C. Clopidogrel works by interfering with platelet aggregation while warfarin works by interfering with the vitamin K–dependent clotting pathway.
   D. Warfarin might turn out to be a better substrate for *CYP2C19*.

Posttest answers are located in the Appendix.

CHAPTER SUMMARY

It is clear that genes contribute to drug-response phenotype. It is also recognized that there is not a single set of genes relevant for all medications. Furthermore, the degree of genetic influence on drug-response variability depends on the medication being considered and on many nongenetic patient factors such as age, other medications the patient is taking, and medication adherence. As a consequence, the utility of a particular PGx test for a particular medication has been difficult to measure, resulting in limited integration of this testing in clinical practice at the time of this writing.

It isn't a question of whether PGx testing will be more commonly used but of when it will be routinely used. This chapter highlighted two medications for which PGx testing is used in some settings. There are other examples, but like tamoxifen and warfarin, not everyone agrees about the routine use of such tests in clinical settings. PGx will be more common once the following two key advances occur: 1) Technology improves the speed, accuracy, and cost efficiency of testing multiple genes that contribute to a medication; and 2) bioinformatics software becomes available to quickly and accurately predict the contribution of each analyzed gene and the important nongenetic factors so that medication selection and dosing can be individualized for the patient.

Nurses need to develop an understanding that PGx can be used for drug selection and dose adjustment to improve patient outcomes. However, pharmacogenomic knowledge and technology is rapidly evolving and integration of testing in clinical settings is inconsistent. A key strategy nurses can use to manage this is to learn whether there are PGx tests available for the medications their patients most commonly use. This chapter described the purpose and limitations of PGx testing so that the reader is able to assess whether his or her patient is making an informed decision when PGx testing is recommended by a prescriber. This chapter also emphasized nurses' important role of closely monitoring and reporting unintended medication responses, as this will remain essential even when PGx testing is more common.

CRITICAL THINKING CHECKPOINT

Jerome is a 14-year-old African-American male who came to the emergency department in sickle cell crisis. Jerome reports that the acetaminophen with codeine his pediatrician prescribed 2 days ago hasn't helped at all. An order is written to draw blood for a codeine PGx test. The hospital's website has brief descriptions of each test. It indicates that codeine is a pro-drug, and metabolism by CYP2D6 is needed to convert codeine to its active metabolite (which is morphine).

1. Based on Jerome's response, what type of CYP2D6 metabolizer do you expect him to be?
2. If Jerome had presented to the emergency department heavily sedated and with parent reports of apnea, what type of CYP2D6 metabolizer would you expect him to be?
3. What type of basic information does the patient need before his blood is drawn?
4. Is there any reason to do a family history in this situation? Why or why not?
5. Once the CYP2D6 result becomes available and the pain medication is selected and dosed based on the result, what genetic/genomics nursing competency should the nurse be able to demonstrate?

Answers are provided in the Appendix

Pearson Nursing Student Resources

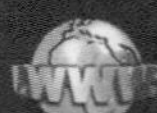

Find additional review materials at nursing.pearsonhighered.com

Prepare for success with additional NCLEX®-style practice questions, interactive assignments and activities, web links, animations, videos, and more!

ONLINE RESOURCES

Genetic Alliance: http://www.geneticalliance.org

Genetics Education Program for Nurses: http://gepn.cchmc.org

Genetics Home Reference: http://ghr.nlm.nih.gov

International Society of Nurses in Genetics: http://www.isong.org

Pharmacogenomics Knowledge Implementation: http://www.pharmgkb.org

REFERENCES

Baggerly, K., & Coombes, K. (2009). Deriving chemosensitivity from cell lines: Forensic bioinformatics and reproducible research in high-throughput biology. *Annals of Applied Statistics, 3*(4), 1309–1334.

Baggerly, K., & Coombes, K. (2011). What information should be required to support clinical "Omics" publications? *Clinical Chemistry, 57*(5), 688–690.

Bluecross Blueshield Association. CYP2D6 *Pharmacogenomics of tamoxifen treatment.* Retrieved July 21, 2012, from http://www.bcbs.com/blueresources/tec/press/cyp2d6-pharmacogenomics-of.html

Becquemont, L., Alfirevic, A., Amstutz, U., Brauch, H., Jacqz-Aigrain, E., Laurent-Puig, P., et al. (2011). Practical recommendations for pharmacogenomics-based prescription: 2010 ESF-UB Conference on Pharmacogenetics and Pharmacogenomics. *Pharmacogenomics, 12*(1), 113–124.

Burmester, J. K., Berg, R. L., Yale, S. H., Rottscheit, C. M., Glurich, I. E., Schmelzer, J. R., et al. (2011). A randomized controlled trial of genotype-based Coumadin initiation. *Genetics in Medicine, 13*(6), 509–518.

Caraco, Y., Blotnick, S., & Muszkat, M. (2008). CYP2C9 genotype-guided warfarin prescribing enhances the efficacy and safety of anticoagulation: A prospective randomized controlled study. *Clinical Pharmacology & Therapeutics, 83*(3), 460–470.

Cashion, A. (2009). The importance of genetics education for undergraduate and graduate nursing programs (editorial). *Journal of Nursing Education, 48*(10), 535–536.

Cincinnati Children's Hospital Medical Center. (2011). *Education at the genetic pharmacology service.* Retrieved June 22, 2011, from http://www.cincinnatichildrens.org/service/g/genetic-pharmacology/education/

Consensus Panel on Genetic/Genomic Nursing Competencies. (2009). *Essentials of genetic and genomic nursing competecies, curricula guidelines, and outcome indicators* (2nd ed.). Retrieved June 22, 2011, from http://www.genome.gov/pages/careers/healthprofessionaleducation/geneticscompetency.pdf

Dang, M. T., Hambleton, J., & Kayser, S. R. (2005). The influence of ethnicity on warfarin dosage requirement. *The Annals of Pharmacotherapy, 39*(6), 1008–1012.

Deverka, P. A., Vernon, J., & McLeod, H. L. (2010). Economic opportunities and challenges for pharmacogenomics. *Annual Review of Pharmacology and Toxicology, 50*, 423–437.

Edwards, I. R., & Aronson, J. K. (2000). Adverse drug reactions: Definitions, diagnosis, and management. *Lancet, 356*(9237), 1255–1259.

Ellis, K. J., Stouffer, G. A., McLeod, H. L., & Lee, C. R. (2009). Clopidogrel pharmacogenomics and risk of inadequate platelet inhibition: US FDA recommendations. *Pharmacogenomics, 10*(11), 1799–1817.

Fargher, E. A., Eddy, C., Newman, W., Qasim, F., Tricker, K., Elliott, R. A., et al. (2007). Patients' and healthcare professionals' views on pharmacogenetic testing and its future delivery in the NHS. *Pharmacogenomics, 8*(11), 1511–1519.

Feucht, C., & Patel, D. R. (2011). Principles of pharmacology. *Pediatric Clinics of North America, 58*(1), 11–19, ix.

Flockhart, D. A., O'Kane, D., Williams, M. S., Watson, M. S., Flockhart, D. A., Gage, B., et al. (2008). Pharmacogenetic testing of CYP2C9 and VKORC1 alleles for warfarin. *Genetics in Medicine, 10*(2), 139–150.

Food and Drug Administration, U.S. Department of Health & Human Services. (2012a). *Draft guidelines for industry, clinical laboratories, and FDA staff-In vitro diagnostic multivariate index assays.* Retrieved June 28, 2011, from http://www.fda.gov/MedicalDevices/DeviceRegulationandGuidance/GuidanceDocuments/ucm079148.htm

Food and Drug Administration, U.S. Department of Health & Human Services. (2012b). *Safety: Paxil (paroxetine HCl) tablets, oral solution and Paxil CR tablets. Detailed view: safety labeling changes approved by FDA Center for Drug Evaluation and Research (CDER).*

Retrieved July 27, 2012, from http://www.fda.gov/Safety/MedWatch/SafetyInformation/ucm233693.htm

Gage, B. F., Eby, C., Johnson, J. A., Deych, E., Rieder, M. J., Ridker, P. M., et al. (2008). Use of pharmacogenetic and clinical factors to predict the therapeutic dose of warfarin. *Clinical Pharmacology and Therapeutics, 84*(3), 326–331.

Goetz, M. P., Knox, S. K., Suman, V. J., Rae, J. M., Safgren, S. L., Ames, M. M., et al. (2007). The impact of cytochrome P450 2D6 metabolism in women receiving adjuvant tamoxifen. *Breast Cancer Research and Treatment, 101*(1), 113–121.

Haga, S., O'Daniel, J., Tindall, G., Mills, R., Lipkus, I., & Agans, R. (2012). Survey of genetic counselors and clinical geneticists' use and attitudes toward pharmacogenetic testing. *Clinical Genetics, 82*(2), 115–120.

Haga, S. B., & Burke, W. (2008). Pharmacogenetic testing: not as simple as it seems. *Genetics in Medicine, 10*(6), 391–395.

Haga, S. B., O'Daniel J, M., Tindall, G. M., Lipkus, I. R., & Agans, R. (2011). Public attitudes toward ancillary information revealed by pharmacogenetic testing under limited information conditions. *Genetics in Medicine, 13*(8), 723–728.

Ingelman-Sundberg, M., Sim, S. C., Gomez, A., & Rodriguez-Antona, C. (2007). Influence of cytochrome P450 polymorphisms on drug therapies: Pharmacogenetic, pharmacoepigenetic and clinical aspects. *Pharmacology and Therapeutics, 116*(3), 496–526.

Jin, Y., Desta, Z., Stearns, V., Ward, B., Ho, H., Lee, K. H., et al. (2005). CYP2D6 genotype, antidepressant use, and tamoxifen metabolism during adjuvant breast cancer treatment. *Journal of the National Cancer Institute, 97*(1), 30–39.

Johnson, E. G., Horne, B. D., Carlquist, J. F., & Anderson, J. L. (2011). Genotype-based dosing algorithms for warfarin therapy: Data review and recommendations. *Molecular Diagnosis & Therapy, 15*(5), 255–264.

Kamali, F., & Wynne, H. (2010). Pharmacogenetics of warfarin. *Annual Review of Medicine, 61*, 63–75.

Kelly, C. M., Juurlink, D. N., Gomes, T., Duong-Hua, M., Pritchard, K. I., Austin, P. C., et al. (2010). Selective serotonin reuptake inhibitors and breast cancer mortality in women receiving tamoxifen: A population based cohort study. *British Medical Journal, 340*, c693.

Kirk, M., Tonkin, E., & Patch, C. (2006). Genetics: Is it part of your role? *Nursing Older People, 18*(8), 22–24.

Kiyotani, K., Mushiroda, T., Imamura, C. K., Hosono, N., Tsunoda, T., Kubo, M., et al. (2010). Significant effect of polymorphisms in CYP2D6 and ABCC2 on clinical outcomes of adjuvant tamoxifen therapy for breast cancer patients. *Journal of Clinical Oncology, 28*(8), 1287–1293.

Klein, T. E., Altman, R. B., Eriksson, N., Gage, B. F., Kimmel, S. E., Lee, M. T., et al. (2009). Estimation of the warfarin dose with clinical and pharmacogenetic data. *New England Journal of Medicine, 360*(8), 753–764.

Lash, T. L., Cronin-Fenton, D., Ahern, T. P., Rosenberg, C. L., Lunetta, K. L., Silliman, R. A., et al. (2011). CYP2D6 inhibition and breast cancer recurrence in a population-based study in Denmark. *Journal of the National Cancer Institute, 103*(6), 489–500.

Lee, C. R., Goldstein, J. A., & Pieper, J. A. (2002). Cytochrome P450 2C9 polymorphisms: A comprehensive review of the in-vitro and human data. *Pharmacogenetics, 12*(3), 251–263.

Lee, K. C., Ma, J. D., & Kuo, G. M. (2010). Pharmacogenomics: Bridging the gap between science and practice. *Journal of the American Pharmaceutical Association (2003), 50*(1), e1–14; quiz e15–17.

Lenzini, P., Wadelius, M., Kimmel, S., Anderson, J. L., Jorgensen, A. L., Pirmohamed, M., et al. (2010). Integration of genetic, clinical, and INR data to refine warfarin dosing. *Clinical Pharmacology and Therapeutics, 87*(5), 572–578.

Lesko, L. J. (2008). The critical path of warfarin dosing: Finding an optimal dosing strategy using pharmacogenetics. *Clinical Pharmacology and Therapeutics, 84*(3), 301–303.

Lubin, I. M., Hilborne, L., & Scheuner, M. T. (2010). *A template for molecular genetic test reports for heritable conditions (abstract #45, platform presentation)*. Paper presented at the American College of Medical Genetics. Retrieved July 25, 2012, from http://submissions.miracd.com/acmg/ContentInfo.aspx?conID=1510

Lubitz, S. A., Scott, S. A., Rothlauf, E. B., Agarwal, A., Peter, I., Doheny, D., et al. (2010). Comparative performance of gene-based warfarin dosing algorithms in a multiethnic population. *Journal of Thrombosis and Haemostasis, 8*(5), 1018–1026.

Medcohealth. Personalized Medicine Programs. Retrieved September 15, 2011, from http://www.medcohealth.com/medco/corporate/home.jsp?BV_SessionID=@@@@2095681981.1316100328-mm4155904223336@@@@&BV_EngineID=ccjkadfejdmdmjmcfklcgffdghfdfjn.0&articleID=CorpPM_PersonalizedMedicine

Miller, F. G., & Pearson, S. D. (2008). Coverage with evidence development: Ethical issues and policy implications. *Medical Care, 46*(7), 746–751.

Novak, B. (2007). Significant pharmacogenetic and molecular factors in prescribing. *Nurse Prescribing, 5*(8), 358–361.

Prows, C. A., & Beery, T. A. (2008). Pharmacogenetics in critical care: Atrial fibrillation as an exemplar. *Critical Care Nursing Clinics of North America, 20*(2), 223–231, vi–vii.

Prows, C. A., & Saldana, S. N. (2009). Nurses' genetic/genomics competencies when medication therapy is guided by pharmacogenetic testing: Children with mental health disorders as an exemplar. *Journal of Pediatric Nursing, 24*(3), 179–188.

Rieder, M. J., Reiner, A. P., Gage, B. F., Nickerson, D. A., Eby, C. S., McLeod, H. L., et al. (2005). Effect of VKORC1 haplotypes on transcriptional regulation and warfarin dose. *New England Journal of Medicine, 352*(22), 2285–2293.

Schroth, W., Goetz, M. P., Hamann, U., Fasching, P. A., Schmidt, M., Winter, S., et al. (2009). Association between CYP2D6 polymorphisms and outcomes among women with early stage breast cancer treated with tamoxifen. *Journal of the American Medical Association, 302*(13), 1429–1436.

Seibert, D., Edwards, Q. T., & Maradiegue, A. (2007). Integrating genetics into advanced practice nursing curriculum: Strategies for success. *Journal of Community Genetics, 10*(1), 45–51.

Seruga, B., & Amir, E. (2010). Cytochrome P450 2D6 and outcomes of adjuvant tamoxifen therapy: Results of a meta-analysis. *Breast Cancer Research and Treatment, 122*(3), 609–617.

Swen, J. J., Nijenhuis, M., de Boer, A., Grandia, L., Maitland-van der Zee, A. H., Mulder, H., et al. (2011). Pharmacogenetics: From bench to byte - an update of guidelines. *Clinical Pharmacology and Therapeutics, 89*(5), 662–673.

Terasawa, T., Dahabreh, I., Castaldi, P. J., & Trikalinos, T. A. (2010). *Systematic reviews on select pharmacogenetic tests for cancer treatment: CYP2D6 for tamoxifen in breast cancer, KRAS for anti-EGFR antibodies in colorectal cancer, and BCR-ABL1 for tyrosine kinase inhibitors in chronic myeloid leukemia* (No. HHSA 290 2007 100551). Rockville, MD: Agency for Healthcare Research and Quality.

Eskreis-Nelson, T. (2000). Nursing case law update: Medication errors and the need for nurses' continuing education. *Journal of Nursing Law, 7*, 49–59; *Journal of Nursing Law, 8*(1), 7–8.

Wu, X., Hawse, J. R., Subramaniam, M., Goetz, M. P., Ingle, J. N., & Spelsberg, T. C. (2009). The tamoxifen metabolite, endoxifen, is a potent antiestrogen that targets estrogen receptor alpha for degradation in breast cancer cells. *Cancer Research, 69*(5), 1722–1727.

Zhou, S. F., Di, Y. M., Chan, E., Du, Y. M., Chow, V. D., Xue, C. C., et al. (2008). Clinical pharmacogenetics and potential application in personalized medicine. *Curr Drug Metabolism, 9*(8), 738–784.

CHAPTER

24 Genetics and Aging

Debra L. Schutte

LEARNING OUTCOMES

Upon completion of this chapter, the reader will be able to

1. Discuss the relevance and role of genetics and genomics to our understanding of aging and common age-related disorders.
2. Discuss the relevance of new genetics and genomics information and technologies to the care of older adults.
3. Describe the components of a comprehensive family health history assessment.
4. Identify older adults and their families who may benefit from specific genetic and genomic information and services.
5. Facilitate referrals for specialty genetics and genomics services.
6. Identify strategies for providing education, care, and support to families experiencing or at risk for experiencing genetic conditions.

The rapidly growing aging population worldwide places growing demands on health care professionals to prevent and manage common chronic diseases and their negative sequelae. An expanding array of genomics technologies provides new approaches for understanding the causes of many chronic age-related conditions as well as the aging process itself. This knowledge, in turn, opens new avenues for nursing assessment and intervention for nurses caring for older adults across settings. The purpose of this chapter is to examine the role of genomics in the care of older adults and to explore the many implications for practicing nurses.

PRETEST

1. A rare change in DNA sequence is called a
   A. mutation.
   B. phenotype.
   C. polymorphism.
   D. single gene disorder.
2. Early onset Alzheimer disease (AD) is characterized by
   A. an autosomal dominant pattern of inheritance.
   B. familial clustering but no clear pattern of inheritance.
   C. no known causative gene mutations.
   D. onset after age 60–65.
3. Diseases that have an autosomal dominant inheritance pattern will
   A. have mutations on the Y chromosome.
   B. have a vertical transmission pattern.
   C. have a mutation on the X chromosome.
   D. not transmit the disease from male to male.
4. The study of individual genes in relationship to health and their impact on relatively rare single gene disorders is the definition of
   A. genetics.
   B. genomics.
   C. genotypes.
   D. phenotypes.
5. An individual's genetic makeup at the chromosome or DNA level is the definition of
   A. genetics.
   B. genomics.
   C. genotype.
   D. phenotype.
6. The observable traits or characteristics of an individual such as height or cognitive status are called
   A. genetics.
   B. genomics.
   C. genotypes.
   D. phenotypes.
7. The following condition is the most common cause of irreversible dementia worldwide:
   A. Parkinson disease
   B. Vitamin B_{12} deficiency
   C. Alzheimer disease
   D. Huntington disease
8. The analysis of human DNA to detect disease-causing mutations for clinical purposes is called
   A. genetic testing.
   B. genomics research.

C. genetic research.
D. phenotypes.

9. Diseases that have an autosomal dominant inheritance pattern will
A. have mutations on the Y chromosome.
B. have a horizontal transmission pattern.
C. have a mutation on an autosome.
D. not transmit the disease from male to male.

10. A decline from a previously attained level of cognition that interferes with occupational and social roles is called
A. depression.
B. dementia.
C. delirium.
D. diabetes.

Pretest answers are located in the Appendix.

SECTION ONE: Genomics and the Care of Older Adults

The ability to integrate genetics and genomics concepts and principles into health care practice is a growing mandate for health care providers caring for clients across the lifespan. Numerous professional organizations provide nurses with the rationale and tools needed to accomplish this mandate. For example, the International Society of Nurses in Genetics (ISONG) states that every nurse plays a role in the identification, referral, and support of clients in relationship to genetics information and technology (ISONG, 2007). The National Coalition for Health Professional Education in Genetics (NCHPEG), an interdisciplinary organization, developed core competencies that cross all health professions' disciplines (NCHPEG, 2007) related to the integration of genetics into everyday practice. Most recently, a consensus panel of nursing leaders developed a set of discipline-specific competencies for our profession, called the Essential Nursing Competencies and Curricula Guidelines for Genetics and Genomics (Jenkins & Calzone, 2007). While these recommendations and competencies are in place, much work remains to be done by nurses in every practice setting and role to implement and test these strategies in real world situations, particularly in the care of older adults.

Playing a role in the integration of genetics into clinical practice for the care of older adults requires that nurses possess a degree of comfort with basic genetics vocabulary, concepts, and principles. Genetics, for example, is the study of individual genes in relationship to health and their impact on relatively rare single gene disorders (Guttmacher & Collins, 2002). In contrast, genomics is the study of all genes in the human genome together—their interactions with each other and with the environment, including physical, psychosocial, and cultural influences (Guttmacher & Collins, 2002). The crux of both of these types of research is to better understand how variations in the human genome sequence influence health and disease. Variations in the human genome sequence occur at different frequencies. **Mutations** are one category of sequence variation and are defined as rare changes in DNA sequence that usually have either no effect or cause a deleterious effect on protein function. A polymorphism is a common change in DNA sequence, usually found in more than 10% of the population. Single gene disorders are diseases caused by mutations in a single gene, such as Huntington disease, sickle cell anemia, and hemochromatosis. Multifactorial disorders are diseases or other health traits that are caused by a combination of genetic and/or environmental factors, including most common chronic conditions such as Type 2 diabetes, obesity, and dementia. Multifactorial disorders are also referred to as complex disorders. In genetics research, scientists are looking at the relationship between a person's genotype (an individual's genetic makeup at the DNA or chromosome level) and phenotype (the observable traits or characteristics of an individual).

Huge strides have been made in genetics and genomics research within the last 2 decades with contributions from scientists across many disciplines, including the nursing profession. The efforts were initially fueled by the Human Genome Project (**HGP**), an international effort launched in 1990 to map and sequence the entire human genome. This goal was largely accomplished in 2001 with the publication of the complete human genome sequence (The International Human Genome Mapping Consortium, 2001; the Celera Genomics Sequencing Team, 2001). Following this milestone, numerous efforts remain underway to better understand the architecture of the human genome and how it is different or the same between individuals. These efforts include the International HapMap Project and the 1000 Genomes Project and Genome-Wide Association Study initiatives. The significance of these research efforts are that they have many actual and potential implications for health care, including the following:

- Improving our ability to identify, isolate, and test for genes that are associated with disease (causative or susceptibility).
- Improving our ability to provide anticipatory guidance about disease risk and/or progression to our clients.
- Providing the capacity to tailor or customize interventions (either pharmacologic or nonpharmacologic) to an individual based upon their genotype or other risk profiles.

Genetics and the Study of Aging

Traditionally, genetic and genomics research was considered the domain of pediatrics and obstetrics, where the emphasis is on identifying the genetic causes of disease in order to inform reproductive decisions. Today, genetics and genomics research intersects the care of older adults in many ways, including contributing to our understanding of the biology of aging as well as our understanding of the etiology of many age-related health problems.

New genomics tools and technology are being applied to the aging process in both animal models and human research. One particular application in humans is to study the genetics of premature aging syndromes. By identifying genetic variations that contribute to these extreme cases of aging, scientists may be able to identify the relevant biologic pathways involved in the aging of cells or even whole organisms. Hutchinson-Gilford progeria syndrome (HGPS) is an extremely rare, autosomal dominant disorder, affecting 1 in 4 million live births resulting in childhood onset of such states as "short stature, early loss of hair, lipodystrophy, decreased joint mobility, osteolysis, and facial features that resemble aged persons" (Online Mendelian Inheritance in Man [OMIM]). A specific mutation in the lamin A/C *(LMNA)* gene causes the disorder (Eriksson et al., 2003), and this discovery has implicated a number of possible molecular mechanisms for the aging process, including defective DNA repair, altered cell proliferation and senescence, and altered stem cell proliferation (Burtner & Kennedy, 2010). Similar goals support research to study the role of genetic variants in human longevity (Chung, Dao, Chen, & Hung, 2010). Studying very long-lived individuals, as the other extreme end of the aging continuum, can inform our understanding of the biology of aging as well. The potential applications of this new knowledge include development of strategies to improve treatment for age-related diseases and delay or slow the aging process.

Genetics and the Study of Common Age-Related Health Problems

Another important application of genetics and genomics in the context of older adults is research to identify genes that contribute to the etiology of common age-related health problems. For example, **Alzheimer disease (AD)** is an increasingly prevalent age-related health problem that has been the focus of considerable attention. AD affects over 5 million persons in United States today (Alzheimer Diseases Association, 2009) and is the leading cause of irreversible **dementia** in persons over age 60–65. In rare cases, AD develops prior to the age of age 60 and may demonstrate autosomal dominant patterns of inheritance in family trees. Mutations in three genes are known to cause AD in a small percentage of families exhibiting early ages at onset and autosomal dominant patterns of inheritance. These three genes include the Amyloid Precursor Protein (*APP*) gene on chromosome 21 (Goate et al., 1991; St. George-Hyslop et al., 1987), the Presenilin 1 (*PSEN1*) gene on chromosome 14 (Mullan et al., 1992; Schellenberg et al., 1992), and the Presenilin 2 (*PSEN2*) gene on chromosome 1 (Levy-Lahad et al., 1992). These discoveries are important in that they point to the biologic pathways that are contributing to AD. In addition, however, it suggests that genetic testing coupled with genetic counseling may be a health care option for persons at risk for early onset AD based upon their family history, providing an opportunity for them to clarify their disease risk status (Bird, 2010; Goldman et al., 2011).

The genetics of the much more common late-onset AD is complex. In the typical late-onset AD, disease onset occurs after the age of 60–65. In addition, the occurrence of the disease in families is sporadic or may exhibit clustering of persons with the disease, but typically a clear pattern of inheritance is not evident. In the case of late-onset AD, research is ongoing to identify genetic factors that might influence one's risk or susceptibility. The strongest risk factor for late-onset AD is age. However, one's risk is likely influenced by a combination of common sequence variations in many genes as well as environmental factors. The Apolipoprotein E (*APOE*) gene epsilon (ε) 4 allele is consistently associated with increased risk of developing AD and earlier ages at onset (Pericak-Vance et al., 1991). However, research is ongoing to identify other gene variations that may increase risk for disease or influence other aspects of the disease progression (Bertram et al., 2007). Nurse scientists are also contributing to our understanding of the role of genes in the complex symptoms experienced in persons with AD, including cognitive losses, increasing inability to manage one's activities of daily living, and behavioral symptoms such as psychopathology, agitation, and mood disturbances (Schutte et al., 2011). Currently, genetic testing for *APOE* status is not recommended clinically, but research findings such as these hold promise for positively impacting our ability to provide improved risk prediction, anticipatory guidance about disease progression, and tailored pharmacologic and nonpharmacologic interventions to improve quality of life in persons with this devastating disorder.

Age-related Macular Degeneration (**AMD**) is another age-related condition, for which our understanding has expanded as a result of genetics research. AMD is the leading cause of irreversible blindness in persons over the age of 50, currently affecting nearly 2 million persons in the United States (Friedman et al., 2004). The prevalence of AMD increases with age; the strongest modifiable risk factor is cigarette smoking (Clemons et al., 2005). Other known risk factors include positive family history, Caucasian ethnicity, obesity, high dietary fat intake, and low dietary intake of antioxidants and zinc (Jager, Mieier, & Miller, 2008; Moroi & Heckenlively, 2008). Several genes have been implicated in the etiology of AMD. For example, DNA variants within the following genes have been consistently

Emerging Evidence

New discoveries about the role of genes in the care of older adults are rapidly emerging. The following resources provide up-to-date information about new genetic studies and their application to clinical practice:

GeneTests

- http://www.genetests.org
- The GeneTests website includes a genetic testing/genetics laboratory resource directory as well as an introduction to genetic counseling and clinical genetic testing.

AlzGene Database

- http://www.alzgene.org
- The AlzGene database provides a comprehensive and regularly updated review of genetic association studies performed in Alzheimer disease, including meta-analyses for those polymorphisms with sufficient data.
- Nurse scientists are playing an important role in learning about the contribution of genes to disease and symptom burden in conditions such as Alzheimer disease. For example, see the following:
- Schutte, D. L., Reed, D. A., DeCranes, S., & Ersig, A. L. (2011). Saitohin and APOE polymorphisms influence cognition and function in persons with advanced Alzheimer disease. *Dementia and Geriatric Cognitive Disorders, 32,* 94–102. doi:10.1159/000329542

replicated to increase the odds of having AMD (Edwards et al., 2005; Gold et al., 2006; Haines et al., 2005; Klein et al., 2005; Francis & Klein, 2011): complement factor H (*CFH*) gene, age-related maculopathy susceptibility 2 (*ARMS2*) gene, complement factor 3 (*C3*) gene, complement factor I (*CFI*) gene, ATP-binding cassette A4 (*ABCA1*) gene, lipase, hepatic (*LIPC*) gene, cholestryl ester transfer protein (*CETP*) gene, lipoprotein lipase (*LPL*) gene and near the tissue inhibitor of metallo proteinase 3 (*TIMP3*) gene. This gene list will no doubt expand, but nonetheless contains valuable clues about the biologic pathways involved in the pathogenesis of AMD towards the long-term goal of preventive or curative interventions. In the short term, scientists are attempting to build predictive risk models for AMD based upon an individual's genetic, clinical, demographic, and environmental information (Seddon et al., 2009).

SECTION ONE REVIEW

1. The initial goal of the Human Genome Project was to
   A. map and sequence the entire human genome.
   B. map and sequence the genomes of nonhuman species.
   C. find the cure for dementia.
   D. find the cure for cancer.
2. All of the following genes are associated with Early Onset Alzheimer disease, EXCEPT
   A. Amyloid Precursor Protein.
   B. Lamin A/C.
   C. Presenilin 1.
   D. Presenilin 2.
3. Which of the following conditions represents an extreme aging phenotype?
   A. Dementia
   B. Age-related macular degeneration
   C. Age-related hearing impairment
   D. Hutchinson-Gilford progeria syndrome

Answers: 1. A; 2. B; 3. D

SECTION TWO: Collecting and Interpreting Family History Data

Nurse providers are in a strategic position to consider the contributions of genetics to the health of older adults by virtue of their often repeated and lengthier contacts with clients. The first-line strategy for assessing genetic risks is the collection and interpretation of family history data.

A comprehensive three- and four-generation family health history is a key goal for health care providers, particularly those working in primary care or long-term care settings. Chapter 13 provides detailed information and tips for collecting and interpreting family history data. To review, the goals for a genetic assessment are to collect information about the biologic relationship of each family member to the client. Then, for each individual identified in the family tree, information is collected about gender, age, current and past health status, age at onset of illnesses (particularly important for common adult and late-adult onset diseases), age and cause of death, and ethnicity. Typically, at the end of a family history interview the interviewee is asked if there is any other information that the interviewee feels would be important for the health care provider to know. Depending on the time constraints of your setting, family history data may need to be targeted to the chief medical diagnosis or complaint (e.g., Alzheimer disease) and may need to be collected in more than one attempt.

Collecting family history data for adult and late-adult onset diseases can present particular challenges. In some cases, individuals at risk for a condition of interest may have died from other causes (e.g., accidents, other diseases) before reaching the age at which they otherwise would have developed a disease. This occurrence is called age-censoring. Another challenge relates to the ability of your client or other family history informant to accurately report family history data. For example, older generations may be less familiar with the health status of younger generations. Finally, historical effects, such as changes in the names of disorders or their diagnostic criteria over time, may occur. The disorder we know today as Alzheimer disease has been referred to as senility, organic brain disorder, and hardening of the arteries of the brain in the past; informants may not realize this connection. All of these factors can limit our ability to accurately collect and interpret family history data.

Once collected, family history data are then used to construct a pedigree, or visual depiction of the family history, using a standard set of symbols and a standard way of depicting biologic relationships (Bennett et al., 1993). The use of a pedigree provides for easier interpretation of how traits or disease (phenotype) are inherited across generations. The pedigree also allows for easier communication of health history data across health care providers and settings.

The pedigree is then interpreted to identify indications for referral to specialized genetic counseling services. Typical indications for referral to specialized services include the presence of a condition that exhibits a recognizable Mendelian pattern of inheritance, such as autosomal dominant, autosomal recessive, and X-linked recessive disorders (see Chapter 7), or the presence of a known genetic disorder (e.g., Huntington disease). An indication that is particularly relevant to nurses caring for adults and older adults is a new diagnosis or family history of an earlier than expected age at onset in common illnesses, such as breast, ovarian, prostate or colon cancer, cardiovascular disease, and Alzheimer disease. Finally, any client or family member with questions about the genetics aspects of a disease, their risk for disease, or the availability of genetic testing for a particular disease should be referred to a specialty genetics provider (Schutte, 2002; Schutte, 2006).

SECTION TWO REVIEW

1. The situation in which individuals at risk for a condition of interest die from other causes before reaching the age at which they otherwise would have developed a disease, is called
   A. historical effects.
   B. premature death.
   C. age-censoring.
   D. phenotype.
2. Which of the following terms is a visual depiction of family health history and biologic relationships using a standard set of symbols?
   A. Pedigree
   B. Phenotype
   C. Genogram
   D. Genotype
3. All of the following things can be assessed through the interpretation of a family history recorded as a pedigree, EXCEPT
   A. patterns in ages of disease onset.
   B. Mendelian patterns of inheritance.
   C. presence of known genetic conditions.
   D. social relationships.

Answers: 1. C: 2. A; 3. D

SECTION THREE: Facilitating Referrals for Specialty Genetics Services

Referral to genetic specialty providers is an important role of any nurse in the 21st century health care environment. In order to make appropriate referrals, nurses will need to identify and develop relationships with specialty genetics services in their practice area. An important first step is to contact the genetics division of a regional tertiary care facility for assistance in identifying local providers or outreach genetics clinics in your area or state. The State Department of Public Health may be another helpful source of information about outreach genetics services in your area. Finally, specialty genetics organizations, such as The International Society of Nurses in Genetics (ISONG) and the National Society of Genetic Counselors (NSGC) may have the capacity to assist in identifying local providers.

Once identified, it may be beneficial to establish and maintain periodic contact with local specialty providers in order to provide anticipatory guidance for your clients in advance of their interactions in a specialty genetics clinic. For example, typically genetics specialists will contact a new referral by telephone to obtain a comprehensive health history and family health history. Genetic specialists may also request the release of medical records in order to verify medical diagnoses as well as any previous screening or diagnostic tests. Following an appointment with genetic specialists, the client and referring provider most often receive a follow-up summary letter of the specialty genetics clinic visit to reinforce information provided in the clinic visit and to facilitate any follow-up actions.

SECTION THREE REVIEW

1. Specialty genetic providers typically provide all of the following services, EXCEPT to
   A. review and refine the comprehensive health and family health history.
   B. request medical records to verify diagnoses.
   C. assume responsibility for ongoing primary care.
   D. provide a follow-up summary letter to primary care providers.
2. All of the following resources may be helpful in identifying local specialty genetics providers EXCEPT?
   A. State Department of Public Health
   B. Local tertiary care facilities
   C. National Society of Genetic Counselors
   D. The Human Genome Project website
3. Which of the following activities is a responsibility of professional practice as a nurse generalist?
   A. Collecting a comprehensive family health history
   B. Providing genetic counseling about recurrence risks for early onset AD
   C. Performing genetic testing
   D. Independently interpreting the results of complex genetic tests

Answers: 1. C; 2. D; 3. A

SECTION FOUR: Interventions Related to Genetics Information and Technology

New genetics and genomics information and technology have implications for nursing interventions both today and tomorrow. Current genetics knowledge allows for the provision of ongoing education and supportive interventions. For example, nurses today can assess client risk for having or transmitting a genetic condition based upon their family health history. Further, nurses can assess their clients' understanding of their individual and family genetic information and follow up with credible, accurate, appropriate, and current information about genetics and genomics clinical information, resources, services, and technologies to facilitate client decision making. Nurses can play an advocacy role by promoting informed consent for genetic testing and/or genetic research that includes a discussion of potential risks and benefits of participation as well as the limitations of participation. Nurse providers can reinforce information and recommendations provided by the genetics specialists. Nurse providers can also offer decision-making support and emotional support as older adults and their families consider if and how they wish to use genetics information and technologies in their health care services. Collaboration in relationship to genetics and genomics care will be an increasingly important role of the nongenetic specialist provider. Multidisciplinary collaboration with other health care professionals in providing genetics and genomics health care will be key. Collaboration with insurance providers/payers to facilitate reimbursement for genomics-based diagnostics or genomics-based interventions may become increasingly important.

Emerging genetics and genomics discoveries and research to evaluate the clinical utility of genetics and genomics information will lay the foundation for tailored or customized interventions based upon one's genetic makeup or risk. For example, nurses may be able to assist clients in implementing health promotion and disease prevention practice that are prioritized or targeted according to the individual's genetic and/or environmental risk factors. Selected examples of these types of nursing interventions include dietary modification, physical activity or exercise prescriptions, and environmental modifications, as well as other nonpharmacologic strategies to improve nursing sensitive outcomes.

Pharmacogenetics research also has important implications for nurse providers, whether practicing in a generalist or advanced practice capacity. Pharmacogenetics is the study of the interaction of genetics with pharmacotherapy towards the goal of tailoring pharmacologic interventions according to genotype to maximize positive effects and minimize adverse effects. One example of research in this area is underway to examine warfarin dosing. The common anticoagulant, warfarin, can be a difficult drug to dose due to its narrow therapeutic range, large degree of interindividual variability in dosing requirements, and serious consequences of inadequate dosing. Scientists are examining the role that genes play in explaining this interindividual variability, particularly the role of DNA variants in the *CYP2C9* isoform and vitamin K epoxide reductase complex subunit 1 (*VKORC1*) genes (Takeuchi et al., 2009; Lane et al., 2011). In 2007, the U.S. Food and Drug Administration updated the warfarin drug label to explain that an individual's genetic makeup may influence how they respond to the drug and approved a genetic test for warfarin sensitivity to be used in conjunction with clinical evaluation and laboratory tests. Subsequently, large scale clinical trials are underway to examine the effectiveness of genotype-guided warfarin dosing in individuals of different ethnicities (Anderson et al., 2007; Do et al., 2011; Gong et al., 2011; Perara et al., 2011).

Warfarin represents one example of genotype-based medication dosing; other examples exist. For example, evidence suggests that functional polymorphisms within the *CYP2D6* gene may help predict the effectiveness of endocrine treatment (such as tamoxifen) in persons with breast cancer (Del Re, Michelucci, Simi, & Danesi, 2011). In the geriatric psychiatry arena, research is underway to examine the effect of DNA variations within dopamine and serotonin pathway genes on effectiveness and adverse outcomes related to psychotropic medication use (Shiroma, Geda, & Mrazek, 2011). As the field continues to advance, other opportunities to tailor a broad range of pharmacologic and biobehavioral interventions to influence nursing sensitive outcomes is likely to expand and is only limited by our imagination and resolve (Schutte, 2004).

SECTION FOUR REVIEW

1. All of the following interventions are appropriate for the nongenetic-specialist nurse provider in relationship to genetic information, EXCEPT
   A. genetic counseling.
   B. education.
   C. emotional support.
   D. decision-making support.
2. Pharmacogenetics is the
   A. study of individual genes in relationship to health and their impact on relatively rare single gene disorders.
   B. study of the interaction between genetics and pharmacotherapy.
   C. academic preparation to become a clinical pharmacist.
   D. study of all genes in the human genome together, including their interactions with each other and with environmental influence.
3. Which of the following medications has an approved genetic test to help guide therapeutic dosing?
   A. Heparin
   B. Warfarin
   C. Insulin
   D. Digoxin

Answers: 1. A; 2. B; 3. B

SECTION FIVE: Evaluation of Care

As the clinical utility of genetics and genomics information continues to emerge, the evaluation of the care we provide, in relationship to genetics and genomics, is a key professional obligation. Nurses will need to evaluate the impact and effectiveness of new technologies and genetic information on client outcomes, such as satisfaction with services and interventions, client knowledge about disease risk and natural history, health outcomes relevant to a particular health problems (such as cognitive status, functional status, presence and severity of behavioral problems, and quality of life in persons with AD), client decision making, and client coping. Modifying plans of care based upon these evaluation strategies closes the loop between assessment, diagnoses, interventions, and outcomes. Collaboration between direct care providers (whether in home, hospital, or long-term care settings) and quality improvement/outcomes/informatics resources will be key to the successful integration of genetics into the care of older adults.

SECTION FIVE REVIEW

1. Evaluation of care is a professional responsibility related to the provision of genetics information and services.
   A. True
   B. False
2. All of the following are key client outcomes related to genetics health care services, EXCEPT
   A. satisfaction with care.
   B. client knowledge.
   C. sleep patterns.
   D. client coping.

Answers: 1. A; 2. C

SECTION SIX: Key Practice Strategies for Gerontological Nurses

The Human Genome Project has fueled amazing strides in our understanding of the evolution, structure, and variation of the human genome. In addition, the identification of the genetic causes of single gene disorders has expanded dramatically over the last 20 years (OMIM). Much work remains to be done in expanding our understanding of the role of genes in common complex disease etiology and symptom progression, many of which are prevalent in older adults. Nonetheless, nurse generalists and gerontological nurses can position themselves to be informed and active participants in the ongoing integration of genomics into health care practice by preparing themselves to achieve competence in these key areas:

- Understand and recognize common Mendelian patterns of inheritance.
- Remember general indications for referral to specialty genetics services.
- Stay current on genetic developments relevant to high-volume populations and health problems.
- Make and maintain connections with local genetic specialists.

- Provide emotional and decision-making support for clients as they consider the role of genetic/genomic information in their current or future health care decisions.
- Participate in the development of documentation systems that will provide for the evaluation of key client outcomes (including nursing-sensitive outcomes) related to genomics health care.

SECTION SIX REVIEW

1. All of the following are key competencies to be achieved by today's gerontological nurse, EXCEPT
   A. collecting and interpreting family history data.
   B. recognizing the key characteristics of Mendelian patterns of inheritance.
   C. ordering a genetic test.
   D. providing emotional and decision-making support for clients who are considering genetic information.
2. All of the following are key competencies to be achieved by today's gerontological nurse, EXCEPT
   A. documenting outcomes of care related to genetics information.
   B. knowing sources of specialty genetics services in your county or state.
   C. recognizing indications for referral to specialty genetics services.
   D. providing risk counseling based on genetic test results.

Answers: 1. C; 2. D

POSTTEST

1. A common change in DNA sequence that occurs in greater than 10% of the population is called a
   A. mutation.
   B. phenotype.
   C. polymorphism.
   D. single gene disorder.
2. Late onset Alzheimer disease (AD) is characterized by
   A. an autosomal dominant pattern of inheritance.
   B. familial clustering but no clear pattern of inheritance.
   C. known mutations in three genes.
   D. onset prior to age 60–65.
3. Using the family history of an 82-year-old female recently diagnosed with Alzheimer disease, what nursing action would provide more family-related information for the registered nurse and the health care team?
   A. Administer the Mini-Mental State Exam to the patient.
   B. Construct a pedigree to display her family health history data.
   C. Develop a plan of care with short- and long-term goals.
   D. Determine who is her medical power of attorney.
4. Diseases that have an X-linked recessive inheritance pattern will
   A. have mutations on the Y chromosome.
   B. have a horizontal transmission pattern.
   C. have a mutation on an autosome.
   D. not transmit the disease from male to male.
5. Emerging genetics knowledge will provide gerontological nurses the ability to individualize (personalize) interventions according to genetic variation or risk. Examples of such interventions include
   A. diet modification.
   B. exercise.
   C. pharmacogenetics.
   D. health screening tests.
   E. All of the above
6. Which of the following genes is consistently associated with increased risk for developing late onset Alzheimer disease (AD susceptibility gene)?
   A. Amyloid Precursor Protein
   B. Presenilin
   C. Apolipoprotein E (*APOE*)
   D. Presenilin 2
7. Clinical genetic testing is not yet available for the genes associated with early onset Alzheimer disease in high-risk families.
   A. True
   B. False
8. Which of the following versions (or alleles) of the *APOE* gene is associated with increased risk for Alzheimer disease?
   A. *APOE-1* allele
   B. *APOE-2* allele
   C. *APOE-3* allele
   D. *APOE-4* allele
   E. None of the above

9. Which of the following genes are being studied for their effects on Warfarin dosing?
   A. Amyloid Precursor Protein
   B. Lamin A/C
   C. Presenilin 1
   D. Vitamin K epoxide reductase complex subunit 1 (*VKORC1*)

10. Which of the following findings is an indication for referral to specialty genetics services?
    A. Client exhibits signs of cognitive impairment
    B. Age of onset before age 60 in persons with Alzheimer disease
    C. Diagnosis of a urinary tract infection
    D. No clear patterns of Alzheimer disease inheritance noted in the pedigree

Posttest answers are located in the Appendix.

CHAPTER SUMMARY

Genetics and genomics is no longer the purview of pediatric and obstetric providers alone, as we learn increasingly more about the role of genes in the aging process, longevity, and common age-related health problems. Nurses providing care for adults and older adults can also play an important role in the identification of persons at risk for genetic conditions, making appropriate referrals, and providing supportive follow-up care. Unlimited possibilities exist for nurse researchers and clinicians to examine the role of genes in interindividual variability in nurse-sensitive outcomes in the care of older adults in order to develop and test tailored, more effective interventions.

Nurses caring for adults and older adults are key liaisons between their clients and genetic specialty providers. By identifying individuals at risk for disease based upon their family history, facilitating referrals to genetic specialists, and providing ongoing educational and emotional follow-up support, clients are best positioned to consider if and how genetic information may be relevant to their current and future health care decisions.

Genetics and genomics information and technology has immediate implications for nursing interventions through the identification of persons at risk, referrals to genetic specialist providers, and ongoing educational and supportive interventions. The emerging role of genes in medication dosing and response impacts nurse providers today and will continue to expand in its importance. Genetics may play a role in the interindividual variability in many nursing sensitive outcomes, suggesting untapped avenues for research and translation for our profession, particularly in the care of older adults.

Satisfaction with care, knowledge about disease risk and natural history as it relates to genetics, disease-specific health symptoms and other health outcomes, decision making, and coping are key client outcomes to be assessed with the translation of genetics research into clinical practice for the care of older adults.

Even though there is much to learn about the human genome, human health, and nursing care, nurse providers can position themselves to competently and confidently access current specialty genetics services, engage in the critique of new genetics research, and engage in multidisciplinary efforts to translate new findings into targeted interventions and services across settings and across populations.

CRITICAL THINKING CHECKPOINT

A.C. is a 41-year-old, Caucasian woman who is admitting her 65-year-old mother, diagnosed with Alzheimer disease, to the memory care assisted living wing in the long-term care facility in which you work. A.C. reports that her mother developed symptoms 8 years ago. She has been the primary caregiver of her mother at home for the last 5 years.

1. What element of this health history represents a red flag in relationship to the AD diagnosis?
2. Is a family history important in this case? If so, what type of information would be particularly relevant?
3. Are there any factors that put A.C. at risk for a genetic problem?
4. What is the role of the assisted living facility nurse in this scenario?
5. What follow-up care would be necessary?

Answers are provided in the Appendix

ONLINE RESOURCES

Center for Disease Control (CDC) National Office of Public Health Genomics: http://www.cdc.gov/genomics/

Gene Tests: http://www.genetests.org

Genome-Wide Association Study Initiatives: http://gwas.nih.gov

International HapMap Project: http://www.hapmap.org

International Society of Nurses in Genetics (ISONG): http://www.isong.org

National Coalition of Health Professional Education in Genetics (NCHPEG): http://www.nchpeg.org

National Human Genome Research Institute (NHGRI): http://www.genome.gov

National Society of Genetic Counselors (NSGC): http://www.nsgc.org

Online Mendelian Inheritance in Man (OMIM): http://www.ncbi.nlm.nih.gov/Omim

The 1000 Genomes Project: http://www.1000genomes.org

U.S. Surgeon General's Family History Initiative - My Family Health Portrait: http://www.hhs.gov/familyhistory

REFERENCES

Alzheimer's Association. (2009). 2009 Alzheimer's disease facts and figures. *Alzheimer's & Dementia, 5,* 234–270.

Anderson, J. L., Horne, B. D., Stevens, C. M., Grove, A. S., Barton, S., Nicholas, Z. P., et al. (2007). Randomized trial of genotype-guided versus standard warfarin dosing in patients initiating oral anticoagulation. *Circulation, 116,* 2563–2570.

Bennett, R. L., Steinhaus, K. A., Uhrich, S. B., O'Sullivan, C. K., Resta, R. G., Lochner-Doyle, D., et al. (1993). Recommendations for standardized human pedigree nomenclature. *American Journal of Human Genetics, 56*(3), 745–752.

Bertram L., McQueen, M. B., Mullin, K., Blacker, D., & Tanzi, R. E. (2007). Systematic meta-analyses of Alzheimer disease genetic association studies: The AlzGene database. *Nature Genetics 39*(1), 17–23.

Bird, T. D. (2010) GeneReviews: Alzheimer disease. Seattle: University of Washington; Retrieved September 16, 2011, from http://www.ncbi.nlm.nih.gov/books/NBK1161/

Burtner, C. R., & Kennedy, B. K. (2010). Progeria syndromes and ageing: What is the connection? *Nature Reviews/Molecular Cell Biology, 11,* 567–578.

Chung, W. H., Dao, R. L., Chenk L. K., & Hung, S. I. (2010). The role of genetic variants in human longevity. *Ageing Research Reviews, 9S,* S67–S78.

Clemons, T. E., Milton, R. C., Klein, R., Seddon, J. M., & Ferris, F. L. (2005). Risk factors for the incidence of advanced age related macular degeneration in the Age-Related Eye Disease Study (AREDS). AREDS report no. 19. *Ophthalmology, 112*(4), 533–539.

Del Re, M., Michelucci, A., Simi, P., & Danesi, R. (2011). Pharmacogenetics of anti-estrogen treatment of breast cancer. *Cancer Treatment Reviews.* Epub ahead of print.

Do, E. J., Lenzini, P., Eby, C. S., Bass, A. R., McMillin, G. A., Stevens, S. M., et al. (2011). Genetic informatics trial (GIFT) of warfarin to prevent deep vein thrombosis (DVT): Rationale and study design. *Pharmacogenomics.* Epub ahead of print.

Edwards, A. O., Ritter, R., III, Abel, K. J., Manning, A., Panhuysen, C., & Farrer, L. A. (2005). Complement factor H polymorphisms and age-related macular degeneration. *Science,* 421–424.

Eriksson, M., Brown, W. T., Gordon, L. B., Glynn, M. W., Singer, J., Scott, L., et al. (2003). Recurrent de novo point mutations in lamin A cause Hutchinson-Gilford progeria syndrome. *Nature 423,* 293–298.

Francis, P. J., & Klein, M. L. (2011. Update on the role of genetics in the onset of age-related macular degeneration. *Clinical Opthalmology, 5,* 1127–1133.

Friedman, D. S., O'Colmain, B. J., Munoz B., et al. (2004). Prevalence of age related macular degeneration in the United States. *Archives of Opthalmology, 122*(4), 564–572.

Goate, A., Chartier-Harlin, M. C., Mullan, M., Brown, J., Crawford, F., Fidani, L., et al. (1991). Segregation of a missense mutation in the amyloid precursor protein gene with familial Alzheimer's disease. *Nature, 349*(6311), 704–706.

Gold, B., Merriam, J. E., Zernant, J., et al. (2006). Variation in factor B (BF) and complement component 2 (C2) genes is associated with age-related macular degeneration. *Nature Genetics, 38,* 458–462.

Goldman, J. S., Hahn, S. E., Catania, J. W., LaRusse-Eckert, S., Butson, M. B., Rumbaugh, M., et al. (2011). Genetic counseling and testing for Alzheimer disease: Joint practice guidelines of the American College of Medical Genetics and the National Society of Genetic Counselors. *Genetics in Medicine, 13*(6), 597–605.

Gong, I. Y., Tirona, R. G., Schwarz, U. I., Crown, N., Dresser, G. K., Larue, S., et al. (2011). Prospective evaluation of a pharmacogenetics-guided warfarin loading and maintenance dose regimen for initiation of therapy. *Blood, 118*(1), 3163–3171.

Guttmacher, A. E., & Collins, F. C. (2002). Genomic medicine-a primer. *New England Journal of Medicine, 347*(19), 1512–1520.

Haines, J. L., Hauser, M. A., Schmidt, S., et al. (2005). Complement factor H variant increases the risk of age-related macular degeneration. *Science, 308,* 419–421.

International Society of Nurses in Genetics. (2007). *Genetics/genomics nursing: Scope and standards of practice.* Washington, DC: American Nurses Association; 2007. ANA Pub. No. 06SSGG.

Jager, R. D., Mieier, W. F., & Miller, J. W. (2008). Age-related macular degeneration. *New England Journal of Medicine, 358*(24), 2606–2617.

Jenkins, J., & Calzone, K. A. (2007). Establishing the essential nursing competencies for genetics and genomics. *Journal of Nursing Scholarship, 39*(1), 10–16.

Klein, R. J., Zeiss, C., Chew, E. Y., et al. (2005). Complement factor H polymorphisms in age-related macular degeneration. *Science, 308,* 385–389.

Lane, S., Al-Zubiedi, S., Hatch, E., Matthews, I., Jorgensen, A. L., Deloukas, P., et al. (2011). The population pharmacokinetics of R and S-warfarin: Effect of genetic and clinical factors. *British Journal of Clinical Pharmacology.* Epub ahead of print.

Levy-Lahad, E., et al. (1995). Candidate gene for the chromosome 1 familial Alzheimer's disease locus. *Science, 269*(5226), 973–977.

Moroi, S. E., & Heckenlively, J. R. (2008). Progress toward personalized medicine for age-related macular degeneration. *Ophthalmology, 115*(5), 925–926.

Mullan, M., et al. (1992). A locus for familial early-onset Alzheimer's disease on the long arm of chromosome 14, proximal to the alpha 1-antichymotrypsin gene. *Nature Genetics, 2*(4), 340–342.

National Coalition for Health Professional Education in Genetics. (2007). *Core Competencies in Genetics for Health Professionals* (3rd ed.). Lutherville MD: Author.

Perera, M. A., Gamazon, E., Cavallari, L. H., Patel, S. R., Poindexter, S., Kittles, R. A., et al. (2011). The missing association: Sequencing-based discovery of novel SNPs in VKORC1 and CYPSC9 that affect warfarin dose in African American. *Clinical Pharmacology Therapeutics, 89*(3), 408–415.

Pericak-Vance, M. A., Bebout, J. L., Gaskell, P. C., Jr., Yamaoka, L. H., Hung, W. Y., Alberts, M. J., et al. (1991). Linkage studies in familial Alzheimer disease: Evidence for chromosome 19 linkage. *American Journal of Human Genetics, 48*(6), 1034–1050.

Schellenberg, G. D., Bird, T. D., Wijsman, E. M., Orr, H. T., Anderson, L., Nemens, E., et al. (1992). Genetic linkage evidence for a familial Alzheimer's disease locus on chromosome 14. *Science, 258*(5082), 668–671.

Schutte, D. L. (2002). Evidence based protocol: Identification, referral, and support of elders with genetic conditions. *The Journal of Gerontological Nursing, 28*(2), 6–14.

Schutte, D. L. (2004). The evolving role of genomics in shaping care for persons with dementia. *Nursing Clinics of North America, 39*(3), 581–592.

Schutte, D. L. (2006) Alzheimer disease and genetics: Anticipating the questions. *American Journal of Nursing, 106*(12), 40–47.

Shiroma, P. R., Geda, Y. E., & Mrazek, D. A. (2010). Pharmacogenomic implications of variants of monoaminergic-related genes in geriatric psychiatry. *Pharmacogenomics, 11*(9), 1305–1330.

Shurin, S. B., & Nabel, E. G. (2008). Pharmacogenomics—ready for prime time? *New England Journal of Medicine, 358*(10), 1061–1063.

St. George-Hyslop, P. H., Tanzi, R. E., Polinsky, R. J., Haines, J. L., Nee, L., Watkins, P. C., et al. (1987). The genetic defect causing familial Alzheimer's disease maps on chromosome 21. *Science, 235*(4791), 885–890.

Takeuchi, F., McGinnis, R., Bourgeois, S., Barnes, C., Eriksson, N., Soranzo, N., et al. (2009). A genome-wide association study confirms VKORC1, CYPSC9, and CYP4F2 as principal genetic determinants of warfarin dose. *PLoS Genetics, 5*(3), e1000433.

The Celera Genomics Sequencing Team. (2001). The sequence of the human genome. *Science*, 1304–1351.

The International Human Genome Mapping Consortium. (2001). A physical map of the human genome. *Nature, 409*, 934–941.

Appendix A

Complete rationales for answers can be found in the Pearson Nursing Student resources at nursing.pearsonhighered.com.

CHAPTER 1 ANSWERS

PRETEST Answers: 1. B; 2. D; 3. C; 4. D; 5. D; 6. B; 7. B; 8. A; 9. C; 10. D

POSTTEST Answers: 1. D; 2. A; 3. A; 4. C; 5. B

CRITICAL THINKING CHECKPOINT ANSWERS

The nurse should be aware that such genetic testing is the current standard of care. The nurse should contact the prescribing physician to determine whether he wishes to order the testing. The hospital pharmacist may be a valuable source of information for the physician.

CHAPTER 2 ANSWERS

PRETEST Answers: 1. A; 2. A; 3. Human Genome Project; 4. E; 5. A; 6. A; 7. A; 8. H; 9. A; 10. E

POSTTEST Answers: 1. Assessment; Policy Development; and Assurance; 2. F; 3. B; 4. D; 5. F; 6. A; 7. A; 8. F; 9. B; 10. A

CRITICAL THINKING CHECKPOINT ANSWERS

1. Arguably, every competency (1–27) listed in Section One, with the possible exception of numbers 1 and 2.
2. Yes, a chromosome study on the baby's blood would have made the correct diagnosis and also suggested the need for additional chromosome studies in this family.
3. Yes, a complete three-generation family history would have strongly suggested that there is a balanced translocation running in Mrs. Smith's side of the family and also that there is a need to perform chromosome studies on Mrs. Smith and many of her relatives.
4. No.
5. Yes.

CHAPTER 3 ANSWERS

PRETEST Answers: 1. D; 2. D; 3. D; 4. A; 5. B; 6. B; 7. C; 8. D; 9. D; 10. D

POSTTEST Answers: 1. A; 2. D; 3. D; 4. D; 5. A; 6. B; 7. D; 8. D; 9. B; 10. C

CRITICAL THINKING CHECKPOINT ANSWERS

1. Yes it is important because of the risk of trisomy 21 due to her advanced maternal age and the positive family history of Fragile X syndrome.
2. The pregnant woman, the health professional giving the woman information so she can make an informed decision, and whoever else she wants to involve.
3. Initially, the nurse midwife or obstetrician and nurse. If the screening tests come back positive, ideally a referral to a genetics counselor should be made. If the woman decides to terminate the pregnancy, grief counseling should be provided if desired.
4. She needs information on the risks of advanced maternal age and on Fragile X syndrome. If she wants information about an abortion she should be given this as well. She should be given any information she requests. In addition, since she is unclear as to whether or not the stage of her pregnancy is too late for genetic testing, she needs information about fetal development and the stages of development.
5. Theoretically the GINA legislation is to protect the woman; however, there are some violations of this law.

CHAPTER 4 ANSWERS

PRETEST Answers: 1. A; 2. B; 3. D; 4. D; 5. C; 6. A; 7. B; 8. A; 9. B; 10. A

POSTTEST Answers: 1. B; 2. A; 3 .D; 4 .B; 5. B

CRITICAL THINKING CHECKPOINT ANSWERS

Spermatogenesis takes approximately 64 days for the entire process. Each phase takes 16 days, so the possibility of environmental insult during the time of meiosis is much less. Since oocytes spend a much longer time in meiosis, the chance of environmental insults is significantly greater and increases with maternal age. While there is some evidence that increasing paternal age plays a role in chromosomal abnormalities, the role is much smaller.

CHAPTER 5 ANSWERS

PRETEST Answers: 1. C; 2. B; 3. B; 4. A; 5. D; 6. C; 7. B; 8. C; 9. C; 10. A

POSTTEST Answers: 1. B; 2. C; 3. D; 4. C; 5. B; 6. A; 7. C; 8. A; 9. A; 10. A

CRITICAL THINKING CHECKPOINT ANSWERS

1. These symptoms are consistent with a history of Down syndrome. Cognitive deficits are often significant and occur concomitantly with congenital cardiac defects, gastroesophageal reflux disease (GERD), and sleep apnea. The presence of recurring chest pain could reflect the presence of GERD or problems associated with a congenital cardiac defect. In terms of physical characteristics, children with Down syndrome exhibit a particular set of facial characteristics that include a protruding tongue, upward slanting (almond shaped) eyes, and a smaller skull than expected for age. These children also display hypotonicity and excessive flexibility due to ligamental laxity. They often have short, stubby fingers and broad hands.
2. Down syndrome is associated with trisomy 21. Trisomy 21 is the presence of an extra 21st chromosome caused by nondisjunction. This can be associated with either an extra full chromosome or a chromosomal segment.
3. The inheritable risk of Down syndrome ranges from 3%–12%, dependent on paternal or maternal risk. The primary risk factor for Down syndrome is maternal age. At the age of 35, the maternal risk of having a child with Down syndrome is 1 in 400. At age 45, the risk rises to 1 in 24 (Resta, 2005).
4. The inheritable risk of Down syndrome ranges from 3%–12%, dependent on paternal or maternal risk. Paternal risk is approximately 3%, primarily due to translocation.

CHAPTER 6 ANSWERS

PRETEST Answers: 1. B; 2. D; 3. A; 4. A; 5. D; 6. C; 7. B; 8. C; 9. C; 10. B

POSTTEST Answers: 1. B; 2. B; 3. A; 4. C; 5. B; 6. A; 7. A; 8. C; 9. A; 10. C

CRITICAL THINKING CHECKPOINT ANSWERS

1. This couple needs to have a detailed, yet simple, explanation of what placental mosaicism is with the use of diagrams. They also need to be given the information that the diagnosis does not necessarily mean the fetus is a trisomic mosaic. Explain to them that amniocentesis may not provide sufficient information to determine if the fetus is affected as well.
2. It is important to stress to this couple that having placental mosaicism does not always correlate with fetal abnormalities, although it can be associated with poor prenatal outcomes. Statistics on placental mosaicism should be provided for their consideration together with all updated information regarding this phenomenon. Review with them the need to know which chromosome is expressed as a trisomy in the placenta as that has implications for the outcome. It could be suggested that percutaneous blood sampling be performed to determine the fetal karyotype. All risks and benefits of each test should be reviewed for their consideration.
3. It would be beneficial for the couple to obtain genetic studies of their individual chromosome karyotypes as well as a family history.
4. As the pregnancy continues, high-resolution ultrasound to determine nuchal translucency together with morphology scans would be beneficial, as would serial ultrasounds to assess appropriate fetal growth and development. The pregnancy should be closely monitored due to the potential for adverse outcomes with biophysical profiles and/or nonstress testing.

CHAPTER 7 ANSWERS

PRETEST Answers: 1. D; 2. A; 3. A; 4. A; 5. C; 6. B; 7. A; 8. A; 9. C; 10. A; 11. D; 12. A; 13. A; 14. D; 15. A; 16. B; 17. A; 18. B; 19. A; 20. C

POSTTEST Answers: 1. C; 2. A; 3. A; 4. C, 5. A, B; 6. B; 7. C, D; 8. D; 9. B; 10. A; 11. D; 12. B; 13. B; 14. A; 15. C; 17. C, D; 18. B; 19. A; 20. E; 21. B

CRITICAL THINKING CHECKPOINT ANSWERS

Case 1

1. Further data should include health history, which includes family history of genetic disorders; perinatal history; changes in developmental status; and history of present illness and treatments.
2. Signs and symptoms of Cystic fibrosis (CF) are seen in the newborn period or at least before 2 years of age with meconium ileus, failure to thrive, and/or frequent respiratory infections. Recurrent infections eventually leads to fibrotic change in the lungs with secondary pulmonary hypertension or cor pulmonale. The characteristic signs and symptoms of cystic fibrosis are recurrent episodes of pneumonia, constipation, weight loss, pale, foul-smelling stools, and diabetes. Infertility is also an issue with both sexes with congenital bilateral absence of vas deferens, and thick secretions of cervix and fallopian tubes. CF is a common autosomal recessive disorder in those with western European ancestry, less common in African-Americans and Asian-Americans.
3. It is autosomal recessive and skips generations; parents and perhaps other family members are carriers.
4. Yes. In most cases of CF, clinical symptoms and an abnormal sweat test confirm the diagnosis. Molecular testing to validate the mutations in the CFTR gene on chromosome 7 is desired to advise relatives regarding their carrier status, as well as prenatal testing or atypical cases.
5. Some sites on gene therapy for CF include:
   - http://www.cfgenetherapy.org.uk/
   - http://www.genome.gov
   - http://www.sickkids.ca/Centres/Cystic-Fibrosis-Centre/

Case 2

1. The history of miscarriages, still births, and infants with congenital malformations in several generations might suggest autosomal dominant condition with reduced penetrance of balance chromosomal structural abnormality (Read & Donnai, 2007).
2. Chromosomal analysis on parents and child.
3. The parents respond with emotions of loss and grief, including shock, anxiety, denial, anger, and confusion. The nurse should be a patient advocate. The nurse needs to keep the family informed about possible findings, information regarding genetic tests, and consultations being arranged. In addition, encourage parent's involvement in the plan of care. The nurse should also identify support systems for the family and community recourses available.

Case 3

1. Clues for DMD are being clumsy and slow to walk; Gower's sign (standing with support and bracing arms against legs because the proximal leg muscles are weak); enlarged calves (pseudohypertrophy); and positive family history (uncle with DMD).
2. X-linked recessive.
3. Muscle biopsy for an absence of dystrophin, DNA genetic testing for the mutation, tests to check whether creatine kinase levels are increased, and an EMG (not neurotransmitter problem).

Case 4

1. Mitochondrial inheritance (maternal mitochondria). Mitochondrial inheritance occurs through maternal lines. Fred will not pass his mtDNA to his children.
2. The nature of the eye problem: rapid progression in the affected males in comparison to the late onset and heart problems in Fred's aunt.
3. Fred is probably in shock or denial. His life goals are altered and there are major changes in his life. The nurse provides an essential role in providing emotional support and referral to appropriate agencies and support groups.

CHAPTER 8 ANSWERS

PRETEST Answers: 1. C; 2. B; 3. D; 4. A; 5. A; 6. C; 7. D; 8. C; 9. B; 10. D

POSTTEST Answers: 1. B; 2. B; 3. C; 4. C; 5. A; 6. A; 7. C; 8. B; 9. D; 10. D

CRITICAL THINKING CHECKPOINT ANSWERS

1. Several factors could have put the fetus at risk including the alcohol and the hot tub. Both can be teratogenic during pregnancy. Also, more questions need to be asked in reference to L.B.'s family's history of cleft lip and Down syndrome.
2. There is no definitive test for cleft lip; however, an ultrasound scan for morphology can be done around 17–19 weeks gestation to determine if the baby has one.
3. In this case, the alcohol consumption is probably not going to have an effect on the fetus; however, if the mother continues to drink alcohol throughout her pregnancy it can cause fetal alcohol syndrome (FAS). A woman who consistently drinks alcohol during pregnancy has a 30% to 46% chance of having a fetus with long-term physical and mental defects (Lewis, 2008). It has never been determined how much alcohol is needed to cause harm so abstaining from all alcohol is recommended in pregnancy.
4. The nurse needs to discuss several topics with the woman about prenatal care and what she should expect during her pregnancy. The woman should be counseled on things such as avoiding hot tubs while pregnant; avoiding people with viral or bacterial infections; abstaining from alcohol, tobacco, or illicit drugs; checking with the physician before taking any medications; avoiding cleaning cat litter pans and bird cages during pregnancy; avoiding eating fish known to contain heavy metals such as mercury; eating a well-balanced diet and taking prenatal vitamins; getting enough exercise and sleep; and scheduling appointments for routine prenatal care.

CHAPTER 9 ANSWERS

PRETEST Answers: 1. D; 2. D; 3. A; 4. B; 5. D; 6. C; 7. B; 8. A; 9. A; 10. D

POSTTEST Answers: 1. B; 2. A; 3. C

CRITICAL THINKING CHECKPOINT ANSWERS

1. Susan is your patient, so your responsibilities are to her.
2. It is up to Susan to share the information about the paternity with her husband. You also should inform Susan that she can elect amniocentesis to determine the genetic status of the baby.
3. The question of insurance coverage for the genetic testing for the nonmarital partner is dependent on his particular coverage and is not easily determined.
4. The question of legal obligation to the fetus may depend on state law determining personhood.

CHAPTER 10 ANSWERS

PRETEST Answers: 1. A; 2. D; 3. D; 4. A; 5. D; 6. B; 7. A; 8. A; 9. B; 10. A

POSTTEST Answers: 1. B; 2. D; 3. A; 4. A; 5. A; 6. B; 7. A; 8. D; 9. B; 10. C

CRITICAL THINKING CHECKPOINT ANSWERS

1. This woman would undergo normal prenatal testing and screening but in addition she may want to consider chorionic villus sampling and/or an amniocentesis.
2. A family history is always important to see what might be revealed about the offspring. In this case it is particularly important as there has been a report of pregnancy losses on both sides of the family.
3. Any woman who is pregnant after the age of 35, especially for the first time, is considered at risk for genetic problems. The other red flag for this woman is the history of pregnancy losses on both sides of the family.
4. The nurse must ensure that the woman and her husband understand what the nurse midwife, nurse practitioner, or physician has told them regarding the need for routine as well as specific prenatal testing and screening. After the tests are done, the nurse must confirm the couple's understanding of the test results and help them to voice any questions or concerns they might have. Even if the test results are fine, the family may need reassurance as they have mostly likely been anxious about the results and may still be anxious about the pregnancy outcome due to the family history of pregnancy losses.
5. The type of follow-up care depends on the test results and the family's needs. This follow-up must be tailored to each individual family.

CHAPTER 11 ANSWERS

PRETEST Answers: 1. A; 2. D; 3. A; 4. A; 5. D; 6. D; 7. C; 8. C; 9. A; 10. D

POSTTEST Answers: 1. B; 2. A; 3. B; 4. C; 5. A; 6. A; 7. B; 8. B; 9. A; 10. B

CRITICAL THINKING CHECKPOINT ANSWERS

1. The United States recognizes parents as the proper surrogates for their children. This viewpoint comes from the presumption that, above all, parents want what is best for their child and understand better than anyone the traditions and conditions of the world in which the child will be raised. Thus, it is not appropriate to simply document that the mother has declined the newborn screen. It is the responsibility of the health care provider to determine the reasons why the mother declined, and to offer education when applicable. Re-education gives the health care provider the opportunity to provide factual information regarding the benefits and limitations of early detection through newborn screening. It also allows the mother a chance to reconsider her decision. Moreover, it is not appropriate to obtain the newborn screen when the mother declines. The traditions and laws of most countries, including the United States, recognize parents as the surrogate decision makers for their own children. Given this widely recognized parental authority, it is rare that anyone is given the authority to bypass the parents' decision or to overrule their decisions.
2. In some circumstances it may be appropriate for the mother to decline newborn screening for her infant based on religious beliefs. Regardless, every attempt should be made to adequately educate the parent about the benefits and limitations of the newborn screen.
3. When the parent declines a newborn screen, nurses and other health care providers should document the following in the infant's medical record:
   a. Discussions between the parent and health care provider, as the discussions pertain to the newborn screen.
   b. Efforts made to provide factual information to the parent, including the use of information sheets or pamphlets about the newborn screen.

Furthermore, some states have special forms that need to be completed when a parent declines the newborn screen.

4. If the parent consents to the newborn screen, the first blood sample is obtained from the infant's heel between 24 and 48 hours of age and the special filter paper is impregnated with the infant's blood. The filter paper is then sent to the newborn screen laboratory for analysis. Additional newborn screens may be required if the infant is ill at the time when the newborn screen is obtained.

CHAPTER 12 ANSWERS

PRETEST Answers:

1. Genetic discrimination is the act of treating an individual differently based on their genetic information. This form of discrimination can occur in any aspect of an individual's life where genetic information may be accessed. However, GINA is applicable to genetic information in employment and health insurance.
2. GINA applies to employment and the health insurance.
3. The DOL, HHS, and DOT regulate the health insurance provisions of GINA. The EEOC enforces the employment provisions of GINA.
4. GINA requires that genetic information is treated the same as medical records, which are normally regulated by HIPAA. In fact, the actual text in GINA makes amendments to HIPAA in order to add these genetic nondiscrimination provisions.
5. Yes. Since the patient's genetic condition is manifest, the genetic information obtained is no longer predictive, and health insurers may use that information to underwrite.
6. No. Since the patient's results are predictive, health insurers are prohibited from using that information to underwrite.
7. No. Employers are not allowed to discriminate based on any genetic information, predictive or reflective of current health status. They may, depending on the job, discriminate based on the individual's ability to do certain aspects of the job. However, the Americans with Disabilities Act may protect the individual with manifest disease.
8. Individuals in the military, federal employees enrolled in FEHB, veterans obtaining health care through the VA, employers with fewer than 15 employees, and individuals covered by the Indian Health Service
9. Life, disability, and long-term care insurance
10. Nurses are often have closer interactions with patients, and it is their responsibility to inform the patients of the protections and limits provided by GINA regarding any genetic tests or services they may be considering. Patients need this complete and accurate understanding of their genetic information protections so that they can make the most informed decision about any genetic test or service.

POSTTEST Answers:

1. The modern world of scientific and medical research opened up the entire field of genomics with the progress of the Human Genome Project. However, the new depth of newly accessible and personal genetic information also created a potential for the misuse of that information, creating the concerns of genetic information discrimination. Read "Introduction to Genetic Discrimination" in Section One.
2. Genetic information includes information about an individual's genetic tests and the genetic tests of an individual's family members, as well as information about the manifestation of a disease or disorder in an individual's family members (i.e., family medical history), participation in genetic research, and use of genetic services. The results of genetic tests can be either (1) predictive, meaning they assess the risk of developing a condition in the future; or (2) they can identify a manifested condition, where the

test has resulted in a positive diagnosis. Thus, Title I's definition does not include the latter tests because these tests include information about current health status, which insurers use to underwrite. Title II's definition includes both predictive tests and those genetic tests that are related to a manifested disease. Read "Definitions in GINA" in Section Three.

3. (1) A health insurance provider may only request genetic information in order to assess the medical need for a test, treatment, or procedure requested by the individual. (2) The health insurance provider may only request that an individual undergo a genetic test for a research study that follows certain specific requirements. Read "Protections in Health Insurance" in Section Three.
4. *Employers* refers to employers at not-for-profit organizations and for-profit corporations with at least 15 employees, employment agencies, labor organizations, and training programs. Read "Protections in Employment" in Section Three.
5. Inadvertent knowledge and publicly available information. Read "Protections in Employment" in Section Three.
6. No. Health insurance providers are prohibited from discriminating based on family members' health information. Read "GINA in Nursing Practice" in Section Four.
7. No, she is not correct. Employers are legally allowed to request genetic information as part of a voluntary health service offered as part of employment. This is one of the five exceptions where employers are legally allowed to request or gain access to genetic information. Read "Protections in Employment" in Section Three.
8. No, the employer is not operating in agreement with GINA regulations. While employers may request genetic information as part of a voluntary health service, they are still prohibited from using the genetic information collected to discriminate against employees. Read "Protections in Employment" in Section Three.
9. Genetic samples taken from military personnel are commonly used for research studies as part of biorepositories. Once a service member leaves the military, he or she can decide to destroy the samples. Read "Military" in Section Five.
10. Not likely. While GINA does not apply to most federal employees, there are other policies and laws that give similar protections. Read Section Five.

CRITICAL THINKING CHECKPOINT ANSWERS

1. Normally, insurance companies use risk assessment in order to estimate the amount of health care services that will be utilized and use this information in order to set premiums and contribution amounts for beneficiaries. Tests that assess the risk for developing a certain condition are considered predictive. The BRCA test is one such predictive test for breast and ovarian cancer. According to GINA, health insurance providers are prohibited from using predictive genetic information in underwriting coverage decisions for individuals.
2. In GINA, the health insurance and employment titles have different definitions of what type of genetic tests are covered. While employers are prohibited from using any genetic test information in making employment-related decisions, health insurers can use genetic information related to current health status (e.g., a manifested disease or condition) for underwriting purposes. Since Debbie's breast cancer was diagnosed, and thus "manifested," GINA no longer applied to Debbie's health insurance provider. However, if Debbie lived in a state with more comprehensive genetic nondiscrimination laws, she might still be protected from changes in insurance coverage.
3. Unfortunately, when Kathleen develops breast cancer, health insurers would likely be able to use this new information about her health status to make underwriting decisions. While health insurers could not previously use her predictive genetic information, the actual diagnosis of breast cancer is now part of her current health status. Thus, GINA is no longer relevant, and health insurers may raise Kathleen's premiums knowing that breast cancer treatments will be needed. However, like her sister's situation described in Question 2, if Kathleen lived in a state with more comprehensive nondiscrimination laws, she might also still be protected from changes in insurance coverage.

CHAPTER 13 ANSWERS

PRETEST Answers: 1. C; 2. B; 3. C; 4. C; 5. A; 6. A; 7. A; 8. A; 9. C; 10. A

POSTTEST Answers: 1. C; 2. C; 3. B; 4. A; 5. B; 6. B; 7. C; 8. B; 9. C; 10. D

CRITICAL THINKING CHECKPOINT ANSWERS

1. Sickle cell disease is an autosomal recessive trait.
2. Characteristics of an autosomal recessive trait are (a) the trait is expressed when two copies (homozygosity) of an autosomal allele are present; (b) individuals who have two different (heterozygous) alleles are carriers of the trait; (c) children born to parents who are carriers of the gene (heterozygous) have a 25% chance of having the disease, a 25% chance of not having the disease and not being a carrier, and a 50% chance of being a carrier; (d) males and females can be affected and can transmit the disease; and (e) the trait can skip generations.
3. Emma's mother has the disease and her father is probably a carrier because his mother has the disease also. Emma's risk of having the disease or of being a carrier can be determined using a Punnett square:

Mother (ss)

Father (Ss)

	s	s
S	Ss	Ss
s	ss	ss

4. Emma could be an Ss = carrier and therefore have a 50% chance of being a carrier for the sickle cell gene. Or, Emma could be ss (affected) and therefore still have a 50% chance of having the disease—which we have already determined she does not.
5. Other possible patterns of inheritance include diabetes and cancer.

To determine risk of other diseases we would need more information. More health and lifestyle information would be needed from all generations of this family before we could determine a true pattern of inheritance.

6. Once the nurse has collected as much individual and family health history as possible and once she identifies a pattern of inheritance or a mode of transmission, she will need to make the proper referrals. In this case, the mother and father may need preconception counseling should they decide to have more children. Otherwise, the nurse should refer the couple and other interested family members for genetic counseling.

CHAPTER 14 ANSWERS

PRETEST Answers: 1. A; 2. D; 3. A; 4. B; 5. C; 6. C; 7. A; 8. C; 9. D; 10. B

POSTTEST Answers: 1. A; 2. D; 3. C; 4. A; 5. D; 6. A; 7. D; 8. B; 9. B; 10. B

CRITICAL THINKING CHECKPOINT ANSWERS

Case 1

1. The Gail model is appropriate because it takes reproductive history AND breast biopsy history into account.

The Claus model is not appropriate because there is no family history of breast cancer.

2. 5-year : 1.93%; lifetime: 11.18%

Case 2

1. Cannot use either model because there is a personal history of breast cancer. There's no point in calculating risk when the individual already has the disease. The abbreviated family history is also a red flag and should generate a referral.

Case 3

1. You cannot use either model. Male breast cancer is an automatic referral (so you can't use the Claus model). The disease is on the paternal side (so you can't use the Gail model).

Case 4

1. You can use either Gail or Claus. There is a family history so you can use Claus. The disease is on the maternal side and the patient has no personal history of breast cancer so you can use Gail.
2. You calculate them both and use the highest estimate.

CHAPTER 15 ANSWERS

PRETEST Answers: 1. C; 2. A; 3. B; 4. A; 5. C; 6. B; 7. A; 8. B; 9. B; 10. B

POSTTEST Answers: 1. B; 2. C; 3. B; 4. A; 5. B; 6. C; 7. D; 8. B; 9. B; 10. B

CRITICAL THINKING CHECKPOINT ANSWERS

1. The significant points regarding CL's history is the fact her fatigue began after the viral syndrome with a high fever; she is a runner who now gets hungry and thirsty after a run; she is especially fatigued at night after dinner; she has a family history of non-insulin-dependent diabetes mellitus.
2. Lab tests that could be of value at this moment would be a blood sugar, hemoglobin A_1C, and urine dipstick because generally all three tests could be done in an office setting.
3. Additional questions to ask would include questions about nocturia, thirst, and weight loss.
4. Suggestions for follow-up would include referral to a diabetes counselor for diet changes and to monitor her blood glucose before and after every meal. If her blood sugars are high after meals, she may need a medication by mouth initially and possibly later insulin. Explain to her that this seems to be a case of autoimmune diabetes. The fact that she had the virus with a high fever and was under stress simultaneously indicates that her body may be attacking itself secondary to the release of stimulators during the fever. Moreover, since it is an autoimmune disease, she could be at risk for other tissue attacks, i.e., thyroid problems. It is important for her to continue her exercise regimen because this improves her circulation and relieves stress.

CHAPTER 16 ANSWERS

PRETEST Answers: 1. B; 2. C; 3. B; 4. C; 5. A; 6. E; 7. D; 8. D; 9. D; 10. E

POSTTEST Answers: 1. B; 2. C; 3. B; 4. C; 5. A; 6. E; 7. D; 8. D; 9. D; 10. E

CRITICAL THINKING CHECKPOINT ANSWERS

1. Adrian developed breast cancer at a very young age. Early age of cancer onset is a red flag suggesting genetic predisposition to breast cancer. In addition, breast cancer is not common in men. When discovered, it is more likely to be associated with a heritable gene mutation. This history suggests there are at least three individuals in the paternal line that have received a breast cancer diagnosis. Multiple primary breast cancers in a maternal or paternal line are a red flag suggesting the need to develop a comprehensive pedigree. It will be also important to assess whether the cancer cases in this three-generation family history reveal bilateral disease. Bilateral disease is a common cancer risk red flag.
2. About 10%–15% of all breast cancers can be associated with a gene mutation. Cancer is the result of a complex interplay between inherited genetic predisposition and environmental and lifestyle exposures. In addition, scientists recently have found that breast tumors that showed mutations in *BRCA2* conferred a survival advantage over disease due to other types of breast cancer associated gene mutations.
3. Breast cancer is not common in men. However, in such instances, a nurse should be alert to the possibility of a *BRCA2* mutation. The *BRCA2* gene is an autosomal dominant mutation that can confer an increased risk for biologic descendants. Each child would have a 50/50 chance of inheriting this gene mutation.
4. There are many benefits to referral for genetic counseling, as discussed in the following:
   - Adrian would have the opportunity for a professional consultation with a geneticist and/or a genetic counselor who could help her to decide on the value of personal genetic testing, as well as discuss the implications of such testing for treatment decisions and possible privacy or insurance discrimination.
   - Other at-risk family members can be identified and genetic counselors could help Adrian strategize ways to share this information with them. These individuals could be offered cancer surveillance options that might include earlier age for specific screening tests and more frequent screening intervals.
   - Adrian would also have the opportunity to discuss the relevance of other breast cancer risk-reduction measures (e.g., prophylactic removal of the other breast or ovaries after child bearing is complete).
   - Gene testing and counseling can provide guidance with new gene-specific treatment options and risk reduction measures as they emerge.

CHAPTER 17 ANSWERS

PRETEST Answers: 1. A; 2. teratogen; 3. A; 4. B; 5. B; 6. A; 7. research; 8. B; 9. F; 10. A

POSTTEST Answers: 1. E; the correct term is *genetic variation;* 2. A; 3. C; 4. A; 5. E; 6. A; 7. A; 8. B; 9. C; 10. D.

CRITICAL THINKING CHECKPOINT ANSWERS

1. No, genetic testing for gout is not included in the standard of care for diagnosing and/or treating the condition. Therefore, it did not need to be done. Genetic testing for research purposes could have been performed and may have been appropriate in this case.
2. The risk factors for developing gout include genetic/genomic risk factors, a positive family history for the condition, gender and age, environmental risk factors, and behavioral and treatment-related factors. Since genetic/genomic testing was not performed (and did not need to be performed in this case) and the past medical history, review of systems, and family history were not significant, making the diagnosis of gout depends on his serum uric acid level (which was suggestive at the time of the attack but cannot be used to make a definitive diagnosis); his age and gender; his borderline hypertension; his being overweight; his taking low-dose aspirin therapy, as well as a diuretic and niacin. These factors all pointed to the diagnosis.
3. No, he did not have a history of chronic gout of at least 10-years duration. An X-ray may have been indicated to rule out a fracture in his right foot, except there was no history of trauma to suggest the need for an X-ray at the time.

CHAPTER 18 ANSWERS

PRETEST Answers: 1. B; 2. C; 3. B; 4. A; 5. B; 6. C; 7. D; 8. D; 9. A; 10. B

POSTTEST Answers: 1. C; 2. B; 3. C; 4. A; 5. A; 6. B; 7. D; 8. A; 9. B; 10. A

CRITICAL THINKING CHECKPOINT ANSWERS

Knowledge about genetic linkages could illuminate understanding of pathophysiology, leading to design of more effective nursing interventions. In addition, it could inform nursing assessment and targeted screening, and influence patient teaching about risk factors and underlying cause of the common disease as well as influence monitoring for complications and side effects of therapies.

CHAPTER 19 ANSWERS

PRETEST Answers: 1.A; 2. A; 3. C; 4. C; 5. D; 6. B; 7. D; 8. A; 9. B; 10. B

POSTTEST Answers: 1. B; 2. D; 3. A; 4. A; 5. A; 6. B; 7. A; 8. D; 9. B; 10. C

CRITICAL THINKING CHECKPOINT ANSWERS

1. The diagnostic criterion for bipolar disorders requires meeting criteria for mania and possibly major depression as well. The criteria for mania must be met, and symptoms need to have lasted for at least a 1-week period. At least three of a set of seven symptoms needs to be observed. In this case, the symptoms have not lasted long enough, even though a decreased need for sleep, increased talking, and a feeling of racing thoughts are present.
2. There is both twin and familial association evidence for bipolar disorder.
3. There is no reliable genetic means of testing for the presence of bipolar disorder. Diagnosis is made through comparison of symptoms with a criterion list and determining symptom duration. The genetic findings in those with bipolar disorder implicate regulation of the circadian cycle as well as serotonergic and dopaminergic pathways.
4. After further evaluation to determine that the symptoms are not due to the use of a substance or medication, then a mental health referral for evaluation should be made. The patient should also be evaluated for depressive symptoms and any plans for self-harm.
5. After a thorough physical examination and assessment, the patient should receive appropriate referrals for mental health evaluation and possible treatment. Information needs to be provided regarding bipolar disorder and the possible genetic links. Should the patient already be on medication, the nurse should evaluate medication adherence and the use of other substances.

CHAPTER 20 ANSWERS

PRETEST Answers: 1. C; 2. A; 3. D; 4. D; 5. B; 6. A; 7. B; 8. B; 9. C; 10. B

POSTTEST Answers: 1. A; 2. A; 3. B; 4. A; 5. B; 6. D; 7. C; 8. B; 9. A; 10. B

CRITICAL THINKING CHECKPOINT ANSWERS

1. While heritability is complex in mood disorders, a three-generation pedigree chart will help to identify the pattern of mood disorders in relatives. It is important to get information about each affected relative, including which mood disorder was present, age at onset, admissions to psychiatric hospitals, and suicidality. Significant numbers of affected relatives may indicate increased heritability in this family.
2. While the genotype of the infant cannot be changed, efforts to control environmental stressors that might produce expression of susceptibility genes are important. The parents should be educated to the importance of making lifestyle changes that will be supportive of their child's physical and mental growth and development. It's important to emphasize that genetics is not destiny and there are many parenting strategies that can be of help to them. Referral to a family therapist or child development specialist may be helpful. Referral to a genetic counselor may be reassuring but at present will be limited to assisting them in estimation of recurrence risk of BPD-I based on the family history. There are no genetic screening or diagnostic tests for mood disorders at this time.
3. The nurse should educate Mr. RS and his family members about the complexity of the genetic contribution to the development of mood disorders and the importance of control of environmental stressors in the development and management of BPD. It is imperative that Mr. RS understand the vital importance of taking his medication regularly. Support groups and various therapy techniques are helpful as supportive measures.
4. It's important that the nurse assist Mr. RS and his family members to identify strategies that will decrease stress; enhance coping skills in potentially difficult situations, such as the birth of a new baby; and improve social interactions between them. Stress-relieving activities such as sports, meditation, yoga, and enjoying family activities together may be recommended. Involvement in community activities will help to foster a sense of involvement and ability to deal with health issues positively.

CHAPTER 21 ANSWERS

PRETEST Answers: 1. B; 2. C; 3. B; 4. D; 5. D; 6. C; 7. A; 8. B; 9. A; 10. D

POSTTEST Answers: 1. B; 2. A; 3. D; 4. A; 5. C; 6. D; 7. A; 8. D; 9. A; 10. A

CRITICAL THINKING CHECKPOINT ANSWERS

1. Alcohol affects a number of areas in Margerie's life. It would be appropriate to suggest alcohol screening and testing. Genetic testing may not be as valuable as a clinical screening for the behaviors of alcohol abuse and substance dependence.
2. Margerie's family history is important as her mother's alcoholism and subsequent death from sequelae and her father's propensity to abuse a substance and distance himself from his responsibilities are both genetic and behavioral influences on her life.
3. Both biologic parents may have contributed genetic predispositions to substance abuse and dependence. Margerie may have a disadvantage in trying to resist using substances of abuse in that her reward circuits, stimulation needs, frustration tolerance, and problem-solving abilities could all be determined by her genetics.

4. Nurses would help Margerie understand the purpose of the tests and translate some of the more unfamiliar language into more understandable terms. Following testing, nurses would be involved in explaining the meaning of the test results on Margerie's day-to-day life.

5. Margerie already demonstrates the need for follow-up care in that she has areas of functioning that are challenged by her substance abuse. Coping skills, perspective, problem solving, group and individual counseling, and therapy would all play a role in competent follow-up care.

CHAPTER 22 ANSWERS

PRETEST Answers: 1. B; 2. A; 3. E; 4. B; 5. D; 6. C; 7. A; 8. E; 9. A; 10. E

POSTTEST Answers: 1. E; 2. C; 3. C; 4. E; 5. E; 6. A; 7. E; 8. B; 9. A; 10. B

CRITICAL THINKING CHECKPOINT ANSWERS

1. Assessment of genetic etiology would begin with a comprehensive health history, a physical evaluation for dysmorphology, and at least a three-generation pedigree of both maternal and paternal relatives. Genetic testing may be conducted to evaluate for syndromes associated with ASD, such as Fragile X syndrome, Angelmen syndrome, mitochondrial disorders, and Prader-Willi syndrome. The parents might be offered chromosomal microarray analysis to test the entire genome for abnormalities. Single-gene testing for specific defects might be offered if the comprehensive health history and record review uncovers other case of autism spectrum disorder among first-degree relatives.

2. There are several good reasons. First, test results will help the medical team design optimal treatment plans. Second, with results in hand, parents can knowledgably join support groups and connect with parents with children with the same diagnoses. Third, certain medical conditions are associated with specific developmental profiles. Knowing the underlying medical cause of the autism will allow tailor-made treatments. Fourth, sometimes knowing the cause offers peace of mind. Fifth, this knowledge will allow parents to make informed choices about family planning. Sixth, results provide families with information they can share with relatives and other offspring to assist them in decision making about family planning.

3. Genetic evaluation seeks to uncover the precise cause but this may not be possible. The risk of ASD in a second child is called *recurrence risk*. Unfortunately, at present this can be estimated only for the 10%–20% of children who have syndromic ASD; in other words, the cause is associated with another disorder such as Fragile X syndrome. Then the recurrence risk is tied to the risk of a second child having the same syndrome, which varies. In the case of Fragile X syndrome, the recurrence risk is 25%–40% in a second child.

CHAPTER 23 ANSWERS

PRETEST Answers: 1. C; 2. A; 3. B; 4. A; 5. A; 6. D; 7. B; 8. A; 9. B; 10. D

POSTTEST Answers: 1. B; 2. D; 3. A; 4. C; 5. D; 6. B; 7. D; 8. B; 9. A; 10. B

CRITICAL THINKING CHECKPOINT ANSWERS

1. A poor metabolizer

2. An ultra-rapid metabolizer, causing an excessive proportion of each codeine dose to be metabolized to morphine

3. Types of information needed is why the test is being ordered, how the results might be used, and what are the limitations of the test.

4. Yes. A brief, targeted family history may identify other family members at risk for having poor response to codeine. Sickle cell is an autosomal recessive disorder. Therefore, Jerome may have a sibling with sickle cell who may require codeine or other opioid pain medications. Hydrocodone, oxycodone, and tramadol are also at least partially metabolized by CYP2D6. If any of Jerome's siblings do have sickle cell, it may be useful to them to have CYP2D6 testing done before crises so a medication plan can be developed ahead of time.

5. The nurse evaluates the impact and effectiveness of genetic and genomic technology, information, interventions, and treatments on a client's outcome.

CHAPTER 24 ANSWERS

PRETEST Answers: 1. A; 2. A; 3. B; 4. A; 5. C; 6. E; 7. C; 8. A; 9. C; 10. B

POSTTEST Answers: 1. C; 2. B; 3. B; 4. D; 5. D; 6. C; 7. B; 8. D; 9. D; 10. B

CRITICAL THINKING CHECKPOINT ANSWERS

1. The ages at onset for a common complex disease that are earlier than usual is a red flag in a personal or family health history. In this case, early onset of Alzheimer disease (before age 60) suggests that the Alzheimer disease *may* have a strong genetic component in this family.
2. Family history is an important part of every nursing assessment. However, in this case, the family history is essential in order to follow up on the early age at onset red flag. The family history should be expanded to include three to four generations in order to answer the following questions: a) Are there other family members who have been diagnosed with Alzheimer disease? b) If so, is there a discernible pattern of inheritance? For example, are there multiple affected individuals across multiple generations? c) What are the ages at onset for other affected family members?
3. The fact that A.C.'s mother has early onset Alzheimer disease, a condition that is known to have a strong genetic component in some families, is a risk factor. Other risk factors would be clarified by obtaining a complete family history.
4. Every nurse, in every role and setting, is responsible for identifying persons at risk for having or transmitting a genetic condition and for making appropriate referrals, if indicated. In this setting, the nurse should complete a comprehensive (or at least targeted) family history in order to gather additional risk information and provide A.C. with knowledge about the availability of specialty genetics services.
5. If this family were to pursue specialty genetics services, the nurse is in a position to play an advocacy role for the family in seeking these services and in providing follow-up decision making and emotional support.

Appendix B

Internet Resources

ABOARD (Advisory Board on Autism & Related Disorders): http://www.aboard.org

A Compendium of Resources on Newborn Screening Policy and System Development: http://www.medicalhomeinfo.org/downloads/docs/NBScategorizedcompend.doc

Alliance of Genetic Support Groups: http://www.geneticalliance.org

Alzheimer's Foundation of America: http://www.alzfdn.org/AboutAlzheimers/research.html

American Academy of Family Physicians CME Bulletin: http://www.aafp.org/online/etc/medialib/aafp_org/documents/cme/selfstudy/bulletins/gout-hyperuricemia.Par.0001.File.dat/Gout.pdf

American Association of Occupational Health Nurses, Inc.: http://www.aaohn.org

American Diabetes Association: http://www.diabetes.org

American College of Medical Genetics: http://www.acmg.net//AM/Template.cfm?Section=Home3

American College of Rheumatology, Gout: http://www.rheumatology.org/practice/clinical/patients/diseases_and_conditions/gout.asp

American Heart Association: http://www.heart.org/HEARTORG/

American Lung Association: http://www.lungusa.org

American Nurses Association: http://www.nursingworld.org

American Public Health Association, Environmental Public Health: http://www.apha.org/programs/environment/

American Public Health Association, Genetics and Public Health: http://www.apha.org/advocacy/policy/policysearch/default.htm?id=1161

American Public Health Association, Occupational Health & Safety: http://www.apha.org/membergroups/sections/aphasections/occupational/

American Society of Human Genetics: http://www.ashg.org

Association of Colleges of Nursing: http://www.aacn.nche.edu

Association of State and Territorial Health Officials: http://www.astho.org

Autism National Committee: http://www.autcom.org

Autism Research Institute: http://www.autismresearchinstitute.com

Autism Resources: http://www.autismsource.org

Autism Speaks: http://www.autismspeaks.org

Autism Support Network: http://www.autismsupportnetwork.org

Behavioral Genetics: http://www.ornl.gov/sci/techresources/Human_Genome/elsi/behavior.shtml

Centers for Disease Control and Prevention: http://www.cdc.gov/ncbddd/pediatricgenetics/newborn_screening.html

Centers for Disease Control and Prevention, Arthritis: http://www.cdc.gov/arthritis/basics/gout.htm

Centers for Disease Control and Prevention Early Hearing Detection and Intervention Program (EHDI): http://www.cdc.gov/ncbddd/hearingloss

Center for Disease Control and Prevention, Family Health History: http://www.cdc.gov/genomics/famhistory/index.htm

Centers for Disease Control Family History: http://www.cdc.gov/genomics/famhistory/resources/fs_web.htm

Centers for Disease Control and Prevention National Center for Environmental Health: http://www.cdc.gov/nceh/

Centers for Disease Control and Prevention Public Health Genomics: http://www.cdc.gov/genomics/default.htm

Centers for Disease Control and Prevention Public Health Organizations and Associations: http://www.cdc.gov/dls/links/links_pa.aspx

Child Health Explanation: http://www.childhealth-explanation.com/genetics.html

Cincinnati's Children's Hospital Genetic Education Program (1999–2011): http://www.cincinnatichildrens.org/education/clinical/nursing/genetics/default/

Coalition for Genetic Fairness: http://www.geneticfairness.org/index.html

Committee on Heritable Disorders in Newborns and Children: http://www.hrsa.gov/advisorycommittees/mchbadvisory/heritabledisorders/

Cystic Fibrosis Foundation: http://www.cff.org/research/ResearchMilestones/

Dor Yeshorium: http://www.modernlab.org/doryeshirum.html

Encyclopedia Of DNA Elements: http://www.nature.com/encode

Environmental Health, Medline Plus: http://www.nlm.nih.gov/medlineplus/environmentalhealth.html

Environmental Health & Toxicology: http://sis.nlm.nih.gov/enviro.html

Fetal Development: http://childdevelopment.howtoinfo-247.com/fetal-developm

First Signs: http://www.firstsigns.org

Genes and Disease: http://www.ncbi.nlm.nih.gov/books/nbk22183

Gene Tests/Gene Reviews: http://www.genetests.org

Genetic Alliance: http://www.geneticalliance.org

Genetic Alliance Collection of Newborn Screening Videos: http://www.youtube.com/geneticalliance#g/c/A6C56724C998F799

Genetic Alliance Family Health History: http://www.geneticalliance.org/fhh

Geneticalliance UK: http://www.geneticalliance.org.uk

Genetic and Rare Diseases (GARD) Information Center: http://rarediseases.info.nih.gov/GARD/

Genetic Counseling: http://www.marchofdimes.com/pregnancy/trying_geneticcounseling.html

Genetics Education Program for Nurses: http://gepn.cchmc.org

Genetics/Genomics Competency Center for Education: http://www.g-2-c-2.org

Genetic Home Reference: Your Guide to Understanding Genetic Conditions: http://ghr.nlm.nih.gov

Genetic Information Nondiscrimination Act of 2008: http://www.eeoc.gov/laws/statutes/gina.cfm

Genetic Nursing Credentialing Commission: http://www.geneticnurse.org

Genetic Services Branch, Maternal Child Health Bureau: http://mchb.hrsa.gov/programs/geneticservices/index.html

GINA or Genetic Information Nondiscrimination Act: http://www.ginahelp.org

Hearing Screening: http://www.medicalhomeinfo.org/how/clinical_care/hearing_screening/

Huntington's Disease Society of America: http://www.hdsa.org

Interagency Autism Coordinating Committee: http://iacc.hhs.org

International HapMap Project: http://hapmap.ncbi.nlm.nih.gov

International Society of Nurses in Genetics (ISONG): http://www.isong.org

International WAGR Syndrome Association (11p Deletion Syndrome): http://www.wagr.org

Johns Hopkins Arthritis Center, Biochemical Causes of Gout: http://www.hopkins-arthritis.org/ask-the-expert/gout-pseudogout-other-009/biochemical-causes-of-gout-928.html

Living with Trisomy 13: http://www.livingwithtrisomy13.org

March of Dimes: http://www.marchofdimes.com

March of Dimes Loss and Grieving in Pregnancy and the First Year of Life Online Course: http://www.marchofdimes.com/nursing/modnemedia/perinataltests/loss_grieving.pdf

March of Dimes Newborn Screening: http://www.marchofdimes.com/baby/bringinghome_recommendedtests.html

March of Dimes Newborn Screening: What Caregivers Need to Know Online Course: http://www.marchofdimes.com/professionals/education_newbornscreening.html

March of Dimes Preconception Health: http://www.marchofdimes.com/pregnancy/getready_indepth.html

March of Dimes Prenatal Screening: http://www.marchofdimes.com/pregnancy/prenatalcare_routinetests.html

Mayo Clinic, Gout: http://www.mayoclinic.com/health/gout/DS00090

Medline Plus, Gout:

- http://www.nlm.nih.gov/medlineplus/ency/article/003476.htm
- http://www.nlm.nih.gov/medlineplus/gout.html

My Family Health Portrait: https://familyhistory.hhs.gov/fhh-web/home.action

National Alliance on Mental Illness: http://www.nami.org

National Association of County & City Health Officials: http://www.naccho.org

National Autism Association: http://www.nationalautismassociation.org

National Cancer Institute: http://www.cancer.gov/cancertopics/pdq/genetics/overview/healthprofessional/page5

National Cancer Institute Angiogenesis Inhibitors Therapy: http://www.cancer.gov/cancertopics/factsheet/Therapy/angiogenesis-inhibitors

National Cancer Institute BRCA1 and BRCA2: Cancer Risk and Genetic Testing: http://www.cancer.gov/cancertopics/factsheet/Risk/BRCA

National Cancer Institute Cancer Genetics Services Directory: http://www.cancer.gov/cancertopics/genetics/directory

National Cancer Institute Targeted Cancer Therapies: http://www.cancer.gov/cancertopics/factsheet/Therapy/targeted

National Cancer Institute Understanding Cancer Series: http://www.cancer.gov/cancertopics/understandingcancer

National Cancer Institute Understand Cancer Series – The Immune System: http://www.cancer.gov/cancertopics/understandingcancer/immunesystem/page1

National Coalition for Health Professional Education in Genetics (NCHPEG): http://www.nchpeg.org

National Conference of State Legislatures (NCSL): http://www.ncsl.org/default.aspx?tabid=14382

National Environmental Health Association: http://www.neha.org/index.shtml

National Fragile X Foundation: http://www.fragilex.org

National Human Genome Research Institute (NHGRI): http://www.genome.gov

National Human Genome Research Institute Epigenomics Fact Sheet: http://www.genome.gov/27532724

National Human Genome Research Institute search results for genome-wide association studies (GWAS): http://www.genome.gov/search.cfm?keyword=GWAS

National Human Genome Research Institute The Genes, Environment and Health Initiative (GEI): http://www.genome.gov/19518663

National Human Genome Research Institute, Online Genetics Education Resources: http://www.genome.gov/10000464

National Human Genome Research Institute Talking Glossary of Genetic Terms: http://www.genome.gov/Glossary/

National Institute of Arthritis and Musculoskeletal and Skin Diseases:

- http://www.niams.nih.gov/Health_Info/Gout/default.asp
- http://www.niams.nih.gov/Health_Info/Gout/gout_ff.asp

National Institute of Child Health and Human Development (NICHD): http://www.nichd.nih.gov

National Institute of Neurological Disorders and Stroke: http://www.ninds.nih.gov

National Newborn Screening and Genetics Resource Center: http://genes-r-us.uthscsa.edu

National Newborn Screening and Genetics Resource Center Parent and Family Resources: http://genes-r-us.uthscsa.edu/parentpage.htm

National Society of Genetic Counselors (NSGC): http://www.nsgc.org

National Toxicology Program: http://ntp.niehs.nih.gov/?objectid=03C9AF75-E1BF-FF40-DBA9EC0928DF8B15

Newborn Screening in Massachusetts: Answers for You and Your Baby: http://www.umassmed.edu/nbs/

Newborn Screening Translational Research Network (NBSTRN): http://www.nbstrn.org

NIH ELSI Research Program: http://www.genome.gov/ELSI/

NIH National Institute of Environmental Health Sciences: http://www.niehs.nih.gov/health/topics/science/gene-env/index.cfm

NIH Genes, Environment and Health Initiative (GEI) Program: http://www.nhlbi.nih.gov/resources/geneticsgenomics/programs/gei.htm

NIH Information on Bipolar Disorder: http://www.nimh.nih.gov/health/publications/bipolar-disorder/complete-index.shtml

NIH information about GINA: http://www.genome.gov/24519851

NIH Issues in Genetics: http://www.genome.gov/Issues/

NIH Senior Health: http://nihseniorhealth.gov/gout/toc.html

Nursing Organization Links: http://www.nurse.org/orgs.shtml

Occupational Safety and Health Administration: http://www.osha.gov

Online Genetics Education Resources: http://www.genome.gov/10000464

Online Mendelian Inheritance in Man (OMIM): http://www.ncbi.nlm.nih.gov/omim

Organization of Teratology Information Specialists: http://www.otispregnancy.org

Pharmacogenomics Knowledge Implementation: http://www.pharmgkb.org

Prenatal Testing: http://www.nlm.nih.gov/medlineplus/prenataltesting.html

Presidential Commission for the Study of Bioethical Issues: http://bioethics.gov/meetings/

Pub Med Health, Gout: http://www.ncbi.nlm.nih.gov/pubmedhealth/PMH0001459/

PubMed Health, Mosaicism: http://www.ncbi.nlm.nih.gov/pubmedhealth/PMH0002294/

Risk Assessment Tools for Colorectal Cancer: http://www.cancer.gov/colorectalcancerrisk/tool.aspx; http://digestive.ccf.org/scores/go

Southeast Regional Newborn Screening and Genetics Collaborative: http://southeastgenetics.org/about.php

Support Organization for Trisomy 18, 13, and Related Disorders: http://www.trisomy.org

Surgeon General's Family Health History Initiative: My Family Health Portrait Tool: http://www.hhs.gov/familyhistory/portrait/index.html

Teratology Society: http://www.teratology.org

The Center for Collaborative Genomic Studies on Mental Disorders: https://www.nimhgenetics.org

The Future of Medicine, Pharmacogenomics: An Online Course: http://www.lithiumstudios.com/fda/Sample_Home.htm

The Parent's Guide to Newborn Screening: These Tests Can Save Your Baby's Life: http://mchb.hrsa.gov/pregnancyandbeyond/newbornscreening

The Prader-Willi Syndrome Association: http://www.pwsausa.org

The Ring Chromosome 20 Foundation: http://www.ring20.org

The Substance Abuse & Mental Health Services Administration (SAMHSA): http://www.samhsa.gov

University of British Columbia, Department of Medical Genetics: http://medgen.ubc.ca

University of Iowa Public Health Genetics Program: http://registrar.uiowa.edu/registrar/catalog/publichealth/publichealthgenetics/

University of Maryland Medical Center; Mosaicism Overview: http://www.umm.edu/ency/article/001317.htm

University of Michigan Public Health Genetics Program: http://www.sph.umich.edu/genetics/

University of Pennsylvania Graduate School Program in Public Health Genetics: http://www.publichealth.med.upenn.edu/course_listing.shtml#Genetics

University of Pittsburgh Graduate Programs in Human Genetics: http://www.hgen.pitt.edu/handbook/handbook_september_2007.pdf

University of Washington Public Health Genetics Program: http://depts.washington.edu/phgen/

U.S. Department of Labor FAQs on the Genetic Information Nondiscrimination Act: http://www.dol.gov/ebsa/faqs/faq-GINA.html

Utah Department of Health Chronic Disease Genomics Program: http://www.health.utah.gov/genomics

Utah Department of Health Chronic Disease Genomics Program Family Reunion Packets: http://health.utah.gov/genomics/familyhistory/familyreunion.html

Utah Department of Health Family Health History Toolkit: http://health.utah.gov/asthma/pdf_files/Genomics/new%20entire%20toolkit.pdf

Welcome Trust organization: http://www.sanger.ac.uk/genetics/CGP/cosmic/

World Health Organization, Environmental Health: http://www.who.int/topics/environmental_health/en/

World Health Organization, Genetics: http://www.who.int/topics/genetics/en/

World of Genetics Societies: http://genetics.faseb.org/genetics/

List of Abbreviations

5-HT 5-hydroxytriptamine (serotonin)
AACN American Association of Colleges of Nursing
AAP American Academy of Pediatrics
ABR Auditory Brainstem Response
ACMG American College of Medical Genetics
AD Alzheimer disease
ADCC antibody-dependent cellular cytotoxicity
ADI-R Autism Diagnostic Inventory-Revised
ADOS Autism Diagnostic Observation Schedule
ADRs adverse drug reactions
AFP alpha-fetoprotein33
AIDS acquired immunodeficiency syndrome
AMA advanced maternal age
AMD Age-related Macular Degeneration
AML acute myeloid leukemia
ANA American Nurses Association
APC antigen-presenting cells
APN advanced practice nurse
APNG Advanced Practice Nurse in Genetics
ARBD Alcohol-Related Birth Defects
ARND Alcohol-Related Neurodevelopmental Disorder
ART assisted reproductive technology
AS Angelman syndrome
ASD autism spectrum disorder
ASTHO Association of State and Territorial Health Organizations
ATP adenosine triphosphate
BAP broader autism phenotype
BCDDP Breast Cancer Detection Demonstration Project
BCR B cell receptor
BDNF Brain-Derived Neutrotrophic Factor
BER base excision repair
BMI body mass index
BPA bisphenol-A
BPD Bipolar Disorder, subdivided as Type I and Type II
BRCA breast cancer susceptibility gene
BRCA1 breast cancer susceptibility gene 1
BRCA2 breast cancer susceptibility gene 2
BRCAPRO breast cancer professional modeling tool
CA-125 cancer antigen-125
CD cluster of differentiation or designation
CDC Centers for Disease Control and Prevention
CDKN2A cyclin-dependent kinase inhibitor 2A gene
CF cystic fibrosis
CGF Coalition for Genetic Fairness
C-H crown to heel (length)
CLOCK Circadian Locomotor Output Cycles Kaput
CMI cell-mediated immunity
CMV cytomegalovirus
CNS central nervous system
CNV copy number variant
COMT catechol-O-methyl transferase
COPD chronic obstructive pulmonary disease
CPM confined placental mosaicism
CRC colorectal cancer
CRY-1 Cryptochrome 1
CRY-2 Cryptochrome 2
CSC cancer stem cell
CTL cytotoxic T lymphocyte
CVD Cardiovascular disease
CVS chorionic villus sampling
DA ductus arteriosus
DALYs Disability adjusted life years
DES diethylstilbesterol
DLBCL diffuse large-B-cell lymphoma
DM diabetes mellitus
DMD Duchenne muscular dystrophy
DNA deoxyribonucleic acid
DOD Department of Defense
DOL Department of Labor
DSM IV-TR Diagnostic Statistical Manual, fourth edition, text revised
DV ductus venosus
DZ dizygotic
ECP eosinophil cationic protein
EDD estimated date of delivery
EDN eosinophil-derived neurotoxin
EEOC Equal Employment Opportunity Commission
EGFR epidermal growth factor receptor gene
EHDI Early Hearing Detection Intervention
ELSI Ethical Legal and Social Implications

EM	extensive metabolizer
EMR	electronic medical record
EPO	eosinophil peroxidase
ER	estrogen receptor
ERISA	Employee Retirement Income Security Act of 1974
FA	Fanconi's anemia
FAP	familial adenomatous polyposis
FAS	fetal alcohol syndrome
FASD	fetal alcohol spectrum disorder
FDA	Food and Drug Administration
FEHB	Federal Employees Health Benefits program
FISH	fluorescent in situ hybridization
FMLA	Family and Medical Leave Act of 1993
FMR1	Fragile X Mental Retardation-1 gene
FO	foramen ovale
FSH	follicle stimulating hormone
GABA	gamma amino butyric acid
GALT	gut-associated lymphoid tissue
GBD	*Global Burden of Disease* study
GCN	Genetics Clinical Nurse
GINA	Genetic Information Nondiscrimination Act
GnRH	gonadotropins releasing hormone
GPCR	G protein–coupled receptors
GSK-3	glycogen synthase kinase-3
GWA	genome-wide association
GWAS	genome-wide association [research] study
hCG	human chorionic gonadotropin
HD	Huntington disease
HER2	another name for the ERBB2 gene
HEV	high endothelial venules
***HGD* gene**	Homogentisate 1,2 dioxygenase
HGP	Human Genome Project
HHS	Department of Health and Human Services
HIPAA	Health Insurance Portability and Accountability Act of 1996
HIV	Human Immunodeficiency Virus
HLA	human leukocyte antigen
hPL	human placental lactogen
HRSA	Health Resources and Services Administration
HSV	herpes simplex virus
ICGC	International Cancer Genome Consortium
IELs	intraepithelial lymphocytes
IFN	interferon
Ig	immunoglobulin
IgA	immunoglobulin A
IgE	immunoglobulin E
IgG	immunoglobulin G
IgM	immunoglobulin M
IHC	immunohistochemistry
IHS	Indian Health Service
IL	interleukin
IM	intermediate metabolism
IMP	integral membrane protein
INH-A	inhibin-A
INR	international normalized ratio
IP	Incontinenta Pigmenti
ISONG	The International Society of Nurses in Genetics
IUGR	intrauterine growth restriction
IVF	in-vitro fertilization
JCIH	Joint Committee on Infant Hearing
KAL	killer-activating ligand
KAR	killer-activating receptor
KIR	killer-inhibiting receptor
L/S	lecithin–sphingomyelin ratio
LAK	lymphokine-activated killer cell
LBW	low birth weight
LD	linkage disequilibrium
LGL	large granular lymphocyte
LH	lutenizing hormone
LMP	last monthly period
MAC	membrane attack complex
MAO	monoamine oxidase
MAOI	monoamine oxidase inhibitors
MBL	mannose-binding lectin
MBP	major basic protein
MCHB	Maternal Child Health Bureau
MDD	Major Depressive Disorder
MECP2	methyl cytosine binding protein 2
MHC	major histocompatibility complex
MLH1	mutL homolog 1 gene
MMR	mismatch repair
MOD	March of Dimes Foundation
MoM	multiples of the median
mRNA	messenger ribonucleic acid
MS/MS	mass spectrometry
MSAFP	maternal serum alpha fetoprotein
MSH2	MutS homolog 2 gene
MSH6	MutS homolog 6 (E. coli) gene
MSI	microsatellite instability
mtDNA	mitochondrial DNA
MZ	monozygotic
NADP	nicotinamide adenine dinucleotide phosphate
NBSC	Newborn Screening Clearinghouse
NCCN	National Comprehensive Cancer Network
NCHAM	National Center for Hearing Assessment and Management
NCHPEG	National Coalition for Health Professional Education in Genetics
NCI	National Cancer Institute

NCSL National Conference of State Legislatures
NDRI norepinephrine dopamine reuptake inhibitor
NEMO Nuclear Factor-kappa β essential modulator gene
NER nucleotide excision repair
NHGRI National Human Genome Research Institute
NICHD National Institutes of Child Health and Human Development
NIDCD National Institutes on Deafness and Other Communication Disorders
NIH National Institutes of Health
NIMH National Institute for Mental Health
NKC natural killer cells
OAE Otoacoustic Emissions
OI osteogenesis imperfecta
OMIM Online Mendelian Inheritance in Man
OTC over the counter
PAMPS Pathogen-associated molecular patterns.
PANDA Prospective Assessment in Newborns for Diabetes Autoimmunity
PARP poly ADP ribose polymerase
PCH public and/or community health
PDD-NOS pervasive developmental disability not otherwise specified
PDF portable document format
PGx pharmacogenetics
PKU phenylketonuria
PM poor metabolizer
PMN polymorphonuclear leukocytes
PMS2 postmeiotic segregation increased 2 gene
PNI psychoneuroimmunology
PROM premature rupture of membranes
PRR pattern recognition receptors
PSA prostate-specific antigen
PTB preterm birth
PTEN phosphatase and tensin homolog gene
PWS Prader-Willi syndrome
RB1 retinoblastoma 1 gene
RFLPs restriction fragment length polymorphisms
RNA ribonucleic acid
RPL recurrent pregnancy loss
RSS Really Simple Syndication
SABO spontaneous abortion
SACGHS Secretary's Advisory Committee on Genetics, Health, and Society
SACHDNC Secretary's Advisory Committee on Heritable Disorders in Newborns and Children
SCD sickle cell disease
SEER Surveillance, Epidemiology, and End Results
SES socioeconomic status
SGA small-of-gestational age
SIDS sudden infant death syndrome
SNPs single nucleotide polymorphism
SNRI serotonin norepinephrine reuptake inhibitor
SSRI selective serotonin reuptake inhibitors
STI sexually transmitted infection
T2DM Type 2 diabetes mellitus
Tc cytotoxic T cells
TCGA The Cancer Genome Atlas
TCR T cell receptor
TEDDY The Environmental Determinants of Diabetes in the Young
Th helper T cells
TLR toll-like receptors
TNF tumor necrosis factor
TP53 tumor protein 53 gene
TPMT thiopurine S-methyltransferase
T_{reg} T regulatory cells
tRNA transfer ribonucleic acid
UPD uniparental disomy
USPSTF U.S. Preventive Services Task Force
VEGF vascular endothelial growth factor gene
VKOR vitamin K epoxide reductase complex subunit 1
WBC white blood cells
WHO World Health Organization
YLDs years of life lived with disability

Glossary

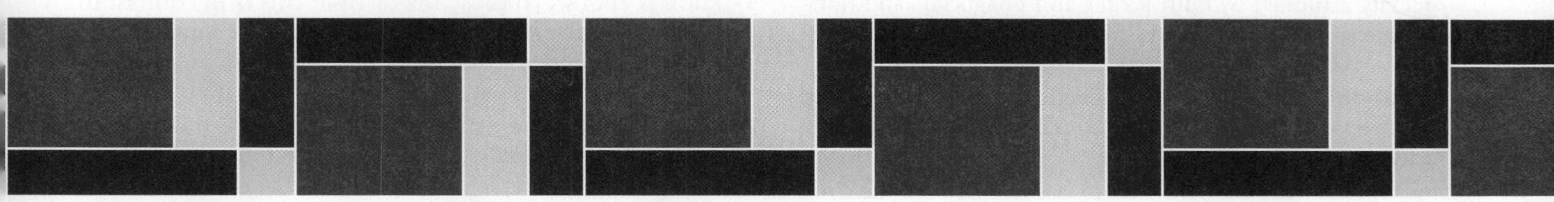

Achondroplasia An autosomal dominant genetic condition that results in dwarfism.

Acrosomal reaction A breakdown of certain enzymes that degrade the outer layer of the ovum (corona radiate) to allow penetration of the sperm into the ovum.

Acrosome A cap-like structure over the anterior half of the head in sperm that produces enzymes necessary for preparation of fertilization.

Active immunity The form of immunity produced by the body in response to stimulation by a disease-causing organism (naturally acquired active immunity) or by a vaccine (artificially acquired active immunity).

Adaptive immunity The augmentation of body defense mechanisms in response to a specific stimulus, which can cause the elimination of microorganism and recovery from disease. Typically, it leaves the host with specific memory (acquired resistance) that enables the body to effectively respond should infection reoccur. It is organized around T and B lymphocytes.

Advanced maternal age Is considered in any woman who is age 35 at the time of delivery.

Adverse drug reaction A dose-related, unintended, noxious response to a medicine. This is a subset of adverse drug events.

Affinity maturation A phase of B cell development in which the cell undergoes somatic hypermutation so that some cells are formed that can achieve high-affinity binding to peptides from a pathogen.

Allele The alternative form or versions of a gene. It is one member of a pair (or any of the series) of genes occupying a specific spot on a chromosome (called locus) that controls the same trait. Originally used to describe variations among genes, it is now also used to refer to variations among noncoding DNA sequences.

Allergen Any substance that causes an allergy.

Allogeneic When placental/umbilical cord blood, referred to as *cord hematopoietic stem/progenitor cells, cord (HPC-C)*, is stored for intended use in recipients unrelated to the donor.

Alpha-fetoprotein A glycoprotein that is produced in the yolk sac in early pregnancy and later by the fetal liver.

Alzheimer's disease A common, age-related, neurodegenerative disorder, representing the most common cause of irreversible dementia.

Amniocentesis A procedure in which a needle is inserted into the amniotic sac to withdraw a small amount of fluid that is used to test for chromosomal abnormalities and other problems and that is later used to test for lung maturity in the fetus. The procedure also may be used to test for fetal lung maturity.

Amnionic membrane A thin, transparent pair of protective membranes that surrounds the fetus and the amniotic fluid.

Amplification A selective increase in the number of copies of a gene coding for a specific protein without a proportional increase in other genes.

Ampulla The outer one-third of the fallopian tube where fertilization usually takes place.

Anaphase lag An error that can occur during cell division where one chromosome fails to get incorporated into the nucleus of a daughter cell.

Anaphase The stage of mitosis where the chromosomes begin to separate.

Anaphylactic shock An often severe and sometimes fatal systemic reaction in a susceptible individual upon a second exposure to a specific antigen after previous sensitization that is characterized especially by respiratory symptoms, fainting, itching, and hives.

Anaphylotoxins The complement components, C3a and C5a, that stimulate release by mast cells of their vasoactive amines.

Aneuploid The presence of an incorrect number of chromosomes.

Aneuploidy The process through which chromosomes are added or subtracted.

Angelman syndrome A genetic disorder that affects the neurologic system and that is caused by deletion of chromosome 15 on the maternal chromosome during meiosis. It is characterized by developmental delays, seizures, speech problems, sleep disturbances, and balance problems (puppet gait).

Angiogenesis The process responsible for the formation of new blood vessels from preexisting blood vessels. It is generally considered an essential process to ensure the supply of nutrients and oxygen to rapidly growing tumors as well as to provide a route for tumor cell metastasis. One important stimulator of angiogenesis is vascular endothelial growth factor (*VEGF*).

Antibody A molecule (also called an immunoglobulin) produced by a mature B cell (plasma cell) in response to an antigen. When an antibody attaches to an antigen, it helps the body destroy or inactivate the antigen.

Antibody-dependent cellular cytotoxicity A cellular activity exhibited by both K cells and phagocytic and nonphagocytic myelogenous-type leukocytes. The target cell in ADCC is coated with a low concentration of IgG antibody.

Anticipation This is when a genetic condition becomes more severe and presents earlier in offspring than in their parents.

Antigen presentation The activity associated with the conveying of an altered antigenic molecule to T and B cells by macrophages, which is necessary for most adaptive responses.

Antigen-presenting cells A functionally defined cell capable of taking up antigens and presenting them to lymphocytes in a recognizable form.

Antigens Substances or molecules that are recognized by the immune system. The antigen can be from foreign material such as bacteria or viruses.

Apoptosis Used to indicate a form of cell death associated with normal physiology, distinct from necrosis, which is associated with acute injury to cells.

Asperger syndrome A neurodevelopmental disorder on the autism spectrum that can affect an individual's behavior, communication, and social interaction.

Ataxia telangiectasia A rare, autosomal recessive disorder that progressively damages the brain and causes motor skill development problems. It is a neurodegenerative disease that eventually leads to death.

Attributes The characteristics of a person that provide information about disease risk.

Audiologic evaluation A screen for hearing loss by Auditory Brainstem Response (ABR) and Otoacoustic Emissions (OAE) testing.

Auditory brainstem response A neurologic test of auditory brainstem function in response to auditory (click) stimuli.

Autism A developmental disorder, usually diagnosed in early childhood, characterized by social and communication impairment and stereotyped or repetitive behaviors.

Autism spectrum disorders The range of pervasive developmental disorders that usually involve impairments in communication and socialization.

Autoimmune diseases Diseases that result when the immune system mistakenly attacks the body's own tissues. Examples include multiple sclerosis, Type 1 diabetes, rheumatoid arthritis, and systemic lupus erythematous.

Autologous When cord hematopoietic stem/progenitor cells are used in a first- or second-degree blood relative.

Autonomy Capacity for self-determination or right to determine what will happen to a person's own body.

Autosomal Chromosomes that are not responsible for the determination of the sex of an individual.

Autosomal dominant Autosomal dominance is a pattern of inheritance characteristic of some genetic diseases. "Autosomal" means that the gene in question is located on one of the numbered, or non-sex, chromosomes. "Dominant" means that a single copy of the disease-associated mutation is enough to cause the disease. This is in contrast to a recessive disorder, where two copies of the mutation are needed to cause the disease. Huntington's disease is a common example of an autosomal dominant genetic disorder.

autosomal recessive An autosomal recessive trait, means that an affected individual inherits two mutated copies of the gene, for example in Cystic Fibrosis or sick cell disease.

Autosomes Chromosomes that are not associated with the development of sex characteristics.

B cell or B lymphocyte A small, white blood cell crucial to the immune defenses. B cells come from bone marrow and develop into blood cells called plasma cells, which are the source of antibodies.

Bandemia An excess of band cells (immature white blood cells); signifies an infection or inflammation.

Barr body The inactivated X chromosome in a female somatic cell that appears as a densely stained mass in the nuclei of those cells.

Basophils White blood cells that contribute to inflammatory reactions. Along with mast cells, basophils are responsible for the symptoms of allergy.

Beneficence To do good or make sure people benefit from the most good.

Biomarker A biologic molecule found in blood, other body fluids, or tissues that is a sign of a normal or abnormal process or of a condition or disease. A biomarker may be used to see how well the body responds to treatment for a disease or condition. Also called molecular marker and signature molecule.

Bipolar I Disorder Characterized by one or more Manic or Mixed Episodes, usually accompanied by Major Depressive Episodes.

Bipolar II Disorder Characterized by one or more Major Depressive Episodes accompanied by at least one Hypomanic Episode.

Blastocyst A very early stage of embryonic development. About 4–5 days after conception, the embryo consists of a circle of cells with fluid in the center and a clump of cells at one end with a thinner layer of cells at the other end.

Blastomeres Cells produced during cleavage of a fertilized ovum during development of the embryo.

Block to polyspermy The process where the zona pellucid undergoes chemical changes to prevent other sperm from entering the ovum once it has been fertilized.

Blood banks Places where blood products are collected, typed, separated, stored, and prepared for transfusion to recipients.

Broader autism phenotype A larger cross section of people with impairments in social or communication skills that do not meet the criteria for diagnosis with autism.

C-activation Alteration of C proteins, enabling them to interact with another component.

Cancer genome The entire set of unique DNA that makes up a specific cancer.

Cancer stem cells Exist within a tumor and possess the capacity to self-renew and generate the heterogeneous lines of cancer cells that comprise a tumor.

Capacitation The deterioration of the acrosomal layer of the sperm head in order to remove an enzyme so that the sperm will be able to penetrate the ovum.

Capacity Ability to make a decision for oneself and to communicate this decision.

Carcinogenesis The molecular process by which cancer develops.

Carrier An individual who transmits a characteristic, a gene, or disease, yet who may not show any signs of the characteristic, gene, or disease.

Cathepsin Any of several intracellular proteases of animal tissue that aid in autolysis in some diseased conditions and after death.

Cell cycle Consists of interphase, mitosis, and cytokinesis.

Cell-mediated immunity The type of immunity dependent on the link between T cells and macrophages.

Centromeres The region of the chromosome where microtubule fibers attach during cell division.

Chemokines Small protein molecules that activate immune cells, stimulate their migration, and help direct immune cell traffic throughout the body.

Chemotaxis The phenomenon in which somatic cells, bacteria, and other single-cell or multicellular organisms direct their movements according to certain chemicals in their environment.

Chorion The outermost of the two fetal membranes, which together surround the fetus. The chorion forms the fetal part of the placenta.

Chorionic villi Tiny vascular hairs of the chorion that embed into the endometrium and help form the placenta.

Chorionic villus sampling Involves the removal of tissue from the chorionic sac and is performed during the first trimester.

Chromatids Strands of a duplicated chromosome.

Chromatin A complex of nucleic acids (DNA or RNA) and proteins that make up chromosomes; located in the cell nucleus.

Chromosomes Threadlike packages of genes and other DNA in the nucleus of a cell.

Chronic sorrow Unresolved grief usually related to having a family member with a life-threatening or chronic illness. The family member may or may not have died.

Circadian rhythm An approximately 24 to 26-hour long cyclical pattern of physiological changes in biochemical and hormonal processes that influence behavior. This rhythm is influenced by a group of cells located in the hypothalamus.

Class switching Change in isotope of antibody produced after a B lymphocyte has encountered an antigen.

Cleavage The process of rapid mitotic division of the zygote producing blastomeres and forming the mass of cells called the morula.

Clonal anergy The process of switching off the ability of potentially harmful T or B cells to participate in immune responses. Clonal anergy is essential for generating the tolerance of T and B cells to the body's "self" tissue antigens.

Clonal deletion The genetically controlled process of eliminating immune cells that could destroy the body's own cells and tissues. The elimination process removes immature T and B lymphocytes that have receptors for cells with "self" Major Histocompatibility Complex (MHC) or Human Leukocyte Antigen (HLA) antigens, and could therefore attack and destroy the body's own cells.

Clonal expansion An enhanced ability to function quickly and effectively as with activated Cytotoxic T lymphocytes (CTLs).

Clonal selection Activation and proliferation of a lymphocyte when an individual lymphocyte encounters an antigen that binds to its unique antigen receptor site.

Cluster of differentiation (cluster of designation) Molecule markers on the cell surface, as recognized by specific sets of antibodies, used to identify the cell type, stage of differentiation, and activity of a cell.

Codon A trinucleotide sequence of DNA or RNA that corresponds to a specific amino acid.

Cognitive Impairment The deficit from what is considered normal thinking ability.

Competent Possession of required skill, knowledge, qualification, or capacity.

Complement A complex series of blood proteins whose action complements the work of antibodies. Complement destroys bacteria, produces inflammation, and regulates immune reactions.

Congenital renal agenesis The absence of one or both kidneys, a condition occurring before birth.

Conjoined twins Identical twins whose bodies failed to separate in early pregnancy.

Consanguinity Descended from the same blood-relative or common ancestor.

Consultand The person who presents for genetic counseling and has requested that a pedigree be created.

Convertase Altered C protein that acts as a proteolytic enzyme for another C component.

Core behavioral characteristics The essential personality attributes and behavioral characteristics.

Core competencies The main strength(s) or strategic asset(s) of an organization or institution.

Core conditions A set of genetically transmittable conditions recommended for uniform screening by the newborn screening programs in every state.

Core functions and health care services 1) Assessment of health and health behaviors including genetics and genomics; 2) development of policies and practices to inform, treat, educate, and empower consumers regarding genetics/genomics; and 3) assurance—i.e., the appropriate integration of genetics and genomics into health care services and strategies for improved public health.

Corona radiata The outer layer of the zona pellucida made up of elongated follicular strata that supply protein to the ovum.

Corpus luteum Develops from a ruptured ovarian follicle and secretes progesterone, a steroid hormone that is essential for establishing and maintaining a pregnancy. If fertilization does not occur, it atrophies into a mass of scar tissue known as corpus albicans.

Co-stimulators The two signals needed by the adaptive immune system to provide a response. The first signal is antigen specific and the second signal is antigen nonspecific.

Cotyledons The separations of the maternal side of the placenta, separated by placental septa, containing villi and fetal vessels and is surrounded by maternal blood.

Cri du chat syndrome A rare congenital disorder characterized by a kitten-like cry.

Critical period The period during the first 8 weeks of embryonic development when the structures are vulnerable to anomalies or birth defects caused by exposure to teratogens.

Crossing over The natural process of breaking and rejoining DNA strands to produce new combinations of genes and, thus, generate genetic variation.

Culture A set of shared attitudes, values, goals, beliefs, and behaviors that are characteristic of a particular social or ethnic group.

Cyclothymia or Cyclothymic disorder A mild form of bipolar disorder in which the degree of mania is less intense than seen with bipolar disorder even while the condition is of longer duration. Characterized by at least 2 years of numerous periods of hypomanic symptoms that do not meet criteria for a Manic Episode and numerous periods of depressive symptoms that do not meet criteria for a Major Depressive Episode.

Cystic fibrosis An autosomal recessive genetic disease characterized by thickened secretions in the respiratory tract and sweat glands. It results in bulky, foul-smelling stool and thickened respiratory secretions contributing to infections and respiratory difficulties. While individuals with CF are living longer than ever, death often occurs in the third decade of life.

Cytochrome p450 enzymes Phase I enzymes in the liver that make small modifications to the chemical structure of drugs. These enzymes are sensitive to physiological changes and are commonly implicated in drug–drug and drug–diet interactions.

Cytokinesis The cleavage furrow of the cell forms and deepens and the cytoplasm divides yielding two daughter cells.

Cytokines Powerful chemical substances secreted by cells that enable the body's cells to communicate with one another. Cytokines include lymphokines produced by lymphocytes and monokines produced by monocytes and macrophages.

Cytotoxic T lymphocyte A subtype of T cells that carries the CD8 marker and can destroy body cells infected by viruses or transformed by cancer.

Cytotrophoblast The inner layer of the trophoblast; also known as the layer of Langhans.

Daughter cell A cell resulting from cell division during mitosis and meiosis.

De Novo mutations Spontaneous, new changes in genes or chromosomes.

Decidua basalis The part of the decidua that connects with the chorion that becomes the maternal side of the placenta.

Decidua capsularis The part of the decidua that covers the blastocyst.

Decidua The lining of the uterus (endometrium) during pregnancy that is shed after giving birth.

Decidua vera The part of the decidua that lines the uterine cavity excluding the placenta.

Deformation An alteration in form or shape resulting from mechanical forces in otherwise healthy tissue.

Degenerative Marked by gradual deterioration of organs and cells along with loss of function.

Deletion A type of mutation involving the loss of genetic material.

Dementia A decline in cognitive ability from a previously attained level to such an extent that it interferes with one's social or occupational roles.

Dendritic cells Immune cells with highly branched extensions that occur in lymphoid tissues, engulf microbes, and stimulate T cells by displaying the foreign antigens of the microbes on their surfaces.

Deoxyribonucleic acid (DNA) The hereditary material in humans that contains the genetic instructions used in the development and functioning of all known living organisms.

Depression A common state of negative mood that does not meet diagnostic criteria for a disorder.

Determinants of health Factors that affect the health of individuals, families, and communities.

Developmental delays Identified in a child who is not meeting developmental milestones at the expected times.

Developmental disability A birth defect that can lead to a problem with neurologic, sensory, or metabolic functioning.

Developmental pediatrician A physician with specialized training to evaluate and treat children with developmental or behavioral difficulties.

Diagnostic criteria The set of symptoms that is used as a guideline for making a diagnosis.

Diagnostic testing A method of examination that can lead to uncovering the cause of a genetic problem or disease state. It is the step that is done after a positive screening test indicates there is a problem.

Diamniotic A set of twins in utero having their own amniotic sac.

Diapedesis Movement through a vessel wall.

Dichorionic A set of twins having separate chorions.

Diploid A cell or organism that has paired chromosomes, one from each parent.

Disruption An interruption of a normal developmental process.

Diversity Differences that distinguish individuals and/or groups from one another.

Dizygotic Fraternal twins originating from two zygotes.

Domain Basic unit of an antibody structure. Variations between the domains of different antibody molecules are responsible for differences in antigen binding and in biologic function.

Dominant Refers to genes that require only one copy in order for a trait or disease to present.

Down syndrome (or trisomy 21) A genetic condition that presents with three copies of the 21st chromosomes when there are normally two.

Duchenne muscular dystrophy A recessive X-linked condition that results in muscle degeneration and ultimately leads to death, usually during the second decade of life. A male child can inherit it from a female carrier, or a daughter can also inherit it from an affected father and a carrier mother or an affected father and an affected mother—although the latter two types of inheritance are not common.

Ductus arteriosus A vascular channel between the pulmonary artery and the descending aorta in the fetal circulation. It becomes a ligament after birth.

Ductus venosus A vascular channel that passes through the liver and joins the umbilical vein with the inferior vena cava in fetal circulation. It closes shortly after birth.

Duplication When part of a chromosome is present twice.

Dysplasia The abnormal growth or development of a structure, e.g., in cells, tissues or organs.

Dysthymia A chronic period of depression that has lasts for a least 1 year. The degree of negative mood found in dysthymia is often less intense than that seen with Major Depression.

Dysthymic disorder Characterized by at least 2 years of depressed mood for more days than not, accompanied by additional depressive symptoms that do not meet the criteria for Major Depressive Episode.

Ectoderm The outer primary germ layer of the early embryo that gives rise to the skin, hair, and nails, central and peripheral nervous system, sensory epithelia of the eye, ear, and nose, and certain glands.

Effector cells Active cells of the immune system that are responsible for destroying or controlling foreign antigens.

Efficacy The capacity of an intervention, medication, or technology to produce a desired effect; it embodies the potential maximum therapeutic response that the intervention or medication (or technology) can elicit.

Elastase An enzyme that digests elastin.

Embryo The time of development in humans that begins with implantation of the fertilized ovum and continues until the end of the eighth week of pregnancy.

Endoderm One of three primary germ layers of the embryo that gives rise to epithelial lining of multiple systems and parts of the liver and pancreas.

Endometrium The lining of the uterus that undergoes monthly shedding and regeneration as a part of the menstrual cycle.

Endoplasmic reticulum A network of membranes inside a cell through which proteins and other molecules move.

Environmental perturbations Environmental factors or agents that can alter the functioning of biologic systems in response not only to the individual characteristics of the factor or agent, but also to the timing, magnitude, frequency and duration of the exposure.

Eosinophils White blood cells containing granules filled with chemicals damaging to parasites and enzymes that affect inflammatory reactions.

Epidemiology The study of the distribution, frequency, and determinants of health-related events and states, and the control and/or prevention of health-related problems.

Epigenetic The study of changes produced in gene expression and the factors that influence them. The development and maintenance of an organism is orchestrated by a set of chemical reactions that switch parts of the genome off and on at strategic times and locations throughout the lifespan.

Epigenome The total epigenetic state of a cell to include a chemical responsible for the activation of a particular gene.

Epilepsy A brain disorder in which clusters of nerve cells, or neurons, in the brain sometimes signal abnormally. The normal pattern of neuronal activity becomes disturbed, causing strange sensations, emotions and behaviors, convulsions, muscle spasms, and loss of consciousness.

Epitopes Also known as antigenic determinant, the parts of an antigen that is recognized by the immune system, specifically by antibodies, B cells, or T cells.

Estimated date of delivery The expected estimated birth date of a baby based on 40 weeks gestation; calculated from the mother's last menstrual period.

Ethics The branch philosophy of that deals with values that pertain to human conduct. It is the examination of moral reasoning about what is right or wrong with regards to personnel and societal actions.

Ethnicity A group of people who identify with each other, often through a common heritage or language and shared cultural traditions such as religion.

Eugenics The proposed improvement of the human species by encouraging or permitting reproduction of only those people with genetic characteristics that are judged desirable.

Eukaryote cells Cells that contain a nucleus and membrane-bound organelles in which specific metabolic activities take place.

Euploid The normal number of chromosomes for a species.

Expansion An increase in the number of nucleotide triplet repeat sequences in a variety of disorders due to unstable mutations.

Expressivity A variation in the severity of a phenotype clinical manifestations of a particular gene or genetic mutation.

Extensive metabolizers Person with two functional alleles at a gene locus, or a functional allele and an allele with reduced function, resulting in a fully functioning enzyme.

Extremely high risk Individuals with a higher chance of developing a disease who are likely to have a genetic component to the risk profile. They will have more than one red flag in their family history and lifestyle/environment.

Factor V Leiden A genetic disorder affecting the factor V that is necessary in blood coagulation. In this instance, there is a hypercoagulability and may lead to clot formation.

False negatives Screening test results that indicate that an individual is disease free or has no genetic problem when in fact he or she does.

False positives Screening test results that indicate that an individual has a disease or genetic problem when in fact he or she does not.

Family (family unit) The members of a social group that may or may not be together; or members of a unit that are considered by that unit to be related and provide caregiving, nurturing, and development to the children or other family members of the unit. Extended family and children who no longer live at home may also be considered part of this family unit. The definition is shaped by cultural values, beliefs, and traditions. For the purposes of a pedigree, a family is referred to as members united by ties of marriage, blood, or adoption.

Family context Consideration of the family unit's cultural beliefs, values, or traditions when caring for any family member.

Family functioning The ability of the persons who make up a family unit to perform expected (or perceived) tasks and roles in that social group.

Family history The taking of information about an individual's relatives for at least three generations in order to determine genetic risks.

Fanconi's anemia An autosomal recessive genetic condition due to a defect or mutation of the DNA that affects the bone marrow, more specifically the blood forming cells, resulting in less cells than normal. The person with Fanconi's may have pancytopenia or rather anemia, neutropenia, and thrombopenia. The skin will have a brown tint. Other anomalies can be present if the person suffers from Fanconi's syndrome (a constellation of anomalies accompanying the anemia). These may include congenital heart disease, genitourinary anomalies, bone deformities, and microcephaly. The lifespan may be reduced to 30 years of age. DNA or gene therapy/repair may be advised.

Fc receptors The portion of an antibody responsible for binding to antibody receptors on cells and a particular component of complement.

Fertilization The fusion of an ovum and sperm (gametes) that lead to the creation of an embryo.

Fetal nuchal translucency An ultrasonic measurement of the fluid located under the skin in the fetal neck region that is done between 11 and 14 weeks of pregnancy to help screen for the presence of a potential genetic problem. Generally, a thickness of this fluid in this region indicates genetic abnormality. This is only a screening test and must be done in conjunction with other screening tests.

Fetus The human being during growth and development starting after the embryonic period and continuing until birth.

Fidelity Stands for the proposition that the health care provider keeps the patients interest first in mind above all others.

Filter paper The primary tool used by the newborn screening program and health care providers for collecting the blood samples obtained from infants following birth.

Fimbria The fringe-like outer third section of the fallopian tube.

First-degree relatives Relatives who share half (50%) of one's genome with an individual; mother, father, brothers, sisters, and children (offspring).

Follicle stimulating hormone A hormone secreted by the anterior pituitary during the follicular phase or first half of the menstrual cycle that stimulates the maturation of the dominant or graafian follicle.

Follicular phase The first phase of the ovarian cycle that includes days 1–4 of a 28-day cycle. During this phase, the maturation of a follicle occurs and the endometrium prepares for implantation of a fertilized ovum.

Foramen ovale An opening between the atria of the fetal heart. It provides a bypass for fetal blood that will later go to the fetal lungs. It closes after birth when the infant takes his first breath and circulation to the lungs begins.

Gametes Cell that joins with another during the process of fertilization.

Gastrulation The process in early embryonic development when the two-layered embryonic disc is reorganized into 3 layers: the endoderm, ectoderm, and mesoderm.

Genes Segments of DNA that contain instructions for the formation of proteins.

Genetics The study of individual genes.

Genetic clinical nurse A designation for a baccalaureate-prepared nurse who has successfully completed a professional portfolio review process in genetic nursing.

Genetic code The order of the nucleotide sequences in DNA or RNA that form the basis of heredity through their role in protein synthesis.

Genetic counseling A communication process that helps individuals, families, and communities understand and adapt to the biological, medical, psychological, financial, ethical, legal, and social implications of the genetic contributions to disease.

Genetic determinism The belief that all human traits are caused solely by genetics.

Genetic discrimination Discrimination, usually by employers or insurance companies, on the basis of a genetic disorder or increased risk of a genetic disorder.

Genetic disorders Diseases caused by an abnormality in an individual's DNA that can be transmitted from the parent to their offspring.

Genetic information Includes information about an individual's genetic tests and the genetic tests of an individual's family members, as well as information about the manifestation of a disease or disorder in an individual's family members (i.e., family medical history).

Genetic locus (pl. loci) The specific physical location of a gene or other DNA sequence on a chromosome.

Genetic monitoring Examination of employees' genetic information to evaluate modifications of their genetic material that might have evolved in the course of employment.

Genetic screening The analysis of a population to determine which individuals are at risk for a genetic disease or for transmitting one.

Genetic susceptibility A predisposition to disease at the genetic level that may be activated under certain conditions.

Genetic testing The analysis of genetic material to determine the presence or absence of specific genetic conditions.

Genetic variation The variation seen as a result of genetic mutation(s) in the genomes of individuals in a species or between different species.

Genetic/genomic bio-banking The collection and storage of biologic materials for research and for other purposes including but not limited to diagnosis, treatment, prognosis of genetic/genomic diseases, and other health-related issues.

Genetic/genomic health care The study of the functions and interactions of genes in the human genome and their interactions with environmental factors in sickness and in health, including the infrastructure necessary to provide genetic/genomic health care, the information and skills required by health care providers and consumers to appropriately offer or act on genetic/genomic information, and the equitable allocation of genetic/genomic services within health care systems.

Genogram An older term for a pedigree. It is a diagram of family relationships and medical history.

Genome The complete biologic makeup of living organisms.

Genome-wide association [research] study The analysis of most or all of the genetic markers in the genomes of different individuals in a particular species or between species to see how much genetic variation exists; to understand how the variation could contribute to different traits (including diseases); to develop strategies that can be used to detect, treat, and prevent diseases; and also to determine prognoses and recurrence risks.

Genomics The study of all genes in an organism, including interactions among genes and interactions between genes and the environment.

Genomic health care Individual or family health care based on the full complement of genetic material, interactions among genes, and interactions between genes and the environment.

Genotype An individual's genetic composition at the gene level.

Germ line mutations Arise in the germ cells that produce sperm and oocytes. They are heritable and passed vertically from generation to generation.

Gonadotropin releasing hormone A hormone secreted by the hypothalamus to stimulate the anterior pituitary to secrete the gonadotropins follicle stimulating hormone (FSH) and luteinizing hormone (LH); GnRH is necessary for successful reproduction.

Graafian follicle A mature ovarian follicle that contains a ripe ovum and ruptures during ovulation to release the ovum; it becomes the corpus luteum after ovulation.

Graft rejection An immune response against transplanted tissue.

Granules Membrane-bound organelles (specialized parts) within cells where proteins are stored before secretion.

Granulocytes Phagocytic white blood cells filled with granules. Neutrophils, eosinophils, basophils, and mast cells are examples of granulocytes.

Haploid A cell or organism that has a single set of chromosomes.

Haplotypes Sets of closely linked genes or DNA polymorphisms inherited as a unit.

Health A state of complete physical, mental, and social well-being, and not merely the absence of disease or infirmity (WHO, 2011).

Health literacy Cultural and conceptual knowledge, listening and speaking skills (oral literacy), writing and reading skills (print literacy), and the ability to understand and work with numbers (numeracy), as they pertain to health and health care.

Helper T cells (Th cells) A subset of T cells that carry the CD4 surface marker that are essential for turning on antibody production, activating cytotoxic T cells, and initiating many other immune functions.

Hemoglobinopathies A term used for a number of disorders causing mutations in the genes for the globin that makes up hemoglobin, such as sickle cell disease and thalassemia.

Hemophilia A (or Factor VIII deficiency) The classic or most common form of hemophilia, an X-linked recessive condition that results in blood coagulation problems.

Heritability The proportion of phenotypic variation in a population that is due to genetic variation between individuals. Phenotypic variation among individuals may be due to genetic and/or environmental factors.

Heterozygous Having two different alleles at a genetic locus; both normal or one faulty or normal copy of the gene.

High endothelial venules Specialized postcapillary venous swellings characterized by simple cuboidal cells as opposed to the usual endothelial cells found in regular venules. HEVs enable lymphocytes circulating in the blood to directly enter a lymph node by crossing through the HEV.

High risk Applies to those individuals who have a red flag for family history and/or lifestyle/environment, but do not fit the criteria for genetic risk.

Homeobox or HOX gene A gene found in almost all animals that controls how and where parts of the body develop. They are active very early in life; they tell other genes when to become active and when to stop.

Homozygous Having two identical alleles at a genetic locus—both normal or both faulty.

Human chorionic gonadotropins A glycoprotein produced in pregnancy by the chorionic villi.

Human genome The entire complement of genes in a human.

Human leukocyte antigen A protein on the surfaces of human cells that identifies the cells as self and, like MHC antigens, performs essential roles in immune responses. HLAs are used in laboratory tests to determine whether one person's tissues are compatible with another person's, and could be used in a transplant. HLAs are the human equivalent of MHC antigens; they are coded for by MHC genes.

Human placental lactogen A placental hormone that functions as an insulin antagonist and breaks down fats to provide fuel for the growing fetus.

Humoral immunity A form of body defense against foreign substances represented by antibodies and other soluble, extracellular factors in the blood and lymphatic fluid.

Humoral Any fluid or semifluid in the body.

Huntington disease An autosomal dominant condition that results in progressive neurologic dysfunction. Its symptoms appear generally in the fourth decade of life.

Hydrocephalus An enlarged infantile head due to an accumulation of fluid in the brain. It is generally associated with other congenital conditions such as neural tube defects.

Hyperthymia A period of sustained mood elevation that does not impair functioning and does not reach diagnostic criteria for mania.

Hyperuricemia Defined as a serum monosodium urate (uric acid) level at or above 6.8 mg/Dl, 6.8 being the limit of urate solubility at physiologic temperature and pH.

Idiotypes The antigenic specificities defined by the unique sequences (idiotopes) of the antigen-combining site. Thus, anti-idiotype antibodies combine with those specific sequences, may block immunological reactions, and may resemble the epitope to which the first antibody reacts.

Immune response (Immunity) Reaction of the immune system to foreign substances. Although normal immune responses are designed to protect the body from pathogens, immune dysregulation can damage normal cells and tissues, as in the case of autoimmune diseases.

Immunogen A large organic molecule that is either a protein or a large polysaccharide and rarely, if ever, a lipid.

Immunoglobulins A family of large protein molecules, also known as antibodies, produced by mature B cells (plasma cells).

Imprinting Refers to when a gene or part of a chromosome is turned off, depending on from which parent it was inherited.

Induction The specialization of one group of cells during embryonic development that causes adjacent groups of cells to specialize.

Inflammation An immune system reaction to foreign invaders such as microbes or allergens. Signs include redness, swelling, pain, or heat.

Inflammatory response Redness, warmth, and swelling produced in response to infection; the result of increased blood flow and an influx of immune cells and their secretions.

Informed consent It is the process of receiving adequate information to make a decision (includes risk, benefit, and alternatives).

Innate immunity An immune system function that is inborn and provides an all-purpose defense against invasion by microbes.

Integral membrane protein A protein molecule (or assembly of proteins) that is permanently attached to the biologic membrane.

Integrins A family of cell adhesion molecules.

Intellectual disability Characterized by a significant limitation in intellectual functioning and adaptive behavior in social and everyday skills. Usually it is characterized by an intelligence quotient (IQ) of 70 or less.

Interconceptual education Education or content offered between pregnancies.

Interferons Proteins produced by cells that stimulate antivirus immune responses or alter the physical properties of immune cells.

Interleukins A major group of lymphokines and monokines.

Intermediate metabolizer Person with two alleles with reduced function, a functional and a nonfunctional allele, or a reduced function allele and a nonfunctional allele. These result in reduced enzyme activity.

International normalized ratio A laboratory test that measures the time it takes for blood to clot compared to an average. The longer it takes for the blood to clot the higher the INR. An INR is useful in monitoring the impact of anticoagulant (blood thinning) medications, like Warfarin (Coumadin).

Interphase The resting stage of the cell cycle, between cell division. This consists of three stages: G1 (gap 1), S (synthesis), and G2 (gap 2).

Intervillous space The space between the placental villi and decidua that contains maternal blood from which the fetus obtains nutrition.

Inversion Refers to a segment of the chromosome being reversed.

Ischemic phase The third phase of the menstrual cycle that takes place if fertilization does not occur. The corpus luteum begins to degenerate and the endometrium prepares for menses.

Isochromosomes Chromosomes with identical arms.

Justice The concept that prescribed actions are fair to those involved.

Karyotype An examination of the chromosomes for the purpose of counting the number and examining the type and structure present.

Key (legend) A diagram of symbols in a remote corner of a pedigree that defines what symbols are used in the pedigree.

Kinship (also Kin, Kindred) Refers to the entire family.

Kinin A small, biologically active peptide.

Lactoferrin A red iron-binding protein synthesized by neutrophils and glandular epithelial cells, found in many human secretions (as tears and milk), that retards bacterial and fungal growth.

Lacunae Hollow spaces that appear in the syncytiotrophoblast and fill with maternal blood to provide nutrition for the embryo.

Lanugo A fine downy hair that covers the fetus after 20 weeks gestation.

Leukocytes White blood cells that function in antigen recognition and antibody formation.

Leukotrienes Any of a group of eicosanoids that are generated in basophils, mast cells, macrophages, and human lung tissue by lipoxygenase-catalyzed oxygenation, especially of arachidonic acid, that participate in allergic responses (as bronchoconstriction in asthma).

Ligamentum venosum A ligament that forms to replace the ductus venosus.

Ligand A group, ion, or molecule coordinated to a central atom or molecule in a complex.

Ligases An enzyme that catalyzes the joining of two large molecules by forming a new chemical bond.

Linkage disequilibrium The nonrandom association of alleles at two or more loci, not necessarily on the same chromosome.

Locus The position of a gene or DNA marker on a chromosome.

Luteal phase The second phase of the menstrual cycle that include days 15–28 in a 28-day cycle. During this phase, ovulation occurs and a corpus luteum is formed.

Luteinizing hormone A hormone secreted by the anterior pituitary during the second phase of the ovarian cycle that triggers ovulation and development of the corpus luteum.

Lymph nodes Small, bean-shaped organs of the immune system, distributed widely throughout the body and linked by lymphatic vessels. Lymph nodes are garrisons of B and T cells, dendritic cells, macrophages, and other kinds of immune cells.

Lymph A transparent, slightly yellow fluid that carries lymphocytes, bathes the body tissues, and drains into the lymphatic vessels.

Lymphatic vessels A bodywide network of channels, similar to the blood vessels, which transports lymph to the immune organs and into the bloodstream.

Lymphocyte A small, white blood cell found in lymph nodes and the circulating blood that is essential to immune defenses. Two major populations of lymphocytes are recognized: T and B cells.

Lymphoid organs Organs of the immune system where lymphocytes develop and congregate. These organs include the bone marrow, thymus, lymph nodes, spleen, and various other clusters of lymphoid tissue. Blood vessels and lymphatic vessels are also lymphoid organs.

Lymphokine-activated killer cell A white blood cell that has been stimulated to kill tumor cells.

Lymphokines Powerful chemical substances secreted by lymphocytes. These molecules help direct and regulate the immune responses.

Macrophages Large and versatile immune cells that devour invading pathogens and other intruders. Macrophages stimulate other immune cells by presenting them with small pieces of the invaders.

Major depression A diagnostic term used to describe when feelings of sadness and negative affect have progressed to level at which social, occupational, or daily function is impaired.

Major depressive disorder Characterized by one or more Major Depressive Episodes (i.e., at least 2 weeks of depressed mood or loss of interest accompanied by at least four additional symptoms of depression).

Major histocompatibility complex A group of genes that controls several aspects of the immune response. MHC genes code for self markers on all body cells.

Malformation A structural defect of an organ or larger body region.

Mania A period of at least 1 week during which there is an abnormal and persistently elevated, expansive, or irritable mood.

Manifestation An indication of the existence, reality, or presence of a genetic condition.

Marker A DNA sequence with a known physical location on a chromosome.

Mass spectrometry The primary instrument used to analyze the blood samples obtained from infants following birth; it works by weighing molecules and sorting them for identification of specific disorders.

Mast cells Granulocytes found in tissue. The contents of mast cells, along with those of basophils, are responsible for the symptoms of allergy.

Megakaryocytes Bone marrow cells responsible for the production of blood thrombocytes (platelets).

Meiosis The process by which germ cells, eggs, and sperm are formed.

Membrane attack complex Typically formed on the surface of intruding pathogenic bacterial cells as a result of activation of the alternative pathway of the complement system. It is one of the effector proteins of the immune system.

Memory cells A subset of T cells and B cells that have been exposed to antigens and can then respond more readily when the immune system encounters those same antigens again.

Menarche The onset of menstrual bleeding, occurring during puberty, in a female human being.

Mendelian A term named after Dr. Gregor Mendel that refers to the laws regarding patterns of passing one characteristic from parent to child. The first law is segregation and the second independent assortment. Mendel also created the classification of dominant and recessive inheritance, the Mendelian inheritance patterns.

Menstrual phase The fourth phase of the menstrual cycle that takes place if fertilization did not occur. During this time estrogen and progesterone drop, the corpus luteum involutes, and the endometrium begins to shed.

Mesoderm One of three primary germ layers of the embryo that gives rise to connective tissue, bone, muscle, blood and lymph vessels, kidneys, genitals, and epithelial tissue.

Metaphase The stage of mitosis where the chromosomes line up on the midline of the dividing cell.

Microarray A process that allows thousands of pieces of DNA that are fixed to a glass slide to be analyzed at one time. It is used to identify the genes (pieces of DNA) in specific cells or tissue that are actively used to make RNA, which then may be used to make proteins.

Microsatellite instability Refers to small segments or sequences of DNA that vary in length, repeated in the human genome. When cellular mutations occur, DNA repair genes attempt to make repairs. A failure in the repair process has occurred when these sequences of DNA appear too long or short, resulting in an unstable condition.

Mitochondria Double membrane organelles located in the cytoplasm outside the nucleus of a cell. They provide energy for the cell converting oxygen and nutrients into adenosine triphosphate (ATP). Mitochondria have their own DNA, which is inherited from the mother.

Mitochondrial DNA The dioxyribosome nucleic acid present in the cell as a structure, mitochondria, or organelles. These structures are responsible for taking food and converting it to energy for cellular life and function.

Mitosis The actual process of chromosomal division, consisting of four fluid phases: prophase, metaphase, anaphase, and telophase.

Mittelschmerz One-sided, lower abdominal pain that occurs during ovulation.

Monoamniotic A set of twins who share the same amnion.

Monochorionic A set of twins who share the same chorion and placenta, although they usually have their own amniotic sac.

Monocytes Large, phagocytic, white blood cells that, when entering tissue, develop into a macrophage.

Monokines Powerful chemical substances secreted by monocytes and macrophages. These molecules help direct and regulate the immune responses.

Monosodium urate A salt of uric acid that is capable of precipitating out in a crystalline form in skin and other tissues as tophi in gout.

Monosomy The loss of a single chromosome.

Monozygotic Identical twins originating from one zygote.

Morbidity A diseased state.

Mortality A fatal outcome.

Morula An embryo as a solid mass of cells at an early stage of development.

Mosaic An organism or part made up of tissues or cells exhibiting mosaicism.

Mosaicism A condition in which an individual can have two different cell population phenotypes.

Multifactorial inheritance Congenital anomalies that are caused by a combination of genetic and environmental factors.

Mutagen Something that can induce a genetic mutation or can increase the rate of mutation—e.g., certain substances, viruses, X-rays, and wave lengths of ultraviolet irradiation.

Mutation Rare changes in DNA sequence that usually have either no effect or cause a deleterious effect on protein function.

Myeloperoxidase A green peroxidase of phagocytic cells (as neutrophils and monocytes) that assists in bactericidal activity by catalyzing the oxidation of ionic halogen to free halogen.

Myotonic dystrophy Part of a group of inherited disorders called muscular dystrophies.

Nägele's rule A method of calculating the expected date of birth. From the first day of the last monthly period, add 7 days and subtract 3 months.

Natural killer cell A large, granule-containing lymphocyte that recognizes and kills cells lacking self-antigens. These cells' target recognition molecules are different from T cells.

Nature versus nurture Refers to the relative importance of the sum of genetic factors (nature) versus the sum of environmental factors (nurture) in the development and/or functioning of living things and, most often, in the causation of human behavior; i.e., a diathesis-stress model.

Neural tube defects Changes that occur within the hollow structure that encases the spinal cord. This structure is called the neural tube. Conditions that arrest the closing or development of the neural tube are generally genetic. However, genomics are involved—environmental factors such as a deficit of folic acid are known to be related to the development of neural tube defects. Thus, folic acid supplementation prior to conception has been linked to a decrease in neural tube defects. They can affect the circulation of the spinal cord and therefore result in an accumulation of fluid or hydrocephalus. Examples are spina bifida, meningomyleocele, or encephalocele.

Neurofibromatosis An autosomal dominant genetic condition that results in benign tumor formation on the nerves.

Neuroligins A Type 1 membrane protein on the postsynaptic membrane that mediates synapse formation between neurons. Neuroligins mediate signaling across the synapse and affect the properties of neural networks by specifying synaptic functions.

Neuropeptides Short sequences of amino acids that function either directly or indirectly to modulate synaptic activity and may also function as primary neurotransmitters.

Neurotransmitter A substance that transmits nerve impulses between nerve cells.

Neutrophils White blood cells that are an abundant and important phagocyte.

New mutation An abrupt, unforeseen condition that appears due to an error occurring in transmission of gene.

Newborn screening The process and procedure of analyzing blood samples obtained from infants following birth for the identification of specific genetic disorders.

Nondisjunction The failure of homologous chromosomes or chromatids to segregate during mitosis or meiosis, which results in one daughter cell having both of a pair of parental chromosomes or chromatids and the other one daughter having none.

Non-maleficence Do no harm.

Nonverbal behaviors Communications through gestures, touch, posture, body language, facial expression, and eye contact.

Normalcy A term used in family management to denote the viewing of a family member with a disease or condition as usual or normal within family life.

Nucleotides Basic building blocks of nucleic acids, RNA, and DNA. It consists of a sugar molecule (either ribose in RNA or deoxyribose in DNA) attached to a phosphate group and a nitrogen-containing base. The bases used in DNA are adenine (A), cytosine (C), guanine (G), and thymine (T). In RNA, the base uracil (U) takes the place of thymine.

Nullisomy A condition in which there is a loss of two chromosomes.

Oligogenic Pertains to hereditary characteristics produced by one or only a few genes.

Oligohydramnios An abnormal decrease in the normal amount of amniotic fluid (< 400 ml).

Oncogene A mutated gene that contributes to the development of a cancer. In their normal, unmutated state, onocgenes are called proto-oncogenes, and they play roles in the regulation of cell division. Some oncogenes work like putting a foot down on the accelerator of a car, pushing a cell to divide. Other oncogenes work like removing a foot from the brake while parked on a hill, also causing the cell to divide.

Oophorectomy The surgical removal of the ovaries.

Opsonins Chemical substances that bind to antigens to promote phagocytosis of particles by phagocytic cells.

Organism An individual living thing composed of one or more cells.

Organogenesis The process whereby the germ layers of the embryo (endoderm, ectoderm, and mesoderm) differentiate into the internal organs.

Organs Parts of the body that have a specific function, such as the kidneys.

Otoacoustic emissions Measure the sounds produced by the cochlea; used to evaluate for hearing loss.

Over the counter Medications, vitamins, and other treatments that do not require a prescription.

Ovulation The process of a mature graafian follicle releasing the ovum midcycle, 14 days before the anticipated start of menses.

Parasites Plants or animals that live, grow, and feed on or within another living organism.

Passive immunity Immunity resulting from the transfer of antibodies or antiserum produced by another person.

Pathogen-associated molecular patterns Molecules associated with groups of pathogens recognized by cells of the innate immune system. These molecules can be referred to as small molecular motifs conserved within a class of microbes.

Pattern recognition receptors Proteins expressed by cells of the innate immune system to identify pathogens.

Pediatric Health Care Home A model of coordinated care that promotes holistic care of children and their families by an identified health provider who manages both acute and chronic health issues.

Pedigree A visual presentation of a family history that uses standardized symbols to represent sex and disease state, and whether a person is alive or not.

Penetrance A proportion of heterozygotes for a dominant gene that expresses a trait mildly to severe in an individual.

Performance measures Objective criteria and methods used to measure performance.

Pervasive developmental disability not otherwise specified A diagnostic category of disorders characterized by delays or impairments in socialization and communication; includes autism, Asperger syndrome, childhood disintegrative disorder, and Rett syndrome.

Phagocytes Large, white blood cells that contribute to immune defenses by ingesting microbes or other cells and foreign particles.

Phagocytosis Process by which one cell engulfs another cell or large particle.

Phagolysosome A digestive vesicle formed within a cell by the fusion of a phagosome containing ingested material and a lysosome containing hydrolytic enzymes.

Phagosome A membrane-bound vesicle that encloses particulate matter taken into the cell by phagocytosis.

Pharmacogenetics The study of how genetic differences among individuals cause varied responses to a medication. Genetic tests specifically targeting genes associated with drug response are refered to as *pharmacogenetics testing*.

Pharmacogenomics The intersection of pharmacology and genomics to enhance knowledge of drug therapeutics and side effects.

Pharmacokinetics Reflects what the body does to the drug.

Phenotype An individual's observable traits, such as height, eye color, and blood type.

Phenotypic An organism's observable characteristics or traits.

Phenylketonuria (PKU) An autosomal recessive disorder in which the affected person completely lacks or is deficient in the enzyme needed to metabolize the amino acid Phenylalanine. When the body cannot break down the amino acid, it will accumulate in the blood and tissues of the body, especially causing toxic effects to the brain.

Phospholipase An enzyme that hydrolyzes phospholipids into fatty acids and other lipophilic substances.

Plasma cells Large antibody-producing cells that develops from B cells.

Plasmin A proteolytic enzyme with the ability to dissolve formed fibrin clots.

Pluripotent The type of stem cell that has the ability to differentiate into any type of tissue.

Point mutation An alteration in DNA sequence caused by a single nucleotide base change, insertion, or deletion. Point mutations can have one of three effects. First, the base substitution can be a silent mutation where the altered codon corresponds to the same amino acid. Second, the base substitution can be a missense mutation where the altered codon corresponds to a different amino acid. Or third, the base substitution can be a nonsense mutation where the altered codon corresponds to a stop signal.

Polyclonal antibody Antibodies obtained from different B cells.

Polyhydramnios An abnormally large amount of amniotic fluid (> 2000 ml).

Polymorphism The existence of a gene in several forms or a variation in a DNA sequence.

Polymorphonuclear leukocytes Related to or formed of cells of several different kinds.

Polyploidy A chromosome with extra sets.

Poor metabolizer Person with two nonfunctional alleles that result in immeasurable enzyme activity.

Population risk Applies to the proportion of the general population who is affected by a certain disorder or carries a certain gene.

Population-based screening Routine genetic tests that are performed on healthy individuals with no history of the disease that the screening test is designed to detect.

Prader-Willi syndrome A disorder caused by deletion of paternally derived chromosome 15 during meiosis. It is characterized by hypotonia, short stature, hypogondasim, hyperphagia, and behavioral abnormalities.

Preconception health counseling Involves giving information about how to maintain a healthy pregnancy and experience a good maternal child outcome. This health information is given prior to a pregnancy and includes examination of the family history to determine genetic risks.

Pre-embryonic development The first 14 days of development of the fertilized ovum.

Pre-implantation genetic diagnosis Involves the creation of an embryo using the technology of in-vitro fertilization (IVF) and then testing each embryo for the condition of concern.

Prenatal testing Genetic testing for conditions in a fetus or embryo before birth.

Prevalence An estimate of how many people have a disease at a given point or period in time.

Primary prevention Refers to efforts aimed at reducing the incidence of specific disorders, injury, and disability, including birth defects.

Primitive streak A structure that forms on the dorsal aspect of the embryonic disc that will establish bilateral symmetry in the developing embryo.

Proband The genetically affected individual through whom a pedigree is created. The proband is identified in the pedigree with an arrow.

Pro-drugs Inactive parent drugs that need to be metabolized to release the active component of the drug.

Proenzymes Precursors of an enzyme that do not have full (or any) function until an inhibitory sequence has been removed.

Proliferative phase The second phase of the uterine menstrual cycle marked by thickening of the endometrium, endometrial glands becoming distended, and blood vessels becoming engorged in preparation for a pregnancy.

Prophase The first stage of mitosis, wherein the chromosomes condense, the nuclear envelope disappears, the centriole divides and migrates to the opposite poles of the cell, and the spindle fibers form and attach to chromosomes.

Proteins Chains of amino acids.

Proto-oncogenes Normal genes that code for proteins that regulate cell growth and differentiation. They have the potential for change into an active oncogene.

Psychoneuroimmunology The study of the interaction between psychological processes and the nervous and immune systems of the human body.

Public health genetics Applies advances in human genetics, genomics, and molecular biotechnology to improving public health and preventing disease. It focuses on increasing knowledge of genetic inheritance in order to better understand common health conditions and how to slow their spread.

Quad screen Prenatal screening that uses maternal blood to determine the levels of human chorionic gonadotropin, alpha fetoprotein, estriol, and inhibin.

Qualitative Impairment An observable deficit in behavior.

Quality assurance The systematic monitoring and evaluation of a project, service, organization, or institution to ensure specific standards are being met.

Quickening Fetal movement felt by the mother for the first time, usually between 16 and 20 weeks gestation.

Race Grouping of people according to various factors including, ancestral background, social identity, or shared set of visible characteristics (such as skin color and facial features).

Recessive Recessive is a quality found in the relationship between two versions of a gene. Individuals receive one version of a gene, called an allele, from each parent. If the alleles are different, the dominant allele will be expressed, while the effect of the other allele, called recessive, is masked. In the case of a recessive genetic disorder, an individual must inherit two copies of the mutated allele in order for the disease to be present.

Reduced penetrance A dominant gene that does not manifest itself in a heterozygote individual with specific disorder.

Registered nurses Treat and educate patients, families, and communities; record medical histories; perform physical examinations; order tests and analyze their results; utilize equipment; administer treatments including medications; and help patients and families with follow-up care.

Reliability Refers to whether or not an instrument, test, or screen consistently measures what it is supposed to measure.

Replication The process by which a DNA molecule is duplicated.

Research A systematic investigation aimed at the discovery of new knowledge including the revision of accepted laws, theories, and facts; and/or the practical application of such new or revised laws, theories, and facts.

Ring chromosomes Chromosomes that form a ring due to deletions in telomeres, which cause ends to adhere.

Risk factors Attributes, exposures, or variables that increase the likelihood of developing a disease or disability—i.e., a negative outcome(s).

Risk The potential that a set of activities (both chosen and not chosen) will result in an undesirable outcome.

Risk models The use of formal techniques to aggregate outcomes.

Screening A method for detecting diseases based on genetic traits. Screening is done on a population-based system and detects potential risks in an otherwise healthy individual.

Secondary prevention Efforts aimed at minimizing the clinical manifestations of specific disorders, injury, and/or disability, including birth defects through disease management.

Secondary target conditions A set of clinically important genetic disorders that are recommended for newborn screening and that are to be obtained when the infant has his or her first newborn screen blood tested or in follow-up testing if indicated.

Second-degree relatives Relatives who share one-fourth (25%) of a genome with each other: grandparents, aunts, uncles, niece, nephew, half-brothers, or half-sisters.

Secretory phase The second phase of the menstrual uterine cycle that follows ovulation. It is characterized by continued preparation of the endometrium in preparation for implantation.

Seizure A sudden attack, often one of convulsions, as in epilepsy. Seizures do not necessarily involve movement or thrashing, some may seem as though they are frozen or unresponsive.

Selectins A family of adhesion molecules.

Self-determination The ability to make a decision for oneself without outside influence or coercion.

Self-tolerance A state of the immune system coexisting peaceably with other body cells in a host.

Sensitivity Refers to the test's ability to identify those who are at risk for the condition, and therefore need more in-depth diagnostic testing.

Sequencing The order in which genes appear or where they are located.

Serine proteases (serine endopeptidases) Proteases (enzymes that cut peptide bonds in proteins) in which one of the amino acids in the active site of the enzyme is serine.

Serotonin A neurotransmitter that is found especially in the brain, blood serum, and stomach lining of mammals.

Sexually transmitted infection A disease or infection that is transmitted by sexual contact between humans; also referred to as a Sexually Transmitted Infection (STI).

Sibship The group of siblings in a family.

Signal transduction The process that occurs when an extracellular signaling molecule activates a cell surface receptor. In turn, the cell surface receptor alters intracellular molecules creating a response.

Single nucleotide polymorphism A type of polymorphism involving variation of a single base pair.

Socioeconomic status An individual's or group's social status based on a combination of variables, including occupation, education, income, wealth, and place of residence.

Somatic hypermutation An enzyme increase in the mutation rate of somatic cells observed in B lymphocytes as they achieve increased bonding affinity for a foreign antigen.

Somatic mutations Arise after conception in any cell of the body except cells that produce sperm and oocytes.

Specificity A test's ability to accurately predict those who are not at risk for a specific condition and who therefore do not need further diagnostic testing.

Spina bifida A genetic condition that is one of several types of neural tube defects. It generally affects the lower spine.

Spinnbarkeit A term associated with the elasticity of cervical mucus during ovulation.

Sporadic cases Disorders that are caused by a new mutation in the proband.

Standard of care practice The diagnostic and treatment process that a clinician should follow for a certain type of patient, illness, or clinical circumstance. In legal terms, the level at which the average, prudent provider in a given community would practice.

Stereotyped patterns of behavior Repetitive or rhythmic movements, postures, or vocalizations, e.g. rocking or hand flapping.

Stroma Connective tissue cells associated with the endometrium.

Substance abuse Repeated use of alcohol and/or drugs with significant adverse consequences.

Substance dependence Maladaptive and regular use of alcohol and/or drugs that causes impairment in important areas of life.

Substance intoxication Reversible syndrome of physiological and behavioral changes due to the effects of the substance on the central nervous system.

Substance withdrawal The development of maladaptive physiological, behavioral, and cognitive changes as a result of reducing or stopping substance use.

Sudden infant death syndrome The unexpected, unexplained sudden death of a child under age 1.

Surrogates Stand in place of one who lacks capacity to decide for themselves.

Surveillance The ongoing scrutiny of a population to determine the frequency of occurrence of a given characteristic or disease of interest.

Syncytiotrophoblast The outermost layer of the trophoblast that invades the endometrium and forms the outermost fetal component of the placenta.

T cell or T cell lymphocyte A small, white blood cell that recognizes antigen fragments bound to cell surfaces by specialized antibody-like receptors. *T* stands for the thymus gland, where T cells develop and acquire their receptors.

T cell receptor Complex protein molecule on the surfaces of T cells that recognizes bits of foreign antigen bound to self-MHC molecules.

Tay-Sachs An autosomally recessive inherited disease that usually affects Askhenazi Jews or those whose parents are from Eastern Europe and that is always fatal. There is an insufficient amount of beta-hexosaminidase A that breaks down gangliosides, a type of lipid that leads to faulty lipid storage. The gangliosides build up in nervous tissue including the brain, affecting brain development and neurologic functioning. Over the first few months of life the infant exhibits increasing neurologic symptoms, eventually leading to death, usually before the age of 4 years.

Telomeres The tips of a chromosome that contain repetitive sequences of DNA that determine how many more mitoses will occur.

Telophase The stage of mitosis where chromosomes migrate or are pulled to opposite poles, a new nuclear envelope forms, and the chromosomes uncoil.

Teratogens Any substances or agents that interfere prenatally with normal growth and development and can cause malformations in the fetus.

Tertiary prevention Efforts aimed at averting and/or preventing social, financial, ethical, and legal burdens and situations including, for example, stigmatization, discrimination, and/or bias against affected patients, families, and communities.

Testing Refers to gene testing either by direct or indirect means. The gene itself may be viewed for alterations or indirectly by examining the byproducts of genes or gene markers.

Tetrasomy Refers to a condition in which there has been an addition of two homologous chromosomes.

Third-degree relatives Relatives who share one-eighth (12.5%) of a genome with an individual: first cousins or great-grandparents.

Tolerance A state of immune nonresponsiveness to a particular antigen or group of antigens.

Toll-like receptors A family of proteins important for first-line immune defenses against microbes.

Tophi The plural of tophus; nodular masses made of monosodium urate crystals in skin and other tissues in gout.

Toxin An agent produced in plants and bacteria, normally very damaging to cells.

Trait A specific characteristic of an individual.

Transcription The process of creating RNA from DNA.

Transition The passage from one stage in life to another; a process of changes and results of life changes on people's health.

Translation The process of creating proteins from RNA.

Triple screen Prenatal screening that uses maternal blood to determine the levels of human chorionic gonadotropin, alpha fetoprotein, and estriol.

Trisomic rescue Occurs with a fertilized egg initially containing 47 chromosomes, as a result of meiotic nondisjunction (instead of the normal 46), that loses the extra chromosome in subsequent cell divisions. The trisomic cell has been rescued and is now a normal, disomic cell.

Trisomy 18 or (Edward's syndrome) A genetic condition where there are three copies instead of two of the 18th chromosome. It results in mental retardation and often very early death.

Trisomy A condition in which an additional chromosome has been added.

Trophoblast Cells that form the outer layer of the blastocyst and provide nutrients to the embryo.

Tumor marker A substance that may be found in tumor tissue or released from a tumor into the blood or other body fluids. A high level of a tumor marker may mean that a certain type of cancer is in the body. Examples of tumor markers include CA 125 (in ovarian cancer), CA 15-3 (in breast cancer), CEA (in ovarian, lung, breast, pancreas, and gastrointestinal tract cancers), and PSA (in prostate cancer).

Tumor necrosis factors A group of the cytokines family that can cause cell death (apoptosis).

Tumorigenesis The transition from normal cells to invasive cancer (Ellisen & Haber, 2010).

Ultra-rapid metabolizers Usually refers to people with more than two copies of functional alleles, resulting in increased enzyme activity.

Ultrasound A test that visualizes structures using sonar or sound pressure with high frequency to create an image.

Underwriting The use of medical or health status information in the evaluation of an application for health coverage by an insurance companies (either life or health insurance).

Uniparental disomy Occurs when both members of a chromosome pair are inherited from one parent rather than one from each parent; may be maternal or paternal.

Validity Refers to whether or not an instrument, test, or screen accurately measures what it is supposed to measure.

Vanishing twin A fetus in a twin, or other fetus in a multifetal pregnancy, that dies in-utero and is partially or completely reabsorbed by the mother or other fetus.

Vernix caseosa A cream cheese–like coating on the skin of the fetus that is made up of fatty secretions from sebaceous glands and epithelial cells and protects the fragile skin from the abrasions, hardening, and chapping that can occur from exposure to the amniotic fluid.

Viral load The amount of a virus present—the more virus present, the higher the load.

Virus A particle composed of a piece of genetic material—RNA or DNA—surrounded by a protein coat. Viruses can reproduce only in living cells.

Wharton's jelly The gelatinous material that surrounds the blood vessels in the umbilical cord and protects it from compression, bending, twisting, or stretching.

White blood cells (or leukocytes) Cells of the immune system involved in defending the body against both infectious disease and foreign materials.

Wild type The most common expression of an allele combination in a population.

Wilson and Jungner Classic Screening Criteria In 1968, Wilson and Jungner published a report titled "Principles and Practice of Screening for Disease" that was based largely upon ethical principles and that provided principles and practices to screen for disease in a clear and simple way.

Withdrawal During or shortly after decreasing or stopping heavy or prolonged substance use, a client develops distress or impairment in an important area of functioning, which can include work or social life.

X-linked A genetic condition that is found on the X chromosome, or the sex chromosome. It is a condition that can be passed on from mother to son but never from father to son—there is no X that is passed by the father in the case of a male offspring.

Yolk sac A membranous sac attached to an embryo that provides nourishment in early pregnancy until the formation of the fetal circulatory system.

Zona pellucid The thick, transparent, noncellular, glycoprotein membrane that encloses a mammalian ovum. This membrane is required to activate the acrosome reaction.

Zygote A fertilized egg from two gametes; considered the first stage in an organism's development.

Index

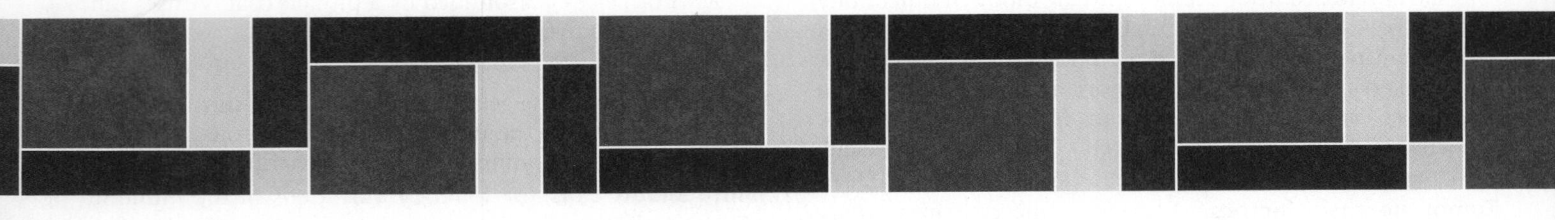

B

C

D

H

I

J

K

L

M

N

O

P

Q

R

S

T